Cardiovascular Eponymic Signs

Steven H. Yale • Halil Tekiner • Joseph J. Mazza
Eileen S. Yale • Ryan C. Yale

Cardiovascular Eponymic Signs

Diagnostic Skills Applied During the Physical Examination

Springer

Steven H. Yale
Department of Internal Medicine
University of Central Florida College of Medicine
Orlando, FL
USA

Eileen S. Yale
Division of General Internal Medicine
University of Florida
Gainesville, FL
USA

Halil Tekiner
Department of the History of Medicine and Ethics
Erciyes University School of Medicine
Melikgazi, Kayseri
Turkey

Ryan C. Yale
The Cooper Union for the Advancement of Science and Art
New York, NY
USA

Joseph J. Mazza
Clinical Research Center
Marshfield Clinic Research Institute
Marshfield, WI
USA

ISBN 978-3-030-67595-0 ISBN 978-3-030-67596-7 (eBook)
https://doi.org/10.1007/978-3-030-67596-7

This Springer imprint is published by the registered company Springer Nature Switzerland AG
The registered company address is: Gewerbestrasse 11, 6330 Cham, Switzerland

To those physicians whose passion about medicine and tireless efforts to better understand and uncover innovative ways to diagnose disease using only their sense of sight, hearing, and touch led the way to improvements in human health and well-being.

Foreword

This book *Cardiovascular Eponymic Signs: Diagnostic Skills Applied During the Physical Examination* is a superb and important contribution to the history of medicine and health sciences. It represents an enormous effort, accurately performed, and seeks the identification of a considerable number of names throughout the centuries of diverse signs related to the cardiovascular system.

This exhaustive research includes illnesses affecting the cardiovascular system such as the heart, not only as a complete organ but also in reference to its internal structures of valves or orifices, the central and peripheral arteries and veins, malformations and developmental defects, pericardium diseases, general affections such as hypertension, and clinical signs associated with pulse, pulsations, and sounds.

The association between medical fundamental documents, diseases, syndromes, anatomical characteristics, specific traits, and clinical signs, including those appreciated only through radiology, and studies derived from technological innovations and descriptors or their discoverers has been a recurrent theme over centuries. Some of these very ancient eponyms survive even today. We recall the Hippocratic Oath, Galen nerve, eponym to the inferior laryngeal or recurrent nerve, Oddi sphincter, or some of the multiple contributions associated with Morgagni's name. In particular, I want to express my pleasure that when I received the text of this book, the sign that immediately came to my mind, Corrigan sign, was found consigned in the book.

Discoverers, authors of primary descriptions, observers of details and signs not seen or described before, creators of new techniques or those who substantively modified existing ones, and inventors of medical devices have the opportunity to associate their names to the facts brought to attention by them. Sometimes the denomination came from disciples honoring their teachers or from medical communities recognizing the importance of the discovered or described fact. Other times, the denomination resulted from the sum of names, product of a sequence of observations, or, in many cases, from the jealousy of different medical schools intending to maintain the names of their representatives aside those of people coming from another school which observed the same phenomenon in a relatively short time.

Related most of the time to western medicine, these long series of names and data constitute a treasure for the history of medicine, because they are the evocation of the long and many times difficult ways to appreciate and identify disease characteristics, and construct the knowledge entities that we can today diagnose and manage. But this richness is not only limited to the history of medicine, but extends its field to medicine itself, medicine as a whole epistemic and practical entity, especially in the clinical or anatomoclinical settings. Scientific knowledge is the slow build product of a sequence of single walks, which goes ahead in a continuous search for better knowledge and solutions, and in a case like this, to cardiovascular health problems.

Eponyms constitute a form to give homage to our predecessors in the building of knowledge and a synthetic way to attribute a name to the person who described the disease. It is evident that for many centuries, eponyms constituted an important means of communication among medical practitioners in an easier manner without having to describe the maneuvers, clinical signs, or exploratory and surgical procedures. In a certain way, it is easy to believe that this method facilitates for students the learning of anatomical structures, abnormalities, and, as a consequence, all clinical realms associating it to their historical figures' names.

Recently, there has been a trend to eliminate eponyms from medical discourse, leaving only short descriptions of signs, syndromes, or diseases to be learned by our students. In anatomical descriptions, there is now a current tendency to eliminate eponyms in lieu of minimal descriptive phrases. Eponyms have been systematically criticized by some actual medical schools and eliminated from many textbooks under the pretext of their aggregated difficulty involved in the learning of names and the loss of reference to medical facts. As a consequence, students now have limited observations and short descriptions without an understanding of the significance of either the observed fact or how the described fact was incorporated in the evolving medical knowledge. In my opinion, accepting that an eponym is one item more to learn falls short of appreciating our most precious tradition; a consciousness of the continuous increasing of medical knowledge and the relationship that exists between these discoveries and the physicians and scientists who made them.

What is the significance of eponyms? As it has been said previously, eponyms are an efficient vehicle to recognize advances in knowledge, exploration, surgical techniques, and invention of instruments or devices. They also attributed a family name to some medicaments or pharmaceutical preparations until half a century ago, and continue today in the denomination of products intended to be employed in traditional or popular medical contexts. Perhaps, the most important information derives from the possibility of establishing a historical narrative. The narrative is based on the recovery of the personages whose names have been recorded, permitting the elaboration of a biographical account, that is, by putting the woman or man and her or his contribution in context of a specific time and place. The result is history reduced to the most relevant data of one's life detached from the implicit elements contained within the eponym. It is important to call attention to the significance aroused by the inclusion of people and their eponyms in one epoch. This approach allows one to ask questions about the setting in which the eponym was derived and relevant conditions of the discovery or invention. In this way, eponyms serve to integrate more general views about the status of medicine as practiced in one place during one's life span. This type of study is conducive towards the writing of a series of biographies, which can be specifically oriented to people whose names are expressed as eponyms. Alternatively, this approach may also introduce the eponym as an important component integrated in the biographical account of its descriptor as included in the *Dictionary of Medical Biography* (2006), a multiple author work in five volumes edited by William F. Bynum and Helen Bynum, or a compilation of medical biographies, as represented by the renowned *The Great Doctors,* published the first time in 1933 and described by Henry E. Sigerist, its author, as "A Biographical History of Medicine." The identification of eponyms could incite the exploration of names of other physicians living at that same time and place with similar characteristics with the intention to capture the image of medicine as expressed through knowledge and practice in a specified period and a geographical definite space. That is, eponyms constitute the first step to materialize the complete figure of medicine in the limits established by the time of their first description.

The second narrative trend derived from the study of eponyms consists of directing attention of the historian towards specific areas of medical knowledge. A good example of this type of approximation is Antonio Rey González and Lorenzo Livianos Aldana's book *La Psiquiatría y Sus Nombres* (Psychiatry and Its Names), defined by its subtitle: *Diccionario de Epónimos* (Dictionary of Eponyms), published in 2000. This book contains the psychiatric eponyms organized in an alphabetical order with the eponym and its content in a first entrance and a short biographical sketch of its name given in a second one.

This book, authored by Steven H. Yale, Halil Tekiner, Joseph J. Mazza, and Eileen S. Yale, could be included in this last type of historical research on eponyms, but has a significant difference. It is organized by chapters dedicated to the discussion of eponyms based on different aspects of the cardiovascular system. The book, as is expressed in the title, is focused solely on clinical eponymic signs. Its structure divides cardiovascular signs according to anatomical structures, certain pathologies, or physical characteristics of elements of clinical diagnoses as sounds, pulsations, observable characteristics, and so on. In each chapter, paragraphs appear expressed as "sign of," with a very concise but complete biographical introduction of the people whose name constitutes the eponym and the description of the sign with a commented reproduction of its original description and remarks on its clinical importance. The central features are the sign and, being its consequence, its clinical significance.

I coincide with the authors in their belief under the deepest sense of the concept, that ideas or knowledge converting into something essential is the most intimate of one's self. The eponyms and their comprehension are the core of an essential part of clinical wisdom. Modern medicine owes its development and proficiency to the incessant growth of clinical knowledge derived from close observation aside the sick person as enumerated by Hippocrates 25 centuries ago. The sick person's bed is enriched with anatomopathological and physiopathological newly recorded knowledge, and the continued practice and establishment of relationships between autopsy and laboratory findings with those facts collected by means of close clinical exploration. The clinic, in this way, continues to be an art, a *techné*, in the ancient sense of the word. It is the ability to know what to do, why it will be done, and how it will be done correctly in the most perfect artistic manner. Clinical activity thus constitutes the most accomplished and essential part of medical practice and the most significant element to make real its substantial compromise to be scientifically sustained.

It is clear that nowadays clinical activity has been modified after the introduction of multiple technical devices, starting with the stethoscope, which from its origins intended to create a space between the patient's chest and the ear of the physician. In a different trend, the employment of "scope" brought a singular ambivalence. At first instance, it provides the possibility to introduce an instrument or in the case of the ophthalmoscope only a light ray. However, it is important to recall that endoscopy signifies an intrusion to the patient's body; in medical anthropology, it denotes an act of an intimate proximity. Hence, this should only be considered an extension of clinical practice. Other devices bring the necessity of including partners in the diagnose or therapeutic team and have a tendency to delude the physician–patient relationship. Ultimately, the most important thing is the continuity of the figure of the clinician, which is, undoubtedly, the person recognized by the patient as her/his physician.

Why this digression? I think, and for me, one of the clues of interest and importance of this book is that the conservation of a well-built relationship between the physician involved in clinical practice, in every possible specialty or subspecialty, not only with her/his patients but between herself or himself and the medical profession, is a primordial constituent of her/his professional identity. The question now is to consider what are the components of this identity? I am deeply convinced that an essential part of it is the recognition of our ancestry, in this concrete case, the clinical tradition which permits the construction of the medical practice as it is today. Medicine without clinics simply is not medicine, but clinics without consciousness of its roots. The evolution of knowledge and its testing in practice, in this case through diagnostic signs, loses value and one of its most precious components of its identity.

It is in these dimensions that eponyms will be recognized as a unique element to arrive to the specific knowledge of how physicians contributed, step by step, to the integration of clinical knowledge and capacity to recognize signs expressing functional or structural alterations in some organ or body part. An element that brings together the appropriation of elements indispensable for a good clinical practice and the recognition of our vinculum with many generations of physicians who were involved, like us, in the task to practice and each day improve medicine and contribute to its advancement.

I congratulate Steven H. Yale, Halil Tekiner, Joseph J. Mazza, and Eileen S. Yale for their splendid effort in the excellent research culminated in this book, and I am sure it will be a multi-dimensional tool for cardiologists, internists, general practitioners, and other medical specialists in their way to excellence.

Carlos Viesca Treviño
President of the International Society for the History of Medicine,
Honorary President of the Academia Panamericana de
Historia de la Medicina,
Mexico City, Mexico

Preface

This book highlights clinicians who identified signs as a method to diagnose cardiovascular, peripheral vascular, and venothromboembolic diseases. Those clinicians refined bedside techniques provided a more in-depth understanding about the pathophysiology of disease. Advances in medical technology have complimented the information acquired through a meticulously performed physical examination. Unfortunately, many basic examination techniques have been compromised and lost by technological advances of modern medicine. We believe that these skills are essential components of medical education and should be passed on to subsequent generations of practitioners.

Our goal in writing this book is to provide biographical information about these astute clinicians and their respective signs and techniques so as to insure that the manuevers are performed exactly as intended. This book was written as a primary resource to be used by medical students and residents as well as teaching and non-teaching physicians alike. Our intent is to provide students and clinical educators an advanced training method when learning cardiovascular physical examination skills. We recognize the potential for the examination, through the use of signs, to be an applied diagnostic tool. We believe that performing these signs will allow a better connection of physicians with patients, and a way to discover disease through the physical examination, allowing for more efficient and cost-effective medical care. We recognize that there are gaps in knowledge regarding the sensitivity and specificity of these signs in clinical practice. With this in mind, there are opportunities to study them further so that we can better understand their role in medical practice.

Steven H. Yale — Orlando, FL, USA
Halil Tekiner — Melikgazi, Kayseri, Turkey
Joseph J. Mazza — Marshfield, WI, USA
Eileen S. Yale — Gainesville, FL, USA
Ryan C. Yale — New York, NY, USA

Acknowledgments

This book represents the combined collaborative efforts among Drs. Steven H. Yale, Halil Tekiner, Joseph J. Mazza, and Eileen S. Yale. It is rare to compile a team of writers who share the same passion and dedication to every detailed aspect of this undertaking. I would like to thank Drs. Carolyn Stalvey and Fan Ye's contribution to the pericarditis inspection and venothromboembolic chapters, two of the most comprehensive parts in this book. We are grateful for Nishanthini Vetrivel, Project Coordinator at Springer Nature, for her guidance and review of each book chapter and Michelle Tam, Managing Editor at Springer Nature, for her support. I would like to acknowledge the reference librarian Melodie Gardner, MLS, at the University of Central Florida and reference librarian staff at the University of Florida Medical Library who have assisted in tracking the obscure papers; without their help, this book would not have been possible. We would like to thank Dr. Mehmet Doganay, Editor-in-Chief, *Erciyes Medical Journal*, for permission to use in part previous published chapters on pericarditis inspection and Elsevier for permission to use in part a previously published chapter on venothromboembolism. The cover design and illustrations throughout the book are the work of Ryan Yale, a senior student at The Cooper Union for the Advancement of Science and Art, New York City, NY, under the aegis of the dean of the School of Art, Mike Essl. Dean Essl was instrumental in supporting Ryan Yale in this project, providing guidance, expertise, and mentorship to him in all aspects of the illustrations and design. For this, I am indebted and truly grateful for his teaching, making Ryan an even better illustrator. I would also like to extend my gratitude to Michelle Wellsandt, executive secretary at the Marshfield Clinic Research Institute, for her work on copyediting chapters of this book and supporting Dr. Joseph J. Mazza and me in this endeavor and throughout a good portion of our careers.

Steven H. Yale, MD, MACP

About This Book

Medical eponyms are widely used and ingrained in medical practice. They are honorific terms bestowed upon individuals for their discovery of a relevant sign, syndrome, test, or medical instrument. This book honors those physicians whose names have been eponymously attributed as signs in the cardiovascular medical literature. We believe that it was important to include, if available, information within their biographies about these peoples' character and their relationship with other students, physicians, and patients. These contributions provide the reader a personalized glimpse of the kind of person they were, how they lead their everyday life, brought honor to the profession, and aspects that make them more than just their discoveries.

This book teaches the physical examination as an applied technique. For each eponymic sign, brief historical background of the person and description of the sign as originally reported is recorded. Some signs within the book are illustrated and serve as a visual reference so that the learner can refer to and ask questions about how to perform the technique. The teacher should demonstrate the technique and later observe the learner to ensure that he/she is performing it correctly. A discussion of the utility of the sign allows the teacher to review the procedure, pathophysiology, and assess the learners understanding regarding what is known about the usefulness of the sign in clinical practice. The application of these bedside signs may promote relevant diagnostic testing that may lead to the delivery of more cost-effective care. This method should engage the learner and teacher in a more meaningful educational experience on how the examination can be used as an important tool for recognizing the pathophysiology of disease. We believe that there should be ample time and opportunity to interpose these historical signs into the medical curriculum to create a more fulfilling learning experience for learners and educators.

We used multiple primary and secondary sources to identify original publications of these signs, identifying 190 medical eponyms in association with cardiovascular, peripheral vascular, and venothromboembolic disease. We attempted to capture all signs that encompass the scope of this book but recognize that there may be some which may have been unintentionally missed. In addition to these signs, there are other names of individuals mentioned in the narrative that represent a fraction of those who have made meaningful contributions to the spectrum of cardiovascular medicine. There are over 40 illustrations contained throughout the book which demonstrate the method of performing the sign. Chapters are organized based on an organ system approach, whereby some are further ordered based on the particular skill of the physical examination (inspection, palpation, percussion, or auscultation). It is of interest that some chapters such as pericarditis, venous thromboembolism, and aortic valve disease are associated with multiple eponyms. Some of the repetition found within these chapters simply reflects the limited accessibility of the medical literature and language from which the papers were written. In other cases, it represents the subtleties identified when performing a meticulous physical examination.

One aspect of eponymic signs that is not recognized is the paucity of information and utility regarding their use in clinical practice. This book will help clarify misconceptions, provide fair and meaningful accounts of an individual or group's contribution to these scientific discoveries, and serve as a vehicle to encourage research on the validity and utility of these signs in clinical practice. We hope that you enjoy these stories as much as we have in telling them.

Contents

Contributors

Carolyn F. Stalvey, MD Division of General Internal Medicine, University of Florida College of Medicine, Gainesville, FL, USA

Fan Ye, MD, PhD Department of Cardiology, Wake Forest School of Medicine, Winston-Salem, NC, USA

Chapter 1
Aneurysm

Introduction

Prior to the advent of advanced imaging methods, physicians relied on the physical examination and their bedside skills to diagnose aortic aneurysms, dissection, and to test the integrity of the collateral vessels to verify if there is adequate blood supply being delivered to the peripheral tissues prior to ligation of an aneurysm. The techniques used and recognized as signs have been eponymously named to honor these physicians' contributions to medicine. We begin our review of signs of aneurysms, aortic dissection, and the collateral circulation by first providing a brief overview of key historical features leading to the recognition of these diseases.

Historical Background

The word "aneurysm" originated from the Greek term "widening." The earliest known description of aneurysms dates back to the Egyptians as written in the Ebers Papyrus in 1550 BC:

> When thou meetest a tumour of the vessels in any part of the body of a person and thou findest it round in form, growing under thy finger, and spread out against the flesh; it is not big and does not protrude; then say thou: 'It is a tumour of the *met* [vessel]. I will treat the disease. The *metu* [injury] causes it and it then becomes a pricking of the *met* [vessel]'. Treat it with the knife and burn it with fire so that it bleeds not too much. Heal it like the cautery heals [1, p. 148].

Galen of Pergamon (130–c.200 CE) was believed to be the first to describe and define traumatic aneurysm, presumably those caused by punctures inflicted by swords from gladiator wounds, of the false (pseudoaneurysm) type involving the outer layers of the arterial wall:

S. H. Yale et al., *Cardiovascular Eponymic Signs*,
https://doi.org/10.1007/978-3-030-67596-7_1

> When an artery is opened, the disease that occurs is called second an aneurism. It happens in consequence of the skin in the neighbourhood of a wounded artery cicatrizing, whilst an ulcer remains in the vessel, which neither becomes agglutinated nor cicatrized, nor filled up with flesh. Diseases of this description are known by their pulsating, and by their disappearing entirely when pressed upon; the contents of the tumour, which we have elsewhere shown to be a thin and bright blood mixed with much subtle spirit, warmer than that contained in the veins, passing back into the artery [2, p. 3].

Oribasius (c.325–403 CE), in the *Iatrikai Synagogai* (Medical Collections), wrote about Galen's and Antyllus's views on the classification of aneurysm types (true and false). They were transcribed by Oribasius as much of Antyllus's works were lost in antiquity:

> Galen and Antyllus both distinguish two kinds of aneurisms; only it is not certain that the classes of these two authors exactly correspond. The identity of the second class of Galen and Antyllus (aneurysm by wound and aneurism by rupture of an artery) seems scarcely doubtful; but the first species (aneurysm anastomosis in Galen and dilatation aneurysm in Antyllus) presents more difficulties. (…) After these preliminaries, we believe we can express the opinion that these small lateral holes were, in Galen's opinion, the seat of the aneurysms by anastomosis, and that, consequently, these tumors corresponded to the true aneurisms of the moderns, it is that is to say, those which really stand at the break of the clean tunic of the arteries. On the other hand, modern surgeons agree that there is no real dilatation aneurysm, except in the nearest parts of the aorta of his anatomy origin, and that it is impossible to admit that in speaking of aneurysms by dilatation, Antyllus had in view these aneurysms alone, one is naturally led to think that Antyllus dilatation aneurysms are still the same as the True aneurysms of the moderns. As a result, the first class of aneurysms, according to Galen, does not differ from the first class of Antyllus, having regard to the tumors which constituted these two classes; only the two doctors explained in a completely different, way the formation of the tumors in question [3, p. 660].

The location and characteristics of aneurysms were first described by Aëtius of Amida (mid-fifth century to mid-sixth century CE):

> A dilatation of the vessels, which the Greeks call an aneurism, may occur in any part of the body. (…) The signs of an aneurism are a tumour, which may be large or small, without discoloration of the skin or pain, soft to the touch, having a loose spongy feel, and yielding in such a way to the pressure of the fingers that it almost disappears, but returning again on the fingers being removed, which is very evident in those aneurisms that have arisen without a wound; but when it has been preceded by a wound of the artery, and the skin then uniting, a dilatation of the vessels has occurred, the tumour is not equally soft: for the blood being in larger quantity than the spirits, coagulates, and thus distends the tumour [4, p. 4].

Achilles Pirmin Gasser (1505–1577), an Augsburg physician, sent a consilium to Andreas Vesalius (1514–1564) about the autopsy findings of Leonard Welser, a patient for whom Vesalius was referred by Gasser to provide medical consultation. Vesalius diagnosed Leonard Welser with a thoracic aortic aneurysm. Vesalius's correspondence to Gasser, written on July 18, 1557 at Brussels, reaffirmed his ability to clinically diagnose thoracic and abdominal aortic aneurysms:

> I am very grateful to you for this, since I am well aware of how we are compelled to deduce the ailments of our patients from various conjectures. It is truly remarkable how the enlargement of an artery of this sort is chiefly distinguished by the closely packed matter contained in the blood, and that which in our patient resembled lard I have found in others to be somewhat similar to the vitreous humor of the eyes; (…). If we frequently discover [an

> aneurysm] lying concealed in the body of the living, how often may it be hidden from us in the brain, in the thoracic cavity, and around the pelvic region. May I perish if, after Master Leonard was seen by me, I did not meet with at least six ailments of this sort, but located in different regions. This condition was first seen by me, as I also informed you in the thoracic cavity near the root of the neck, and it shaped the upper ribs of the chest just as you write that the ribs and transverse processes of the vertebrae were gradually shaped in Master Leonard rather than attacked by caries and putrefaction [5, p. 395–396].

Ambroise Paré (1510–1590) in 1582 acknowledged Galen's observations regarding the formation of atherosclerotic changes within an aneurysm, recognized that not all aneurysms are pulsatile, and postulated the mechanism for the formation of atherosclerotic lesions and thrombosis within the aneurysm:

> [t]his hardness is owing to the cold and repercussing applications constantly made to such tumours, which may harden and thicken them. (…) Besides, in very large aneurisms there is frequently no pulsation; and on pressing upon them, the blood cannot be forced back into the artery, both because it is in too large quantity, and because it concretes into a thrombus [6].

It was Richard Wiseman (1622–1676) who was the first to believe that aneurysms arise from rupture of all the layers (coats) of the vessel wall with blood extravasating into the surrounding tissues:

> [b]ut not having been able by my practice to discover one aneurisma made by dilatation or relaxation of the outward coat, I am apt to believe that there is no such thing, but that it takes its rise from the blood bursting quite through the artery into the interstices of the muscles, where it raiseth a tumour suitable to the cavity it findeth, growing bigger or less, of this or that shape, as the muscles give way. (…) Those which I have met with did all come from downright eruption through both the coats; and those that come from external punctures must of necessity begin with a breach of the external coats first, it being next the lancet or other weapon that made the division [7, p. 70–71].

Later, Donald Monro (1727–1802) in 1760 described the case of John Parker, a 40-year-old man with multiple aneurysm where all three layers of the vessel wall were identified on macroscopic dissection within the aneurysmal sac reaffirming Wiseman's impression:

> For in the three smaller ones of the right side, the circular fibres, and all the other coats, were traced distinctly over the whole circumference of the tumours: In the one in the left ham they were seen on the fore side; and, although they could not be traced on the back part, nor be at all observed in the large sac of the right ham, it is most probable that these two aneurisms were originally formed in the same manner as the others; though the violent stretching, and the mixture of other substances with the coats of the sac, confounded all the parts so much, as to make such a demonstration impracticable. And we may presume, that so many good anatomists, who have given us histories of what they call true aneurisms, were not deceived in the nature of the disease, although they have not described minutely the texture of the aneurismal sacs, corresponding to that of the arteries in a natural sound state [8, p. 239–240].

Giovanni Maria Lancisi (1654–1720), in *De Motu Cordis et Aneurysmatibus* published posthumously in 1728, proposed a general definition of aneurism, recognized that weakness of the arterial wall occurs prior to its dilation and the congenital nature of some aneurysms:

> In the first place, then, I will divide aneurysms into the genuine and the spurious: I call genuine those that arise from causes close at hand when they weaken the tissue and powers of resistance of the arteries and heart; I mean those that in a short time destroy or at least enfeeble the firm strong web of the villi; and moreover there are some that belong to this class which arise from external causes, wounds, for instance, or contusions; others again, from internal causes, that is now from a natural deficiency and slackness of the villi [9, p. 15].

Jean-Louis Petit (1674–1750) in 1736 was the first to recognize the tendency for aneurysm to undergo recurrent episodes of rupture and bleeding [10].

We conclude our discussion by acknowledging the contributions by Pierre Bourdelot (1610–1685) and Giovanni Battista Morgagni (1682–1771) who were the first to recognize and describe arteriovenous and dissecting aneurysm, respectively. Bourdelot in his description of arteriovenous aneurysm wrote, "He will see sufficiently large pulsating arteries pouring all their blood into veins that do not pulsate. The veins and arteries of which he speaks as opening into other veins and arteries have the same orifice, and one often performs the functions of the other (…)." [11, p. 212]. Morgagni described the autopsy findings in a 60-year-old man with a dissecting aneurysm:

> The pericardium was distended with a large quantity of blood. (…) On the internal surface of the great artery, not far from the heart, a foramen large enough to admit the finger originated, and passing between the coasts in an oblique direction, for about the space of three digits, it opened on the external surface of the artery, within the pericardium [12, p. 362].

Great strides in understanding the pathogenesis, diagnosis and surgical management of aneurysms continued into the nineteenth century to the present. These advanced can be attributed to the development of the microscope and radiography. A variety of signs have been identified as mechanisms to diagnose aneurysms and dissection particularly during the nineteenth and early twentieth century. Our goal in this chapter is to provide a brief historical background of the person who described signs of aneurysms, dissection, and the collateral circulation and to record their original description. The lack of studies evaluating sensitivity, specificity, and predictive value limits the ability to draw meaningful conclusions regarding their utility in clinical practice. The signs are described chronologically from the date they were first reported.

Signs

Corrigan Sign

Sir Dominic John Corrigan (1802–1880) was born in Dublin, Ireland, and graduated from medical school from University of Edinburgh, Scotland, in 1825 [13–16]. After graduation, he served as a medical assistant in the dispensary on Meath-street, Dublin, followed by appointments at Fever Hospital and House of Recovery,

Cork-Street, and Jervis Street Charitable Infirmary, Dublin [14]. He was appointed consulting physician to the Whiteworth and Harwicke Hospitals (House of Industry Hospitals) in Dublin from 1840 to 1856 [14, 17]. The title baronet of Cappagh and Inniscorrig in Dublin was granted to Corrigan in 1866 [16, 18]. Corrigan was Fellow of the Royal College of Physician, Ireland in 1856, President of the King and Queen's College of Physicians from 1859 to 1864 and President of the Royal Zoological Society, Ireland [16]. He served as Member of Parliament from 1868 to 1874, Physician-in-Ordinary to her Majesty the Queen in Ireland, Senate and Vice-Chancellor of Queen's University in 1871 and corresponding member of the Academy of Medicine [13, 14, 16, 18].

He is best recognized for his work titled "Permanent patency of the aortic valve" published in the *Edinburgh Medical and Surgical Journal* in 1832, which he provided the most thorough description of the clinical and pathological features of aortic insufficiency, a name referred to by Armand Trousseau (1801–1867) as "Maladie de Corrigan" [14, 19, 20]. In a description of his character as described in a memoriam:

> He was a man of great physical energy; his feats of activity and strength in his youthful days were most surprising; his powerful frame is well preserved in the grand statue of him by Foley which was presented by numerous friends and admirers to the College of Physicians-no doubt the most appropriate place for it to rest [17, p. 271].

Corrigan identified a "visible pulsation of the arteries of the upper extremities" in three cases of aneurysm of the ascending aorta or its arch [21, p. 589]. Regarding the significance of this finding, he stated that:

> The arteries are empty, and, of course not at their full caliber, as in the living body. If the eye be kept on the situation of even comparatively minute branches at the moment when the injection is sent in, these vessels are seen thrown out in strong relief, presenting precisely the same appearance which the larger trunks present in a case of aneurism. (…) Whether this singular pulsation of the arteries be a constant accompaniment of aneurism of the ascending aorta, it will remain for further observation to ascertain but from what I have seen, were a patient to be presented to me with this symptoms with constant *bruit de soufflet* and *frémissement cataire* in the larger trunks, I would not hesitate to pronounce on the case [21, p. 590].

Thus, Corrigan sign refers to the visible pulsation of the arteries of the upper extremity in patients with an aneurysm of the ascending aorta or aortic arch (Table 1.1).

Hope Sign

James Hope (1801–1841) was born in Stockfort, Cheshire, England, and received his medical degree from the University of Edinburgh, Scotland in 1825 [22, 23]. He studied surgery at St. Bartholomew's Hospital, London in 1826 qualifying for the diploma from the Royal College of Surgeons [23, 24]. In 1827, he was a clinical clerk to Auguste-François Chomel (1788–1858) and also studied under Gabriel Andral (1797–1876), Pierre Charles Alexandre Louis (1787–1872), and Alexis

Table 1.1 Aneurysm signs

Name	Year	Description of sign	Method of examination
Corrigan [21]	1829	Visible pulsation of the arteries of the upper extremities (subclavian and brachial).	Observation
Hope [29]	1832	The first aneurysm sound coincides with the pulse and is louder than the first heart sound. The second aneurysm sound is diastolic. Both sounds decrease in intensity as one moves from its source toward the heart. The sounds are a deep hoarse tone of short duration yet louder than most murmurs with an abrupt onset and termination. Compared to a murmur the sound is rasping, soft, prolonged with a gradual crescendo-decrescendo.	Auscultation
Jaccoud [37]	1873	A hard mass, a tumor, situated in front of the aorta is raised such that it is projected isochronously with the arterial beats at the second intercostal space. Heard are two normal aortic clicks. There is a sudden and direct uplift without expansion or undulation with the second pulsation being completely absent. A solid tumor situated more deeply behind the aorta and pushing this vessel forward may cause a vibrating tremor with a single pulsation. A murmur is caused by the posterior-anterior compression of the artery and the diminution of its caliber.	Observation Auscultation Palpation
Cardarelli [43]	1878	Palpable throbbing pulsation is felt when pressure is applied using the finger tips to the right side of the trachea. The pulsation is less obvious when the same technique is applied to the left side of the trachea.	Palpation
Oliver [47]	1878	Place the patient in a standing position. Ask the patient to close his mouth and to fully elevate his/her chin. Grasp the cricoid cartilage between the finger and thumb and apply gently upward pressure. If an aneurysm present, the pulsation of the aorta will be distinctly felt transmitted through the trachea to the hand.	Palpation
Drummond [52, 53]	1882	Expiration is interrupted at each heart beat by a whiff. In some cases, it is very loud, while in others, it is only detected at the end of expiration. For large aneurysms, a diastolic as well as systolic whiff is heard. In cases in which the sign is well marked, it can be plainly heard in the trachea during quiet expirations, or when the patient is holding his breath with the mouth open and the tongue depressed. In very well marked cases, the whiff is audible in the trachea with the mouth closed, but disappears when the nostrils are compressed by the fingers. In searching for this sign, it is most important to avoid cardiac excitement. Thus, it should only be sought for after the patient has laid in the recumbent position for a short while and after the reasons for inserting the binaural stethoscope into the patients mouth have been fully explained.	Auscultation
Bozzolo [59]	1887	Pulsation of the arteries within nostrils in patients with thoracic aortic aneurysms.	Observation
Delbet [66]	1888	In patients with a popliteal aneurysm palpate the posterior tibial artery. If a pulse is present then there is collateral blood flow to the leg and foot.	Palpation

Table 1.1 (continued)

Name	Year	Description of sign	Method of examination
Cheesman [69]	1888	Breath sounds, particularly in expiration, are intermittent and interrupted by a puff at each heartbeat. The expired air instead of leaving the mouth in an even prolonged current, comes in a series of whiffs which are represented quite accurately by the sounds huh, huh, huh, huh. These sounds were loudest at the start of expiration, becoming fainter toward its end. Inspiration was similarly broken, but the interruptions were less marked. As the heart's action quieted down, the pulsation of the breath became less and less noticeable, until it finally ceased. If the puff is absent at rest, ask the patient to run up and down the stairs several times. The sound is now plainly heard about a foot from the patient's open mouth. The sound is absent over the chest but was loudest when the stethoscope is placed along the trachea.	Auscultation
Potain [77]	1889	1. An area of increased dullness is present to the right of the sternum when percussing starting lateral and moving medially. 2. Two auscultatory aortic sounds are present. The first aortic sound is sometimes loud. The second aortic sound is loud, sometimes brilliant and clangorous comparable to a high-pitched tympanic tone.	1. Percussion 2. Auscultation
Broadbent (William Henry) [78]	1890	Aneurysms involving the anterior aspect of the arch may present as a pulsating mass in the second or third intercostal space close to the margin of the sternum. Dullness on percussion over the manubrium sterni and immediately to the left of it may be found before the pulsation is visible. It is only when the aneurysm is located on the upper and anterior aspect of the arch, and attains a considerable size, that physical signs such as dullness over the manubrium sterni and to the left of it, or pulsation in the second left intercostal space may occur prior to the presence of symptoms.	Observation Percussion
Sansom [83]	1892	The patient places within his mouth the small chest-piece of the binaural stethoscope and asked him/her to close the lips over it. On auscultation, the observer hears a distinct or loud systolic murmur. This maneuver may be useful in cases were the murmur is either absent or barely heard on auscultation of the thorax.	Auscultation
Glasgow [89]	1895	Extend the arm and auscultate over the brachial artery for a systolic sound or thud synchronous with the cardiac systole. An arterial murmur may be heard.	Auscultation
Castellino [94, 96]	1896, 1897	The laryngotracheal pulsation is observed while the patient breaths normally and after deep inspiration. If an aneurysm is present, there will be an increased heartbeat and laryngotracheal beats.	Observation
Porter [100]	1899	(1) Double pulsation heard at the right sternal–costal junction at the second or third ribs. (2) Tracheal tugging and tracheal pulsation.	Auscultation Palpation
Hall [107]	1901	Auscultatory finding of accentuation of the aortic second sound sometimes described as a distinct thud or shock.	Auscultation

(continued)

Table 1.1 (continued)

Name	Year	Description of sign	Method of examination
Steell [113]	1901	Anterior heave of the chest wall occurring during systole in patients with a solid tumor located posterior to the heart. In patients with a descending thorax aneurysm located posteriorly to the heart, a double impulse may be present although most physicians will only perceive a single heave.	Observation Palpation
Dorendorf [115]	1902	The pit overlying the left clavicle is protruded in aneurysms involving the aortic arch. Downward pressure temporarily removes the soft supraclavicular protrusion. The left external jugular vein is more dilated compared to the right external jugular vein.	Palpation
Bryant [119]	1903	Ecchymoses of the anterior abdominal wall with unilateral involvement of the spermatic cord and scrotum.	Observation
D'Amato [124]	1909	Percuss the exposed part of the trachea and auscultate in the vicinity of the oral cavity by asking the patient to open his mouth. A very clearly transmitted resonance, the laryngotracheal resonance, is heard. If a neoplastic tumor or aneurysm is located between the trachea and manubrium sterni, then a tracheal tone is heard on percussing the sternum and manubrium.	Percussion
Quénu-Muret [129]	1910	Expose during surgery the dorsalis pedis artery and apply direct compression above the popliteal aneurysm to determine whether bleeding or increased blood flow occurs.	Observation
Henle-Coenen		Above (central) and below (peripheral), close to the aneurysm, the artery is compressed so that there is no blood flow. Now place a Höpfner clamp, below the peripheral ligature and cut between this and the peripheral ligature of the artery. If this Höpfner clamp is released and bright red bleeding occurs from the clamped peripheral arterial trunk, then there is sufficient collateral circulation (positive collateral sign), and the ligature can safely be made. If, however, no blood is emptied from the peripheral stump, no collateral circulation has formed (assuming no thrombus is present) ("negative collateral sign").	Observation
Henle [137]	1912		
Coenen [134]	1913		
von Frisch [139]	1914	When the main artery is clamped, the peripheral part of the main vein becomes enlarged. If venous stasis occurs each time compression is repeated, then this indicates that there are secondary pathways through which arterial blood flows extensively into the extremity.	Observation
Chalier [142]	1923	Metallic suction cups are placed close together at the painful site on the chest wall. A clicking sound is repeatedly heard as the two cups contact each other.	Auscultation
Shennan [146]	1934	In dissecting aortic aneurysm, a delayed pulse compared with the apical heart beat may be present in all arteries.	Palpation

Table 1.1 (continued)

Name	Year	Description of sign	Method of examination
Sabathié [151]	1934	The patient is initially placed in the left or right dorsal decubitus position with the head and upper chest exposed and head rotated to the side opposite to the one being examined. Comparing the right and left sides allows one to appreciate the exclusive or predominant engorgement of the jugular vein. Asking the patient to expire completely accentuates the venous engorgement particularly in picnicos or obese subjects.	Observation
Roesler [154]	1937	Rapidly expanding area of pulsation starting 6 cm from the spinous process at the level of the eight interspace extending to 9 cm. Over this pulsating area, the aortic second sound was accentuated.	Palpation
Nissim [156]	1946	Reduplication on the right and single pulsation on the left carotid artery without a coexisting noticeable difference in the intensity of the pulsations on the two sides. There were two almost equal beats in quick succession on the right carotid for every single beat on the left carotid artery.	Palpation
Logue [161]	1952	Pulsating sternoclavicular joint.	Observation

Boyer (1757–1853) at the Charité, Paris followed by additional studies in Switzerland, Rome and Florence [23, 25, 26]. He returned to London to practice medicine in 1828 and from 1829 to 1831 operated a private dispensary. After a brief appointment as a physician at Marylebone Infirmary, he became a student and governor at St. George's Hospital, London in order to enhance his future station and appointment in the English University [25]. In 1831, he completed his book *Diseases of the Heart and Great Vessels* and in 1832 was elected Fellow of the Royal Society of Medicine [27]. He was appointed assistant physician in 1834 and full physician in 1839 at St. George's Hospital [22, 25]. In a letter to Mrs. Hope, Dr. George Julius spoke of her husband's character:

> Having once made up his mind to do a thing, however arduous, however remote the accomplishment, nothing could check, or interrupt his course. Every energy was bent towards that one object; he never lost sight of it; every daily task had a direct reference to it; every occupation bore upon it; every attainment was regarded but as a step towards the honourable prize he held in view. It was this loftiness of aim that gave a largeness to his design: he rejected all competition for mediocrity: nothing short of success, and eminent success in the highest sphere, would satisfy his desires [28, p. 325–326].

Hope described the auscultatory double beat which he believed to be a pathognomonic sign for detecting aortic aneurysm and explained how this sound can be distinguished from the normal heart beat:

> 1st: The first aneurismal sound, coinciding with the pulse, is invariably louder than the healthy ventricular sound, and generally than the most considerable bellows-murmurs of the ventricles. 2nd: On exploring the aneurismal sound from its source towards the region of the heart, it is found to decrease progressively, until it either becomes totally inaudible, or is lost in the predominance of the ventricular sound. Now, if the sound emanated from the heart alone, instead of decreasing, it would increase on approximating towards the precordial region.
>
> 3rd: The second sound actually does sustain this progressive augmentation on advancing towards the heart; and as its nature and rhythm are found to be precisely similar to those of the ventricular diastole heard in the precordial region, it is distinctly identified as the diastolic sound. The second sound, therefore, corroborates, rather than invalidates the evidence of aneurism afforded by the first; for, if both sounds proceeded from the heart, both would, on approximating towards it or receding from, it, sustain the same progressive changes of intensity.
>
> 4th: Another distinctive characteristic of the aneurismal pulsation is, the peculiar nature of its sound. It is a deep, hoarse tone, of short duration, with an abrupt commencement and termination, and generally louder than the most considerable bellows-murmurs of the heart. It accurately resembles the rasping of a sounding-board heard from a distance; whereas, the sound occasioned by valvular disease of the heart has more analogy to the bellows-murmur, being somewhat soft and prolonged, with a gradual swell and fall [29, p. 425–426].

Thus, Hope sign refers to the presence of the double sound heard on auscultation of the thorax in patients with aortic aneurysms (Table 1.1).

Jaccoud Sign

François Sigismond Jaccoud (1830–1913) was born in Geneva, Switzerland, and received his medical degree from the University of Paris in 1860 [30, 31]. He was appointed physician to the "Central Bureau" in 1862 and agregé in 1863. Jaccoud served as hospital physician at Lourcine, Cochin, Saint Antoine (1867), La Maison Municipale de Santé (1868) and Lariboisière (1870), Paris [30, 31]. He was appointed Professor of Internal (Medical) Pathology in 1877 and later appointed Professor of Clinical Medicine at Faculty of Medicine in Paris at the Pitié-Salpêtrière Hospital in 1883 [31, 32]. Jaccoud was a member of the French Académie de Médecine (Academy of Medicine), section of medical pathology in 1877, served as its President in 1898 and life secretary from 1901 [31, 33, 34]. He was honorary professor in 1901 and honorary doctor of the hospital in 1902 [30]. He was the recipient of the Order of Saint James of the Sword of Portugal, Knight of the Légion d'honneur and the Royal Crown of Prussia [35]. Among his best known works he published *Traité de Pathologie Interne* in 1871, *Leçons de Clinique Médicale* (1867 to 1888), and served as editor of a 40-volume set titled *Nouveau Dictionnaire de Médecine et de Chirurgie Pratique* (1864 to 1886), collegially referred to as "Jaccoud's Dictionary" [31, 32, 36].

In his book titled *Traité de Pathologie Interne,* under the discussion on cancer, he stated:

> I have shown in several examples in my *Leçons de Clinique*, that the diagnosis of aneurysms compared with other thoracic tumors can be confirmed based on physical signs. I have dwelt with this question at length and studied aortic aneurysm in order to avoid having to return to it at this moment. I recalled that voluminous cancers that exceed the ordinary limits of the lung are found by the beating of the great vessels on which they extend and by compression may cause systolic murmur sounds (the case of Graves and Stokes). These beats as well as the murmurs are always simple and there is never any sound of closure of the cardiac valves as to giving the impression of a second cardiac sound [37, p. 126].

In his discussion on aortic aneurysm in his book titled *Leçons de Clinique Médicale,* Jaccoud wrote:

> Suppose a hard mass, a tumor, situated in front of the aorta is raised by it so as to project isochronously with the arterial beats. Its soft parts are found at a limited point at the second intercostal space. You hear two normal aortic clicks which are transmitted and exaggerated by an interposed mass acting as if it were pushing with support. You have a sudden and direct uplift without expansion or undulation with the second pulsation being completely absent. It would be similar to a thrill or vibrating tremor but which in this case would be absent. A solid tumor situated more deeply behind the aorta and pushing this vessel forward may cause a vibrating tremor with a single pulsation. Moreover, there would be a murmur as a result of a membranous cleft caused by the posterior-anterior compression of the artery and the diminution of its caliber. Finally, in either of these varieties because of their anatomical relations there would be signs of compression either on the side of the superior vena cava or right bronchus [38, p. 235].

Thus, Jaccoud sign refers to displacement of a solid tumor by aortic pulsation for tumors located anterior to aorta. For tumor located posterior to the aorta, a vibrating tremor with a single pulsation is present (Table 1.1). Other authors refer to this sign as a prominence of the aortic arch in the suprasternal notch or fullness of the sternal notch in patients with leukemia [39–41]. We were unable to identify the passage where he described such a phenomenon although a chloroma, or a solid mass of leukemic cells within the superior mediastinum, could be displaced by an aneurysm involving the aortic arch in the suprasternal notch.

Cardarelli Sign

Antonio Cardarelli (1831–1927) was born in Civitanova del Sannio, Italy, and completed his medical studies at the Collegio Medico di Sannio Aniello, University of Naples, Italy, in 1853 [42]. After graduation, he served as an assistant, achieving the rank of physician at Ospedale degli Incurabli, Naples. At the University of Naples, he was appointed Professor of Medical Pathology in 1890, and Professor of Clinical Medicine and Director of the First Medical Clinic [42]. He also served as Senator of the Kingdom of Italy. A description of his character:

> From the story of his pupils, Cardarelli had to be a man with a strong and decisive character, confident, but not vain, unwilling to rethink and to be contradicted. (…) However, he was much loved by his students because the activity to which he devoted himself with the greatest passion was precisely teaching. In fact, all his experiences that were gradually obtained were transmitted to his students (as opposed to many university students today). His classroom was always packed with a considerable number of students who had chosen him as their teacher… [42].

Cardarelli published in 1879 in *Movimento Medico-Chirurgico* (Medical-Surgical Movement) his observation and palpatory finding involving the posterior portion of an aortic arch aneurysm (Fig. 1.1):

> [I] have above all recognized a throbbing pulse of the trachea which is felt by applying the finger tips to the right side especially if one presses with some force. The pulsation is less obvious when the same observation is made on the left side of the trachea. In this case, it seemed to me that the aneurysm is located far left to the arch, at a point where the aorta crosses the left bronchus. Alteration of the left chest wall is felt due to pressure exerted on the left bronchus and at the same time the impulse emanating from the left side is felt, using the other hand, to the right of trachea as well as observing the neck [43, p. 488].

He accounted for the pathogenesis of the condition:

> When the anatomical relationship is present, in which the trachea is adjacent to the aortic arch, it is easy to understand that an aneurysm particularly in its posterior aspect causes compression against the trachea. It is all the more valid as it is easily seen that the aneurysmal sac contractions are caused by more or less dense adhesions extending to the trachea. In conditions other than stenosis, the tracheal tube can in part undergo a more or less remarkable displacement and receive the aneurysm impulse. This deviation and impulse of the endothoracic portion of the trachea can be observed and therefore serves as an important sign of aortic aneurysm. Since this fact is true, as in our case, even for a very small aneurysmal sac it must have important diagnostic value since no other objective signs are present [43, p. 489].

Thus, Cardarelli sign refers to the palpable pulsation felt to the right of the trachea in patients with aneurysm of the aortic arch (Table 1.1). A variation of this sign was also described by General William Silver Oliver in 1878, Pietro Francesco Castellino in 1896, and William Henry Porter in 1899.

Oliver Sign

General William Silver Oliver (1836–1908) was born in Kilfinane, Ireland, received his medical degree from Halifax, Nova Scotia, and ascended to the ranks from an assistant surgeon in 1857 to Brigade Surgeon in 1882 [44, 45]. On his retirement in

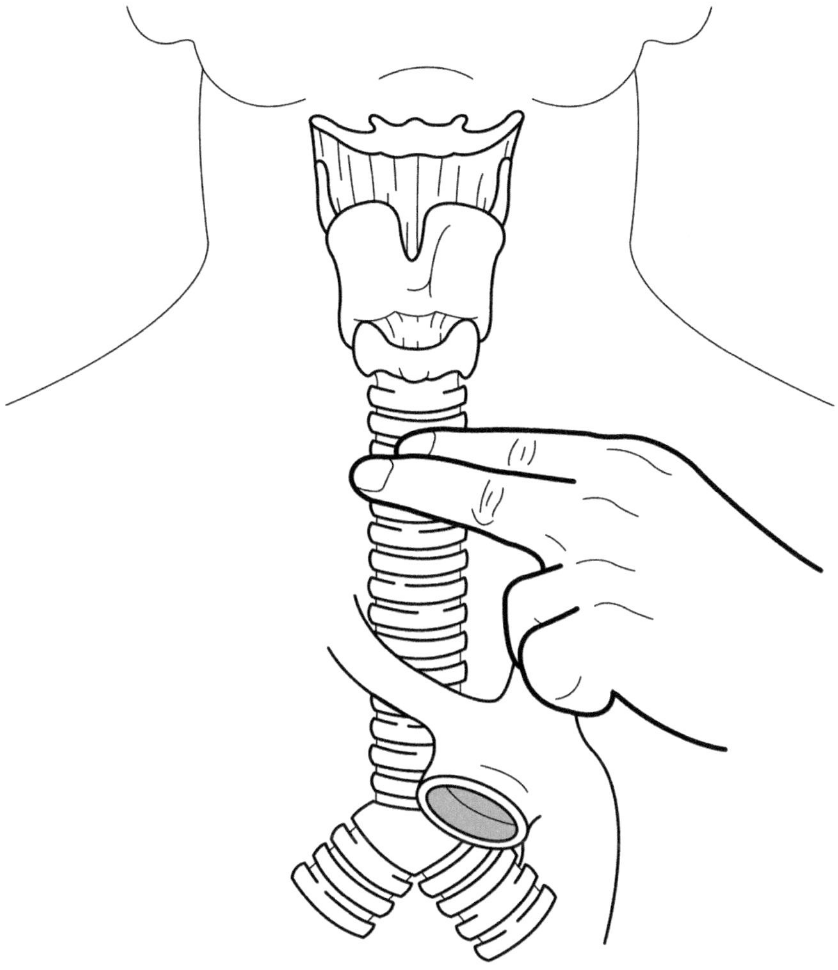

Fig. 1.1 Cardarelli sign (by Ryan Yale)

1883, he was named Honorary Deputy Surgeon-General [44]. As Deputy Surgeon in Halifax, he designed and patented the Canadian army accoutrement, designed to redistribute the load weight in order to avoid spinal injuries [46]. Oliver described the diagnostic method for detecting a thoracic aneurysm as follows (Fig. 1.2):

> Place the patient in the erect position, and direct him to close his mouth and elevate his chin to the fullest extent, then grasp the cricoid cartilage between the finger and thumb, and use gently upward pressure on it, when, if dilation or aneurism exist, the pulsation of the aorta will be distinctly felt transmitted through the trachea to the hand. The act of examination will increase laryngeal distress should this accompany the disease [47].

Howard noted that in addition to aortic aneurysm, the "tracheal tug" has also be reported to occur in "certain cases of indurative mediastinitis where the trachea and aorta are firmly bound together" [48, p. 143]. A variation of this sign was described by Antonio Cardarelli in 1878, Pietro Francesco Castellino in 1896, and

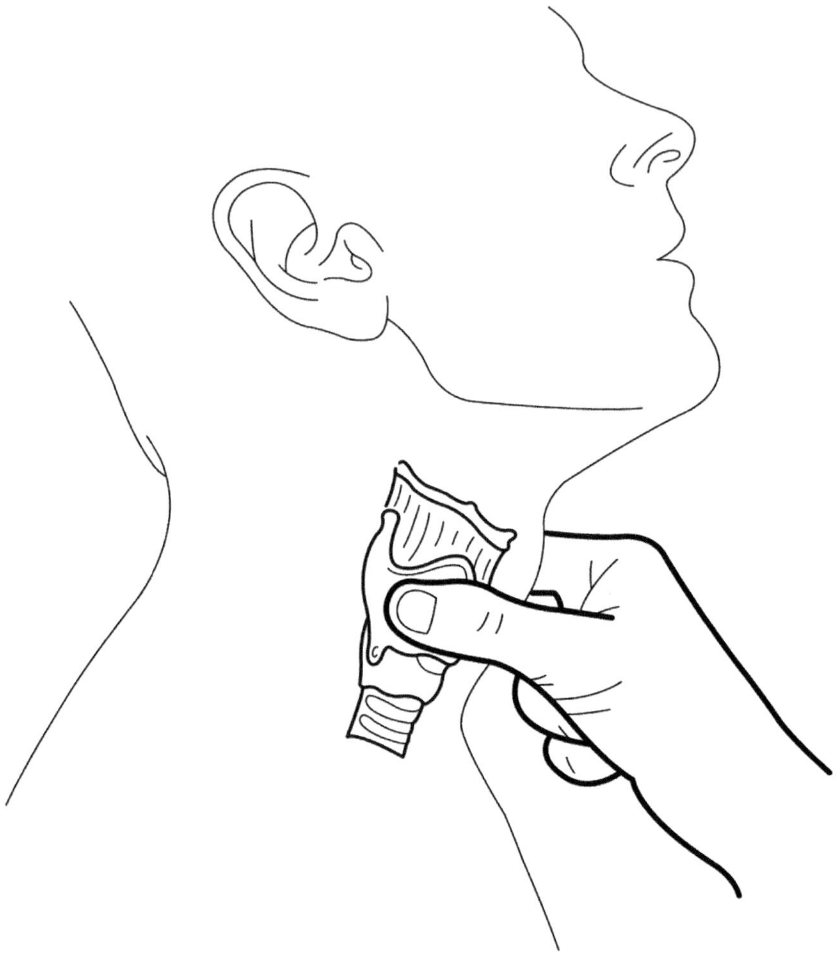

Fig. 1.2 Oliver sign (by Ryan Yale)

William Henry Porter in 1899 (Table 1.1). The presence of this sign in other disease states suggests that it lacks sufficient specificity to confirm a diagnosis of aortic aneurysm.

Drummond Sign

Sir David Drummond (1852–1932) was born in Dublin, Ireland, and received his Bachelor of Medicine and Bachelor of Surgery degrees from Trinity College, Dublin. He continued his studies in Prague, Vienna and Strasbourg prior to receiving his medical degree [49]. Drummond was subsequently appointed assistant physician to the

Children's Hospital in Newcastle-on-Tyne and next as pathologists and assistant physician to the Royal Victoria Infirmary from 1878 to 1912 [49]. At the University of Durham College of Medicine Newcastle, he served as a Lecturer in Physiology, Pathology, and Therapeutics, Professor of the Principles and Practice of Medicine (1911–1924), and Vice-Chancellor of the University and President of the College of Medicine [49]. In 1920, he received the title Commander of the Order of the British Empire for his services as a physician at the Northumberland War Hospital and knighted in 1923 [49, 50]. He was the recipient of honorary degrees from the University of Durham College of Medicine (DCL), Ireland and University of Glasgow (LLD), Scotland. He was appointed Fellow of the Royal Academy of Medicine, Ireland. He served as President within the British Medical Association (1921–1922) as well as the Association of Physicians of Great Britain and Ireland [49]. As a pathologist, his name is also recognized in association with the identification of the marginal artery of the colon (artery of Drummond), the anastomotic branch connecting the superior mesenteric with the inferior mesenteric artery [51]. A description of his character:

> No appreciation of "Physician Drummond," as he was known throughout the North, would be adequate without a reference to his invariable and unstudied courtesy, his consideration for others, his genuine sympathy, and generous help to all in need of it. Apart from the justified confidence in his professional attainments, these qualities won for him the respect and love of many friends. No man consistently held to higher ideals of the duty of a consulting physician in relation to medical ethics none had greater pride in his profession [49, p. 865].

As described by Professor Grey Turner:

> Sir David Drummond will always be gratefully remembered by a numerous succession of men, now scattered all over the world, who came under his influence either as students or house-physicians or young practitioners, and each will remember him for his sound teaching, genial personality, and kindly influence and timely help rendered in one way or another. Drummond was a great clinician and clinical teacher, who constantly taught and urged the importance of actual contact with patients. (…) In dealing with patients he was habitually courteous and kindly, but on occasion he could be-to say the least of it unmistakably emphatic, and by observing his methods of handling difficult situations young practitioners gained a great insight into the conduct of their work [49, p. 866].

Drummond in a paper read before the Northumberland and Durham Medical Society in 1880 and British Medical Association in 1882 [52], and published in the *British Medical Journal* that same year, described a sign found in patients with aortic aneurysm:

> Briefly, the oral whiff, which I may call the sign I am now referring to, can be detected in the following manner in cases of aortic aneurysm. The patient is directed, whilst lying on his back, to breathe as quietly as possible through the widely open mouth; the oval piece of the binaural stethoscope is then introduced into the mouth to receive the expired air. Should, then, the sign be present, the expiration will appear to be interrupted at each beat of the heart by a whiff, which, in some cases, is very loud, whilst, in others, it is only detected at the end of expiration, an indication that it is but feebly marked. In certain cases, especially if the aneurysm be large, a diastolic whiff can be heard as well as a systolic. In cases in which the sign is well marked, it can be plainly heard in the trachea during quiet expirations, or when the patient is holding his breath, with the mouth open and the tongue depressed, so as to allow the gaping glottis to communicate freely with the buccal cavity. In very well marked cases, the whiff is audible in the trachea with the mouth closed, but it at once disappears when the nostrils are compressed by the fingers. In seeking for the sign,

> it is most important to avoid cardiac excitement; hence it should only be sought for after the patient has lain in the recumbent position for a short while, and after the reasons for inserting such a formidable looking instrument as the binaural stethoscope into the mouth have been fully explained. It is well, indeed, to school the patient accurately before commencing the examination, for nervous, interrupted respiration on the one hand, and forcible or nasal breathing on the other, will defeat the object of the examination [53, p. 773].

Drummond in his assessment of 24 patients with thoracic aneurysm (23 involving the aorta and 1 of the innominate artery) found:

> Of the 23 aortic aneurysms, the whiff was present in 17; in some of which it was well marked, and in others but feebly so; it was entirely absent in 3; in 1 it was not sought for; and in 2 stridor and *râles* were so loud as to interfere with its development. The sign was altogether absent in the case of innominate aneurysm. In 3 cases, the whiff only developed after the patients had been observed in hospital from six to eight weeks [53, p. 773].

Thus, Drummond sign refers to the soft interrupted whiff heard during expiration when the mouth is open in patients with an aortic aneurysm (Table 1.1).

Bozzolo Sign

Camillo Bozzolo (1845–1920) was born in Milan, Italy, and received his medical degree from the University of Pavia in 1868. After graduation in 1871, he furthered his studies in Vienna, Austria under the auspices of Johann Ritter Oppolzer (1808–1871), Salomon Stricker (1834–1898) and Carol von Rokitansky (1804–1878), and in Berlin under Rudolf Virchow (1821–1902) and Ludwig Traube (1818–1876). After returning to Milan in 1871, he was appointed Assistant to the Office of Pathological Anatomy at the Ospedale Maggiore under Achille Visconti (1836–1911) [54]. In 1872, he worked in the branch of Pathological Anatomy with Giulio Bizzozero (1846–1901) in Torino [54, 55]. He returned to Milan and served as an Assistant Physician at Maggiore Hospital and Prosecutor of Anatomy and Pathology from 1873 to 1876 [55]. Bozzolo served as Senator of the Kingdom beginning in 1910 [56]. In 1877, he directed the Medical Clinic at the University of Torino, was chair of the newly formed Propaedeutic Medical Clinic from 1878 to 1883, and appointed ordinary Professor and Chair of the new General Medical Clinic in Torino in 1833, a position which he held for 37 years. His noteworthy honors include Knight, Commander, and Grand Officer of the Order of the Crown of Italy [56]. He was one of the first physicians in Italy to apply radiology as diagnostic and therapeutic tools used as radiotherapy for leukemia [57]. In addition to the sign which bears his name, other notable accomplishments include the discovery that the parasite *ancyclostoma duodenale* was the cause of anemia in workers at the St. Gothhard railway and recognized thymol as a treatment for this condition [58].

A description of his character as described by Sen Prof. E. Maragliano, "Camillo Bozzolo was a character that never broke in the face of difficulties; tenacious in defending his own convictions; inflexible, who never capitulated to everything that did not persuade him: but he was always honest, always correct, always right" [1, p. 234]. As described by G. Satta:

> Subtlety and sharpness of observation and genius of views were the main qualities of his teachings. His objective and conscientious lessons devoid of any form of courage and any display of eloquence, were not always rightly appreciated by the novices, but for the student and the attentive doctor, it was the sources of precious lessons [54, p. 234].

Bozzolo building on the studies of Giulio Ceradini (1844–1894) and Angelo Mosso (1846–1910), regarding the movements which the column of air in the cavities of the nostrils undergoes in relation to the cardiac moments, applied this phenomenon to the diagnosis of intrathoracic aneurysms:

> This is based on the following four facts: 1. The positive pulse of the open glottis nostrils. 2. The nostrils pulse is positive when the glottis is open, but is preceded by a slight negative pulse corresponding to systole. A more or less strong positive nostril pulse follows this towards the end of systole. 3. When the pulse of the heart in the chest is negative, the pulse of the open glottis nostrils is positive. 4. The pulse of the nostrils remains negative during the systole.
>
> Here are the conclusions: 1. The presence of an endothoracic aneurysm can be suspected by changes occurring in the pulse of the nostrils. 2. The pulse of the nostrils can become positive when the glottis is open due to an aneurysm. 3. The negative open glottis pulse in thoracic aortic aneurysms, when not due to an extended elevation of the ribs, may signify filling of the aneurysmal sac with clot and therefore a greater tendency to heal. 4. From the examination of the pulse of the nostrils you can draw important conclusions regarding the pathological mechanisms of the heart [59, p. 962].

Thus, Bozzolo sign refers to the visible pulsation of arteries within the nasal mucosa (Table 1.1).

Delbet Sign

Pierre Louis Ernest Delbet (1861–1925) was born in La Ferté-Gaucher, Seine-et-Marne, France, and received his medical degree from the University of Paris in 1899. He served as agrégé at the University of Paris in 1892, surgeon at des Hôpitaux de Paris in 1893, and Full Professor of the Surgical Clinic at the faculty of Medicine of Paris in 1909 [60, 61]. He was a member of the Academy of Medicine (Operative Medicine Section) from 1921 to 1957 and founding member, along with Dr. Charles Jacques Bouchard (1837–1915) and Henri de Rothschild (1872–1947), of the French Association for the Study of Cancer (currently Société Française du Cancer or French Society of Cancer) [61].

He is perhaps best recognized for his work on the use of magnesium chloride as an antiseptic and for identifying the relationship between low magnesium levels and the development of cancer [62]. He is also credited for establishing that magnesium halide salts enhance phagocytosis of white blood cells and was the first to use rubber as a hip prosthesis in the finger joint and as an abdominal-like mesh [62–64]. Arrou in his description of the management of absent pulsation in a popliteal aneurysm stated:

> When the useless malleable piece of the sac is removed, the arterial circulation continues to function as it has been doing so by way of the collaterals. This point is not new and was established exactly twenty years ago by our colleague Delbet. I have been able to appreciate its value in the six observations I have already published and here is a seventh, of recent date, which seems to me rather suggestive. (…) In closing, I will repeat my opening sentence: look for the pulse of the posterior tibial artery, and remain confident as it signifies that the circulation is not affected by the aneurysm. On the contrary, the dilated collateral circulation is providing blood flow to the leg and foot [65, p. 868].

Delbet further discussed the role of mechanical and elastic compression:

> Indeed, indirect compression that acts as an incomplete and temporary ligature prepares for the development of the collateral circulation by dilating the vessels which must take part in opening the way beyond the ligature. On the other hand, elastic compression flattens all of the arterioles and thus cannot in any case favor the collateral circulation [66, p. 557–558].

Delbet sign describes the method for determining the integrity of the collateral circulation in patients without pulsation of a popliteal aneurysm (Table 1.1). There is sufficient collateral circulation to the distal lower extremity if the posterior tibial arterial pulse is palpable in patients with absent pulsation of a popliteal artery aneurysm.

Cheesman Sign

Williams Sanderson Cheesman (1853–1912) received his medical degree from the College of Physicians and Surgeons, New York in 1879 [67]. He served at Bellevue Hospital in New York City from 1879 to 1884 and practiced in Auburn New York in 1881 [68]. Cheesman served as President of the Central New York Medical Association, Fellow of the New York Academy of Medicine and Member of the Committee on Experimental Medicine, New York Medical Society [67]. A description of his character:

> It may readily be seen, therefore, that Dr. Cheesman's preparation for the life work he had chosen was thorough and complete. His constitution was not strong, however, while his ambition to work and achieve was almost without limit. Thus he labored against a grievous hindrance, yet, he made notable progress in his profession and gained a reputation that was state wide. (…) As a physician, surgeon and friend, Dr. Cheesman won a place in the community and in the state that will remain on record during the years to come. (…) As a citizen of Auburn, Dr. Cheesman had the confidence and honor of everybody. He was interested in good works and gave time and money to further the causes [68, p. 259–260].

Cheesman reported the auscultatory finding of respiratory puff or whiff in five patients, thoroughly describing the symptoms conveyed by a 33-year-old man who:

> [o]bserved that the sound of his breathing, particularly in expiration, was intermittent, giving a puff at each beat of the heart. The expired air, instead of leaving the mouth in an even, prolonged current, came in a series of whiffs which may be represented quite accurately by the sounds huh, huh, huh, huh. These were loudest at the commencement of expiration, and became fainter toward its close. Inspiration was similarly broken, but the interruptions were less marked. As the heart's action quieted down, this pulsation of the breath became less and less noticeable, till it finally ceased. A second run, however, reproduced it exactly as before [69, p. 235].

When he examined the chest, the puff was absent at rest but when he asked the patient to run up and down the stairs several times:

> The sound was then plainly heard by the ear held about a foot distant from the patient's open mouth. I listened with the stethoscope over the chest, but could not distinguish it there at all. When the instrument was applied along the trachea, however, it came out loudly, and had the characters already described. Drummond's "oral whiff" as a sign of thoracic aneurism came to my mind, and therefore, though there were neither symptoms nor physical signs of this disease, I re-examined for it carefully and repeatedly, but with an entirely negative result [69, p. 235].

Based on his observations in these patients, he concluded:

> The only account which I can find is in descriptions of Drummond's "oral whiff," where it seems to be looked upon as a familiar fact. But, considering the sort of men who have professed to me their ignorance, it certainly cannot be an every-day matter. To them, as well as to myself, it was a puzzle—which is my reason for describing it here. Why it occurs in so few subjects and not in others I cannot explain. In my small experience it has usually been associated with a distinctly neurotic constitution [69, p. 236].

He proposed two mechanisms for the pathogenesis of this finding:

> Two explanations have occurred to me. When one listens to the sound along the trachea, it seems as if it must certainly be due to interruptions of the column of in-going and out-going air by the intermitting pressure of some part of the circulatory apparatus; the entering current being simply retarded at each systole, the emerging current being alternately obstructed, and then liberated under accumulated pressure. This is the explanation sometimes given of the "whiff" in cases of thoracic aneurism. No such compression of the air-passages could take place, however, without dyspnoea. Both in health and in aneurismal disease it seems more likely that the sign described is due to the fact that each rise of intra-thoracic pressure attending the aortic expansion so increases the expulsive force of expiration that the sound of the air rushing through the narrow *rima glottidis* is momentarily intensified into a puff [69, p. 236].

Cheesman clarified the significance of the whiff sign in intrathoracic aneurysms:

> The value of this whiff as a sign of intrathoracic aneurysms must depend on its association with other physical signs of that disease. It would certainly seem that any physician accepting the usual statement that the "oral whiff" occurring during physical mental quietude is of itself evidence of aneurism (see *Pepper's System of Medicine*, vol. iii, p. 811) would inflict needless alarm his patient [69, p. 236].

Thus, Cheesman sign refers to the presence of an interruption of expiration or whiff sound. He clarified its presence in conditions other than aneurysm such as in otherwise healthy persons or those with neurosis (Table 1.1).

Potain Sign

Pierre Carle Édouard Potain (1825–1901) was born in Paris, France, and received his medical degree from the University of Paris in 1853. Following graduation, he served in the Ivry Insane Asylum until 1856 when was named *chef de Clinique* under Jean-Baptist Bouillaud (1796–1881) in 1856 [70]. He was appointed Physician to the Bureau Central and staff physician at Hospice des Ménages, Hôpital Saint Antoine, and Hôpital Necker, Paris [70, 71]. In 1861, he qualified with the title Professeur agrégé (adjunct professor) and was appointed Physician to the Hospital of Paris [71]. Potain served briefly as Professor of Medical Pathology followed by an appointment as chair of Clinical Medicine at Necker Hospital in 1887, and from 1886 to 1900 was chief of Bouillad's clinic at la Charité [70, 72, 73]. He received numerous honors including being elected Member of the National Academy of Medicine in 1883, National Academy of Science in 1893, Member of the Institute of France and Commander of the Légion d'honneur [70, 73, 74].

In addition to the sign which bears his namesake, Potain made a number of important contributions to the field of medicine. These included among others refinements in Marey's sphygmograph, a device used to measure the pulse, collapsotherapy for the treatment of pulmonary tuberculosis, thoracentesis device for removable of pleural fluid, further description of the gallop rhythm and distinguished a split first heart sound (S_1) from a presystolic sound (S_4 gallop), and a hemocytometer, a device to count red blood cells [74–76]. A description of his character as described in his obituaries:

> In his devotion to his profession, to his pupils, and to those who sought counsel of him, in his scorn of everything savouring of advertisement or self-seeking in his constant effort to relieve suffering and do good. Professor Potain was the model of a true physician. The history of his life may be summed up in the words, *Pertransiit benefaciendo* [70, p. 121]. (…) His kindness to the pupils, his gentleness to his poor patients, his justice in the examination of students, which was always tempered with kindness, made him one of the most beloved of all the teachers in the faculty of medicine. (…) In the death of Professor Potain France has lost one of her noblest sons, the medical profession one of its most illustrious members, the world a good and noble man [72].

Potain described three patients with severe aortitis and dullness on percussion of the thorax:

> [t]here is an increase in the extent of dullness to the right of the sternum. The precise limits of this deep dullness must be carefully traced and great care should be taken to strike the chest wall hard, because if the lung is slightly emphysematous superficial percussion provides no information. To conduct a good examination, it is necessary to strike around the region of proposed dullness starting peripherally and moving in a medial direction. If we suddenly find a low pitch tone, when percussing under the clavicle in person with a normal lung, this signifies the presence of a tumor of the mediastinum whose nature remains to be determined through a differential diagnosis [77, p. 750].

Potain further described a high pitched tympanic tone on auscultation in patients with an aortic aneurysm:

> The first aortic sound can be loud. It results, as we know, from the tension of the vessel, and usually merges with the first heart sound. Sometimes the aortic component of the sound is much louder when the less elastic artery stretches more abruptly causing the first heart tone to lag behind the rest of the sound. According to Marey, this delay is about 1/10th of a second and the timing probably does not always occur at exactly the same. In the ear, it seems that we are dealing with a kind of duplication of the first noise. The second aortic sound is loud, sometimes brilliant, and clangorous. According to the expression of Guéneau de Mussy, it can be exactly compared to the sound of the *darbouka* of Turkish music. This

> character of the noise indicates that there is induration of the aortic valves. This induration may be caused by endocarditis; however, the noise is louder and does not assume the particular tone as it does in aortitis [77, p. 751].

Thus, Potain described two signs in patients with aortic aneurysms. An area of dullness on percussion located to the right of the sternum and a high pitched tympanic second sound on auscultation indicating aortic valve involvement (Table 1.1).

Broadbent [Sir William Henry (W.H.)] Sign

Sir William Henry Broadbent (1835–1907) was father to Sir John Francis Harpin Broadbent (1865–1946) and Walter B. Broadbent (1868–1951). Historical information regarding Sir William Henry Broadbent and John Francis Harpin Broadbent is found within the chapter pericardium where his name is eponymously associated with another sign described with his son John Francis Harpin in 1897. In Sir William Henry Broadbent's book, *The Pulse*, he described a finding seen in ascending aortic aneurysms:

> The ascending aorta is freely movable, and does, in fact, move up and down—or, to speak more exactly, down and up—with each beat of the heart; it probably expands and contracts also more than any other part of the vessel. Accordingly, provision exists for its free play; it is not closely attached to surrounding parts, and is not in close relation with the nearest important structures, the root of the lung and the vena cava superior and the pneumogastric nerve. In this way it comes to pass that an aneurism of the ascending aorta may attain a considerable size before pressure-effects, or, in other words, symptoms, are produced. On the other hand, this part of the aorta is near the surface of the chest, an expansion of the vessel here very often takes a superficial direction upwards and outwards, and in whatever direction takes place can scarcely fail to produce actual contact with the chest-wall; the aneurism, therefore, reveals itself by dullness, pulsation and characteristic auscultation signs [78, p. 229–230].

In Sir William Henry and John Francis Harpin Broadbent's book *Heart Disease and Aneurysm of the Aorta with Special Reference to Prognosis and Treatment* on their discussion of aneurysm of the transverse portion of the aortic arch, they described a physical finding:

> When it springs from the anterior aspect of the arch, the sac may present as a pulsating tumour in the second or third intercostal space close to the margin of the sternum [2, p. 461]. (…) Dullness on percussion over the manubrium sterni, and immediately to the left of it, may often be made out before pulsation is visible. It is a valuable sign when it occurs in conjunction with characteristic symptoms, though the possibility of it being due to enlarged glands or other mediastinal tumour must be borne in mind. (…) It is only when it is situated on the upper and anterior aspect of the arch, and attains a considerable size, that the physical signs such as dullness over the manubrium sterni and to the left of it or pulsation in the second left intercostal space may precede the appearance of symptoms [79, p. 462].

Thus, Broadbent (W.H., J.F.H.) sign is left lateral pulsation or percussion dullness occurring at the second or third parasternal intercostal space in patients with an aneurysm involving the anterior portion of the aorta arch (Table 1.1).

Sansom Sign

Arthur Ernest Sansom (1838–1907) was born at Coraham, Wiltshire, England, and received his medical degree from the University of London in 1866 [80]. He was appointed assistant physician, then physician at the London Hospital and North-Eastern Hospital for Children [80]. His other positions included physician at the Royal Albert Orphan Asylum and Hospital for Diseases of the Chest, City-Road [80]. He was elected Fellow of the Royal College of Physicians, London in 1878, and served as an examiner in medicine for the Royal College of Surgeons England, and Universities of London and Durham, as well as to the physicians of the Royal Hospital for Diseases of the Chest [80, 81]. In 1885, he was appointed Chairman of the Council of The Medical Society of London [82]. As a tribute to Sansom's character as described in his obituary published in 1907 in the *Lancet*:

> Dr. Sansom was possessed of a most charming personality. His kindness and geniality made him beloved by all who knew him. No one can forget the warmth of his greeting and his true friendliness towards those who were privileged to have a close acquaintance with him. He was a staunch and in a quiet unostentatious manner performed countless acts of charity and was willing to lend a helping hand to those who required assistance by money, time, and advice. When he retired from practice he caused a gap which was difficult to fill and he left Harley-street amidst the sincere sympathy and regret of his numerous friends [80, p. 845].

Sansom described an auscultatory finding for detecting a thoracic aneurysm:

> I have found valuable auscultatory evidence in some cases of aneurysm, when a murmur has been absent, or very feebly heard, over the thorax, by causing the patient to place within his mouth the small chest-piece of the binaural stethoscope, and to close his lips over it. On auscultating thus, the observer may hear a distinct or loud systolic murmur in the case of a thoracic aneurysm, the vibrations being communicated to the trachea, and thence directly by the air-column to the ears [83, p. 250].

Thus, Sansom sign refers to the presence of a systolic murmur heard with head of the stethoscope place within the patient's closed mouth when the sound is not discerned over the chest in patients with an aortic aneurysm (Table 1.1).

Glasgow Sign

William Carr Glasgow (1845–1907), son of William Glasgow Jr. (1813–1882), was born in St. Louis, Missouri, and received his medical degree from St. Louis Medical College in 1869 [84, 85]. After graduation, he continued his training abroad in Vienna where he devoted his studies to the fields of laryngology and diseases of the chest [85]. Glasgow was appointed Lecturer on Physical Diagnosis at St. Louis Medical College in 1872 and Professor of Disease of the Chest and Laryngology at St. Louis Post-Graduate Medical School in 1890 [85]. He was a member of the Faculty at the Missouri Medical College (later with St. Louis Medical College became known as Washington University) [85]. At Washington University, he

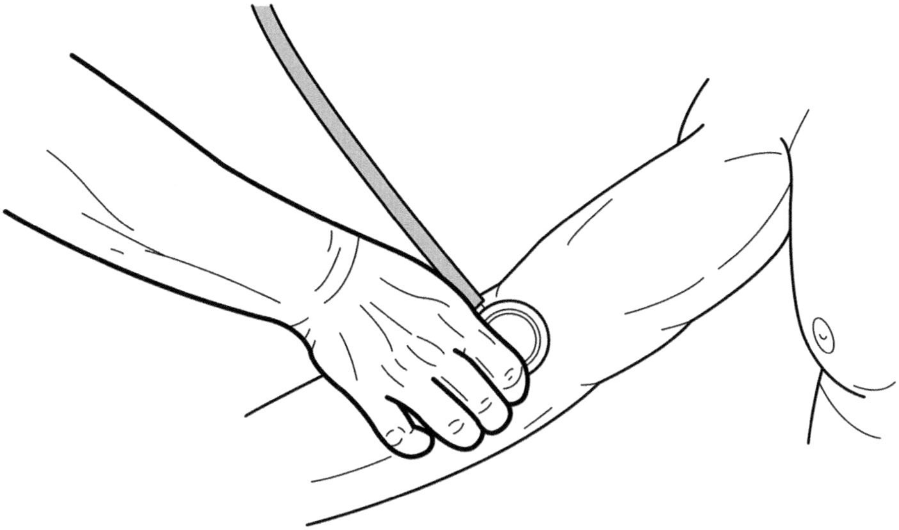

Fig. 1.3 Glasgow sign (by Ryan Yale)

served as Chair, Professor of Medicine and Laryngology, and practiced medicine at St. Louis City Hospital and Martha Parsons Hospital for Children, St. Louis, Missouri [84–86]. He served on the council of the Bates County Medical Society in St. Louis and was a co-founder of the American Laryngological Association in 1878, serving as its president in 1890 [86–88]. A description of his character as described by his friend D.B.D:

> As a scholar and as a man, Dr. Glasgow represented the highest and best type of the American physician. Through his character, breeding, and temperament his high social standing was everywhere assured. As a physician he was devoted to the welfare of all classes needing his aid. He was enthusiastic in his love for the scientific side of his calling. Personally, with unusual temptations to the contrary, he possessed a singular modesty of disposition and a large appreciation of the good work of other men. Notoriety of any kind was especially repugnant to him. Easily the first authority of his department in a section of the United States geographically larger than that occupied by any of his contemporaries living in other cities, he held the field without the semblance of a rival from the beginning to the end of his long and useful career. He was a delightful companion, an ideal physician and a widely appreciated and dearly loved friend [86].

Glasgow described a sign found over the brachial artery in five patients with an aortic aneurysm as a method for confirming the diagnosis. The maneuver is performed by extending the arm (Fig. 1.3):

> [t]o allow the free, unimpeded vibration of the brachial artery [89, p. 326]. [t]he presence of a systolic sound, or thud, in the brachial artery, synchronous with the systole of the heart. This sound is sometimes accompanied by an arterial murmur. When this sound can be heard and aortic regurgitation can be excluded, I claim that a positive diagnosis of aneurism can be made, even in the absence of all other signs or symptoms [89, p. 325].

He believed that "a forcible ventricular contraction" and "a free an unobstructed flow of blood through the aorta" were required in order to generate this sound. In patients whose aneurysm is present beyond the aortic arch, "[I] would explain the sign through the syphon action, which would draw the blood from the brachial artery, produced by the flow of blood into the dilated portion of the aorta." [89, p. 326]. This sign is not pathognomonic of aortic aneurysm and it may also be found in pure aortic regurgitation as reported by Josef Škoda (1805–1881) in 1869 [89]. The presence of this sign in other disease states suggests that it lacks sufficient specificity to confirm a diagnosis of aortic aneurysm. Thus, Glasgow sign refers to the presence of a systolic murmur auscultated over the brachial artery in patients with an early aortic aneurysm (Table 1.1).

Castellino Sign

Pietro Francesco Castellino (Castelino) (1864–1933) was born in Montevideo, Uruguay, and received his medical degree from the Clinic of Genoa in 1889 [90]. At the University of Genoa, he served as an assistant in medical propaedeutic followed by an appointment as ordinary assistant in the chair of the medical clinic [91]. This was followed by appointments at Pisa then Padua as Professor of Medical Pathology in 1894 [90–93]. At the University of Naples, Italy, he was Professor of the General Medical Clinic in 1899 [92]. He was elected deputy to the Parliament in the College of Foggia from 1904 to 1921 [93]. Castellino supported Fascism and in 1925 received a membership card from the National Fascist Party, serving as President of the National Institute of the Fascist Culture founded in 1926 [90]. Castellino reported to the Congress of Rome in 1897, as described in *Bulletin Medical*, the following finding:

> It consists of observing the laryngotracheal pulsation while the patient breaths normally or by asking him to take a deep inspiration. If an aneurysm is present, there will be a change in the heartbeat as expressed in the laryngotracheal beats. It is known that deep inspiration causes a variation in intrathoracic pressure and that this variation affects the pressure of blood within the aneurysmal pocket and therefore the intensity of its beat [94].

Castellino believed that this was a method for differentiating thoracic aneurysm from a solid intrathoracic tumor since the latter is not affected by changes in intrathoracic pressure and therefore, laryngotracheal pulse [95]. In fact, at the Seventh Congress of the Italian Society of Internal Medicine in 1896, he reported two patients with esophageal carcinoma extending to the second dorsal vertebrae and near the aortic arch with:

> [a] pulsation of the laryngotracheal tube which was not changed by deep inspiration. (…) [t]he malignant tumor had pressed the larynx and trachea forward to the aortic arch which communicated pulsations to them. In a given case this pulsation may be used as a diagnostic symptom [96].

The laryngo-tracheal pulsation in these cases were not affected by deep inspiration and were caused by an esophageal cancer pushing the tracheal forward against the aorta [96]. A similar phenomenon was described by Antonio Cardarelli and General William Silver Oliver in 1878 and William Henry Porter in 1896 (Table 1.1).

Porter Sign

William Henry Porter (1790–1861) was born in Dublin, Ireland, and received his medical degree from Trinity College in 1842 [97]. He assisted Sir Philip Crampton (1777–1858) (first surgeon Extraordinary to the King in Ireland) and conducted his professional training at College School and Meath Hospital beginning in 1809 [97]. Porter was elected member of the Royal College of Physicians, Ireland, in 1814 [97]. He was a surgeon at Meath Hospital and Consulting surgeon to Dublin Hospital in 1819, taught anatomy and surgery at the Park-Street School in 1826, and was appointed Professor of Surgery to the College of Surgeons in 1837 [97]. He published two books, one in 1826 titled *Observations on the Surgical Pathology of the Larynx and Trachea* and the other in 1840 titled *Observations on the Surgical Pathology and Treatment of Aneurism* [97]. He was elected President of the Royal College of Surgery, Ireland, in 1838 [97]. In his book *Observations on the Surgical Pathology and Treatment of Aneurism,* Porter described the following finding:

> Occasionally, a distinct double pulsation, as the contraction of two cavities, is heard toward the superior part of the thorax-at the junction of the second or third rib with the sternum on the right side-or corresponding to the junction of the first and second pieces of the breast bone. (…) All the other symptoms of thoracic aneurism have reference to the degree and direction of the *pressure* exercised on one or other of the organs within the chest. Few tumor could exist in the neighbourhood of the arch of the aorta without compressing the trachea or bronchial tubes more or less, and hence there may be difficult or imperfect respiration of every possible character and intensity, from a slight feebleness to a total absence in some part or portion of the lung [98, p. 66].

Joseph Winston et al., in their 1897 paper "Signs and symptoms of aortic aneurism" published in the *American Medico-surgical Bulletin* (edited by William Henry Porter and colleagues), reported that:

> Even a small aneurism, if so situated as to press upon the left bronchus, will cause rhythmic downward excursion of this tube. This movement can be appreciated as a distinct downward "tug" of the thyroid cartilage when the finger is placed below the beak of the larynx [99, p. 561].

William Henry Porter in his 1899 paper "The early diagnosis of aneurysm of the arch" described the clinical signs and symptoms found in thoracic aneurysm:

> Tracheal tugging and tracheal pulsation as well as dysphagia may appear, the latter varying in intensity at times but generally at a stage when there is other and more positive evidence, and thee have received as much prominence in our books and journals as, in the present state of our knowledge, they are entitled to [100, p. 4].

Park in his chapter on aneurysm stated that detecting this pulsation is a method for distinguishing innominate from aortic aneurysms [101]. Thus, Porter sign like Cardarelli and Oliver signs refers to the presence of tracheal tugging in patient with aortic aneurysms. General William Silver Oliver and Antonio Cardarelli published their finding of the "tracheal tug" seen in aortic aneurysm in 1878 and Castellino in 1896 (Table 1.1).

Hall Sign

Francis de Havilland Hall (1847–1929) was born in Hatfield, England, and received his medical degree from St. Bartholomew Hospital Medical School, London, in 1872 [102, 103]. Throughout his career, he was stationed at Westminster Hospital, London, beginning as a medical registrar and tutor in 1875, followed by appointments in the laryngeal department as assistant physician, full physician in 1896, and consulting physician in 1912. He also was appointed vice-president, and member of the house committee [102, 104]. In the Royal College of Physician, London, he was elected Fellow in 1881, examiner in medicine for the conjoint Board (as well at Durham University, London), member of the council (1901–1903) censor (1908–1910), and Lumleian Lecturer (1913) [102, 104]. In 1901, he also served on the council and was President in the Chair of the Laryngological Society of London, which he cofounded with Sir Henry T. Butlin (1845–1912) and Felix Simon (1849–1921) [102, 105]. In addition, he was as honorary staff physician at St. Luke's Hostel and St. Mark's Hospital, London, and consulting physician to Brentfor, Eltham and Mottingham Hospitals [104, 106]. A description of his character as described by C.B.G., a friend whom he knew for 50 years:

> Dr. Hall had a signally gracious and happy style and manner, so transparently sincere, high-minded, and true that friends and patients alike trusted him through and through, and as a result he was rightly rewarded with a fine consulting practice of high order, which his painstaking and always up-to-date scientific knowledge amply merited. Although saturated with the love of his profession, Dr. Hall, like all wise men, had many and great interests outside it. His reading was wide and extensive: all historical and biographical and much theological matter was keenly read, English literature of a hundred or so years ago especially appealing to him. (…) He was a capital talker, with a large range of general information, and also a good listener and a most acceptable and congenial companion [102, p. 272].

De Havilland Hall, in describing the clinical findings of aneurysms involving the first part of the aortic arch in 1900, identified, "By far the most reliable auscultatory sign is the accentuation of the aortic second sound, sometimes amounting to a distinct thud or shock. This when present, affords very strong evidence in favour of an aneurysm." [107, p. 38–39]. Sir William Broadbent found in discussing this case also seen by him and presented by Hall:

> When that diastolic shock was present he regarded it as absolutely diagnostic, if well marked. But its absence, and more especially in aneurysm of the second and third part of the arch, must not be allowed to interfere with a diagnosis based on other physical signs because it might entirely disappear when consolidation had taken place to any considerable extent [107, p. 47–48].

Thus, this sign refers to the presence of an accentuated aortic component to the second heart sound or diastolic shock present in aneurysm involving the first part (proximal) portion of the aorta (Table 1.1).

Steell Sign

Graham Steell (1851–1942) was born in Edinburgh, Scotland, and qualified (MB) at the University of Edinburgh in 1872 [108]. After completing postgraduate training in Berlin, London, and Leeds, he returned and served as house-physician to George Balfour (1823–1903) in 1873 followed by appointments in Edinburgh Royal Infirmary, Stirling Infirmary, the Dispensary at Leeds Fever Hospital, and London Fever Hospital [108–110]. He received his medical degree in 1877 and from 1877 to 1878 was assistant in the Department of Materia Medica and Therapeutics at Edinburgh University [108]. From 1878 to 1883, he served as Resident Medical Officer, Honorary Assistant Physician beginning in 1883, and in 1889, full staff physician and Professor and Chair of Clinical Medicine to the Manchester Royal Infirmary (Manchester University) [110]. Additionally, he had staff appointments at Monsall Fever Hospital, Hospital for Diseases of the Skin, and Christie Cancer Hospital [110]. He was elected Fellow to the Royal College of Physicians in 1889, served as President of the Manchester Medical Society, Vice-President of the Section of Medicine in 1902, and member of the British Medical Association [110, 111]. His character as described by Bramwell:

> The present writer, who had that privilege thirty years later, can find no words that would more aptly describe his character: in fact, his modesty and courtesy would have been almost embarrassing to his younger friends had they not realized the truehearted kindness that lay below [108, p. 115].

In an obituary written in 1942, "He was a first-rate bedside teacher-best when demonstrating the physical signs of intrathoracic disease and considering their interpretation" [111].

Graham Steell in his lecture presented at the Royal College of Physicians on November 2, 1911 on the topic "Intrathoracic tumors and aneurysms in their clinical aspect," described two patients, one caused by an aneurysm in front of the heart and the other caused by a posterior intrathoracic mass. In both cases, the heart was thrusted forward during systole. In the patient with aneurysm there also were "two apex beats-if I may so say-one including and not extending much beyond the normal apex situation and the other quite separate and approach the left mid axillary line" [112, p. 22]. In the patient with the posterior mediastinal mass:

> The peculiar thrusting forwards of the heart in systole that occurs even when a solid tumour is situated behind the heart, no doubt depends on the ventricles of the heart becoming a solid mass of rigid muscle in systole, with its adjoining cartilages. The spine cannot yield backwards, therefore the sternum has to yield forwards. What may be called the special impulses of the heart are quite lost in *general* heave forwards. No doubt the instruments of precision we now possess may distinguish a dual pulsation in the case of an aneurysm situated behind the heart, but my old fashioned ideas make me apprehensive of such blending of the two impulses in the case I refer to as would make their distinction one of peculiar difficulty. Of one thing I am convinced; it is that to the eye, at any rate, the two very different conditions a solid tumour and a large aneurysmal sac behind the heart-occasion to the clinical observer a very similar condition, while I doubt if the most sensitive hand could convey the double impulse that must, one would think theoretically, be present in front in the case of aneurysm of the descending thoracic aorta [112, p. 22].

It is of interest that Steell, in fact, first published this finding of a forward thrusting pulsation of the precordium in cases of tumors of the posterior mediastinum in 1901 in the *Medical Chronicle* (Table 1.1) [113]. His name is best recognized in association with the sign Graham-Steell murmur described and published in the *Medical Chronicle* in 1888 while he was a staff member at the Royal Infirmary in Manchester [109]. He is also credited for recognizing the association between alcoholic cirrhosis and cardiac failure and beriberi later recognized as caused by thiamine deficiency [109].

Dorendorf Sign

Hans Dorendorf (1866–1943), at the time of the publication of the sign which bears his namesake in 1902, was an Assistant Surgeon at the Second Medical University Clinic of the Charité of Professor Carl Adolf Christian Gerhardt (1835–1902), a position which he held from 1899 to 1902 [114]. From 1909 to 1937, he served as head and chief physician of the Internal Department at Diakonissenkrankenhaus Bethanien (Deaconess Hospital Bethanien) [114]. He was appointed Professor in 1917 and, from 1939 to 1943, served as war representative at Bethanien Hospital [114]. Dorendorf described a previously unrecognized finding identified in six cases of aneurysms involving the aortic arch:

> The symptom observed in aortic arch aneurysms is that the pit overlying the left clavicle is absent. This area is commonly missed or tumor-like in appearance. The left external jugular vein shows considerably more filling than the right external jugular vein. Pressure applied superiorly removes the soft supraclavicular protrusion. The protrusion is due to the difficulty of blood draining from the root area of the innominate vein. The innominate vein runs from the top left to the bottom right to the superior vena cava crossing the aortic arch anteriorly. Thus, an aneurysm of the aortic arch could exert pressure on the vein causing it to be narrowed [115, p. 554].

Thus, Dorendorf sign refers to the absence of fullness or prominence of the supraclavicular fossa in aortic arch aneurysms (Table 1.1). He believed that the finding was caused by pressure exerted by the aneurysm of the aortic arch on the left innominate vein.

Bryant Sign

John Henry Bryant (1867–1906) was born in Somerset, England, and received his medical degree in 1891 from Guy's Hospital [116–118]. At Guy's Hospital, he served as house-physician, resident obstetric assistant, and Medical Registrar from 1892 to 1898, assistant physician in 1898, and Demonstrator of Morbid Anatomy from 1899 to 1903 [116, 117]. He was elected fellow to the Royal College of Physicians, London, in 1901, and appointed Lecturer on Materia Medica and Therapeutics at Guy Hospital in 1903 [116, 117]. He also served as editor of the Guy Hospital Reports [116]. A description of his character as written in an obituary:

> Apart from his profession, he had a nature that all who knew him loved. Always strenuously opposing deceit in any form, he said freely what he thought, perhaps sometimes to his own detriment, and he always pursued the course which he considered right. It would be hard to find a man of more upright character, who ran straight at all times, and thus endeared himself to everyone who really knew him. He accordingly made and retained a very large circle of real friends [117].

Bryant described the cases of a 28-year-old male with a rupture abdominal aortic aneurysm where on postmortem examination he found:

> In one cases blood was effused into the right spermatic cord, and the corresponding half of the scrotum was much ecchymosed [119, p. 75]. (…) When blood is extravasated into the anterior abdominal wall ecchymoses may appear, and in one case which I have already mentioned in which blood was effused into the spermatic cord, the scrotum on the same side became much ecchymosed [119, p. 79].

Thus, Bryant sign refers to the presence of scrotal ecchymosis in cases of ruptured abdominal aortic aneurysm (Table 1.1).

D'Amato Sign

Luigi D'Amato (1874–1951) was born in Campochiaro (Campobasso), Italy, and received his medical degree in 1897 from the University of Naples [120]. He served as assistant in the Second Medical Clinic in 1899, Lecturer in Special Medical Pathology in 1902, and Lecturer in Medical Clinic in 1905. He was appointed Full Professor of Medical Pathology in 1923 and Director of the Medical Clinic from 1923 to 1925 at the University of Messina, Italy [121, 122]. He returned to the University of Naples and in 1928 was appointed Full Professor of Special Medical Pathology and Full Professor of General Medical Clinic and Medical Therapy in 1935 [120]. In collaboration with Luigi Zoja (1866–1959), they founded the *Diagnostica e Tecnica di Laboratorio* (Diagnostic and Laboratory Techniques), a monthly international journal published between 1930 and 1941 [123]. He was Resident Member of the Royal Society of Naples in 1933 and served as Member of the Governing Council of the Italian Society of Internal Medicine, Ordinary Member of the Academy of Internal Medicine and Surgery at Naples and appointed

Senator of the Kingdom of Italy, serving as Minister of National Education in 1939 [120].

D'Amato, a student of Cardarelli, described in the beginning of 1870 two diagnostic signs to detect pathological conditions such as neoplastic tumors and aneurysms in the mediastinum (Table 1.1):

> I would like to literally reproduce the words with which he described the phenomenon in a brilliant lecture on latent and obscure aneurysms of the aorta: If you put the stethoscope to your throat, i.e. on the extrathoracic part of the trachea, you will hear very clear laryngotracheal breathing. If however, you place the stethoscope on the higher part of the manubrium sterni, close to the upper edge of the sternum, from this point downwards, you will no longer perceive this breathing, because the intrathoracic trachea is distant from the manubrium sterni by the abundant connective tissue. What I have said about auscultation also applies to percussion: if you percuss on the exposed part of the trachea and auscultate in the vicinity of the oral cavity by letting the patient open his mouth, you will perceive a very clearly transmitted resonance: laryngotracheal resonance. On the other hand, if you percuss the sternum on the manubrium, even vigorously, you will not hear that resonance. Therefore, the law is that the intrathoracic part of the trachea does not allow its tracheal breathing to be heard, nor does it disclose the resonance of the percussion. However, if a neoplastic tumor, or the most common tumor-an aneurysm is located between the trachea and manubrium sterni then a tracheal tone similar to extrathoracic auscultation is heard. If you percuss the manubrium sterni the tumor picks up the percussion sound and transmits it to the trachea [124, p. 316].

His name is also associated with two other signs. First, a pulmonary sign for pleural effusion which is the presence of percussion dullness in the paravertebral region moving to the cardiac border after the patient assumes the contralateral decubitus position [6]. Second, an abdominal sign which involves retraction of the right upper quadrant abdominal wall in cases of inflammation of the gallbladder or liver [38].

Quénu-Muret Sign

Edouard André Victor Alfred Quénu (1852–1933) was born in Marquise, Pas-de-Calais, France. He completed an internship in medicine at Desnos and three years of surgical training with Armand Després (1834–1896), Paul-Jules Tillaux (1834–1904), and Alfred Richet (1816–1891) [125, 126]. He was subsequently named prosector, and in 1883, hospital surgeon [125]. In 1886, he served as aggrégé to the sections of histology, anatomy, and physiology, and in 1890, was appointed professor and director of the amphitheater of the Cochin Hospital [125, 126]. He was appointed to the Academy of Sciences from 1917 to 1933, President of the National Academy of Surgery, Vice-President of the Anatomical Society of Paris, and Member of the Surgical Pathology Section in 1908 as well as President of the National Academy of Medicine in 1929 [126]. He was the awarded Commander of the Légion d'honneur in 1933 [126, 127]. A description of his character as described by Bernard Cunéo:

> Quénu was certainly a bit cold at first, and had the reputation of a rather rough man. I have, however, preserved from my reports with him the memory of perfect courtesy. Perhaps he was so because he knew me little and reserved his severity for those whom he had the task of educating. I believe, indeed, that if Quénu inspired any fear to his pupils, it was because he was convinced that a somewhat distant authority was the indispensable condition for the maintenance of discipline. All those who knew him well agreed that he was very kind. I talked about him with some of his patients. All had kept their surgeon the memory of a man very sweet and very compassionate. Quénu, it is true, had a very whole character. He defended what he believed to be the truth, without worrying about the consequences of his attitude. He showed it well during the war. I do not think he had a great indulgence for certain moral failings that we may be too ready to forgive today. A long existence of probity and honor gave him after all the right. I have not known Quénu well, and it is difficult for me to show him outside his official life, in the intimacy of his family. It is to the piety of one of his pupils who will be the person to portray his more personal traits and saw that the figure of this man had a great character and very good-hearted background hid under his apparent roughness [125, p. 143].

There is limited historical information on Louis Muret (1878–?). He served as a former intern of Hôpitaux de Paris in 1902 [128]. Edouard André Victor Alfred Quénu and Paul Louis Muret described in their paper "Sur le traitement moderne des anévrismes poplités", a method for testing the integrity of the collateral circulation prior to performing reconstructive or obliterative surgery on a popliteal aneurysm:

> If indeed the peripheral blood pressure is maintained after the main trunk has been compressed it is probable that one can apply the obliterative aneurysmogram. But if this pressure falls to zero, chances are that the collateral circulation is insufficient and that the obliterative operation leads to the same disasters as ligation or extirpation. To verify that there are sufficient collaterals which is so important, there would be in our opinion no disadvantage in exposing the dorsalis pedis artery during surgery to verify if direct compression of the popliteal above the sac causes bleeding or blocks the circulation within this artery [129, p. 287].

Matas in his 1914 paper entitled "Collateral circulation" described the limitation of this method:

> The fallacy underlying this test is that the pedal pulses (dorsalis pedis and posterior tibial) are often totally absent in popliteal and other aneurysms of the lower extremities and that scant, if any, hemorrhage occurs from the peripheral vessels. Yet, the nutrition and circulation of the foot is well preserved, even though weeks and months may have elapsed after the pulses have been lost. In these cases the circulation and nutrition of the peripheral parts are well preserved by impalpable collaterals after the main channels of the circulation have been blocked by pressure, thrombosis, embolism or atheroma. Furthermore, apart from the importance of avoiding open trauma in the peripheral parts, in which the circulation is most likely to suffer, it is desirable that the sufficiency or insufficiency of the collateral circulation should be determined long before an operation on the aneurysm is performed in order that suitable measures may be applied to develop the insufficient collaterals. Finally, this mode of demonstrating the persistence of the collateral circulation is unnecessary, as there are other means of determining quite clearly the collateral circulation without injuring or sacrificing the peripheral vessels [130, p. 1442].

Thus, Quénu-Muret sign refers to the method of determining the collateral circulation by the presence of increased blood flow and bleeding within the dorsalis pedis artery occurring after compressing the popliteal artery proximal to the arterial sac (Table 1.1).

Henle-Coenen Sign

Adolf Henle (1864–1936) was born in Dortmund, Germany. He was the father of Fritz Henle (1909–1993, photographer) and Werner Henle (1910–1987, described the Loop of Henle in the kidney), and AnneMarie (Pope) Henle (1907–2001, Founder and President of the International Exhibition Foundation) [131, 132]. Prior to 1908, Coenen served as Assistant to the Berlin Surgical Clinic under Professor Ernst von Bergmann (1836–1907). That same year, he was appointed Associate Professor of Surgery in Breslau (Wroclaw, Poland) [133]. During World War I, he served as Surgeon General for the German Army [131]. He also served as Director of Städtische Krankenanstalten (State Hospital in Heidelberg) [131]. At the time of his publication of the sign which bears his namesake in 1913, he was Senior Physicians at the Breslau Clinic [134]. In 1915, he was awarded by the King of Greece two souvenir medals in gratitude for his medical care provided for wounded soldiers rendered during the Greek-Turk and Greek-Bulgarian campaigns [135]. He was appointed Professor of the Surgical Department at the University of Münster from 1923 to 1945 [136].

Henle, in a brief commentary written in 1914 regarding Professor H. Coenen's report published in *Zentralblatt für Chirurgie* in 1913, stated that:

> The collateral sign given by Coenen, i.e. The determination of whether there are enough collaterals besides an injured or aneurysm-diseased artery, or whether the formation of the secondary tracts requires a suture or plastic, corresponds exactly to my opinion at the Congress of Surgeons in 1912 (Verh, p. 134). A more detailed communication on the same subject in the papers on clinical surgery was written by my assistant Stolz is in press [137].

Carl Stolz, a medical assistant of Dr. Henle, published a short report on a series of six aneurysms cases treated by Dr. Henle by "double ligation and extirpation of the sac" as well as a surgical technique for management of aneurysm involving the femoral artery [138]. He further noted that:

> Professor Henle has already written on two femoral aneurysms and elsewhere briefly reported (7 and 8) and commented on the question which operation method should be used in each case and on what indications. Whether to stop, sew or graft an aneurysm during surgery depends on the circulation in the peripheral parts of the extremity after ligation. It is possible to formulate how the circulation will respond during an operation after an occlusion if one proceeds in the following way: Before resection of the aneurysm sac, one looks for the leading and trailing arterial end and compresses them using Höpfner clamps [138, p. 452].

Coenen described the "collateral sign" for testing the collateral circulation during operations for aneurysm and management of injuries involving large arteries:

> When the blood flows, i.e. without Esmarch's blood deficiency, the aneurysm sack is completely dissected free of the vessels. The artery is compressed above (central) and below (peripheral), close to the aneurysm, so that there is no blood flow from the arterial vessel pathway. Now place a Höpfner clamp, below the peripheral ligature and cut between this and the peripheral ligature of the artery. (...) If this Höpfner clamp is released and hemorrhage of bright red blood occurs from the clamped peripheral arterial trunk, then there is

> sufficient collateral circulation (positive collateral sign) and the ligature can safely be made. If, however, no blood is flowing from the peripheral stump then no collateral circulation has formed (assuming no thrombus is present) ("negative collateral sign") [134, p. 1914].

Henle-Coenen sign refers to the intraoperative method for determining whether there are sufficient collateral circulations during repair of an aneurysm (Table 1.1).

Von Frisch Sign

We were unable to identify any historical information on O. Von Frisch. Von Frisch described a method for testing the integrity of the collateral circulation during surgery on vascular injuries and aneurysms which involved compressing the artery at the proximal side of injury and observing for the following:

> l) Normal or near normal coloration of the periphery. 2) Arterial bleeding from the peripheral opening of the injured artery. 3) Venous stasis behind the clamped main vein. If the latter is present, then this phenomenon is significant. When, the main artery is clamped, the peripheral part of the main vein becomes enlarged and if this phenomenon of stasis recurs each time compression is repeated then this indicates with certainty that there are secondary pathways through which arterial blood flows extensively into the extremity [139, p. 90].

He found that "If point 1 is clearly positive, then the other phenomena are not required. Point 3 may be used alone if the other manifestations are not clear; but only if the finding is positive" [139, p. 90]. Von Frisch believed that of these three observations that:

> [I] think I can attach more importance to the phenomenon of the veins, for the following reason: l) Not infrequently, in most varied operations, we see that there is bleeding from the peripheral end of the divided artery. 2) A moderate arterial hemorrhage from the peripheral stump of the vessel does not yet prove that the blood entering through the collateral route also penetrates into the periphery of the extremity; indeed in most aneurysms I found no peripheral pulse before the operation. In contrast, a visible stasis of blood distally to the clamped main vein indicates that blood flows in from the capillary area of the extremity, that is, blood is flowing collaterally up to the final branching. This provides further evidence that venous reflux is a much more certain sign of peripheral perfusion than arterial hemorrhage from the peripheral stump [139, p. 90–91].

Thus, Von Frisch sign refers to the method of testing the integrity of collateral circulation in patients with aneurysm after clamping the peripheral portion of the primary vein and assessing for the presence of venous reflux (Table 1.1).

Chalier Sign

Joseph Chalier (1884–1942) was born in Mende, France, and completed his thesis in Medicine from Hospital of Lyon in 1909 [140]. He served as head of the adjoint laboratory, medical clinic in the Hospital of Lyons in 1919 [141]. In 1920, he was head of the Infectious Disease service at the hospital at Croix-Rousse followed by an appointment as Professor of Medical Pathology from 1937 to 1938 and Professor Infectious Disease from 1938 to 1942 [140, 141].

In his discussion on aortic aneurysm, Chalier emphasized the importance of recognizing pulsation in diagnosis. He reported that:

> Most often palpation is negative. Even then a particular phenomenon is suggestive when pulsatility is not seen. It is the sign of the suction cup, which one of our patient's posed. On examination no pulsatility of the thorax was recognized. X-ray revealed the aneurysm. The patient's wife was made aware of the nature of the lesion and ask us why when she applied suction cups close together at the painful site she repeatedly heard them clink each other. As we have not personally looked for this symptom, we believe it prudent to express some reservations about its meaning; perhaps it was a noise related only to breathing movements [142, p. 80].

Thus, Chalier sign refers to a double-click when two metal cups are placed on the chest wall (Table 1.1) [38].

Shennan Sign

Theodore Shennan (1869–1948) was born at Bathgate, West Lothian and received his medical degree from the University of Edinburgh, Scotland, in 1895 [143, 144]. In 1896, he was a pathologist at Leith Hospital followed by an appointment at the Royal Edinburgh Hospital for Sick Children and the Edinburgh Royal Infirmary [144]. He was appointed Fellow of the Royal College of Surgery, Edinburgh, in 1898, Lecturer in Pathology and Bacteriology in Surgeons Hall in 1899, pathologist and conservator of the museum of Surgeons Hall to the Edinburgh Royal Infirmary, and Chair of Pathology at the Royal Infirmary [143–145]. From 1914 to 1936, he was appointed Professor of Pathology at Aberdeen University, Scotland, and served as Dean of the Faculty of Medicine from 1915 to 1919 and from 1925 to 1927 at Aberdeen University. He was Chairman of the House Committee of Marischal College (merged with King's College to form University of Aberdeen in 1860) and appointed to the University court [143]. He was one of the founding members of the Pathological Society of Great Britain and Ireland [143]. A description of his character:

> His lively interest in the student body never flagged; he served for many years on the committee of management of the Union and did much to encourage social and athletic pursuits. Shennan will be remembered for his work as a morbid anatomist. The first edition of his textbook on *Post Mortems and Morbid Anatomy* appeared in 1912, the second in 1927, and the third in 1935. They embody the personal experience of a keen and accurate observer and contain a great store of useful information for the more mature pathologist as well as for the students for whom they were designed [143].

He found that "In dissecting aneurysm of the aorta delay of the pulse beat, when compared with the apical beat, can occur in all arteries, resulting from delay and weakening of the blood stream entering or passing through the involved artery or arteries" [146]. Thus, Shennan sign refers to the delayed pulse compared to the apex heart beat occurring in patients with aortic dissection (Table 1.1).

Sabathié Sign

Luis González Sabathié (1905–1957) received his medical degree from the Faculty of Medical Science of Rosario graduating with a gold medal in 1931 [147, 148]. In 1932, he published his book *Clasificación Clínica de la Arteria Pulmonar - La Esclerosis Primitivas Latentes* (Clinical Classification of the Pulmonary Artery - Latent Primitive Sclerosis), for which he was awarded first prize by the Rosairo Medical Circle in 1932, and in 1935 and 1939, he published the first and second volumes of his book titled *Temas de Cardiología* (Cardiology Issues) [147]. In 1937, at the National Centennial Hospital, he developed the first Dispensary of the Cardiac Aid Organization in Rosario, Argentina, and later was instrumental in serving as founder and full member of the Argentine Society of Cardiology [147, 148].

In 1939, he published the book *Las Cardiopatías y el Problema Médico Social* (Heart Disease and the Social Medical Problem), highlighting the social aspects of heart disease in Argentina [147]. In 1946, he resigned due to political reason from the National Government and was reinstated in 1954. He founded the Rosario Institute of Cardiology I at San Lorenzo y Corrientes in 1954. In recognition of his accomplishment, the institute was later named Instituto de Cardiología de Rosario Dr. Luis González Sabathié [147]. He was appointed Full Professor in 1957 [147–149], Foreign Correspondent Member of the French Society of Cardiology, and founder and first President of the Rosario Cardiology Society in 1956 [147, 148, 150]. Additionally, he was founder and member of the first board of director of the Rosarina Association of English Culture, member of Friends of Art Association, and President of the Cultural Association of El Circulo [149].

Among his many accolades, he was awarded in 1939 the Municipal Culture Commission of Rosario for his works on "Temas de Cardiología" (Cardiology Issues), and "Las cardiopatías y el problema médicosocial" (Cardiopathies and the Medical-Social Problem) [148, 149]. As a description of his character:

> Finally, there is no semblance of the figure of González Sabathié if one does not include a memory from all of his friends. He was the one who eased turbulent times by bringing out a smile even during the toughest times in life. His discussion among friends, his vivacious smile, and his talents as a category narrator had us pending his words sometimes for hours in all the acts of comradeship at the Society which he accompanied us. It is our most sincere feeling during this hour in time where understanding and tolerance are oddities of daily living that when we know that his disappearance leaves a void which will be difficult to fill [148, p. 6].

Sabathié reported a new sign involving the left external jugular vein in patients with diseases involving the thoracic aorta:

> As a pathological index, unilateral distention of the jugular is of great importance. Despite a thorough literature search we did not find that it has been previously reported as an important sign indicating an aortopathy. We have found this sign particularly in four aortic conditions: arterial hypertension with somewhat pronounced changes in the aortic, aortic sclerosis, aortitis, and aneurysms. The engorgement, which ranges from being hardly perceivable to grossly evident, is isolated, or predominantly on the left side. Looking for it systematically in healthy and ill patients we found it around sixty times. In two cases it was not just an aortopathy. One was a cancer of the left pulmonary vertex that caused other alterations of the supraclavicular fossa and the other in a subject apparently free of cardiovascular disease. The rest corresponded preferably to hypertensive patients with more or less pronounced radiological alterations of the aorta and aortitis [151, p. 270].

I observed in one patient marked engorgement of the left external jugular vein when the patient was standing and dressed. He described the technique for identifying left jugular vein distention in cases where this finding is not apparent:

> The patient is placed in the left or right dorsal decubitus position with the head and upper chest exposed. The head is rotated to the side opposite to the one being examined. The comparative observation allows one to appreciate the exclusive or predominant engorgement. In certain not so obvious cases, especially in picnicos or obese subjects it is possible to accentuate the engorgement by asking the patient to take a deep expiration [151, p. 271].

He described the proposed pathogenesis of the findings:

> Because of the anatomical relationships of the left brachiocephalic trunk and the highest part of the arch, this sign should be interpreted as being caused by the elevation and pathological elongation of the aortic arch. The pathogenesis is more likely if subjects with this sign have increased venous pressure and decreased blood velocity on the same side [151, p. 273].

Thus, Sabathié sign refers to dilation of the left external jugular vein (more predominant if bilateral or unilateral) in patients with diseases involving the aorta (arterial hypertension with changes in the aortic, aortitis, sclerosis, and aneurysm) (Table 1.1).

Roesler Sign

Hugo Roesler (1899–1961) was born in Vienna, Austria, and received his medical degree from the University of Vienna School of Medicine in 1931 [152]. In 1931, he served as a Research Fellow at New York and Harvard Universities [152]. He was appointed Faculty to Temple University School of Medicine, Philadelphia Pennsylvania in 1932 and rose to the rank of Associate Professor of Medicine. Roesler published three books including *Clinical Roentgenology of the Cardiovascular System* in 1937 [153].

Roesler, Gifford, and Betts reported and described a diagnostic sign in a 76-year-old male patient with dissecting aortic aneurysm at, "[t]he level of the eighth interspace, the center being 6 cm. from the spinous processes. Three days later it was found to be 9 cm. out. Over this pulsating area the aortic second sound was very accentuated." [154, p. 426]. They indicated that a rapidly increasing area of pulsation as well as radiological change in the aortic shadow to be diagnostic of dissecting aneurysm. Thus, Roesler sign refers to a rapidly shifting area of pulsation in the interscapular area over which the aortic second sound was accentuated (Table 1.1).

Nissim Sign

Joseph Abraham Nissim (1907–1966) was born in Iraq and received his medical training at Guy Hospital, London, beginning in 1938 [155]. He was a resident medical officer at County Hospital, Dartford and Queen Mary's Hospital, Sidcup, from 1943 to 1944, graduating with a Medical Degree (MB) from Guy's Hospital, London, in 1944 [155]. From 1944 to 1946, he was appointed resident medical officer at North Staffordshire Royal Infirmary [155]. At Guy Hospital, he spent his medical career in the Pharmacology Department first as a demonstrator in 1947, lecturer in 1950, senior lecturer in 1954, and reader in 1957 [155]. He is credited for developing the first intravenous iron preparation [155]. A description of his character as described by J.M.R:

> On the surface Nissim appeared shy and retiring, but he had a strong and unusual personality, highly sensitive and somewhat eccentric, yet uncompromising to the extent of obsession. His life was based entirely on his work, and literally nothing else counted. He worked day and night, without break and without holidays, like a monk worshipping his mystic religion of scientific idea and discovery [155].

Nissim reported the case of a 71-year-old male with dissecting aortic aneurysm and a:

> [d]ifference between the right and left carotid pulsations. They were reduplicated on the right and single on the left, without a coexisting noticeable difference in the intensity of the pulsations on the two sides. There were two almost equal beats in quick succession on the right carotid for every single beat on the left [156, p. 204].

He believed that this unilateral finding within the right carotid artery was caused by "the difference of the rate of propagation of the pulse wave through the lumen of the artery and through its dissected coats where the blood was probably partly clotted" [156, p. 205]. Thus, Nissim sign refers to the double beat palpated over the right carotid artery in patients with aortic dissection (Table 1.1).

Logue Sign

Bruce Logue (1911–2007) was born in Augusta, Georgia, and received his medical degree from Emory University Medical School Atlanta, Georgia, in 1937 [157]. He served during World War II in the Army Medical Corps from 1941 to 1946, was

Chief of Cardiology at Lawson General Hospital from 1941 to 1943, and Chief of Medicine (248th General Hospital, Philippines from 1945 to 1946, achieving the rank as Lieutenant Colonel) [158, 159]. In 1946, he was appointed Instructor in the Department of Medicine at Emory University School of Medicine [159]. He founded the Emory University Clinic in 1953, served as Chief of the Medical Section of Emory Clinic from 1955 to 1980, and Chief of Medicine at Emory University Hospital from 1957 to 1980 [157–159]. From 1980 to 1986, he served as Director of the Carlyle Fraser Heart Center [159].

Dr. Longue established the cardiology fellowship program at Emory University and Grady Hospital [157, 158]. From Emory University, he is the recipient of the Medical Alumni Award of Honor in 1970 and Master Teacher Award in 2005. The Chair of Cardiology at Emory was named in his honor in 1986 [157]. He served on a number of national committees including President of the American Federation for Clinical Research, Vice-President of the American Heart Association, Chairman of the Subspecialty Board of Cardiovascular Disease of the American College of Physicians and American Board of Cardiology [157, 159]. He coedited along with Willis Hurst the first seven editions of the book *The Heart*. He received a number of awards from the American College of Cardiology including the Master Teachers Award in 1969, Presidential Citation Award in 1999, and in 2000, the Bruce Logue Award established to honor those physicians who best display humanitarian and ethical aspects of medicine [157].

As described by Charles R. Hatcher, Jr. a cardiology surgeon in an obituary written by Derrick Henry:

> Bruce was one in a million. He was a very dynamic physician, very dedicated to his patients. And he was an extremely good teacher and diagnostician. Bruce was very good with a stethoscope. He could make a diagnosis in seconds and was extremely accurate. He tried to make exams as economical as possible for his patients [160].

R. Bruce Logue and Clayton Sikes reported in five cases the method to further confirm the diagnosis and distinguish dissecting aortic aneurysm from an acute myocardial infarction as a causes of chest pain, "If present, pulsation of either the right or left sternoclavicular joint may be vigorous or minimal. This sign depends on the sudden fluctuating increase in superior mediastinal pressure resulting from acute expansion of the aorta" [161, p. 1209].

Logue and Sikes noted the absence of sternoclavicular pulsation in cases of chronic aortic enlargement and hypertension and "syphilitic aortic insufficiency with chest pain due to coronary ostial disease" [161, p. 1210]. Based on their experience, they concluded, "The presence of a pulsating sternoclavicular joint with aortic insufficiency, hypertension and a dilated aorta has proved diagnostic of dissecting aneurysm"[161, p. 1209–1210]. Thus, Logue sign refers to the presence of pulsation of the sternoclavicular joint in the case of aortic dissection (Table 1.1).

Conclusion

The majority of patients with aortic aneurysms are asymptomatic and hence they are not detected during the physical examination. Symptoms when present depend upon the location and may include pain and the presence of a pulsatile soft mass. Aortic dissection typically presents acutely with symptoms referable to the site of dissection. Physician prior to the development of imaging studies identified signs found on physical examination in order to aid in diagnosis. These techniques or maneuvers were attributed after their namesake to honor their contributions. We call attention to the name Castellino who was a member of the Fascist party, as eponyms represent honorific names and therefore should not be used if there is connotation to beliefs that represent hatred, bigotry, or crimes against a race. Many of these signs were identified in patients with advanced disease. They have not been studied and thus their utility in clinical practice is unknown providing opportunities in some cases for further investigation. Nonetheless, they are important as they provide insights and reinforce the importance of taking a detailed history and physical examination and to consider aneurysm and dissection in the differential diagnosis.

References

1. Bryan CP. Diagnosis. In: Ancient Egyptian Medicine – The Papyrus Ebers. Chicago: Ares Publishers; 1974. p. 133–51.
2. Erichsen JE. Galen - Symptoms, pathology and causes. Observations on Aneurisms, Selected from the Works of the Principal Writers on that Disease from the Earliest Period to the Close of the Last Century. Translated and edited by John E. Erichsen from Claudii Galeni Opera omnia, tom. viii, 1609. vol. v, p. 84, De Tumoribus pneter Naturam, cap. 11, De Aneurysmate et Sydratione. London: Sydenham Society; 1844. p. 3.
3. Daremberg B. Oeuvres d'Oribase: Collationné sur les manuscrits. Tome quatrième. Paris: Imprimerie Impériale; 1862. p. 660.
4. Erichsen JE. Aëtius - On dilation of the vessel. In: Observations on Aneurisms. Selected from the works of the principal writers on that disease from the earliest period to the close of the last century. Translated and edited by John E. Erichsen from Aëtii, Contracts; ex Veteribus Tetrabiblos; fol. Basiliae, 1542. Serrno 3, cap. x, De Vasorum Dilatatione. London: Sydenham Society; 1844. p. 4.
5. O'Malley CD. Translations of Vesalius's medical opinions. In: Andreas Vesalius of Brussels, 1514–1564. Berkeley: University of California Press; 1964. p. 378–402.
6. Erichsen JE. Petit – Symptoms, pathology and causes. In: Observations on Aneurisms. Selected from the Works of the Principal Writers on that Disease from the Earliest Period to the Close of the Last Century. Translated and edited by John E. Erichsen from Paré A. De Aneurisme Le. vii, Liu Des Tum. En general. chap. 34. In: Les oeuvres d'Ambroise Paré A., conseiller et premier chirurgien du Roy. Dixième édition. Lyon: Chez Claude Prost; 1641. p. 184.

7. Wiseman R. Chap XVI of an Aneurisma. In: Several Chirurgical Treatises. London: Norton and J. Macock; 1686. p. 70–7.
8. Monro D. Cafes of aneurisms, with remarks by Dr. Donald Monro, physician to St. George's Hospital, London. In: Essays and Observations, Physical and Literary, vol. III. Edinburgh: Printed for John Balfour; 1771. p. 178–291.
9. Wright WC. Aneurysms in general. In: Giovanni Maria Lancisi 1654–1720. Aneurysms: The Latin Text of De Aneurysmatibus, Rome 1745. Wright WC, translator. New York: The MacMillian Company; 1952. p. 3–18.
10. Erichsen JE. Petit – Symptoms, pathology and causes. Observations on Aneurisms. Selected from the works of the principal writers on that disease from the earliest period to the close of the last century. Translated and edited by John E. Erichsen from Par M. Petit. Observations Anatomiques et Pathologiques au sujet de la Tumeur qu'on nomme Anevrysme. Memoires de l'Academie Royale des Sciences. Paris, 1736. p. 244–55. London: Sydenham Society; 1844. p. 89–98.
11. Erichsen JE. Bourdelot – Symptoms, pathology and causes. Observations on aneurisms. Selected from the works of the principal writers on that disease from the earliest period to the close of the last century. Translated and edited by John E. Erichsen. London: Sydenham Society; 1844. p. 207–13.
12. Morgagni JB. Aneurism of the heart, and dilation of the aorta; the aorta ruptured into the pericardium by an indirect canal. In: The Seats and Causes of Diseases, Investigated by Anatomy; Containing a Great Variety of Dissections, and Accompanied with Remarks, vol. 1. Abridged, and elucidated with copious noted by William Cooke. Boston: Wells and Lily and HC Carey and I. Lea; 1824. p. 362.
13. Dawes SL. Little biographies and the eponymic diseases: Dominic John Corrigan. Albany M. Ann. 1908;29:363–5.
14. [No author]. Obituary: Sir Dominic John Corrigan, Bart; M.D. Med Times & Gaz. 1880;1:164–6.
15. Stephen L. Corrigan Sir Dominic John, M.D. (1802–1880). Dictionary of National Biography, vol. 12. London: Smith, Elder, & Co.; 1887. p. 252.
16. Debrett J. Corrigan, creation 1866, of Cappagh and Inniscorrig, Dublin. In: Debrett's Peerage, Baronetage, Knightage and Titles of Courtesy. London: Dean & Son; 1878. p. 111.
17. [No author]. In Memoriam Sir Dominic John Corrigan, Bart, M.D. Dublin J M Sc. 1880;69:268–72.
18. [No author]. Titular distinctions for medical men. Med Press & Circ. 1883:38.
19. Zacek P. Corrigan sign. In: Vojacek J, Zacek P, Domink J, editors. Aortic Regurgitation. Cham: Springer; 2016. p. 67–8.
20. [No author]. Obituary: Sir Dominic John Corrigan. Med News & Abstr. 1880;38:254.
21. Corrigan DJ. Aneurysm of the aorta; singular pulsation of the arteries: necessity of the employment of the stethoscope. Lancet. 1829;1:586–90.
22. Hope J. Sketches of Eminent Medical Men. London: The Religious Tract Society; 1790. p. 166–92.
23. Wilius FA, Keys TF. James Hope (1801–1841). In: Classics of Cardiology. New York: Dover Publications, Inc. 1941. p. 403–4.
24. [No author]. James Hope (1801–1841). JAMA. 1965;191:1076–7.
25. Major RH. James Hope. In: Classic Descriptions of Disease. 3rd edition. Illinois: Charles C. Thomas; 1945. p. 349–51.
26. Fye WB. James Hope. In: Hurst JW, Conti CR, Fye WB, editors. Profiles in Cardiology. New Jersey: Foundation for Advances in Medicine and Science; 2003. p. 109–10.
27. [No author]. Dr. James Hope. Nature. 1941;147:605–6.
28. Hope J. Memoir of the Late James Hope, M.D., Physician to St. George's Hospital. Grand K, editor. London: J. Hatchard & Son; 1842.
29. Hope J. General signs of aneurism of the aorta. In: A Treatise of the Diseases of the Heart and Great Vessels, Compromising a New View of the Physiology of the Heart's Action. London: William Kidd; 1832. p. 414–31.

30. Fresquet JL. Sigismond François Jaccoud (1830–1913). Biographies. Historia del a Medicina. 2008. https://www.historiadelamedicina.org/jaccoud.html. Accessed 20 Jun 2019.
31. [No author]. Death of Sigmond Jaccoud. JAMA. 1913;60:1650.
32. RHPST. Fonds Sigismond Jaccoud (1830–1913). https://rhpst.huma-num.fr/items/show/274. Accessed 20 Jun 2019.
33. Perier C. Jaccoud François Sigismond. Comité des travaux historiques et scientifiques Institut rattache à l'Ecole nationale des chartes. http://cths.fr/an/savant.php?id=3879#. Accessed 15 Apr 2019.
34. Colby FM. Necrology: Jaccoud François Sigismond. In: The New International Year Book: A Compendium of the World's Progress for the Year 1913. New York: Dodd, Mead and Company; 1914. p. 481.
35. Sigismond Jaccoud. Académie royale de Médecine de Belgique. http://www.armb.be/index.php?id=4294. Accessed 12 Feb 2019.
36. Collective. The Encyclopedia Americana: A Library of Universal Knowledge. New York: The Encyclopedia Americana Corporation; 1923. p. 572.
37. Jaccoud S. Cancer: Traité de pathologie interne. Troisième éd. Paris: Adrien Felahaye; 1873. p. 123–7.
38. Jaccoud S. De l'anevrysme aortique au début. In: Leçons de clinique médicale faites a l'Hôpital de la Charité. Troisième éd. Paris: Adrien Delahaye; 1874, p. 224–50.
39. Williams ME. The neck. In: Geriatric Physical Diagnosis: A Guide to Observation and Assessment. Jefferson: McFarland & Company, Inc.; 2009. p. 129.
40. Birrer RB, Birrer CD. Medical Diagnostic Signs: A Reference Collection of Eponymic Bedside Diagnostic Signs. Springfield: Charles C. Thomas Publisher; 1982. p. 49.
41. White FA. Physical Signs in Medicine and Surgery: An Atlas of Rare, Lost and Forgotten Physical Signs. Ocala: Museum Press Books; 2009. p. 131.
42. Antonio Cardarelli. Cose di Napoli Apt Napoli. 2017 Associazione di promozione turistica e culturale. http://cosedinapoli.com/culture/antonio-cardarelli/. Accessed 14 Jun 2019.
43. Cardarelli A. Sulla pulsazione de tubo laringo-tracheale come segno di certi aneurismi dell'arco aortico. Gior Internaz d Sc Med. 1894;16:481–91.
44. [No author]. Surgeon-General William Silver Oliver, MD. Br Med J. 1908;1(2474):1337.
45. [No author]. Oliver, Dr. W.S., formerly of Ireland (-1908). The Evening Mail (Halifax, Nova Scotia). 1 May 1908. p. 10.
46. Patent no. 45782. Filing year 1894. Army Accoutrement, William Silver Oliver. Made in Canada Patents of Invention and the Story of Canadian Innovation. http://www.collectionscanada.gc.ca/innovations/023020-2220-e.html. Accessed 20 Aug 2019.
47. Oliver WS. Physical diagnosis of thoracic aneurysm. Lancet. 1878;2:406.
48. Howard CP. The diagnosis of mediastinitis. Bull Johns Hopkins Hosp. 1915;26:140–4.
49. [No author]. Obituary: Sir David Drummond MD, DCL. Br Med J. 1932;1(3722):865–6.
50. [No author]. Central chancery of the orders of knighthood. Lond M Gaz. 1929;5:1237.
51. Bhat S. Colonic surgeries. In: SRB's Surgical Operations: Text & Atlas. New Delhi: Jaypee Brothers Medical Publishers Ltd; 2014. p. 938–78.
52. [No author]. Drummond on auscultation of the mouth and trachea. London Med Rec. 15 Dec 1882. p. 499.
53. Drummond D. On auscultation of the trachea and mouth in thoracic disease. Med Press and Circular. 1882;2:773–4.
54. [No author]. Necrologio: Camillo Bozzolo commemorato dal Sen prof. E. Maragliano. Riforma Med. 1920;36:243–4.
55. Dianziani MU. Camillo Bozzolo (1845–1920).TorinoScienza Sito di informazione scientifica del Sistema scienza Piemonte 2016. https://www.torinoscienza.it/personaggi/camillo-bozzolo. Accessed 20 May 2019.
56. Bozzolo Camillo. Senato della Repubblica. http://notes9.senato.it/web/senregno.nsf/5cf68b34c7af786ac12571140059a4cb/388880b235e31a424125646f005949d3?OpenDocument. Accessed 10 Jun 2019.
57. [No author]. Notiziario: la morte di Camillo Bozzolo. Radiol Med. 1920;7:293–4.

58. Bozzolo C. L'anchilostomiasi e l'anemia che ne conseguita (anchilostomanemia). Gior Internaz d Sc Med. 1879;1:1054–69.
59. [No author]. XII. Congresso dell'Associazione Medica Italiana in Pavia. Gior Internaz d Sc Med. 1887:9:956–66.
60. Pierre Delbet (1861–1957). BnF Data. Last update 2029-05-16. https://data.bnf.fr/en/14629849/pierre_delbet/. Accessed 28 Feb 2019.
61. François M, Dosso D. Delbet Pierre Louis Ernest, Docteur. Comité des travaux historiques et scientifiques. Institut rattaché à l'École nationale des chartes. Fiche créée le 27/12/2012-Derniére mise à jour le 5/12/2018. http://cths.fr/an/savant.php?id=112306. Accessed 12 Jun 2019.
62. Professor Pierre Delbet. Institut Pierre Delbet 2014. http://en.institutpierredelbet.org/prof-pierre-delbet.html. Accessed 10 Jul 2019.
63. Gomez P, Morcuende JA. Early attempts at hip arthroplasty. Iowa Orthop J. 2005;25:25–9.
64. Tag Archives: Pierre Delbet. Paris Surgeon Grafts rubber on human body. New York Times. 11 Mar 1914. https://juxtintime.wordpress.com/tag/pierre-delbet/. Accessed 10 Jul 2019.
65. [No author]. Extirpation d'un anevrisme poplite. Bull et Mém Soc de Chir. 1909;35:865–80.
66. Delbet P. Du traitement des anevrysmes externs. Rev de Chir. 1888;8:533–58, 789–828, 869–913.
67. [No author]. Dr. William S. Cheesman of Auburn died May 7, 1912. Buffalo Med J. 1912;67:654.
68. Monroe JH. William S. Cheesman, M.D. In: Historical Records of a Hundred and Twenty Years. New York: F. Humphrey; 1930. p. 259–60.
69. Cheesman WS. The oral whiff. Med Rec. 1888;33:235–6.
70. [No author]. Obituary: Pierre Karl Edouard Potain, M.D. Br M J. 1901;1:121.
71. Beeson RB. Potain: his life and works. Bull Soc M Hist Chicago. 1923–1925;3:142–50.
72. Knopf SA. Obituaries: Professor Potain. N York M J. 1901;73:162.
73. [No author]. Pierre-Carl Potain (1825–1901), cardiovascular physician. JAMA. 1966;196:1086.
74. Pierre-Carl-Édouard Potain. The free dictionary by Farlex. http://encyclopedia2.thefreedictionary.com/Pierre-Carl-Edouard+Potain. Accessed 21 Mar 2019.
75. Pump aspirating (1) by Potain. Museum Sybodo. Medizinische Instrumente und Geräte der Krankenpflege. https://www.kugener.com/en/humanmedizin-en/chirurgie/50-artikel/8577-pump-aspirating-1.html. Accessed 25 Feb 2019.
76. Carpentier A, Filsoufi F. Pierre Charles Edouard Potain (1825–1901). Mitral Valve 2013. http://www.themitralvalve.org/mitralvalve/pierre-charles-edouard-potain. Accessed 14 Jun 2019.
77. Potain CE. De l'aortite. Union méd. 1889;48:746–51.
78. Broadbent WH. The pulse in aneurism. In: The Pulse. London: Cassell & Company; 1890. p. 227–35.
79. Broadbent WH, Broadbent John FH. Heart Disease and Aneurysm of the Aorta with Special Reference to Prognosis and Treatment. 4th ed. New York: William Wood & Company; 1906.
80. [No author]. Obituary: Arthur Ernest Sansom M.D. Lond. F.R.C.P. Lond. Lancet. 1907;1:842–5.
81. [No author]. Obituary: Arthur Ernest Sansom M.D. Lond; F.R.C.P. Med Press & Circ. 1907:134:319–20.
82. [No author]. Officers and Council of the Medical Society of London: Arthur Ernest Sansom, MD. Proc M Soc Lond. 1885;8:12.
83. Sansom AE. Systolic murmurs in aneurysm of the thoracic aorta-murmurs heard over the arteries and veins of the neck: their causes and associations. In: The Diagnosis of Diseases of the Heart and Thoracic Aorta and the Pathology which Serves for the Recognition of Morbid States of the Organs of Circulation. Philadelphia: P. Blakiston, Son & Company; 1892. p. 247–55.

84. Dr. William Carr Glasgow. Find A Grave. Created by Laura Added: 3 Jun 2005. https://www.findagrave.com/memorial/147356806/william-carr-glasgow. Accessed 6 Jul 2019.
85. W.A.H. Alumni necrology: William Carr Glasgow. The Bulletin of the Washington University Association. 1907;5:255–6.
86. [No author]. Obituary: William C. Glasgow, MD. of St. Louis. N York M J. 1907; 85:705.
87. [No author]. Bates County Medical Society: meeting of the Council. St Louis M & S J. 1878;35:51.
88. Rutkow IM. William Carr Glasgow (1845–1907). In: The History of Surgery in the United States, 1775–1900, vol. 2. San Francisco: Norman Publishing; 1992. p. 251–2.
89. Glasgow WC. A new and distinguishing sign of latent aneurism of the aorta. Trans Am Climatol Assoc. 1895;10:324–31.
90. [No author]. Pietro Castellino. Gior di Med Mil. 1933;81:907–9.
91. Castellino, Pietro. Treccani. http://www.treccani.it/enciclopedia/pietro-castellino_(Dizionario-Biografico)/. Accessed 20 May 2019.
92. Castellino P. Foreign university intelligence: medical news. Lancet. 1899;1:735.
93. [No author]. Necrologio: Pietro Castellino. L'Università Italiana Rivista dell'istruzione Superiore. 1933;29:193.
94. [No author]. Valeur séméiologique des pulsations laryngo-trachéales. Bull méd. 1897;5:1026.
95. [No author]. M. Castelino. Arch Internat de Laryngol. 1896;9:779.
96. P.K. Ueber das Pulsiren des Laryngotrachealrohres bei Oesophaguskrebs. (Les pulsations laryngotrachêules dans le cancer de l'oeso phage.) Von Dr. Castelino. (Septième Congrès de la Société italienne de médecine interne, October 1896 und Semaine médicale 1896, no. 55.) Monatsschr Ohrenheilkd Laryngorhinol. 1897;31–32:188.
97. Cameron CA. William Henry Porter, President in 1838. In: History of the Royal College of Surgeons in Ireland and of the Irish School of Medicine Including Numerous Biographical Sketches. Dublin: Fannin; 1886. p. 392–4.
98. Porter WH. Observations on the Surgical Pathology and Treatment Aneurism. Being the substance of a course of lectures on that disease. Delivered in the School of the Royal College of Surgeons in Ireland during the session 1839–1840. Part I. Dublin: Joshua A Porter; 1841.
99. Winston JP, Robinson WJ, West GE, Schöney L. Signs and symptoms of aortic aneurism. Am Med-Surg Bull. 1897;11:561–2.
100. Porter W. The early diagnosis of aneurysm of the arch. New York Med J. 1899:1–7.
101. Park R. Aneurism. In: The Principles and Practice of Modern Surgery. Philadelphia: Lea Brothers & Co.; 1907. p. 339–49.
102. [No author]. Obituary: F. de Havilland Hall M.D., F.R.C.P. Br Med J. 1929;1(3553):271–2.
103. Hall FDH. Who's Who 1923: An Annual Biographical Dictionary with which is Incorporated "Men and Women of the Time" Seventy-Fifth Year of Issue. London: A & C Black Limited; 1923. p. 1187–8.
104. Brown GH. Francis De Havilland Hall. Lives of the fellows. Royal College of Physicians 2009 Royal College of Physicians of London. http://munksroll.rcplondon.ac.uk/Biography/Details/1973. Accessed 12 Jul 2019.
105. Collective. Proceedings of the Laryngological Society of London, 1900–1901. London; 1901.
106. [No author]. Medical Sickness and Accident Society. Med Press & Circ. 1909;138:229.
107. Hall H. The diagnosis and treatment of intrathoracic aneurysm. Tr M Soc Lond. 1901;24:32–64.
108. [No author]. Graham Steell BC. Br Heart J. 1942;4:115–9.
109. [No author]. Graham Steell (1851–1942): Graham Steell murmur. JAMA. 1965;191:671.
110. Brown GH. Graham Steell. Lives of the fellow. Royal College of Physicians. http://munksroll.rcplondon.ac.uk/Biography/Details/4229. Accessed 12 Sep 2019.
111. [No author]. Obituary: Graham Steell MD, F.R.C.P. Br Med J. 1942;1:129.
112. Steell G. The Bradshaw Lecture on Intrathoracic Tumours and Aneurysms. Delivered before the Royal College of Physicians of London. Reprinted from the Lancet. 9 Dec 1911. p. 1–28.

113. Steell G. On a sign of intrathoracic tumor involving the posterior mediastinum. Med Chron. 1901;1:11–6.
114. Dorendorf, Hans. Edition Luisenstadt, 2002. Last updated 7/09/2009. Berliner Bezirkslexikon, Friedrichschain-Kreuzberg. https://berlingeschichte.de/lexikon/frkr/d/dorendorf_hans.htm. Accessed 4 Jan 2020.
115. Dorendorf S. Ueber ein bisher wenig beachtetes Aneurysmensymptom. Dtsch med Wochenschr. 1902;28(31):554–5.
116. [No author]. Obituary: John Henry Bryant. Lancet. 1906;167(4318):1575.
117. [No author]. Obituary: John Henry Bryant MD, Lond, FRCP. Br Med J 1906;1:1319.
118. John Henry Bryant. Munk's Roll, vol. IV. http://munksroll.rcplondon.ac.uk/Biography/Details/627. Accessed 28 Mar 2019.
119. Bryant JH. Two clinical lectures on aneurysm of the abdominal aorta: lecture 1. Clin Jour. 1903;23:71–80.
120. D'Amato Luigi. Senato della Repubblica. http://notes9.senato.it/Web/senregno.NSF/4038162380009750c125703d004eed42/f8448c75688adabb4125646f005aa7dd. Accessed 15 May 2019.
121. Luigi D'Amato (medico). Wikipedia L'enciclopedia libera. 2019. https://it.wikipedia.org/wiki/Luigi_D%27Amato_(medico). Accessed 3 Mar 2019.
122. Luigi D'Amato. Himetop. The History of Medicine Topographical Database. http://himetop.wikidot.com/luigi-d-amato. Accessed 4 Mar 2019.
123. G. Dall'Olio. 1930: nasce una Rivista di Laboratorio Clinico. Schegge di Storia della Medicina. RiMeL. p. 59–64. https://www.sipmel.it/it/riviste/articolopdf.php/102745. Accessed 23 May 2019.
124. D'Amato L. Die Auskultation des Bronchialatmens auf dem Thorax als Zeichen einiger Mediastinalaffektionen (Tumoren, Aneurysmen). Ztschr f klin Med. 1909;68:315–44.
125. Cunéo B. Notice nécrologique sur M. Edouard Quenu (1852–1933). Bull Acad de méd. 1933;110:131–44.
126. Quénu Édouard André Victor Alfred. Comité des travaux historiques et scientifiques. Institue rattaché à l'École nationale des chartes. Fiche créée le 28/01/2013-Derniére mise à jour le 02/07/2019. http://cths.fr/an/savant.php?id=112829. Accessed 5 Jun 2019.
127. Quénu Légion d'honneur. Archives Nationales 1933. p. 1–17. http://www2.culture.gouv.fr/LH/LH185/PG/FRDAFAN83_OL2246035V001.htm. Accessed 25 Jun 2019.
128. Muret, Paul-Louis. Association Amicale des Anciens Internes en Médicine de Hôpitaux de Paris. (AAIHP). http://www.aaihp.fr/AIHP.php?Lettre=M. Accessed 5 Jun 2019.
129. Quénu EA, Muret PL. Sur le traitement moderne des anévrismes poplités. Rév de Chir. 1910;41:282–94.
130. Matas R. Testing the efficiency of the collateral circulation as a preliminary to the occlusion of the great surgical arteries. JAMA. 1914;63:1441–7.
131. Flukinger R. Fritz Henle: In Search of Beauty. Austin: University of Texas Press; 2009.
132. [No author]. Paid notice: Deaths Pope, Annemarie Henle. The New York Times. 11 Nov 2001. p. 48.
133. [No author]. Foreign university intelligence: Dr. Hermann Coenen. Lancet. 1908;2:775.
134. Coenen H. Zur Indikationsstellung bei der Operation der Aneurysmen und bei den Gefaßverfetzungen. Zentralbl f Chir. 1913;40:1913–6.
135. [No author]. Medal for Coenen. JAMA 1915;64:676.
136. Fink BR, Morris LE, Stephen CR. The history of anesthesia. In: Third International Symposium: Proceedings, Atlanta, Georgia, March 27–31, 1992. Schaumburg, IL: Wood Library-Museum of Anesthesiology; 1991, p. 467.
137. Henle. Zur Indikationsstellving bei der Operation der Aneurysmen und, bei den Gefäsßverletzungen. Centralbl f Chir. 1913;41:913.
138. Stoltz C. Eine Indikation zur Wahl der Operationsmethode bei Aneurysmen, erläutert an zwei Fällen von Aneurysma der Arteria femoralis. Beitr z klin Chir. 1914;88:452–65.
139. Von Frisch. Zur Indikationsstellung bei der Operation der Aneusmen und bei den Gefassverletzungen. Zentralbl f Chir. 1914;41:89–91.

140. Chalier, Joseph-Fortuné (1884–1942). Identifiants et Référentiels pour l'enseignement supérieur et la recherche. https://www.idref.fr/150178379. Accessed 25 Jun 2019
141. Chalier J. La Presse Médicale. 12 Sep 1942, 41. https://www.biusante.parisdescartes.fr/histoire/images/index.php?refphot=med100000x1942xartorigx0589. Accessed 25 Jun 2019.
142. Chalier J. Les anévrysmes de l'aorte thoracique descendante. Rev de Méd 1923;40:65–85.
143. [No author]. Obituary: T. Shennan MD, FRCS Ed, LLD. Br Med J. 1948:839.
144. [No author]. Obituary notices of deceased members: Theodore Shennan, 9th March 1869-21st October 1948. Jour Path. 1950;62:461–8.
145. [No author]. Theodore Shennan MD. Royal College of Surgeons of Edinburgh. In: Oliver and Boyds Edinburgh Almanac and National Repository for 1902. Glasgow: D. Robertson and Co.; 1902. p. 883.
146. Shennan T. Dissecting Aneurysms, M.R.C. Report No. 193, H.M. Stationery Office, London. Medical Research Council Special Report Series No. 193, London His Majesty's Stationery Office, 1934.
147. Luis González Sabathié, un modelo a seguir. Fundación Ciencias Mėdicas de Rosario. https://www.fucimed.org/index.php?runComponent=actividades-ampliada.php&id=332. Accessed 2 Aug 2019.
148. [No author]. Dr. Luis R. Gonzalez Sabathie Falleció en Rosario (R.A.) el 2 de julio de 1957. Rev Argent Cardiol. 1957:5–6.
149. Algo par recorder: Instituto de Cardiología: Dr. Ljuis González Sabathie. Fundacion Ciencia Medicas Rosaio. https://www.fucimed.org/index.php?runComponent=actividades-ampliada.php&id=330. Accessed 2 Aug 2019.
150. Luis González Sabathie. Rosario Cardiology Society. https://www.cardiorosario.org.ar/expresidentes/. Accessed 2 Aug 2019.
151. Sabathie LG. Un neuvo signo periférico en las aortopatías. Rev Argent Cardiol. 1934;1:267–75.
152. [No author]. Obituary: Hugo Roesler, 62, a heart specialist. New York Times. 28 Apr 1961, p. 31.
153. Roesler H. Clinical Roentgenology of the Cardiovascular System. Illinois: Charles C. Thomas; 1943.
154. Roesler H, Gifford UG, Betts W. Dissecting aneurysm of the aorta, correctly diagnosed. Am Heart J. 1937;13:426–30.
155. [No author]. Obituary: J.A. Nissim, M.D. Br Med J. 1966;1:549.
156. Nissim JA. Dissecting aneurysm of the aorta: a new sign. Br Heart J. 1946;8:203–6.
157. R. Bruce Logue Sr. The Atlantic Journal-Constitution on March 2, 2007. Legacy.com. https://www.legacy.com/obituaries/atlanta/obituary.aspx?n=r-bruce-logue&pid=86662242&fhid=4911. Accessed 2 Mar 2019.
158. R. Bruce Logue. Pioneering Cardiologist 1934C 1937M. Emory University History and Traditions. http://www.emoryhistory.emory.edu/facts-figures/people/makers-history/profiles/logue.html. Accessed 3 Mar 2019.
159. Hurst JW. Profiles in cardiology: R. Bruce Logue. Clin Cardiol 1992;15:931–3.
160. Henry D. Dr. Bruce Logue: News Obituary Article. Atlanta. Dr. Bruce Logue, 95, expert on matters of heart. https://www.legacy.com/obituaries/atlanta/obituary.aspx?n=bruce-logue&pid=86669392. Accessed 2 Mar 2019.
161. Logue RB, Sikes C. A new sign in dissecting aneurysm of aorta: pulsation of a sternoclavicular joint. JAMA. 1952;148:1209–12.

Chapter 2
Atherosclerotic and Ischemic Heart Disease

Introduction

Angina pectoris is the term used to describe the constellation of symptoms occurring in the heart caused by conditions that result in a mismatch between coronary arterial supply and tissue demand. The word "angina" is derived from Latin, a chocking from *angere* and Greek *ankhonē* (strangling) [1], while the word "pectoris" is derived from Latin, genitive of *pectus* "chest" [2]. Some of the earliest descriptions of this disease were made by Giovanni Battista Morgagni (1682–1771) in 1707 [3], Giovanni Maria Lancisi (1654–1720) posthumously in 1728 [4], and Edward Hyde (1609–1674) in 1759 [5]. Both Morgagni and Lancisi correlated the clinical history of exertional chest pain relieved with rest and other associated symptoms to autopsy findings [3, 4]. William Heberden (1710–1801) is credited for coining the term "angina pectoris" as well as defining and providing a detailed description of the disease:

> There is a disorder of the breast, marked with strong and peculiar symptoms, considerable for the kind of danger belonging to it, and not extremely rare, of which I do not recollect any mention among medical authors. The seat of it and the sense of strangling and anxiety with which is attended, may make it not improperly to be called Angina pectoris [6, p. 59]. (…) that it has not yet, as far as I know, found a place or a name in the history of diseases [6, p. 67].

His contributions were significant in that he was the first to carefully describe the symptoms, differentiate them from other conditions, and assign a name to this disease [6].

The advent of the clinical electrocardiogram by Willem Einthoven (1860–1927) in 1901, as further refined based on the earlier work by Augustus Desiré Waller (1856–1922) in 1887, provided a tool to assist in the diagnosis of myocardial infarction [7]. Fred M. Smith (1888–1946) under the aegis of James B. Herrick (1861–1954) observed electrocardiographic findings after ligation of coronary

S. H. Yale et al., *Cardiovascular Eponymic Signs*,
https://doi.org/10.1007/978-3-030-67596-7_2

arteries in dogs [8]. He found that after ligation of any branch of the left coronary artery, the electrocardiographic findings:

> [w]ere among the most consistent and most remarkable, and we have not, we believe, been previously recorded by others. (…) The early exaggeration of the T-wave, its marked negative drop below the line within twenty-four hours and its more gradual return to its positive position and its final iso-electric or negative location were so characteristic in dogs watched for several days, that similar changes in the wave in man might reasonably be supposed to be due to similar lesions. In fact, one case in man, will be reported later, was observed in which a clinical diagnosis of coronary thrombosis was made by James B. Herrick which was verified later at necropsy [8, p. 27].

Herrick described the case of a 42-year-old man with chest pain, and electrocardiograms taken during his clinical course, later found at autopsy to have acute occlusion of the left coronary artery in the ramus descendens anterior and first descending branch of the circumflex [9]. These electrocardiograms were compared to those obtained earlier by Smith. He concluded that "there seems to be fairly constant variation in the electrocardiogram following the ligation of a particular branch of the coronary" [9, p. 390]. Herrick concluded based on this preliminary findings declaring that:

> There is some hope that the work may assist in interpreting abnormal human electrocardiograms. The thought has been that if it can be proved that with a certain artery obstructed there is a definite lesion in the heart muscle or in the conducting system, and if that lesion there is a definite electrocardiogram, may we not, when we encounter that abnormal electrocardiogram in the human being, particularly if he has had symptoms suggestive or coronary thrombosis, be able to state with a reasonable degree of certainty that the patient has had obstruction in a particular portion of the coronary system? May it perhaps be possible to localize a lesion in the coronary system with an accuracy comparable to that with which we locate obstructive lesions in the cerebral arteries? [9, p. 390].

The goal of this chapter is to review signs reported for the bedside diagnosis of atherosclerosis and its ischemic consequences—angina pectoris and myocardial infarction, electrocardiographic signs associated with myocardial infarction, as well as the precordial gestures or postures assumed by some patients with myocardial ischemia and infarction. Reported is the historical backgrounds of the person who described the sign, its original description, and accuracy in clinical practice, if known. The signs are divided into atherosclerotic and ischemic heart disease subcategories and presented chronologically based on the year they were first reported.

Signs

Beaumé Sign

Lucien Jules Beaumé (1865–1918) received his doctorate of medicine in 1892 based on his thesis *Contribution à l'Étude des Myocardites: Évolution, Étiologie, Pathogénie* (Contribution to the Study of Myocardites: Evolution, Etiology,

Pathogenesis) [10]. During that time, he was former intern of the Hôpitaux de Paris and physician of the Reserve Aides Majors [11]. He was knighted by the Légion d'honneur [12]. Lucien Beaumé described the case of a 47-year-old man with a prior clinical diagnosis of mitral insufficiency with:

> [s]igns of sclerosis (very hard arteries, senile arc of the cornea, signs of interstitial nephritis without albumin, etc.). A jolt was located at the fifth intercostal space. The first sound was muffled, while the second sound was clearly heard at the base. There was no murmur or duplication sign on repeat monthly examinations to suggest a diagnosis of a valvular lesion. The pulse was rapid with a slight arrhythmia. Finally there were some retro-sternal pains radiated to the cervical region. We thought we should report this observation because it seems to us to that it shows evolution of sclerosis [13, p. 54–55].

He acknowledged Peter M. Huchard's prior studies whereby he described the five varied types of arteriosclerosis heart disease, one type being, "A painful type with all the modalities of retrosternal pain" [13, p. 18]. Thus, Beaumé sign is the presence of retrosternal pain radiating to the cervical region in patients with angina pectoris (Table 2.1).

Osler Sign

William Osler (1849–1919) was born in Bond Head, Ontario, Canada, and received his medical degree and Chirurgia Magister of Master of Surgery from McGill University, Montreal, Canada, in 1872 [14, 15]. After graduation, he pursued post-graduate training abroad in physiology and pathology in Dublin, Glasgow, London, Berlin, and Vienna [15]. In 1874, he was appointed Lecturer, followed by Professor in the Institutes of Medicine, McGill University [14]. He was involved in teaching physiology, pathology, and clinical medicine as an attending physician from 1878 to 1883 at Montreal General Hospital [14, 16]. Osler was appointed Professor and Chair of Clinical Medicine at the University of Pennsylvania between 1884 and 1889 and Professor of Medicine and Physician-in-Chief at Johns Hopkins University, Baltimore, in 1889 [14, 17]. In 1892, he published his medical textbook titled *The Principles and Practice of Medicine* [16]. As Chair and Regius Professor of Medicine at Oxford University in 1905, he developed the departments of pathology and physiology, cultivating an academic atmosphere of scientific pursuits and clinical inquiry [14, 15, 17]. His work was instrumental in reformatting medical education to incorporate the clinical laboratory and teaching medicine at the patient's bedside on the medical wards, mirroring the English methods of instruction.

Osler described the palpatory appearance of the radial and temporal artery in patients with atherosclerosis (Fig. 2.1):

> A high-tension pulse may exist with very little arterio-sclerosis; but, as a rule, when the condition has been persistent, the sclerosis and high tension are found together. The pulse wave is slow in its ascent, enduring, subsides slowly, and in the intervals of the beats the vessel remains full and firm. It may be very difficult to obliterate the pulse, and the firmest pressure on the radial or the temporal may not be sufficient to annihilate the pulse wave

Table 2.1 Ischemic heart disease signs

Name	Year	Description of sign	Method
Beaumé [13]	1892	Retrosternal pains radiating to the cervical region.	Observation
Livierato [21]	1906	Patient in supine position on bed. Chest percussion delineates the heart borders with dullness located at the median line of the sternum, the vertical papilla where the apex beat is detected, the upper border of the fourth left rib along the left sternal margin which curves gradually downward until it reaches the cardiac apex and the sixth rib. The pulse is frequent but regular. Repeatedly tap on the midline of the abdomen from the epigastrium and to the umbilicus. Again delineate the area of dullness of the heart. Its limit extends considerably to the right. The inner limit reaches the margin to right of the sternum, while the upper and the outer margins are modified slightly. The cardiac dullness extends to the right for about 3 cm. The pulse is increased somewhat in frequency, and the pulmonary component of the second sound is accentuated. Patient is asked to rise from the bed and walk quickly around the room several times, and the area of cardiac dullness is again delineated. This area is now considerably narrowed. The internal limit reaches the margin to the left of the sternum, the upper area is slightly lowered, almost unchanged, and the left one remains the same. The pulse is stronger and more frequent than previously. Following this movement, the patient does not experience any problems with breathing or palpitations.	Palpation percussion
Pardee [31]	1920	ST-segment elevation found at the thickening of the descending limb of the R wave at its notch in limb leads II and III.	Electrocardiogram
Libman [37, 38]	1926	Press the thumb against the tip of the mastoid bone and then move the finger forward and push it against the styloid process. Pressure on the normal mastoid bone causes no pain and therefore serves as a control. It is important not to rub the bone because rubbing the periosteum is likely to evoke pain. Pressure in the direction of the styloid process is painful to some individuals. When the styloid test is performed, it is important not to press on the lower jaw. A sensitive point is present around the middle of the ramus, and when this is pressed, in addition to the sensitive point behind it, a summation pain occurs, which may be misleading. According to the response to the test, individuals are classed as follows: 1. 0 sensitive, 2. + sensitive, 3. + + + sensitive. Group 1: Gives no evidence of pain and state that they feel none. Group 2: Give little evidence of pain and show none but in response to questioning say that they feel a little pain or give some such answer as "I feel a little pain when you press" or "It hurts when you press" or "I feel your pressure." Groups 1 and 2 are classified as hyposensitives. Group 3: Gives evidence of marked pain and while patients may control the expression of pain, they admit that the test is definitely painful. Patients with angina pectoris in whom pain is always on the right side are hyposensitives.	Palpation

Bürklen [39]	1940	Temperature differences of up to 1–2° are present and prominently differ especially at the time of the resolution of the fever. Later although the temperature decreases, the differences continue to persist albeit to a lesser extent. The temperature of the left axilla is always lower than that of the right axilla and reaches a maximum of 37° at a time when 38.2° is measured in the right axilla.	Thermometer
Dressler-de Winter [61, 62]	1947, 2008	The ST segment showed a 1- to 3-mm upsloping ST-segment depression at the J point in leads V1 to V6 that continues into tall, positive symmetrical T waves. The QRS complexes were usually not widened or were only slightly widened, and in some, there was a loss of precordial R-wave progression. In most patients, there was a 1- to 2-mm ST elevation in lead aVR.	Electrocardiogram
Robertson [66]	1947	Maculopapules dull pink to purple in color, according to their age, occurring chiefly on the trunk and rarely on the upper extremities.	Observation
Cabrera [74]	1953	Notch with a duration of 0.05 sec. Or more observed in the terminal portion of QRS in the precordial leads that show a morphology rS or QA (usually V_3 and V_4).	Electrocardiogram
Levine (carotid sinus test) [45]	1958	Slowing of the heart by carotid pressure in a patient with angina causes the pain to disappear or lessen almost instantly. When the patient has his customary pain or distress, the physician should stop everything and auscultate the heart. The patient is not told what to expect. A nurse or another physician, if present, is asked to hold the stethoscope in place so that auscultation is clear. If not, the patient holds the stethoscope. The patient is asked whether he is still having distress. If so, the right carotid sinus is massaged for a few seconds. If this does not produce appreciable cardiac slowing, the left side is massaged. As soon as the heart slows for several beats, the pressure over the carotid is released. The patient is now asked whether the pain is worse. If the heart has been slowed, almost invariably the patient pause for a second or two, seem to be looking into himself, and reply, "the pain is gone" or "its letting up." The disappearance or lightening of the pain occurs in seconds not minutes.	Palpation
Levine (substernal oppression, or Cossio-Levine) [52]	1965	Clenched hand over the sternum as a description of cardiac ischemia.	Observation
Chapman [78]	1957	Early notching of the R wave in leads I, aV_L, and V_6 and the S wave in leads aV_F and V_4.	Electrocardiogram
Oram [53]	1981	Fist clenched and pressed into the center of the sternum.	Observation
Wellens [86]	1982	ST-T wave segments in leads V2 and V3 are isoelectric or minimally elevated (1 mm) from the takeoff of the ST segment of the QRS complex. A concave or straight ST segment passes into a negative T wave at an angle of 60–90 degrees Symmetrically inverted T waves. Most patients also have in lead V1 an isoelectric or minimally elevated (1 mm) takeoff of the ST segment and a concave or straight ST segment passing into the first part of the T wave at an angle of approximately 135 degrees followed by T wave inversions.	Electrocardiogram

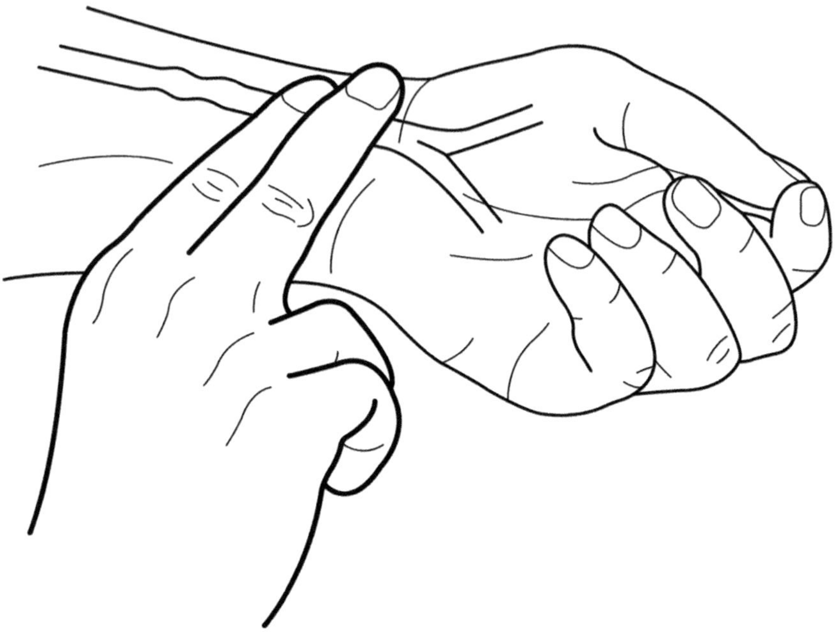

Fig. 2.1 Osler sign (by Ryan Yale)

> beyond the point of pressure. This is not always a sign of high tension. (…) The sphygmographic tracing shows a sloping, short up-stroke, no percussion wave, and a slow, gradual descent, in which the dicrotic wave is very slightly marked. It may be difficult to estimate how much of the hardness and firmness is due to the tension of the blood within the vessel, and how much to the thickening of the wall. If, for example, when the radial is compressed with the index-finger the artery can be felt beyond the point of compression, its walls are sclerosed [18, p. 704].

Thus, Osler sign is a bedside method for determining the presence of atherosclerosis in the radial artery (Table 2.2).

Livierato Sign

Panagino Livierato (1860–1936) was born in Kefalonia, Greece, and received his medical degree in 1886 [19]. He was appointed Ordinary Professor of Special Medical Pathology in Genoa, Italy, in 1890 and served at the Medical Clinic of Palermo, Italy, in 1895 [19, 20]. Livierato described the case of a 35-year-old man with postprandial chest heaviness and occasional shortness of breath. The symptoms resolve with activity and were otherwise absent while walking upstairs or a hill. Physical examination revealed an increased pulse rate with the right heart border extending to the midline of the sternum.

Table 2.2 Atherosclerosis signs

Name	Year	Description of sign	Method
Osler [18]	1897	When the radial artery is compressed with the index finger, it is felt beyond the point of compression if its wall is sclerosed.	Palpation
Hertzell [26]	1913	While the patient is recumbent in bed, a rubber cuff is placed around each limb. The cuff of one arm is used for measuring the blood pressure, while an assistant pumps air into the cuffs on the three other extremities by means of a three-piece hose connection. After the circulation in completely interrupted, fluctuation in the blood pressure is controlled during the following 3 minutes. The prevailing blood pressure in the cuffs is related to stasis observed and recorded by means of a second manometer, while the column of the manometer used for measuring the systolic blood pressure is continuously being recorded in the cubital artery.	Sphygmomanometer
Frank [82]	1973	Bilateral prominent crease in the lobule portion of the auricles.	Observation

He identified and described a palpatory technique that involves tapping the abdominal wall to detect right ventricular failure prior to the onset of cardiac symptoms:

> We can now delineate the area of absolute dullness of the heart after the patient is placed in a supine position on the bed. As seen it has limits: internally the median line of the sternum, externally the vertical papilla where the apex beat is detected, superiorly the upper border of the fourth left rib along the left sternal margin which curves gradually downward until it reaches the cardiac apex, and inferiorly the sixth rib. The pulse is frequent and regular. Now let's repeatedly tap on the midline of the abdomen beginning in the epigastrium and extending to the navel, that is, along the path of the abdominal aorta. We will see which cardiac area, if any, is modified and can be defined. By delineating the area of dullness of the heart again, it is obviously seen that its limit has extended considerably to the right. The inner limit reaches the margin to the right of the sternum while the upper and the outer margins are slightly modified. The cardiac dullness extends to the right for about three centimeters. The pulse is increased somewhat in frequency and the pulmonary component of the second sound is accentuated. I now asked the patient to rise from the bed and walk quickly around the room several times and again delineated the area of cardiac dullness. As is seen, we find this area considerably narrowed. The internal limit reaches the margin to the left of the sternum, the upper area is slightly lowered almost unchanged, and the left one remains the same. The pulse is stronger and more frequent than beforehand. Moreover, as seen following this movement, the individual from the subjective point of view does not experience any problems with either his/her breathing or palpitations [21, p. 5].

He accounted for the proposed pathogenesis for which he named the abdominocardiac reflex:

> In our case we have seen schematically that irritation of the abdominal nerves gives rise to the expansion of the right ventricle in an obvious and perceptible way [21, p. 6]. (...) Usually there is no subjective feeling that the individual experiences because the normal right ventricle makes up for the increase in energy. However, as soon as the myocardium

> due to any cause is compromised the impediment that causes reduced pulmonary blood flow causes right ventricle dilation. Thus, we understand why all individuals suffering from stomach, liver, or other diseases do not present with dilation of the heart. It is necessary for the tonicity and strength of the myocardial fibers to be decreased in order for dilatation to occur. Therefore, in our case by tapping on the abdomen we produced an excitement which, due to the sympathetic nerves, causes constriction of the pulmonary vessels. In fact, we detected the strengthening of the tones of the lung and the extension of the dullness of the heart to the right. Our observation is so simple and brings with it the proof that we did not excite the vagus because the pulse not only did not slow down but rather increased in frequency [21, p. 7].

Livierato explained his patient's symptoms on the basis of the abdominocardiac reflex:

> The ingested foods produce an excitement which starts from the stomach mucosa and causes constriction of pulmonary vessels by the sympathetics. The semiological artifice used by us and which we call the abdominal-cardiac reflex enables us to explain the bothersome sensation experienced by our patient and to rationally cure him. This simple artifice shows that the myocardium of this individual has little strength and tone [21, p. 7].

It is of interest that Albert Abrams described a reflex (heart reflex) in 1898 which involves the left ventricle. The reflex is elicited and determined as follows:

> If we irritate the skin at the precordial region by vigorous rubbing with a blunt instrument a contraction of the myocardium is observed. The myocardial contraction is as a rule more manifest in the left than in the right ventricle. (…) The degree of myocardial recession (heart reflex) varies greatly. In some persons it is scarcely perceptible while in other individuals the heart may recede fully an inch on either side upon the first application of the cutaneous irritant. (…) The heart reflex can be observed only with the Roentgen rays, the fluorescent screen approximating the anterior chest wall [22, p. 10].

Based on his observations, he found that friction on the skin induced by rubber such as a pencil eraser near the precordial region was the best irritant to elicit the reflex. He found that the reflex was more prominent in patients with dilated hearts compared to those of normal size and served as a method for distinguishing cardiac dilation from pericardial effusion [22]. According to Barton, Livierato and Abrams reflex should not be performed on the same patient the same day [23].

Thus, Livierato sign refers to increased right ventricular dullness elicited by vertically tapping on anterior abdominal wall between the epigastrium and umbilicus with the patient in the supine position (Table 2.2). It is a method for detecting early right ventricular failure in heart disease regardless of its cause.

Hertzell Sign

There is limited historical information on Carl Hertzell (1881–1940). He devised several instruments including an "opthalmodiaphanoscope" that illuminates the orbit and sinuses by placing the light source within the patient's mouth for visualization [24] and an "ectropionator," a tool used for everting the upper eyelid [25]. As an assistant, published under the aegis of Dr. L. Brieger, Head Council of Professor at the Clinical Department of the Hydrotherapeutic Institute of the University of Berlin, he described a method for detecting atherosclerosis using pneumatic compression:

> The experimental setup was designed as per the Recklinghausen method in that a rubber cuff was placed around each limb while the patient was in a bed. The cuff of one arm was used for the usual measurement of the blood pressure while three others limbs served the purpose of suddenly interrupting the circulation in the extremities by establishing an air pressure considerably exceeding the individuals blood pressure. (…) An assistant pumps air into the cuffs of the three extremities by means of a three-piece hose connection. After the circulation is completely interrupted, fluctuation in the blood pressure was controlled over the following three minutes. In this case the prevailing blood pressure in the cuffs is related to stasis observed and recorded by means of a second manometer, while the column of the manometer used for measuring the blood pressure was continuously being obtained at a height close to the respective blood pressure. (…) We determined the systolic blood pressure by means of auscultation of the sounds of the cubital artery according to Korotkov and Fellner [26, p. 536].

Using this design, Hertzell identified that if the blood circulation in normal individuals is occlude in the legs and arms by pneumatic compression at rest, the systolic blood pressure in the free arm is on average 5 mmHg higher. In contrast, in patients with atherosclerotic disease, the systolic blood pressure may rise as high as 60 mmHg (Table 2.2). Hertzell postulated that the abnormally high systolic blood pressure found in patients with atherosclerosis was the result of increased rigidity (altered vasculature) preventing normal expansion in the uncompressed extremity. The height of the blood pressure thus depends on the severity of atherosclerotic lesions [26].

Pardee Sign

Harold Ensign Bennet Pardee (1886–1973), son of Ensign Bennett Pardee MD (1853–1917), received his medical degree from the College of Physicians and Surgeons (Columbia University) New York City in 1909 [27, 28]. He completed an internship at New York Hospital in 1912, served in the Medical Clinic at New York Hospital, and followed by an appointment as instructor in physiology in 1913 [28]. He served as attending physician at New York and Polyclinic Hospitals, consulting cardiologist at Women's Hospital in New York, Methodist Hospital Brooklyn, New York, and the New York Infirmary. He was an Associate Professor of Clinical Medicine at Cornell University Medical College, New York [29].

Pardee was president and founder of the Association of Cardiac Clinic of the New York Heart Association as well as founder of the Scientific Council of the American Heart Association [29]. He authored the book *Clinical Aspects of the Electrocardiogram* in 1924 and was editor of *The Nomenclature and Criteria for the Diagnosis of the Heart and Blood Vessel,* first published in 1928 [4]. Also in 1928, he published the book written for the general public titled *What You Should Know about Heart Disease* [30].

Pardee was the first to record the electrocardiographic pattern seen in a three standard limb lead in a 38-year-old man during the course of a transmural myocardial infarction. He recorded the findings in a patient with what he believed to be an acute coronary occlusion involving the left coronary artery:

> The characteristic changes appearing a day or two after the obstruction are as follows: The QRS group is usually notched in at least two leads, and usually shows left ventricular predominance. The T wave does not start from the zero level of the record in either Lead I or Lead III though, perhaps, from a level not far removed from it, and in this lead quickly turns away from its starting point in a sharp curve, without the short straight stretch which is so evident in normal records preceding the peak of the T wave. The T wave is usually of larger size than customary and accordingly shows a somewhat sharper peak. The T wave is usually turned downward in Lead II and in one other lead. Not all of these changes are to be found in every record, but enough of them are present to give it a characteristic appearance [31, p. 257].

By the third day, there were changes in the electrocardiogram (EKG):

> The T wave has changed considerably, so that in Lead I it no longer has a downward but an upward direction. In leads II and III the former upward direction is retained but the amplitude is much smaller and at the end of this wave at the same time interval after the QRS group as in the peak of the upward T wave in Lead I, there appears a small downward wave in Lead III [31, p. 257].

These EKG changes continue to evolve resulting in persistent upright T wave and T wave inversion in leads II and III persisting for months after the myocardial infarction [31, p. 249]. He believed that this electrocardiographic sign:

> [i]ndicates the presence of a rather large area of muscle degeneration, and when it is obtained from a patient who gave a history of precordial pain coming either in attacks or upon exertion, that it will complete the diagnosis of obstruction of a branch of a coronary artery [31, p. 257].

Thus, Pardee sign refers to the electrocardiographic findings occurring during a myocardial infarction and includes ST-segment elevation found at the thickening of the descending limb of the R wave at its notch in limb leads II and III [31, p. 249] (Table 2.1).

Libman Sign

Emanuel Libman (1872–1946) was born in New York City, NY, and received his medical degree from the College of Physicians and Surgery of Columbia, New York, in 1894 [32–34]. He completed his internship at Mount Sinai Hospital in 1896, followed by additional postgraduate studies for 1 year in Graz and Vienna, Austria; Berlin and Munich, Germany; and Prague, Czechoslovakia [32, 34, 35]. At Mount Sinai Hospital in New York City, he was appointed assistant pathologist in 1897, associate pathologist from 1898 to 1923, followed by appointments in clinical medicine as an adjunct physician in 1903, attending physician from 1912 to 1925, and consulting physician from 1925 to 1940 [32, 33, 35]. He was a staunch supporter for continued medical education at Mount Sinai and served as a member of the Committee on Medical Education at the New York Academy of Medicine [32, 34]. His other appointments included serving as a consulting physician within and near New York City and Clinical Professorship at Columbia University, New York [35].

He served as a member of the Board of Governors beginning in 1925 at Hebrew University New York, and he was President of the American Friends at this same institution [35]. At Hebrew University, he founded the American Physicians Committee which was responsible for establishing the Post Graduate and Research Institutes at this institution [35]. He was successful in securing endowed funds to support the Edward Gamaliel Janeway and William Henry Welch lectureships at Mt. Sinai Hospital, Hideyo Noguchi at Johns Hopkins Hospital and Humphry Rolleston at Royal College of Physicians London, Herbert Celler Fellowship Fund, and Henry Dazian Foundation for Medical Research [32, 33]. The Emanuel Libman Fellowship Fund was established in his honor providing postgraduate research scholarship [32].

His name is eponymously associated with his discovery of *Streptococcus enteritis* (*Streptococcus Libman*) which he identified while conducting research in the laboratory of Theodor Escherich (1857–1911) in Graz, Austria, atypical verrucous endocarditis (nonbacterial endocarditis or Libman-Sacks endocarditis) in collaboration with Benjamin Sacks (1896–1971) at Mt. Sinai Hospital, New York, in 1924, and Libman phenomenon or the precipitation and whitening of glucose-serum agar by acid-producing bacteria [32, 35, 36]. He comprehensively defined and described what he referred to as subacute infective endocarditis later named subacute bacterial endocarditis [32]. He can best be considered as an applied pathologist where postmortem findings are correlated to clinical diagnosis [32]. For his work on endocarditis, he received the Gold (1911) and Silver (1942) Medal from the American Medical Association. As a description and tribute to his character, Oppenheimer wrote:

> Throughout his professional career he had devoted himself whole-heartedly to medical science and research, to medical practice of a high order, to the study of medical literature, to medical education and to promoting in others those ideals which had inspired his own life. (…) The outstanding characteristic of Libman was his ability to stimulate, to inspire, to quicken others to work and study with something of his own enthusiasm [33, p. 116]. (…) In addition to his formal work in medical education, he was tireless in his efforts to help younger physicians and scientists by his sound advice, his stimulation and his financial aid. As a result he built up a school of disciples and gathered a host of personal friends both here and abroad with whom he kept in touch to the end of his life [33, p. 117].

Libman reported a maneuver in 1926 for determining a person's sensitivity to pain:

> I have found in the last few years that there is a simple method for gauging a person's sensitiveness to pain, and I believe that a study carried out with this or similar methods will be of the greatest importance to us in showing us the necessity of re-writing the clinical picture of disease. (…) These patients who belong in the hyposensitive group very often have more of the reflex symptoms of disease than of the local symptoms. They are the patients who are more apt to radiate pain to the wrong side of the body, and if you have a patient who is hyposensitive at this test point that I use, or any other test point, it is important always to take into consideration what conditions may produce a similarly located pain on the other side [37, p. 62].

In his paper "Observations on individual sensitiveness to pain with special reference to abdominal disorders" published in 1934, he further elaborated on this bedside maneuver to determine sensitivity to pain:

> The simple test that I employ is carried out by first pressing the thumb against the tip of the mastoid bone and then slipping the finger forward and pushing against the styloid process. Pressure on the normal mastoid bone causes no pain and therefore serves as a control. (...) The sensitive point is really not the styloid process but a branch of the auricularis magnus nerve [38, p. 335].

He described the different responses that may occur and their significance when pressure is exerted upon the mastoid and styloid process:

> According to the response to the test, individuals are classed as: 1. 0 sensitive 2. + sensitive 3. + + + sensitive. The first group comprises those who give no evidence of pain, and who state that they feel none. The second includes those who evidence little pain, and also those who show none, but who in response to questioning say that they feel a little pain or give some such answer as "I feel a little pain when you press" or "It hurts when you press" or "I feel your pressure." For practical purposes it is desirable to classify groups 1 and 2 as hyposensitives. I do not refer to those in group 1 as "insensitive" because, given sufficient provocation, pain is manifested by some of them at least. Group 3 represents those who give evidence of marked pain and those who, while they may control the expression of pain, admit that the test is definitely painful. In order to indicate that there is a sharp division between hyposensitivity and sensitivity, a + + group is not made. There is apparently no practical advantage in making any groups of those so sensitive that they might be designated ++++ sensitive, and so on [38, p. 335].

He further explained the significance of pain at the mastoid bone or control site, how to interpret those patients who response to pressure with complaints of being sensitivity, which in fact they are actually hyposensitive, and interpretation of pain on unilateral styloid pressure:

> If the patient experiences pain when the control pressure is exerted on the (normal) mastoid bone, it must be concluded that central (cerebral) sensitization is present. (...) The point that I have chosen has several advantages. It is accessible and the test is easily carried out without the patient realizing what is being done. It is important to note that there are individuals—fortunately small in number—who, though really hyposensitive, react to the test as though they were sensitive. In such subjects, if one reverses the test by employing the styloid before the mastoid pressure, it elicits but little or no response, whereas the mastoid pressure proves painful. In other not naturally sensitive parts of the body, they act in the same way. In other words, any second stimulus gives a reaction. Because of this observation it is wise in all cases in which the styloid pressure is found sensitive to employ it again after a short interval. In the peculiar group under consideration, the reaction will now be that characteristic of hyposensitivity. Clinical experience has revealed that individuals who are sensitive to the styloid pressure on only one side react clinically like those who are hyposensitive on both sides [38, p. 335].

Libman described the application of this maneuver in patients with angina pectoris, "We have found, for instance, that the patient with angina pectoris in whom the pain is always on the right side are hyposensitives." [37, p. 63]. He also found that moderate pain and dyspnea were the predominant symptoms in hyposensitive patients with angina pectoris [38]. Thus, Libman sign refers to the presence of rights sided anginal pain and dyspnea in hyposensitive patients based on the mastoid pressure pain test (Table 2.1).

Bürklen Sign

We were only able to identify limited historical information on Roland Bürklen (1908–1992). At the time of the publication that described his sign titled "Ein Beitrag zur Symptomatologie der Koronarthrombose" (A Contribution to the Symptomatology of Coronary Thrombosis) he served in the Medical Department of the Rudolfstiftung Hospital under Karl Hitzenberger (1893–1941) in Vienna [39]. In 1973, he was the Federal President and Medical Director of the Specialist Assessment Station of the Pensions Insurance Company of Employees [40]. Bürklen graphically recorded axillary temperatures in patients with coronary thrombosis and found:

> It turns out that temperature differences of up to 1 to 2° are present. They differ predominantly, especially at the time of the resolution of the fever. Later although the temperature decreases, the differences continue to persist albeit to a lesser extent. The temperature of the left axilla is always lower than that of the right axilla and reaches a maximum of 37° at a time when 38.2° is measured in the right axilla. We have now followed this remarkable fact in other cases of coronary thrombosis in order to determine whether it is a behavior specific to this condition and have consistently found the same result [39].

He described the method for taking the temperatures, "The temperatures were measured simultaneously in both axillas with two calibrated thermometers in order to remove any possible sources of error such as abnormal sweat secretion" [39]. Thus, Bürklen sign refers to the differences in axillary temperature in cases of coronary thrombosis (Table 2.1).

Levine Sign

Samuel Albert Levine (1891–1966) was born in Lomza, Poland, graduated from Harvard Medical School in 1914, and completed an internship at Peter Bent Brigham Hospital and fellowship at the Rockefeller Institute [41]. After World War I, he joined the staff at Peter Brent Brigham Hospital as a physician and consultant in 1919, earning the rank of Clinical Professor of Medicine at Harvard Medical School in 1948 and emeritus physician in 1958. He published the monograph *Coronary Thrombosis: Its Various Clinical Features* in 1929, several books including *Clinical Heart Disease* in 1936 and with Watkins Proctor Harvey *Clinical Auscultation of the Heart* in 1949 [41]. In commemoration of his contributions to cardiology, the Samuel A. Levine Professorship endowed chair was named at Harvard in 1954 and a cardiac intensive care unit at Peter Bent Brigham Hospital in 1965 [41, 42]. He is the recipient of a number of awards and honors including the Gold Heart Award from the American Heart Association, honorary Doctor of Humane Letters degree from Yeshiva University (1959), and American-Israel Freedom Award (1960) [41]. In addition to the sign which bears his name, other eponymous contributions include the Lown–Ganong–Levine syndrome and Levine Scale – a method for grading the severity of cardiac murmurs [43].

Reevan I. Levine (no known relationship to Samuel A. Levine) in a letter to the editor referred to "the Levine sign" as relief of acute angina through carotid sinus pressure [44]. S. Levine described the "carotid sinus test" as a method to assist in the diagnosis of myocardial ischemia (Table 2.1):

> It has been found that if a patient is having angina pain, slowing of the heart by carotid pressure will make the pain disappear or lessen almost instantly. I have employed this test hundreds of times without any mishap and frequently found it helpful to prove or to rule out the diagnosis of angina [45, p. 111,112]. (…) When the patient has his customary pain or distress the physician should stop everything and auscultate the heart. The patient is not told what to expect. A nurse or another physician, if present, is asked to hold the stethoscope in place so that auscultation is clear. If not, the patient holds the stethoscope. Then he is asked whether he is still having distress. If so the right carotid sinus is massaged for a few seconds. If this does not produce appreciable cardiac slowing, the left side is massaged. Just as soon as the heart slows for several beats pressure is released and the patient is asked whether the pain is worse. The purpose is not to ask a leading question but, on the contrary, to try to misdirect him. If the heart has been slowed, almost invariably the patient pauses for a second or two, seem to be looking into himself, and reply, "the pain is gone" or "its letting up." The disappearance or lightening of the pain occurs in seconds, not in minutes [45, p. 112].

It is of historical interest that Sigismund Peller initially reported in his paper "Zur Kenntnis der Amylnitrit und Atropinwirkung mit besonderer Berücksichtigung der Stenokardie" [The effect of amyl nitrite and atropine with special consideration of stenocardia (angina pectoris)] published in 1922 on carotid sinus pressure applied during an angina attack:

> Finally, it should be emphasized that short-lasting vagal pressure (Tschermak) had no affected on either the pulse rate (sphygmographically controlled) or attack in this patient. A pressure applied between 5-12 min was required. Once the pain resolved and the pulse and pressure decreased, the patient was able to sleep [46, p. 128].

Levine in his paper titled "Carotid sinus massage: a new diagnostic test for angina pectoris" published in 1962 acknowledged prior clinical use of the carotid sinus massage in 1928 by Wasserman and in 1933 by Wayne and Laplace for relief of angina pain [47]. Levine is credited for stressing the value of this test in the diagnosis of angina. Alan Leviton in his letter to the editor published in 1965 wrote (Table 2.1, Fig. 2.2):

> I would like to add another "Levine sign" also attributed to Dr. Samuel A. Levine. (…) This "Levine sign" is the use of a clenched fist by the patient to describe his substernal pain. Proponents of this sign, and I am one, consider it almost diagnostic of acute myocardial infarction [48].

Costeas and Katsareas described "Levine's sign for substernal oppression," a marker of coronary insufficiency as "[t]ransient or long continued, with or without radiation to the arms, may be an eponymous as well as topographic descriptive sign" [49, p. 282]. We were unable to identify in Samuel Levine's book *Clinical Heart Disease* or monograph *Coronary Thrombosis: Its Various Clinical Features*, any reference to the "clench fist on the chest" as a sign of myocardial ischemia [45, 50].

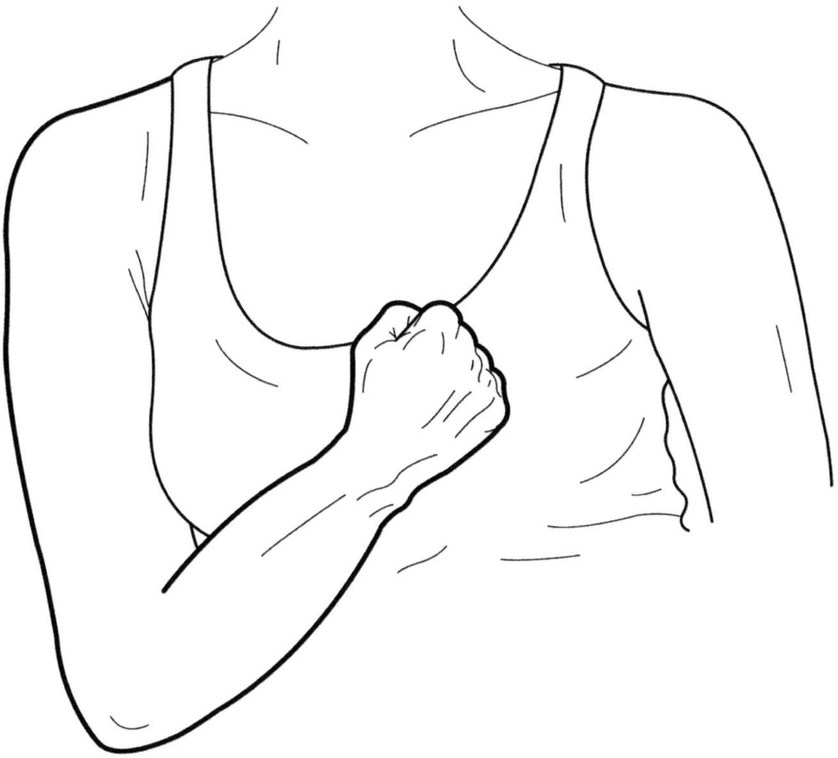

Fig. 2.2 Levine-Cassio sign (by Ryan Yale)

Richard Asher in his paper "Clinical sense: the use of the five senses," published in 1960, described a movement diagnostic of coronary artery disease "[t]he sponge-squeezing hands approaching the sternum of patients describing the pain of cardiac ischemia. Dr. Byron Evans first called my attention to it" [51, p. 988].

Pedro Alurraide Cossio (1900–1986) in 1965 described a position assumed by patients with angina pectoris:

> The patients keep completely still, as if he were nailed to the floor. (…) Often the hand is placed over the precordial area or the midchest, with the fingers closed in the form of a claw (*main en griffe*). If this occurs while the patient is walking on the street, he hides his inability to continue walking by pretending to wait for a bus or stopping to look through a show window (Vasquez) [52].

This hand movement has been referred to as the "palm sign" or by some authors as Cossio-Levine sign [43].

Samuel Oram described in the second edition of his book titled *Clinical Heart Disease* published in 1981 what he referred to as the "fist sign" or "the gesture that the patient makes whilst describing his pain may be virtually diagnostic if he clenches his fist and presses it into the centre of his sternum" [53, p. 417] (Table 2.1). Given Drs. Evans and Oram's contribution to this infamous sign, we felt that it was fitting to provide brief historical information about each of these cardiologists.

Rees Byron Evans (1912–1990) was born in Llanon, Cardiganshire, and received his medical training at London Hospital and medical degree in 1939 [54]. During World War II, he served as officer leading the Royal Air Force Medical Division [54]. After the war, he served as consultant, achieving the ranks of Senior Physician at the University Hospital in Wales, Cardiff. He was appointed Fellow of the Royal College of Physicians, London, in 1957 [54]. As a testimony to his accomplishments, he was awarded Her Majesty's Silver Jubilee Medal in 1977 and honorary doctorate (LLD) from the University of Wales for his "distinguished contribution to medial education and the promotion of health" [54].

Samuel Oram (1913–1991) was born in Camberwell, London, and received his medical training at King's College Hospital Medical School, London, receiving his medical degree in 1941 [15]. During World War II, he served in the Royal Army Medical Corps (RAMC) [55]. On return from the war, he served as chief assistant at the National Heart Hospital, and at King's College Hospital consultant in 1947 and Senior Physician Director, Department of Cardiology, from 1958 to 1978 [55, 56]. His name is perhaps best known in association with the rare familial syndrome characterized by congenital heart disease and upper limb deformities which he described in collaboration with Mary Holt, Holt-Oram syndrome, in 1960 [55, 56]. His book, *Clinical Heart Disease* first published in 1971, is considered the last single author textbook of cardiology [55, 56]. In the British Cardiac Society, he served as secretary, treasurer, and council member and on the board of *The British Heart Journal* [56].

Marcus et al. compared four gestures: the Levine sign (clenched fist to the chest), palm sign (palm of the hand to the chest), arm sign (touching the left arm), and pointing sign (pointing with one finger) in 202 patients presenting with chest pain or chest discomfort [57]. Using elevated troponin in the myocardial infarction range as the criterion standard, a positive predictive value ranging from 13% (Levine sign) to 88% (pointing sign) and negative predictive value ranging from 33% for pointing sign to 78% for arm sign were found [57]. These findings overall suggest that the presence or absence of these gestures is not useful to either rule in or rule out myocardial ischemia or infarct. The high positive predictive value of the pointing sign, however, suggests that it may be a useful marker in diagnosing nonischemic chest pain.

Dressler-de Winter Sign

Historical information for William Dressler (1890–1969) will be described in the chapter on pericarditis: percussion. Robbert Jan de Winter (1958–) received his medical degree from the University of Amsterdam, the Netherlands, in 1988 [58].

He was elected Fellow of the European Society of Cardiology in 2002 [58]. He is currently a Professor in Clinical Cardiology, Acute Coronary Syndrome in the Academic Medical Center, Meibergdreef, Amsterdam; a deputy editor of the *Netherlands Heart Journal*; and a member of the editorial board of *Coronary Artery Disease* journal [59].

Hugo Roesler (1899–1961) was a member of the Departments of Medicine and Radiology at Temple University Hospital and Medical School, Philadelphia, Pennsylvania. He published in 1937, *Clinical Roentgenology of the Cardiovascular System*, one of the earliest book on cardiovascular imaging [60]. William Dressler and Hugo Roesler in 1947 described the evolution of electrocardiographic findings occurring in 27 instances of myocardial infarction in 25 cases:

> In twenty-five cases the earliest electrocardiographic signs of infarction were high 'T' waves, the majority of which became inverted in the healing stage of infarction. In most of the cases the high T waves were no longer present twenty-four hours after the attack. (...) The high T waves are thought to be part of the injury pattern. They were accompanied by abnormal elevations of S-T in twenty-one cases. In five instances elevation of S-T was either absent or within normal range. In one instance huge upright T waves were associated with marked depression of S-T. In the majority of the cases high T waves preceded the development of significant changes in the QRS complex. The latter usually appeared within twenty-four hours after the onset of symptoms, when the high T waves were already in the regressive stage. In one instance characteristic changes in QRS did not appear until six days after the attack, and in two instances they failed to develop at all. In five cases high T waves were not associated with abnormal elevation of S-T, nor with significant changes in QRS. Thus, they represented the leading diagnostic sign in the early stage of myocardial infarction [61, p. 644–645].

One case (case 4), with an anterior wall myocardial infarction was unique in that the initial EKG taken 3 hours after the development of symptoms showed, "[h]igh T waves in Lead I and especially in the chest leads. Instead of elevation, marked depression and upward concavity of S-T is noted, notably in Leads CR3 through CRe. No significant changes in QRS are present." [61, p. 644]. He described the pathophysiology mechanisms believed to account for this finding:

> Downward displacement of S-T in limb and chest leads is sometimes observed in patients in whom repeated anginal attacks constitute, a prolonged "prodromal stage" prior to the appearance of classical signs of myocardial infarction. In such patients, depression of S-T is thought to indicate marked coronary insufficiency which has caused injury primarily to the subendocardial muscle layers. We believe that the first tracing in Case 4 depicts a transitional stage which was the result of an extension of injury from the subendocardial to the subepicardial muscle layers, possibly due to progression from incomplete to complete coronary occlusion [61, p. 644].

De Winter et al. identified in 30 of 1532 (2%) patients with an anterior myocardial infarction electrocardiographic features taken on average 1.5 hours after the onset of symptoms:

> Instead of the signature ST-segment elevation, the ST segment showed a 1- to 3-mm upsloping ST-segment depression at the J point in leads V1 to V6 that continued into tall, positive symmetrical T waves. The QRS complexes were usually not widened or were only slightly widened, and in some there was a loss of precordial R-wave progression. In most patients there was a 1- to 2-mm ST-elevation in lead aVR [62, p. 2071].

This series was significant in that based on percutaneous angiographic findings the pattern correlated with occlusion of the proximal left anterior descending artery. They were unable to identify either patient or coronary angiographic factors to account for this unique electrocardiographic pattern.

Littman suggested that the sign originally described by Dressler in 1947 also be credited to de Winter as he further elucidated the frequency of this electrocardiographic occurrence and correlated angiographically the electrocardiographic pattern of anterior myocardial infarction to proximal LAD occlusion [63]. Furthermore, he identified that this distinctive phenomenon was more commonly found in younger male patients with hypercholesterolemia compared to those with ST-segment elevation [64] (Table 2.1).

Robertson Sign

William Egbert Robertson (1869–1956) was born in Camden, New Jersey, and received his medical degree from the University of Pennsylvania in 1892 [65]. He completed several months of internship at Episcopal and Cooper Hospitals in Philadelphia and Camden, New Jersey, respectively and travelled abroad for additional training in Heidelberg, Germany, and Vienna, Austria [65]. He returned to the University of Pennsylvania and from 1893 to 1896 served as an Instructor in Medicine and Assistant in the outpatient department [65]. He was a pathologist (1897–1904) and Instructor of Bacteriology and Microscopic Pathology at the Episcopal Hospital, Philadelphia, PA, followed by an appointment as Instructor in Physical Diagnosis at the Medico-Chirurgical College and Hospital (known as the University of Pennsylvania Graduate School of Medicine) beginning in 1897. From 1904 to 1931, he was Visiting Physician to the Episcopal Hospital with subsequent positions as Instructor in Medicine and Assistant Professor of Clinical Medicine at the Medico-Chirurgical College and Hospital [65]. He was appointed Professor of Medicine and Chairman of the Department in the School of Medicine at Temple University and Visiting Physician to Samaritan Hospital, Philadelphia, PA, from 1916 to 1933 [65]. Robertson served as visiting physicians to a number of hospitals including Philadelphia General Hospital, Garretson, St. Luke's and Children's Hospital Medical Center and Consultant at Rush, Northeastern and Kensington Hospital for Women, Philadelphia, PA [65].

He was an active member of a number of local and national organizations including the Philadelphia Medical Society and College of Physician of Philadelphia [65]. He served as President from 1937 to 1938, member of the Board of Censor, and Board of Directors in the Philadelphia Medical Society [65]. He was appointed Fellow of the College of Physicians, Philadelphia in 1903. Within the College of Physicians of Philadelphia, he served as Chairman of the Sections of General Medicine from 1927 to 1928, medical historian in Medical History Department from 1934 to 1935, member of the Library Committee from 1934 to 1955, Chairman and Member of Council from 1940 to 1944, and Honorary Librarian from 1945 to 1955 [65]. As a description of his character:

> [h]is charm of personality, his grace of manner, his steadfastness of purpose, the deliberate thoroughness with which he did things, his meticulous attention to detail. He was soft-spoken and courteous, patient and forbearing, but let no one think that his mildness of manner betokened any weakness of resolution or vacillation in action [65, p. 57].

Robertson described several signs associated with the heart and aorta at Philadelphia General Hospital. In patients with myocardial degeneration secondary to advanced heart failure (Table 2.1):

> [m]aculopapules of dull pink to purple, according to their age, occurring chiefly on the trunk, rarely on the upper extremities in myocardial degeneration. When viewed with a hand lens, they appear to be made up of many discrete prints. Microscopic sections reveal numerous capillaries, some thickening of the collagen, and more or less edema. In luetic cardiac conditions they may disappear with recovery of the patient, but they are less apt to disappear in the nonluetic [66, p. 214].

He identified prior to death that there is seen over the heart in the preagonal state due to advanced cardiac disease the presence of "a rapid fibrillary contraction of the pectoral muscle" [66, p. 287]. He believed that the aortic diameter was a useful method for distinguishing syphilis from hypertension in that the transverse diameter of the aorta as determined by percussion in patient with syphilitic aortitis is greater than 8 cm while in patients with hypertension does not exceed 8 cm [66].

Thus, Robertson sign refers to the following sign in patients with heart failure: 1) maculopapular dull, pink to purples skin lesions in various stages on the upper extremities, and 2) fibrillary contraction of the pectoral muscle in those in eminent death. The other sign which bears his name is in refer to the aortic diameter in patients with syphilitic aortitis which exceeds 8 cm.

Cabrera Sign

Enrique Cabrera Cossío (1918–1964) was born in the Federal District of Mexico and received his medical degree with honors in 1942 from National Autonomous University of Mexico [67–70]. Beginning in 1943, he pursued training in internal medicine at Presbyterian Hospital, New York, and subsequently received a doctorate in cardiology and electrocardiography in France [71, 72]. At the National Institute of Cardiology in Mexico, he served as an assistant physician in 1944 and from 1946 to 1962 as deputy head in the Department of Electrophysiology [69, 70]. He emigrated to Cuba in 1962 during the Cuban revolution and was a staunch supporter of socialism and the Cuban government [68]. Here, he served as Director of the Department of Cardiology at the National Hospital of Altahabana, William Soler Hospital, and Professor of Internal Medicine and Faculty of Medicine at University of Havana [3, 4]. He also served as Ministry of Public Health of Cuba [73].

Cossío and Charlotte Friedland described the following electrocardiographic findings in a series of 45 patients with preexisting anteroseptal myocardial infarction with left bundle branch block (LBBB):

> The sign consists of a notch with a duration of 0.05 sec. or more, observed in the terminal portion of QRS in the precordial leads that show a morphology rS or QA (usually V_3 and V_4). [T]he new sign has a high incidence (91%) in LBBB with myocardial infarction, and a low incidence (6 to 9%) in LBBB not complicated by infarction. (...) [i]n a case of complete LBBB, the presence of the sign is a clue of infarction with 87% of probabilities in favor and 17% against such a diagnosis [74, p. 458].

A sensitivity between 29% and 47% and specificity of 87–91% have been reported by other authors for this sign [75, 76]. Barold and Herweg found that this sign had a sensitivity of 23–50%, which varied based on the size of the myocardial infarction, and specificity of 97–100% depending on whether notching is identified [77]. Hence, Cabrera sign is mildly sensitive and highly specific for the presence of prior anterior-septal myocardial infarction in LBBB. The sign is thus useful for diagnosing anteroseptal myocardial infarction, but its absence should not exclude the diagnosis (Table 2.1).

Chapman Sign

There is limited historical information on Myron G. Chapman. At that time of his publication, he served at the Veterans Administration Center and the Department of Medicine, University of California School of Medicine, Los Angeles, California. Chapman and Pearce studied 50 cases in patients with confirmatory locations of myocardial infarction and LBBB, and 18 patients with LBBB and no evidence for myocardial infarction. They found (Table 2.1), "[t]hat the early notching of the R wave in leads I, aV_L, and V_6 and the S wave in leads aV_F and V_4 are different from the usual notching in uncomplicated LBBB, and are related to myocardial infarction" [78, p. 569].

Thus, they identified an electrocardiographic method of diagnosing acute myocardial infarction in the setting of left bundle branch block. Chapman's sign is a specific (91%) but nonsensitive sign (21%) in this setting [79]. Thus, the presence of this sign is helpful to rule in the diagnosis of myocardial infarction in the setting of LBBB. Its absence does not exclude the diagnosis.

Frank Sign

Sanders T. Frank (1938–1997) was born in Middletown, Connecticut, and received his medical degree from New York Medical College [80]. He was Associate Clinical Professor and Director of Respiratory Medicine at Garfield Medical Center, Monterey Park, California [80, 81]. In 1973, he observed and described an ear lobe sign believed to be present in patients with premature coronary artery disease, "It is characterized by a prominent crease in the lobule portion of the auricle and is

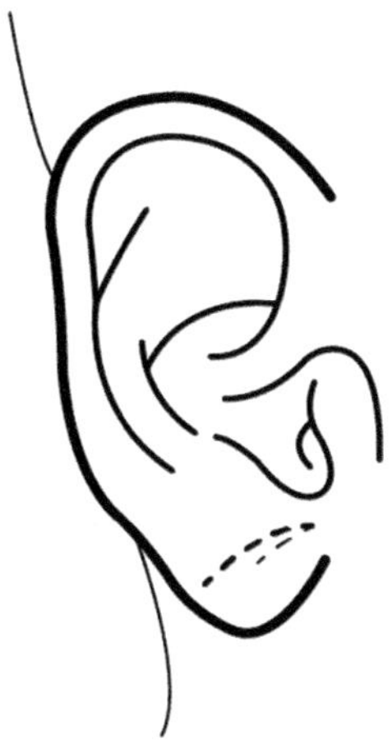

Fig. 2.3 Frank sign (by Ryan Yale)

usually bilateral" [82, p. 328] (Table 2.2, Fig. 2.3). In an uncontrolled observational study of 20 patients 60 years of age or younger with an ear lobe sign, 19 had one or more risk factors for coronary artery disease (elevated cholesterol, triglycerides and blood sugar, hypertension, cigarette smoking, and a family history of premature cardiovascular disease). Among the 20 patients, 33% had a cholesterol level ≥ 250 mg/100 ml, average triglycerides of 293 mg/100 ml, and diabetes (as defined by a 2-hour glucose tolerance test of >150 mg/100 ml). Seventy-five percent of patients had hypertension, 61% were current smokers (>1 pack/day), and 40% had a family history of premature cardiovascular disease. Coronary or peripheral vascular disease was confirmed in 3 (15%) patients [82].

Wellens Sign

Henrick Joan Joost (Hein) Wellens (1935–) was born in The Hague, the Netherlands, and received his medical degree from the University of Leiden. He completed his internal medicine and cardiology training at the University of Amsterdam at the Wilhelmina Gasthuis Hospital [83, 84]. He served as Professor of Cardiology at the University of Amsterdam from 1973 to 1977 [83, 84], and Professor and Chair of Department of Cardiology of Academisch Ziekenhuis at Maastricht University Amsterdam from 1978 to 2002 [85]. He was Professor and Director of the Interuniversity Cardiology Institute of the Royal Netherlands Academy of Arts and Sciences of the Netherlands from 1993 to 2003.

De Zwaan et al. described electrocardiographic findings occurring within 24 hours after hospital admission in 26 of 145 (18%) consecutively admitted patients with unstable angina at risk for an impending and extensive anterior myocardial infarction (Table 2.1):

> [a]ll 26 patients showed a typical pattern of ST-T wave segments in leads V_2 and V_3 consisting of an isoelectric or minimally elevated (1 mm) takeoff of the ST segment from the QRS complex, a concave or straight ST segment passing into a negative T wave at an angle of 60 to 90 degrees, and a symmetrically inverted T wave. Twenty-five of the 26 patients also had a typical pattern in lead V_1; an isoelectric or minimally elevated (1 mm) takeoff of the ST segment and a concave or straight ST segment passing into the first part of the T wave at an angle of approximately 135 degrees, followed by a T wave inversion. In addition 22 had an ST-T segment pattern in lead V_4, and sometimes V_5 and V_6, consisting of a takeoff of the ST segment from the QRS complex below the isoelectric line and a convex ST segment passing into a negative T wave at an angle of about 120 degrees with a deep symmetrical inverted T wave [86, p. 730].

They reasoned that these electrocardiographic findings were presumably caused by "a critical lesion in the proximal portion of the left anterior descending artery" [86]. They recommended that these patients undergo urgent coronary angiography. Morris and Howard in their review identified two retrospective studies which reported the sensitivity, specificity, and predictive value of this sign in patients with suspected acute coronary syndrome and stenosis of the left anterior descending artery. They found that the sensitivity, specificity, and positive predictive value (PPV) decreased as the severity of the stenosis of the LAD artery lesion decreased. A sensitivity, specificity, and positive predictive value of 76%, 89%, and 61%, respectively, were reported at 50% stenosis. At 70% stenosis, the sensitivity, specificity, and positive predictive values were 65.4%, 69.2%, and 51.5%, respectively [87]. These findings suggest that Wellens sign is moderately specific for LAD lesions of 50% stenosis. Its absence, however, does not exclude the diagnosis.

Conclusion

A variety of signs related to atherosclerosis and ischemic heart disease were described during this time period using the physical examination skills of observation, palpation, percussion, maneuvers, and instruments such as sphygmomanometer, thermometer, and EKG. The signs have either not been further studied, are neither sensitive nor specific, or in the case of electrocardiographic findings are relatively specific which may be helpful in diagnosis if present, although their absence should not exclude underlying disease.

Signs used to diagnose atherosclerosis were enumerated prior to the development of methods to image atherosclerotic plaques within the coronary vessels. This chapter highlights some of the controversies regarding medical eponyms [88]. First, eponyms may not include all of the names of the authors whom collaborated and contributed to the publication, for example, Chapman and Pearce, and Chapman sign. Second, the eponym may be named after the last or presumably senior author, for example, Wellen sign. Third, the sign may have been previously described and therefore may not reflect scientific accuracy from when and by whom it was discovered, for example, Levine sign. Understanding these eponymous signs provides insights into the pathophysiology of disease and perhaps provides a useful method for recalling their significance. Their findings were honored as signs to recognize these physicians' accomplishments.

References

1. Skinner HA. Angina pectoris. In: The Origin of Medical Terms. Baltimore: The William & Wilkins Company; 1949. p. 24.
2. Random House: unabridged dictionary. Angina. C2019. https://www.dictionary.com/browse/angina. Accessed 12 Mar 2019.

3. Morgagni JB. Letter the twenty-fourth: treats of preternatural pulses. In: The Seats and Causes of Diseases Investigated by Anatomy in Five Books, vol. 1. Alexander B, translator. London: A. Millar and T. Cadell; 1769. p. 708–69.
4. Lancisi GM. Hypertrophy of the heart with prolapse upon diaphragm: case histories. Malpighi's opinion. In: Aneurysms - The Latin text of De Aneurysmatibus, Rome 1745. Wright WC, translator. New York: The MacMillian Company; 1952. p. 213–60.
5. Earl of Clarendon EH. The Life of Edward Earl of Clarendon, Lord High Chancellor of England and Chancellor of the University of Oxford. Oxford: Clarendon Printing House; 1759.
6. Heberden W. Some account of a disorder of the breast. Med Tr Roy Coll Phys Lond. 1772;2:59–67.
7. AlGhatrif M, Lindsay J. A brief review: history to understand fundamentals of electrocardiography. J Commun Hosp Intern Med Perspect. 2012;2(1):14383.
8. Smith FM. The ligation of the coronary arteries with electrocardiographic study. Arch Intern Med. 1918;22(8):8–27.
9. Herrick JB. Thrombosis of coronary arteries. JAMA. 1919;72(6):387–90.
10. Beaumé L. Thèse pour le doctorate en médecine: contribution à l'étude des myocardites. Paris: G. Steinheil; 1892.
11. Beaumé L. Médecins aides-majors de 2e classe. In: Annuaire de l'Armée Française. Paris: Berger-Levrault et cie; 1897. p. 744–58.
12. [No author]. Nouvelles: Le Dr. Lucien Beaumé. Paris méd. 1918;30:294.
13. Beaumé L. Contribution à l'étude des myocardites: évolution, étiologie, pathogénie. Paris: G. Steinheil; 1892.
14. [No author]. Obituary: Sir William Osler. Boston M & S J. 1920;182:232–6.
15. McCall N. Celebrating the contributions of William Osler. Biography 12 July 1849–29 December 1919. The portrait collection of Johns Hopkins Medicine: A catalog of paintings and photographs at The Johns Hopkins University School of Medicine and The Johns Hopkins Hospital. Baltimore. 1993. http://www.medicalarchives.jhmi.edu/osler/biography.htm. Accessed 14 Mar 2019.
16. Profiles in Science. US National Library of Medicine. The William Osler Papers Biographical Information. Bethesda, MD; National Institutes of Health, Department of Health & Human Services USA.gov. https://profiles.nlm.nih.gov/ps/retrieve/Narrative/GF/p-nid/348. Accessed 22 Feb 2019.
17. McGill Library. About William Osler. McGill University; 2019. https://www.mcgill.ca/library/branches/osler/oslerbio. Accessed 22 Jan 2019.
18. Osler W. Diseases of the arteries arterio-sclerosis (arterio-capillary fibrosis). In: The Principles and Practices of Medicine. 2nd ed. New York: D. Appleton and Company; 1897. p. 700–6.
19. [No author]. Obituary: Dr. Panagino Livierato. Br Med J. 1936;12(128):1278.
20. [No author]. Necrologio: Panagino Livierato. L'Università italiana rivista dell'istruzione superior. 1936;2(5):48.
21. Livierato P. Riflesso abdomino-cardiaco. Gior di Biol e Med. 1906:3–8.
22. Abrams A. The clinical value of the heart reflex. Med Rec. 1901:59:10–12.
23. Barton WM. Manual of Vital Function Testing Methods and Their Interpretation. Boston: Richard G. Badger; 1911.
24. De Schweintz GE. Ophthalmodiaphanoscopy. In: Diseases of the Eye: A Handbook of Ophthalmic Practice for Students and Practitioners. 7th ed. Philadelphia: W.B. Saunders Company; 1913. p. 141–2.
25. Wood CA. Ectropionater. In: The American Encyclopedia and Dictionary of Ophthalmology, vol. 6, Dioptric System to Exophthalmitis. Chicago: Cleveland Press; 1915. p. 4145.
26. Hertzell C. Die Stauungreaktion bei Arteriosklerose. Berlin klin Wochschr. 1913;50:535–8.
27. [No author]. Deaths: Ensign Bennett Pardee MD. JAMA. 1918;70:113.
28. [No author]. Harold Ensign Bennet Pardee. Catalogue of Officers and Graduates of the Columbia University from the Foundation of King's College in 1754. New York: Published for the University; 1916.

29. [No author]. Dr. Harold E.B. Pardee dies; electrocardiographic pioneer. New York Times. 2 March 1973. p. 38.
30. Klingfield P. Profiles in cardiology: Harold Ensign Bennet Pardee. Clin Cardiol. 2005;28:396–8.
31. Pardee HEB. An electrocardiographic sign of coronary artery obstruction. Arch Intern Med. 1920;26:244–57.
32. Oppenheimer BS, Friedberg CK. In memoriam Emanuel Libman. Mt Sinai J Med. 1946–1947;13(5):215–21.
33. Oppenheimer BS. Emanuel Libman, 1872–1946. Bull N York Acad M. 1947;23:116–7.
34. Nevins M. Master diagnostician. In: More Meandering in New Jersey's Medical History. Bloomington: iUniverse; 2011. p. 130–5.
35. Baehr G. Emanuel Libman, 1872–1946. AJYB. 1947–1948;49:81–4.
36. Libman E, Sacks B. A hitherto undescribed form of valvular and mural endocarditis. Trans Ass Am Phys. 1924;38:46–61.
37. Libman E. Method of physical examination with special reference to painful diseases of the thorax and abdomen. Proc Int Postgrad M Ass N America. 1926;3:60–6.
38. Libman E. Observations on individual sensitiveness to pain with special reference to abdominal disorders. JAMA. 1934;102:335–41.
39. Bürklen R. Ein Beitrag zur Symptomatologie der Koronarthrombose. Med klin. 1940;36:709.
40. [No author]. Personalnachrichten: Titelverleihungen. Soziale Sicherheit. 1973;26–27:426.
41. [No author]. Samuel Albert Levine, MD, dies. JAMA. 1966;196:38.
42. Dr. Samuel A. Levine dead at 75: Cardiologist was medical innovator. The Harvard Crimson The University Daily, Est. 1873. 1 Apr 1966. https://www.thecrimson.com/article/1966/4/1/dr-samuel-a-levine-dead-at/. Accessed 25 Apr 2019.
43. Zhang G. Samuel Albert Levine. Life in the fastlane. https://litfl.com/samuel-albert-levine/. Accessed 25 Apr 2019.
44. Levine RI. Levine sign. N Engl J Med. 1964;271:1425.
45. Levine SA. Angina pectoris and coronary thrombosis. In: Clinical Heart Disease. 5th ed. Philadelphia: W.B. Saunders Co; 1958. p. 89–163.
46. Peller S. Zur Kenntnis der Amylnitrit und Atropinwirkung mit besonderer Berücksichtigung der Stenokardie. Wien Arch Inn Med. 1922;4:121–8.
47. Levine SA. Carotid sinus massage: a new diagnostic test for angina. JAMA. 1962;182:1332–4.
48. Leviton A. Another Levine sign. N Engl J Med. 1965;272:264.
49. Costeas F, Katsareas P. Further comments on the Levine sign. N Engl J Med. 1965;272:282.
50. Levine S, Brown CL. Coronary thrombosis: it's various clinical features. Medicine. 1929;8:245–418.
51. Asher R. Clinical sense: the use of the five senses. Br Med J. 1960;1(5178):989–93.
52. Cossio P. Inspection, palpation and low-frequency tracings. In: Luisada AA, editor. Examination of the Cardiac Patient. New York: McGraw-Hill Company Book; 1965. p. 3–17.
53. Oram S. Clinical Heart Disease. London: Heinemann Medical; 1981.
54. [No author]. Obituary: Evans B. Br Heart J. 1990;63:374.
55. Samuel Oram MD, FRCP (1913–1991): eminent cardiologist. Monday 20 Aug 2012. Ivall One-Name Study Blog. http://ivall.blogspot.com/2012/08/samuel-oram-md-frcp-1913-1991-eminent.html. Accessed 29 Jul 2019.
56. Luniewska VC. Samuel Oram. Lives of the fellows. Royal College of Physicians. http://munksroll.rcplondon.ac.uk/Biography/Details/3382. Accessed 29 Jul 2019.
57. Marcus GM, Cohen J, Varsosy PD, Vessey J, Rose E, Massie BM, Chatterjee K, Waters D. The utility of gestures in patients with chest discomfort. Am J Med. 2007;120:83–9.
58. Curriculum Vitae Prof. Dr. J de Winter. https://www.ecri-trials.com/files/cv-rjdewinter.pdf. Accessed 29 Jul 2019.
59. R.J. De Winter, Amsterdam. Deputy editors. Netherland Heart J. https://www.springer.com/journal/12471/editors. Accessed 31 Dec 2009.

60. Temple Health Magazine 2017. https://issuu.com/templehealth/docs/th_magazine_summer2017/27. Accessed 31 Dec 2009.
61. Dressler W, Roesler H. High T waves in the earliest stage of myocardial infarction. Am Heart J. 1947;34:627–45.
62. de Winter RJ, Verouden NJW, Wellens HJJ, Wilde AAM. A new ECG sign of proximal LAD occlusion. N Engl J Med. 2008;359:2071–3.
63. Littmann L. The Dressler - de Winter sign of acute proximal LAD occlusion. J Electrocardiol. 2018;51:138–9.
64. Verouden NJ, Koch KT, Peters RJ, Henriques JP, Baan J, van der Schaaf RJ, et al. Persistent precordial "hyperacute" T-waves signify proximal left anterior descending artery occlusion. Heart. 2009;95:1701–6.
65. Kern RA. Memoir of William Egbert Robertson (1869–1956). Trans Stud Coll Physicians Phila. 1958;26:56–8.
66. Robertson WME, Robertson HF. Diagnostic Signs, Reflexes, and Syndromes. 3rd ed. Philadelphia: F.A. Davis Company Publishers; 1947.
67. Wikipedia: La encyclopedia libre. Enrique Cabrera Cossío. 2018. https://es.wikipedia.org/wiki/Enrique_Cabrera_Coss%C3%ADo. Accessed 10 Apr 2019.
68. Palma López FM, Barreto OA, Álvarez LR, Ballester DS. Dr. Enrique Cabrera Cossío: personalidad de la historia, el arte y la medicina. Revista Habanera de Ciencias Médicas. 2014;13:657–63.
69. Lirys Maria Garica Argüello Information Technology. Biografia. Enrique Cabrera Cossio. Somos Solidarios Con El Ser Humano Que Sufre. Fidel Castro Ruz. la Habana Cuba; National Medical Sciences Information Center 1999–2019. https://instituciones.sld.cu/hec/biografia/. Accessed 5 May 2019.
70. Biografia Enrique Cabrera. FCM Enrique Cabrera. https://instituciones.sld.cu/fcmec/biografia-enrique-cabrera/. Accessed 5 May 2019.
71. Vilma Alvarez Benitez. Biography Enrique Cabrera. La Habana, Cuba: Infomed National Medical Sciences Information Center1999–2019. https://www.ecured.cu/Enrique_Cabrera. Accessed 5 May 2019.
72. [No author]. En vísperas del "50 aniversario" de la muerte de Enrique Cabrera Cossio. Revista Cubana de Cardiologia y Cirugia Cardiovascular. 2013;19:117–8.
73. Servico Medicos Cubanos Para El Mundo Hospital General Docente "Enrique Cabrera Cossio". https://www.paho.org/cub/index.php?option=com_docman&view=download&alias=1483-hospital-general-docente-enrique-cabrera-cossio&category_slug=servicios-medicos-cuba&Itemid=226. Accessed 6 May 2019.
74. Cabrera E, Friedland C. La onda de activacion ventricular en el bloqueo de rama izquierda con infarto: un nuevo signo electrocardiografico. Arch Inst Cardiol Mex. 1953;23:441–60.
75. Wackers FJ. The diagnosis of myocardial infarction in the presence of left bundle branch block. Cardiol Clin. 1987;5:393–401.
76. Hands ME, Cook EF, Stone PH, Muller JE, Hartwell T, Sobel BE, Roberts R, Braunwald E, Rutherford JD. Electrocardiographic diagnosis of myocardial infarction in the presence of complete left bundle branch block. Am Heart J. 1998;116(1):23–31.
77. Barold SS, Herweg B. Electrocadiographic diagnosis of myocardial infarction during left bundle branch block. Cardiol Clin. 2006;24:377–85.
78. Chapman MG, Pearce ML. Electrocardiographic diagnosis of myocardial infarction in the presence of left bundle-branch block. Circulation. 1957;16:558–71.
79. Piccolo E, Zuin G. What is the clinical and prognostic significance of atrioventricular and intraventricular conduction defects? In: Raviele A, editor. Cardiac Arrhythmias 1997 - Proceedings of the 5th International Workshop on Cardiac Arrhythmias. Milano: Springer Verlag; 1998. p. 175–82.
80. Up/Closed. STF Sanders T. Frank. American Pulmonologist. https://upclosed.com/people/sanders-t-frank/. Accessed 1 Apr 2019.

81. Firkin BG, Whitworth JA. Frank sign. In: Dictionary of Medical Eponyms. 2nd ed. New York: Parthenon Publishing Group; 1996. p. 130–1.
82. Frank ST. Aural sign of coronary-artery disease. N Engl J Med. 1973;289:327–8.
83. Jim Maloney. Biography of Hein JJ Wellen. Heart Rhythm Society. Boston. 19 May 1995. https://web.archive.org/web/20120526000637/http://www.hrsonline.org/News/ep-history/notable-figures/heinwellens.cfm. Accessed 12 Mar 2019.
84. Hein JJ, Wellens MD, FACC. FESC member of the scientific advisory board. Inc. Health Care Equipment and Supplies. Company Overview of Vicor Technologies. Bloomberg: Vicor Technologies; 2019. https://www.bloomberg.com/research/stocks/private/person.asp?personId=8329410&privcapId=8031884&previousCapId=21813672&previousTitle=Biowatch%20Medical,%20Inc. Accessed 12 Mar 2019.
85. Guest researchers. School for Cardiovascular Disease. Carim self-evaluation 2007. 2012 Faculty of Health, Medicine and Life Sciences, Maastricht University. Maastricht University Medical Centre. https://carim.mumc.maastrichtuniversity.nl/sites/intranet.mumc.maastrichtuniversity.nl/files/carimmaastrichtnl/carim_erc_part_1.pdf. Accessed 12 Mar 2019.
86. Zwaan C, Bar FEHM, Wellens JJ. Characteristic electrocardiographic pattern indicating a critical stenosis high in left anterior descending coronary artery in patients admitted because of impending myocardial infarction. Am Heart J. 1982;103:730–6.
87. Morris N, Howard L. Bet 1: In patients with suspected acute coronary syndrome does Wellens' sign on the electrocardiograph identify critical left anterior descending artery stenosis? Emerg Med J. 2017;34(4):264–6.
88. Woywodt A. Should eponyms be abandoned? Yes. BMJ. 2007;335(7617):424.

Chapter 3
Endocarditis

Introduction

Names used to describe peripheral physical examination findings in endocarditis are descriptive and referred to as a node (Osler), lesion (Janeway), spot (Roth), or categorically as splinter hemorrhage. In fact, the only eponymously named sign in endocarditis is ascribed in honor of Moritz Litten (1845–1907) as Litten sign. Although not named a "sign," we included the eponymous descriptions by William Osler (1849–1919), Edward Gamaliel Janeway (1841–1911), Moritz Roth (1839–1914), and George Blumer (1872–1962) in order to provide a historical perspective of the significance of their contributions to the physical diagnosis of endocarditis. These signs and findings are typically absent and thus lack sufficient sensitivity or specificity to be used alone in diagnosis. Nevertheless, their presence in the appropriate clinical setting provides clues to consider endocarditis in the differential diagnosis. This chapter highlights those signs and findings reported in endocarditis. We begin our review of the signs of endocarditis by first providing an overview of the key historical aspects of endocarditis which lead to the recognition of this disease.

Historical Background

The earliest description of endocarditis dates back to seventeenth century when Lazarus Riverius (1589–1655) published the description he identified in 1646 on autopsy that "round carbuncles were found like the substance of the lungs, the larger of which resembled a cluster of hazelnuts and filled up the opening of the aorta, which I judged caused the failure of pulsations in the aorta." [1, p. 459].

S. H. Yale et al., *Cardiovascular Eponymic Signs*,
https://doi.org/10.1007/978-3-030-67596-7_3

René Laënnec (1781–1826) acknowledged Riverius as being the first to publish what was later named "valvular excrescence" (vegetation) by Jean-Nicolas Corvisart (1755–1821). Laënnec differentiated two types of vegetations-verrucal and globular forms:

> There are two very distinct varieties of this affection. The one, first noticed by Riverius (...) has been described by M. Corvisart under the name of excrescence of the valves; the other, which does not appear to have been hitherto described, I shall notice under the name of globular excrescence. The first might very well be named warty excrescences, in as much as they are extremely like warts, especially those of venereal origin on the parts of generation. Like these, the excrescences in the heart sometimes resemble small strawberries, in their form and tuberous surface; at other times they are elongated into the form of a small cylinder or cord, and, occasionally, they are so short and so crowded together, as merely to give to the parts on which they are situated a rough or rugged surface; more frequently, however, they are either isolated or ranged in a single line along the loose or the attached border of the valves. I have never observed any longer than three or four lines. But we occasionally meet with them sufficiently numerous and voluminous to present a rough resemblance to the comb of a cock. The colour of these excrescences is sometimes whitish like that of the valves, and hardly so opaque; more commonly they are either wholly or in part tinged with a reddish or light violet colour. Their texture is fleshy, like venereal warts, only of somewhat less firm consistence; although this is variable. They adhere immediately to the subjacent parts; sometimes so strongly as to be only separable by incision; more commonly, they are removable by scraping with the blade, or even the handle of the scalpel. In the latter case, the excrescences are soft, of a yellowish white colour, very humid, and somewhat resembling fat. The venereal origin of these excrescences, entertained by Corvisart, appears to me very improbable, when we consider their rarity and the frequency of venereal complaints, and when we meet with them, as we do, in individuals who, in all probability, never had this disease. Whatever may be the remote cause of these bodies, the manner of their formation seems to me more explicable. In dissecting the more voluminous excrescences, it has always appeared to me that their texture was exactly like that of the more compact polypous concretions, only firmer. Frequently, we observe in their centre a purple or sanguineous tint; and sometimes I have even found a very small but distinct coagulum of blood. From these circumstances, I am led to consider such excrescences as merely small polypi organized by the same process which transforms the false albuminous membranes into true adventitious membranes, or into cellular substance. In like manner as Corvisart, I have only met with these excrescences in the following situations; viz. the mitral, tricuspid, and sigmoid valves, and (much more rarely) the interior of the auricles, especially the left. In general, they are more common in the left than the right side of the heart [2, p. 716–717].

Giovanni Battista Morgagni (1682–1771) in *Delle Sedi e Cause Delle Malattie Anatomicamente Investigate* (On the Locations and Causes of Anatomically Investigated Diseases) reported the case of a 36-year-old miller servant with gonorrhea, found at autopsy to have vegetation on the aortic valve and inflammatory changes on the mitral valve:

> The aortic valves were occupied by short and irregular excrescences, and were so approximated as to leave a very narrow orifice for the transmission of blood. When examining them individually with more attention, I found that the border of the right valve was shorter than usual, and that the left was ruptured, through the middle from the border to the base; and from the lips of the ruptured valve other excrescences sprouted. Although the general tex-

ture of these was more flaccid than natural, yet, when they were rubbed between the fingers, some particles like cartilage could be perceived. This disease had originated in ulceration, and the internal surface of the contiguous ventricle participated in it. The borders of the mitral valves, in places, were somewhat thickened and indurated [3, p. 393].

Jean-Baptiste Bouillaud (1796–1881) is credited for coining the term "endocarditis" to describe the inflammation involving the inner layer of the heart and cardiac valves. In the second volume of his book *Traité Clinique des Maladies du Coeur* (Clinical Treatise on Heart Diseases), he wrote:

The disease whose history we are attempting to sketch here is common. It is at least as frequent as pericarditis or pleurisy, and yet it was so little known prior to us that it had not even received a specific name. That name *endocarditis*, which I assigned to the inflammation of the internal membrane of the heart in general, seems to me in all respects to be in conformity with nomenclature principles universally adopted today. I will propose *cardio-valvulitis* to designate specifically the inflammation of the valves of the heart which are as everyone knows essentially formed by a fibrous tissue on which the *endocardium* or internal membrane of the heart is reflected. This *partial* phlegmasia can also be called *valvular endocarditis* [4, p. 1].

He provided a comprehensive description on the evolution or stages of the inflammatory process, correlating pathological and cardiac auscultatory findings:

But before reporting on these new observations, some of which have already been included in my *Clinical Treatise on Joint Rheumatism,* allows me to recall here that which I have already recorded in the first volume of this *Treatise* under the number 14. In this case collected by me from the year 1832 *the mitral valve thickened and adherent to the internal surface of the heart, dotted and overloaded with multiple vegetations similar to leeks, cauliflower, or warts, was composed of a fibrinous friable material, easily crushed under the blade of the scalpel, etc. A sound of heart murmurs had accompanied the valve lesion.* Before 1832 such a complete observation of endocarditis had not yet been published [4, p. 19].

Rudolf Virchow (1821–1902) in "Ueber die akute Entzündung der Arterein" (Concerning the acute inflammation of the arteries), published in 1847, described several cases of cardiac embolism caused by valvular vegetation including a 27-year-old man with "Thickening and narrowing of the mitral valve with fibrous softening clot on the valve. Emboli in the cerebral carotid artery, left femoral artery and right iliac artery. Hemorrhagic splenic infarctions." [5, p. 338].

In 1856, Virchow recognized that valvular vegetation represented fibrin deposition as well as a new growth on the valve surfaces:

At this point I have already explained the important difference between deposits within the blood vessels and the outgrowths of the inner wall of heart and arteries. In Germany at that time, it was fairly common to believe that the changes in the heart valves were all due to endocarditis and those within the arteries were caused by an atherosclerotic processes from the blood. My early examinations showed agreement of both of these changes. I therefore described the diseased parts of the heart valves as atheromatous. I also found that the atheromatous and semi-cartilaginous areas of the heart and arterial wall, which result from diseases inside the inner layer, are different from the deposits that are more frequently found on the heart and less often on the arteries from the blood [6, p. 142].

Emanuel Winge (1827–1894) in 1870 described the autopsy findings in a 42-year-old man with a foot abscess and bacterium in the heart valves and thus was the first to recognize the bacterial origin as a cause of endocarditis:

> In the present case it is possible to show an infectious process, the illness progressing with the picture of a pyemic fever with striking intermittent chills. The endocarditis could with some reason also be considered as a pyemic secondary process, and certainly can be considered the point of origin for the later pathological process (in the lungs from the right heart, in the kidneys, heart muscle, synovial membrane and skin from the left heart) [7, p. 473].

On microscopic examination of the heart valves, kidneys and heart using oil immersion Winge found:

> Short, rod-shaped or round bodies, they were partly branched also the grains of the short rods had the appearance of small bacteria, while the threads appeared like the mycelium of leptothrix. (…) As far as I know no one has definitively shown any parasite in pyemia especially that form associated with endocarditis, and it is therefore certainly of interest that in the present case there appears to be a parasitic process [7, p. 473].

Edward Gamaliel Janeway (1841–1911) in his 1899 paper "Certain clinical observations upon heart disease" described a finding observed in bacterial endocarditis:

> In trying to determine whether a given case is more probably due to endocarditis or to another malignant process I have found that attention to the position of the hemorrhages is at times very helpful. Several times I have noted numerous small hemorrhages with slight nodular character in the palms of the hands and in the soles of the feet, when possibly the arms and the leg had but a scanty crop in malignant endocarditis, whereas this has not been my experience with the processes likely to be mistaken for it [8, p. 260].

It was Emanuel Libman (1872–1946) who assigned the name "Janeway lesion" to this characteristic finding in honor of his teacher Dr. Janeway: "Another characteristic skin lesion, which one of us has stressed, and which was demonstrated to him by his teacher, E.G. Janeway, was termed the Janeway lesion." [9, p. 35].

William Osler (1849–1919) on his description of the features of chronic endocarditis reported the findings presented at the Association of Physicians of Great Britain and Ireland, Edinburgh on June 12, 1908, "One of the most interesting features of the disease and one to which very little attention has been paid is the occurrence of ephemeral spots of a painful nodular erythema, chiefly in the skin of the hands and feet, the *nodosités cutanées éphémères* of the French." [10, p. 222]. Osler recorded the description of these lesions made by Dr. J.A. Mullen:

> The spots came out at intervals as small swollen areas, some the size of a pea, others a centimeter and a half in diameter, raised, red, with a whitish point in the centre. I have known them to pass away in a few hours, but most commonly they last for a day, or even longer. The commonest situation is near the tip of the finger, which may be slightly swollen [10, p. 222].

He identified the findings of painful nodular erythema in a case as early as July 1888 and shed further light on this phenomenon:

> They are not beneath but in the skin and they are not unlike an ordinary wheal of urticaria. The pads of the fingers and toes, the thenar and hypothenar eminences, the sides of the fingers, and the skin of the lowest part of the arm are the most common localities. In one case they were present in the skin of the flank. I have never seen them hemorrhagic, but always erythematous, sometimes of a very vivid pink hue, with a slightly opaque centre [10, p. 222].

Osler nodes have been reported to be blue, purple, or hemorrhagic and may rarely ulcerate [11]. It is of interest that Étienne Lancereaux (1829–1910) in 1873 reported in a patient with endocarditis that "the right middle finger is the seat of a small ulcer." [12, p. 674]. It was Parkes Weber who first used the term "Osler sign" in the title of his paper titled "Osler's sign" and certain cutaneous phenomena sometimes associated with heart disease to describe the cutaneous finding in patients with chronic or subacute malignant endocarditis:

> I have here used the short terms, "Osler's spots" and "Osler's symptom", because, although I am not sure who first described the spots in question, it was, as far as I know, Sir William Osler who first called general medical attention to their full diagnostic importance and distinguished them from the ordinary purpuric eruptions not rarely met with in cases of malignant endocarditis [13, p. 385].

Osler nodes have been identified in a variety of other conditions including systemic lupus erythematosus, disseminated gonococemia, typhoid fever, bacteremia, septic endarteritis, and infected vascular grafts [14, 15]. They are believed to be caused by microembolism [15].

George Blumer (1858–1940) in his review of subacute bacterial endocarditis included his analysis and observation of 150 autopsies of patients with the disease, describing on the toes or fingernails:

> [c]urious subungual linear hemorrhages which look exactly like a splinter under the nail. I have seen these in but one patient and can find no reference to exactly similar cases though Horder describes a vivid linear splash at the side of the nail bed and Lerebollet and Mouzon speak of subungual ecchymoses [16, p. 142].

Splinter hemorrhages have been described in other diseases such as malignancy, renal failure, minor trauma, vasculitis (e.g., rheumatoid arthritis, systemic lupus erythematosus), antiphospholipid antibody syndrome, left atrial myoma, and thrombosis, and thus lack sufficient sensitivity or specificity in the diagnosis of endocarditis [14, 15].

In a series of 80 patients with native valve endocarditis, Osler nodes were found in 7 (9%), Janeway lesions in 2 (2.5%), Roth spots in 2 (2.5%) of patients [11]. Thus, these peripheral signs of endocarditis are distinctively uncommon [11]. Their presence, however, may provide clues to earlier diagnosis.

We continue our discussion of the signs found in patients with endocarditis including historical information of the person who described the sign and its original description. The signs are presented chronologically from the date they were first published.

Signs

Roth Sign

Moritz Roth (1839–1914) was born in Basel, Switzerland and studied medicine in Basel, Berlin, and Würzburg under Albert von Kölliker (1817–1905) and Friedrich Wilhelm Scanzoni von Lichtenfels (1821–1891), respectively, and in Göttingen under Friedrich Gustav Jacob Henle (1809–1885) and Karl Ewald Hasses (1810–1902). He received his doctorate summa cum laude for Doctor Medicinae from the University of Basel in 1864 [17, 18]. That same year he worked in Berlin at Virchow Institute and in 1865 served as a physician at the Auxiliary Hospital under the auspices of Fritz Müller (1834–1895) [17]. He received venia docendi from the Faculty of Medicine at the University of Basel in 1865. In 1866, he worked as an assistant with Rudolf Virchow (1821–1902) in Berlin and lectured as an adjunct professor from 1866 to 1868 at the University of Basel. He habilitated as a first assistant under Friedrich Grohl at the pathological institute in Greifswald from 1868 to 1872 [18]. He was appointed Associate Professor of Pathological Anatomy at the University of Basel in 1872 and in 1874 full Professor, a position which he held until 1898 [17, 18]. He served the faculty as Dean in 1875, 1884, and 1896 and rector in 1885, as well as president in the Basel Medical Society in 1875 and honorary member in 1897. He received his doctorate honoris causa from the philosophy faculty of Basel for his work on the history of medicine, in particular, his study of Andreas Vesalius [17]. As a description of his character:

> [h]is most striking traits were a sense of duty, conscientiousness, truthfulness, and "intellectual honesty". (…) [h]is character was noble and kind, unselfish, modest, and undemanding. He fearfully guarded his independence, but allowed others in. He was grateful for all the good things that personally happened to him, thankful for the beauties and riches of earthly existence, an idealist and enthusiasm in literature and art, especially music. (…) To us remaining in gratitude and admiration, his outstanding personality will be unforgettable, guiding, correcting and encouraging. Even succeeding generations will be able to learn and benefit from Roth's life's work [18, p. 328–329].

Roth recognized that in some cases of endocarditis, emboli involve the retina and choridea and may rapidly progress to involve other portions of the eye causing a purulent panopthalmitis. He found that in addition to this severe panopthalmitis in retinitis septica (Table 3.1, Fig. 3.1):

> [t]here are also minor affections of the fundus of which those of the retina are of general interest. One sees in such cases near the optic papilla and the macula lutea small white spots of various numbers, usually on both sides, or even red spots. The latter consist of clusters of red blood cells which are extravasated into the optic layer or the deeper layers of the retina while the white spots consist of groups of thickened (hypertrophic) nerve fibers, which are also connective-tissue-cells, partly in a state of asphyxiation (granular cells). Furthermore, fatty degenerated capillaries and pigment granules may be added [19, p. 475].

Table 3.1 Sign of endocarditis

Name	Year	Signs	Method
Roth [18]	1872	Small white and red spots of various numbers are typically located on both sides of the optic papilla and macula lutea.	Observation
Litten [24]	1878	Massive hemorrhages scattered over the retina which are usually round without sharply defined borders. Many of them have a bright white spot in their center.	Observation
Duclos [31]	1889	Asynchrony between the auscultated ventricular contraction and palpable radial pulsation. This delay of the radial pulsation was not accompanied by any abnormal cardiac or extra-cardiac sound.	Auscultation palpation

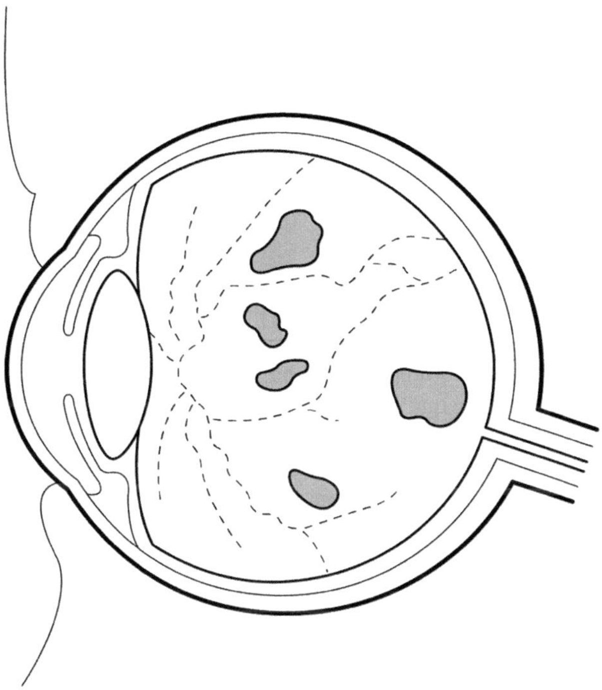

Fig. 3.1 Roth sign (by Ryan Yale)

Roth acknowledged that Virchow in 1856 identified in the retina of a 69-year-old laborer who sustained a fracture of the pelvis and right shoulder complicated by a suppurative infection that:

> Throughout the course of the arteries small foci extend on both sides with the largest being about 1 mm. in diameter. These foci are found partly alongside and over to the left of the artery so that in the latter case the vessel disappeared below. Some of these spots were brownish-red, slightly washed, not quite round, slightly raised, others flat, all white and opaque. (…) In the spots of the retina were found pigmentary granules, hypertrophic nerve fibers, and granule cells [19, p. 478].

Roth listed three features that distinguish "retinitis septica" (septic retinitis) from embolic panopthalmitis:

1. It is more common than the panopthalmitis, which not to speak of other pyemic processes is a very rare phenomenon even in puerperal fever;
2. It is characterized by being relatively benign. The retinal foci are very small, circumscript, sometimes numerous, and have no tendency to diffuse onto the adjacent parts. Rarely is the choroid hyperemic or is there discoloration of the epithelium. Only once did a circumscribed purulent infiltration of the choroid lead to retinal changes (Case 2). Also, the vitreous is rarely affected by the proliferation of its cells and partial opacities.
3. The fact that this form of retinitis does not occur on an embolic basis. Vascular blockages of the retina have not so far been found in any of the cases observed. The capillaries in the white spots are either normal or have fatty degeneration and do not produce abnormal contents. Also, the heart valves were found without deposits [19, p. 476].

Roth originally thought that the white spots were caused by disseminated foci of bacterial abscess but later they were recognized to represent fibrin-platelet plugs.

Litten Sign

Moritz Litten (1845–1907) was born in Elbing, Germany, studied medicine in Heidelberg, Marburg, and Berlin, and received his medical degree in 1868 [20]. He completed his postgraduate studies in Vienna, Prague, Paris, London, and Edinburgh [20]. He served as an assistant to Julius Friedrich Cohnheim (1839–1884) at the Allerheiligen Hospital in Breslau and from 1872 to 1876 senior physician to Friedrich Theodor von Frerichs (1819–1885) at the Charité in Berlin. Litten habilitated in Berlin as an adjunct professor in 1876 and titular professor in 1884 [20]. His name is eponymously associated with "diaphragmatic phenomenon," the normal excursion of the diaphragm during respiration [21]. He was also the first to introduce the centrifuge into the clinic and to describe vitreal bleeding in patients with subarachnoid hemorrhage [20, 22, 23]. A description of his character, "Here the deceased, with whom I was allowed to share a close seat next to him for almost twenty years at the executive table, has so fairly proved his incorruptibility and conviction." [24, p. 1055].

Litten observed in the fundus of the eyes in patients with endocarditis, "On the retina of both eyes massive hemorrhages were visible. These are scattered over the retina, usually round, without being sharply defined. Many of them have a bright white spot in their center." [25, p. 138]. He acknowledged the previous reported findings identified by Moritz Roth and Hjalmar Heiberg:

> Analogous cases of embolic-purulent panopthalmitis with retinal bleeding in the puerperium are described by Roth and Heiberg. In the cases from both authors valvular affections existed; in the former (Roth's case) on deposits on the Mitralis, in the latter (Heiberg's case) diphtheritis of the same valve [25, p. 159]. (…) M. Roth (1d c.) describes changes of the retina, which occur in the setting of wound diseases, under the name "retinitis septica."

> These consist partly in white and red patches on the retina occurring near the optic papillae and the macula lutea. The latter which alone are of interest to us are according to him composed of piles of red corpuscles extravasated into the optic layer or the deeper layers of the retina. He believes he excluded an embolic occurrence of these haemorrhages and attributes them to chemical changes of the blood. Roth observed "retinitis septica" most frequently in putrid-diseased states with widespread exudations and multiple suppurations in pronounced septicemia. Among the cases of septic retinitis which he describes, there are two in which retinal changes are present without other ocular changes occurring in endocarditis [25, p. 159–160]. (…) Therefore, two distinct groups of retinal hemorrhages occur in septic conditions. One which forms as part of a widespread and severe systemic disease including the eye and the others in which the retinal bleeding is confined to the eye. In both groups, the general symptoms may be equally severe and pernicious. Most of the time you will find in both an acute endocarditic processes [25, p. 160].

Thus, Litten referred to the current designation of "Roth spots" as seen in the retinal fundus in patients with bacterial endocarditis (Table 3.1). Roth found white spot as well as retinal red spots (scattered retinal hemorrhages) in endocarditis as well as other acute and chronic pyemic diseases which he referred to as retinitis septica. As to the etiology and pathophysiology of the finding Litten proposed (Fig. 3.2):

> The possibility that the white centers signify sclerosis of the retina around which the nucleus haemorrhagia had developed, is to be ruled out, since those white spots by no means correspond to the changes of the ganglion layer described by Virchow in the tenth volume of his archives. I am thus unable to say anything conclusive about the meaning of

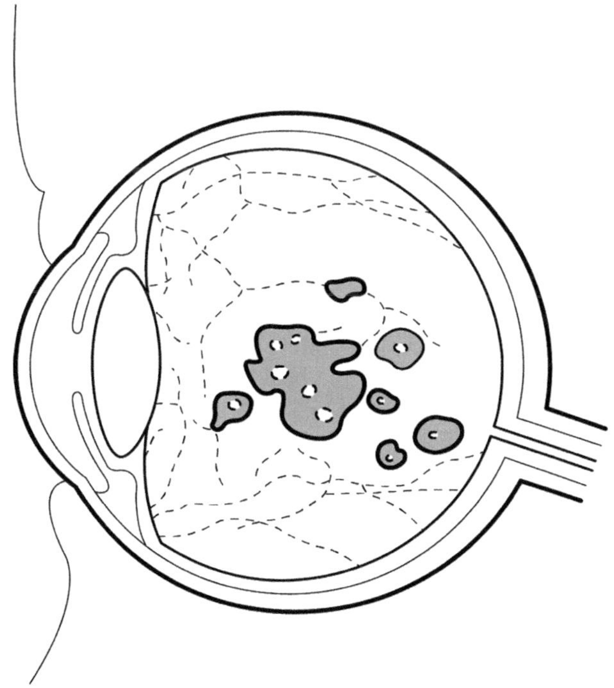

Fig. 3.2 Litten sign (by Ryan Yale)

> these white central other than mentioning that the same formations occur in other affections especially leukemia and pernicious anemia and here, as I have said in the 14th Bd the *Berl. Klin. Wochenschrift* No. 20., had to be attributed to various pathological processes. So much is certain that these retinal hemorrhages with white centers are not characteristic for any certain disease picture [25, p. 166].

These white spots, with the exception of cases of leukemia, represent leukocytes from the fibrin-platelet plugs. They are believed to result from the disruption of the retinal capillary caused by a variety of conditions, in addition to bacterial endocarditis, including anemia, thrombocytopenia, collagen vascular disease, hypertensive and diabetic retinopathy, pre-eclampsia, human immunodeficiency virus, anoxia, and shaken baby syndrome in response to elevated intravascular pressure, ischemia, and/or increased capillary fragility [26, 27]. Thus, Litten recognized that the white retinal spots although commonly seen in endocarditis are not pathognomonic for this disease.

Duclos Sign

Michel Duclos (1822–1900) was born in Tours, France, and received his medical training under Pierre Bretonneau (1778–1862) at l'Ecole de Médecine de Tours and in Pallau, France, under Parisian physicians Armand Trosseau (1801–1867), Jean-Gaston-Marie Blache (1799–1871), and Charles Lasègue (1816–1883) [28]. In 1846, he defended his thesis *Les Convulsions de l'enfance* (Convulsion in Childhood) which earned him the title of Laureate of the Faculty [28, 29]. He received his medical degree with gold medal distinction from the hospital of Paris in 1849 and was appointed Chair of Pathology in 1867, a position which he held for 18 years. He was also Professor of Clinical Medicine at l'Ecole de Médecine de Tours from 1874 to 1896 and appointed honorary professor in 1895 [28–31].

He was the recipient of the Knight's Cross of the Légion d'honneur in 1850 and in 1871 the rosette of officer from the Légion d'honneur by General Ernest Courtot de Cissey (1810–1882) for the medical care which he provided for wounded soldiers [28]. He was appointed a corresponding member of the Academy of Medicine in 1882 and served as a member of the health council and President of Indre-et-Loire Medical Society and Society of Medicine [28, 29]. As a description of Duclos character as delivered at the commencement session of the Tour School of Medicine by R Mercier, Professor and predecessor of Duclos for Chair of Medical Pathology at the School of Medicine:

> I at least want to evoke before you the memory of the one who knew how to be a true master. The one who never stopped sharpening my clinical sense during my studies. The one who at the start of my career guided me with his advice and honored with a friendship of which I have grateful memories [28, p. 6]. (…) He excelled in fact in putting the questions within the reach of the pupil and in letting them resolve it. Never substituting authority in his mind

> for reason he did not teach him science, but let him invent it. Admirably served by an infallible memory, he knew how to extract the immutable truth from general laws from a whole series of facts borrowed from his daily practice. The rigorous analytical method which he brought into the study of diseases allowed him to uncover the cause and by a skillful deduction suggest the appropriate medication. We know that in medical practice, the art is to move from the science of diagnosis through symptoms to the science of drugs [28, p. 8]. (...) Duclos was one of the men most able to highlight it. In a word, he knew how to inspire confidence in his patient and by the seductions of his spirit, aided by the kindness of his heart, drive away the dismal despair. In the dark dramas of life, which no one can avoid, who does not appreciate the alms of a little pity? Psychologist emeritus, he quickly acquired a great deal of medical notoriety. It belonged, in fact, to the kind so easily overlooked by doctors of the tears of a mother at the bedside upset of a dying child and the ingratitude of a sick patient wounded in the heart like betrayal. In the cruel hours when his science became powerless, he knew how to find speech that calmed and the discreet clasp of hands that encouraged. It is, in fact, the doctor's sad privilege to participate less in the ephemeral joys than in the lasting sorrows of all those whom he approaches, and no one better than Duclos was longer able to console the bruises of life [28, p. 8].

Duclos described in 1889 an auscultatory and palpable sign for the early detection of endocarditis in rheumatic fever:

> At the morning daily visit while examining the heart of a rheumatic patient with my ear placed on the cardiac region and fingers on the radial artery, as it is always useful to do in any auscultation of the heart, I was struck by the lack of synchronism between the ventricular contraction and the radial pulsation. This fact interested me deeply. In the normal physiological state the dyschronism between the ventricular contraction, that is to say the cardiac pulsation and the radial pulsation, is almost nil. Appraised with a watch that marks thirds of a second, it certainly lasts less than a quarter of a second. My patient reached more than a third and almost two-thirds of a second. This delay of the radial pulsation was not accompanied by any abnormal cardiac or extra-cardiac sound. (...) Thus, dyschronism of the cardiac and the radial pulse constituted by a delay of the radial pulsation found the next day, as discovered through auscultation of the heart by the stethoscope and finger placed on the radial artery, was consistent with the classical pathognomonic sign of endocarditis. (...) It was possible to ascertain with certainty a relatively significant number of cases in which the synchronism failure of the contraction and radial pulsation occurred 24 to 30 hours in advance of the inflammatory changes within the endocardium [32, p. 33].

Duclos attempted to account for the proposed pathogenesis recognizing the limitations of his conclusions:

> This question cannot be answered decisively unless death and an accurate autopsy, revealing the state of the endocardium, myocardium, and arteries, is performed in a short interval after the dyschronism. This condition has not yet been recognized and therefore remains difficulty to elucidate. However, it must be considered, as shown by the unexpected and sudden decrease in the force of the pulsation, that the ventricular contraction seems lessened. It is suggested that the cardio-radial dyschronism is due to a weakening of the myocardial fibers immediately underlying the endocardium. It would be of great interest to know if the sign in endocarditis, on which I draw attention, is found incidentally during the course of other diseases [32, p. 34].

Thus, Duclos sign refers to the dyssynchrony between the auditory cardiac apex beat and palpable radial pulse (Table 3.1).

Conclusion

There are four primary peripheral phenomenon that have been described in patients with endocarditis with only one, reported by Moritz Litten, as being an eponymous sign. These findings lack sufficient sensitivity and specificity to be used alone in diagnosis. Their presence along with an appropriate history supported by echocardiographic and blood cultures are used to confirm the clinical diagnosis of endocarditis. Hence, it is imperative that physicians learn these peripheral findings, understand their limitations, differential diagnosis, and utility in clinical practice.

References

1. Riverius L. Palpation of the heart and unequal pulse. Opera Omnia, Venice, Viezzeri. 1723. In: Classic Descriptions of Disease with Biographic Sketches of the Authors. Major RH, translator. 3rd ed. Illinois: Charles C. Thomas; 1945. p. 457–9.
2. Laënnec RTH. Of excrescences on the valves and internal walls of the heart. In: A Treatise on the Diseases of the Chest and on Mediate Auscultation. Forbes J, translator. New York: Samuel Wood & Sons; 1830. p. 716–24.
3. Cooke W. Excrescence and ulceration of the aortic valves, case 1. In: The Seats and Causes of Diseases Investigated by Anatomy Containing a Great Variety of Dissections by John Baptist Morgagni, vol. 1. Boston: Wells and Lilly; 1824. p. 393–4.
4. Bouillaud J. De l'endocardite (inflammation de la membrane interne et des valvules du coeur) et de ses suite: considérations préliminaire. In: Traité clinique des maladies du coeur, vol. 2. Paris: Chez J.-B. Baillière; 1841. p. 1–19.
5. Virchow R. Ueber die Akute Entzündung der Arterien. Arch f Path Anat u Physiol. 1847;1:272–378.
6. Virchow R. Vegetationen der Herzklappen und Auflagerungen der Arterein. In: Gesammelte Abhandlungen zur Wissenschaftlichen Medicin: Ueber den Faserstoff. Frankfurt: Verlag von Meidinger Sohn & Comp; 1856. p. 57–146.
7. Winge EFH. Mycosis Endocarditis. Hygiea. Medicinsh och Formaceutisk Manadskrift. 1870, xxxii. In: Major RH, editor. Classic Description in Disease. Carlson HE, translator. Springfield: Charles C. Thomas Publisher; 1945. p. 471–4.
8. Janeway EG. Certain clinical observations upon heart disease. Medical News Phila. 1899;75:257–62.
9. Libman E, Friedberg CK. Subacute Bacterial Endocarditis. London: Oxford University Press; 1948.
10. Osler W. Chronic infectious endocarditis. Q J Med. 1908–9;2:220–30.
11. Sandre RM, Shafran SD. Infective endocarditis: review of 135 cases over 9 years. Clin Infect Dis. 1996;22:276–86.
12. Lancereaux E. De l'endocardite végétante ulcéreuse et de ses rapports avec l'intoxixation palustre. Arch Gén Méd. 1873;21:672–92.
13. Weber FP. "Osler's sign" and certain cutaneous phenomena sometimes associated with heart disease. Q J Med. 1912–13;6:384–90.
14. Chong Y, Han SJ, Rhee YJ, Kang SK, Hyeon J, Na MH. Classic peripheral signs of subacute bacterial endocarditis. Korean J Thorac Cardiovasc Surg. 2016;49:408–12.
15. Long B, Koyfman A. Infectious endocarditis: an update for emergency clinicians. Am J Emerg Med. 2018;36:1686–92.
16. Blumer G. Subacute bacterial endocarditis. Medicine. 1923;2:105–70.

17. [No author]. Moritz Roth (1839–1915). Br Med J. 1915;1(2841):662.
18. Burckhardt A, Roth M. Nekrolog von A Burckhard. Cor Bl f Schweiz Aertze. 1915;45:321–31.
19. Roth M. Über Netzhautaffectionen bei Wundfiebern. I. Die embolische Panophthalmitis. Deutsche Ztschr f Chir. 1872;1(5):471–84.
20. Pagel J. Biographisches Lexikon-Hervorragender Arzte des neunzehnten Jahrhunderts. Berlin: Urban und Schwarzenberg; 1901.
21. [No author]. The diaphragm phenomenon. Am M Rev. 1895;4:1–2.
22. [No author]. Death abroad: Moritz Litten MD. JAMA. 1907;49:68.
23. Litten M. Ueber einige vom allgemein-klinischen Standpunkt aus interessante Augenveränderungen. Berl klin Wochenschr. 1881;18:23–7.
24. [No author]. Nekrolog von Fürbringer. Deutsche med Wchnschr 1907;33:1055.
25. Litten M. Ueber akute maligne Endocarditis und die dabei vorkommenden Retinalveranderungen. Charite Ann. 1878;3:137–90.
26. Fred H. Little black bags, ophthalmoscopy, and the Roth spot. Tex Heart Inst J. 2013;40(2):115–6.
27. Ruddy SM, Bergstrom R, Tivakaran VS. Roth spots. In: StatPearls. Treasure Island, FL: StatPearls Publishing; 2019.
28. [No author]. Michel Duclos (1822–1900). Gaz méd du Centre. 1908:6–9.
29. [No author]. Décés de MM Duclos et Bêranger-Féraud, correspondants nationaux. Bull Acad de méd. 1800:46:789–90.
30. Gautier É. Duclos. In: L'Année scientifique et industrielle, vol. 44. Paris: Libraire Hachette et c.; 1901. p. 391.
31. [No author]. Ecole de Médecine de Tours. Union méd. 1895;1:384.
32. Duclos M. Sur un signe prémonitoire de l'endocardite dans le rhumatisme. Rev Gen de Clin et de Thérap. 1889;3:33–4.

Chapter 4
Hypertension

Introduction

The development and redesigns of the sphygmomanometer were revolutionary in that it provided an indirect and portable method to measure blood pressure. Using this device, physicians identified a method to distinguish normal from abnormal blood pressure and define hypertension. The ophthalmoscope provided an image of the retinal vessels and the identification of vascular signs in patients with uncontrolled hypertension and atherosclerosis. The electrocardiogram further provided evidence of the systemic effects of uncontrolled hypertension. These findings were collectively later recognized as sign of end-organ damage and enumerated as medical eponyms to honor these physicians' accomplishments. This chapter first provides a brief historical overview of innovations that lead to the development of the modern-day sphygmomanometer, the quintessential tool for diagnosing hypertension, followed by a description of the physicians who described these signs and their original description.

Historical Background

The first recorded method to determine blood pressure was performed by Stephen Hales (1677–1761), a clergyman, who in 1708 used a long glass tube inserted directly into the carotid artery of horses and found:

> There had been before the tube was fixed to the artery, about seventy cubic inches of blood. The blood rose in the tube in the same manner as in the case of the two former horses, till it reached to nine feet six inches height. I then took away the tube from the artery, and let out by measure sixty cubic inches of blood; and then immediately replaced the tube to see how high the blood would rise in it after each evacuation [1, p. 15].

S. H. Yale et al., *Cardiovascular Eponymic Signs*,
https://doi.org/10.1007/978-3-030-67596-7_4

Jean Faivre (1824–1871) was the first to record blood pressure in humans, also using the direct method, in 1856 by applying the mercury manometer designed by Jean Léonard Marie Poiseuille (1797–1869) in 1828:

> Nothing is easier than to arrive in man knowledge of the arterial blood pressure. It suffices to take advantage of an amputated arm or the thigh and to adapt to the arteries of these limbs the hemodynamometer of M. Poiseuille. Desgranges and Barrier had been nice enough to promise me that I would be apprised of the first occasions of this kind, which appeared in the rooms of the Hôtel-Dieu de Lyon. It was in the service of Mr. Barrier that they met me as soon as possible. Thanks to his complacency I was able, without imposing additional suffering on the sufferers, to carry out this experiment twice. The first time was on the radial artery of a man of sixty years of age who had developed a chronic lesion on the elbow which was in a certain degree of adynamy. The difference between the two mercurial columns was exactly 12 centimeters. The second experiment was made on the femoral artery of a man thirty years of age with extraordinary vigor; the mercurial ascending column exceeded the other with perfect accuracy by 12 centimeters. A third experiment was made later in the service of M. Desgranges. The patient, a porter aged about twenty-three, had a white swelling of the right wrist and elbow. His condition was rather unsatisfactory. The pressure on the humeral artery was eleven and a half centimeters [2, p. 727].

Etienne-Jules Marey (1830–1904) is credited to be the first to develop a portable sphygmographic instrument for recording the pulse wave and arterial pressure. He acknowledged the instrument constructed by Karl von Vierordt (1818–1884) who named it "sphygmograph," defined its limitations, and described the improvements that he made to his device:

> The considerable mass of the instrument specifically prevents it from being used as indicated for its greatest value. The weighted sphygmograph oscillates as a balanced scale whose two plates are very loaded; the lever up and down movements are substantially isochronous. The number of pulsations, their more or less regularity and amplitude, are therefore the only characters provided by Vierordt's sphygmograph. It is the inadequacies of these findings as well as to the inconvenience of the device, not very portable because of its volume, that we have sought to remedy by constructing a new one which has in common with the German apparatus the use of the lever as a means of transmitting and amplifying the pulsation. Our first concern was to give the new instrument all the necessary sensitivities, which could only be achieved with an extreme lightness of the lever. Because it was necessary to exert a fairly considerable pressure on the artery to obtain the pulsation, we used a completely independent piece formed by a long steel spring R, which applies a force through a small ivory plate to the artery, that can be graduated as desired using an adjustment knob. The movements that this plate receives from arterial pulses are transmitted to the lower part of the lever, fairly close to its center of movement, so that the free end can move to a sufficient extent [3, p. 7]. (...) The whole device is established on a kind of cuff BB, which adapts to the forearm to ensure its perfect fixation. Finally, the tracing is received on a small glass or metal plate P, and moves in a clockwise direction with a known speed H, parallel to the lever recording the pulse rate. The instrument is only 18 cm long, weighs 240 gram and is portable [3, p. 8].

Samuel Siegfried von Basch (1837–1905) is credited in 1880 for devising the first indirect method for obtaining blood pressure by a device he constructed and referred to as a "sphygmomanometer." This device became the forerunner for the more modern-day instruments designed by Riva-Rocci and Hill and Barnard. Von Basch's device used both a mercury column and water, the latter filled a very thin rubber membrane. The blood pressure recorded the point when the arterial pulse palpably disappeared:

> If it were possible to determine the limit at which the changes in the volume of the arm associated with the pulses disappeared, one would be able to obtain an indirect value for the blood pressure. (…) It would be different if it were possible to pass it through a column of liquid. As it is known, when fluid pressure is used, ever part of the pressed surface experiences the same pressure corresponding to the height of the column of fluid. It can be measured provided that the surface pressed is greater than the cross-sectional area of the artery [4, p. 86].

Scipione Riva-Rocci (1863–1937) mercury manometer, an adoption of von Basch's instrument, was presented at the Reale Accademia di Medicina di Torino (Royal Academy of Medicine of Turin, Italy) and published under the title "Un nuovo sfigmomanometro" (A new sphygmomanometer) in *Gazzetta Medica di Torino* in 1896 [5]:

> The instrument which I present is a true sphygmomanometer, that is, an apparatus intended to measure the total load in the arterial vasculature. Being intended to measure the stress of the heart it is applied on the sleeve of the arm, a large arterial trunk, as close as possible to the heart itself. (…) For technical simplification, the principle of manometric measurement is applied in this type of instrument independent of the compressed surface introduced by Marey. (…) The new sphygmomanometer is essentially composed of an armband and a large rubber tube covered with a sleeve of inextensible fabric. It is designed so that through the use of a clamp, it can be adjusted to any arm circumference. Based on the Richardson model, the inside of the tube connects to an insufflator apparatus by means of a rubber duct. On this is interposed a manometer, which for convenience of experimentation is a metal barometer pressure gauge. The apparatus is used in the following way: the armband is applied to about half of the arm so that the clamp is on the outside. The examiner feels the wrist for the radial pulse and blows air into the armband by means of the Richardson ball until the palpated radial pulse disappears. The reading at this time records the pressure marked by the pressure gauge which is the required pressure to compress the major vascular trunks of the arm - the humeral - to the point of intercepting the blood flow. It is necessary when obtaining this measurement that the arm and forearm is flexed, almost at a right angle on the arm [6, p. 180].

Riva-Rocci using palpation was able to measure the systolic blood pressure, which corresponded to the point at which the radial pulse disappeared. It is of interest that unbeknownst to Riva-Rocci a similar device was built by L. Rabinowitz in 1881:

> The suitably modified Roy and Brown method was also used for determining blood pressure in humans. A Herisson sphygmometer was attached to the periphery of the compression site to indicate the disappearance of the pulse. The Basch apparatus was less useful for the author. The experiments show the good usage of the device for relative pressure determinations in the same individual. The pressure difference between the brachialis and radialis was 10-30 mm Hg [7, p. 204].

It was Leonard Erskine Hill (1866–1952) and Harold Leslie Barnard (1868–1908) whom in 1897 substituted a needle pressure gauge in lieu of a mercury manometer, a modification which became the basis for the present-day portable sphygmomanometer:

> [a] vertical glass tube about 12 cm in length. Above, the tube ends in a small bulb which is closed at the top by a tap. To the base of the tube there is affixed, by a special mechanism, a small rubber capsule filled with fluid. The fluid used is a dilute solution of glycerine acidulated with chromic acid. On pressing the rubber capsule down over the radial artery the fluid rises in the tube and compresses the air in the bulb. The air acts as an elastic spring. At a certain height the fluid meniscus exhibits maximal oscillation. The tube is empirically graduated in divisions which correspond to mmHg pressure. The pressure is read at the point where maximal pulsation is obtained. Before each observation the valve is opened and the fluid set at the zero of the scale, thus errors due to barometric or thermal changes are avoided. This instrument is of pocket size and can be used clinically with great ease [8, p. 67].

This device was significant in that it now allowed diastolic blood pressure to be measured by the oscillatory method.

Although the focus of this discussion has been on instruments devised for the measurement of blood pressure it is apropos to include the auscultating finding identified over the brachial artery on release of the air-pressure cuff identified by Nikolai Sergeyevich Korotkov (1874–1920). He presented this finding at the meeting of the Imperial Military Medical Academy, St. Petersburg, Russia in 1905 and published it in *Izestiya Imp Voiennomedicinskoi Akademii* (Bulletin of the Imperial Military Academy) in a short paper titled "On methods of studying blood pressure" we included Korotkov's discussion as translated by William Hall Lewis, Jr.:

> On the basis of his observation, the speaker came to the conclusion that a perfectly constricted artery, under normal conditions, does not emit any sounds. Taking this fact into consideration, the speaker proposes the sound method for measuring blood pressure on human beings. The sleeve of Riva-Rocci is put on the middle third of the arm; the pressure in this sleeve rises rapidly until the circulation below this sleeve stops completely. At first there are no sounds whatsoever. As the mercury in the manometer drops to a certain height, there appear the first short or faint tones, the appearance of which indicates that part of the pulse wave of the bloodstream has passed under the sleeve. Consequently, the reading on the manometer when the first sound appears corresponds to the maximum blood pressure; with the further fall of the mercury in the manometer, there are heard systolic pressure murmurs which become again sounds (secondary). Finally, all sounds disappear. The time of the disappearance of the sounds indicates the free passage or flow of the bloodstream; in other words, at the moment of the disappearance or fading out of the sounds, the minimum blood pressure in the artery has surpassed the pressure in the sleeve. Consequently, the reading of the manometer at this time corresponds to the minimum blood pressure. Experiments conducted on animals gave positive results. The first sound tones appear (I0-12 mm.) sooner than the pulse which (1. ar. radialis) can be felt only after the passage of the major portion of the blood stream [9, p. 877].

We continue our discussion of eponymous sign of hypertension including brief historical information of the persons who described the sign and its original description. The sensitivity or specificity of these signs has not been studied and thus their utility in clinical practice is unknown. The signs are presented chronologically from the date they were originally discovered.

Signs

Gunn Sign

Robert Marcus Gunn (1850–1909) was born in Rattar, Dunnet; Caithness, Scotland (Dunnet, Sutherlandshire) and received his MB and CM degrees from Edinburgh University in 1873 [10–12]. In 1873, he worked under John Couper (1835–1918) at the Moorfields Eye Hospital in London and studied the comparative anatomy of the eye under Edward Albert Schäfer (1850–1935) at the University College, London in 1874 [10–12]. From 1874 to 1875 he continued his studies under Eduard Jáger von Jaxthal (1818–1884) in Vienna and then returned to Moorfields Hospital where he ascended to the ranks of Senior House Surgeon, a position which he held from 1876 to 1879 [10–12]. He received his FRCS (Eng.) in 1882. Gunn was elected assistant surgeon in 1883 and full surgeon at the Moorfields Hospital in 1888. He also served as an Ophthalmic Surgeon to the National Hospital for the Paralyzed and Epileptic Queen Square and to the Hospital for Sick Children in 1886 [11, 12]. Later he was an Assistant Ophthalmic Surgeon to the University College Hospital and Visitor for the King's Hospital Fund [10, 11].

He served as President in the Section of Ophthalmology of the British Medical Association in 1906 [10]. In addition to the sign which bears his name other eponyms include the Marcus Gunn pupil, Marcus Gunn jaw-winking phenomenon, Gunn's dots, and inverted Marcus Gunn syndrome (reverse jaw-winking, inverted Marcus Gunn Phenomenon or Marin-Arnat Syndrome) [13]. His character as recorded in an obituary by J.B.L:

> Of Marcus Gunn's character we can say that he was courageous and pure in body and mind, modest to a degree, but clear and strong in his convictions, sweet of temper, and if sometimes intolerant never aggressive, ready to see the better side, and scrupulous in giving credit wherever due, but sensitive and quick to resent, without respect of persons, anything he thought an infringement of dignity. He had no desire for wealth, as such, and valued it even for what it brings less than many. His influence, alike with colleagues, students, and patients, depended on their conviction that he was true and loyal always, was never satisfied with slipshod examination or half knowledge, and although himself guileless, was no mean judge of character and motives in others [10, p. 1720].

As described by one of his colleagues:

> Gunn was greatly beloved, and respected in an equal degree, by those who knew him. Mr. Nettleship to whom we are indebted for much of the information in this notice, writes in these words: "Marcus Gunn's character might be described as little removed from that of the perfect knight—courageous and pure in mind and body, modest, but clear and strong in his convictions, sweet of temper, ready always to see the better side, scrupulous in giving credit where credit was due. He was a man of considerable intellectual gifts and brain power and an exceedingly keen and accurate observer; his mental grasp was strong, his judgment careful and well-balanced: a certain matter of fact simplicity was set off by a ready sense of humor. His influence with colleagues, students, and patients depended largely on the conviction that he was true and loyal to the core and never satisfied with slipshod methods or imperfect knowledge. Himself singularly guileless he was a good judge of character and motives in others" [12, p. 51].

Table 4.1 Signs of hypertension

Name	Date	Signs	Method
Gunn [14]	1892	Where an artery crosses over a retinal vein, the circulation in the latter is impeded and in some cases appears as being tapered and distended peripherally from the point where it is crossed.	Observation
Huchard [21]	1901	The is no difference or increased pulse when moving from the standing to supine positions.	Palpation
Pende [34]	1926	Large difference between the systolic blood pressure and the diastolic blood pressure (pulse pressure).	Palpation Auscultation
Wood and Selzer [46]	1939	The p wave is widened, of low voltage, and bifid or flat-topped.	Observation
Salus [49]	1939	Change in course and indentation of the vein. In the nicking sign, the vein is slightly indented by the crossing artery which causes the "nicking" or even a very small arch (S-shaped curing or deflection) corresponding to the width of the crossing artery. In other instances, the vein deviates in a more or less obtuse angle in an attempt to avoid the crossing artery.	Observation
Cunningham [55]	1946	The sphygmomanometer cuff is inflated slowly until the first sound (diastolic reading) is audible. It is again inflated more rapidly but smoothly until the sounds disappeared (systolic reading). After raising the mercury column 30–40 mm higher, the pressure was then determined in the usual manner with the mercury falling. Thus, the first sound to appear when the cuff was inflated corresponded to the last sound when it was deflated, and the last sound during inflation corresponded to the first sound on deflation. In hypertensive patients, (1) the sounds might disappear at a certain level during inflation of the cuff, only to return if the inflation were stopped at that level, or (2) the sound might disappear on further inflation and reappear at a higher level until a maximum point was reached beyond which there was no further rise.	Auscultation
Bonnet [59]	1951	A collateral vein when approaching an artery is stopped at the crossing of its branch. The vein upstream of the crossing is dilated, inflated, and abutting, like the "head of a snake," at the arterial wall.	Observation

Gunn described the appearance of the retinal veins in patients with hypertension:

> Attention is also directed to the effect produced on the veins by arteries overlying them. Where an artery, even a small twig, passes over a retinal vein, the circulation in the latter is much impeded. In some cases the vein is indistinguishable, just at the spot where it is crossed, and is evidently distended for some distance peripherally from this point. There is a liability to the occurrence of haemorrhages from a vein thus distended with blood. The appearance is interpreted as an evidence of high arterial tension [14, p. 125].

Thus, Gunn sign refers to the tapering of the retinal vein at an arterial-venous crossing in patients with hypertension caused by compression of the retinal vein by the retinal artery (Table 4.1, Fig. 4.1).

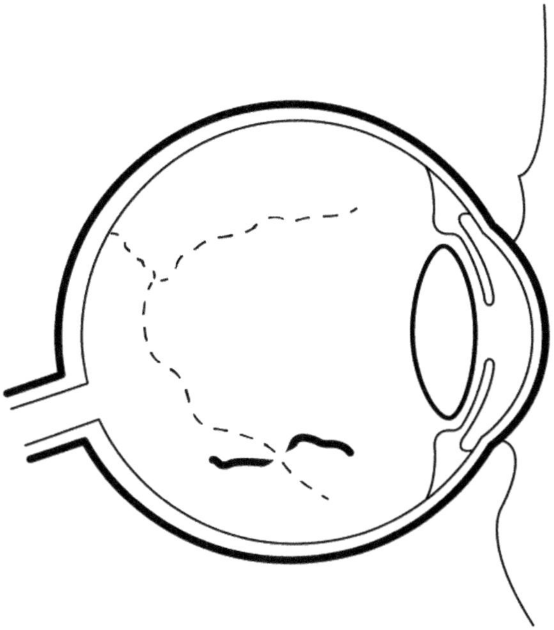

Fig. 4.1 Gunn sign (by Ryan Yale)

Huchard Sign

Henri Huchard (1844–1910) was born in Auxon (Aube), France and received his medical degree from the University of Paris. He practiced medicine at Bichat and Necker Hospitals, Paris [15]. He was an honorary member of the Academy of Medicine (Belgium), honorary President of the Medical-Surgical Society, Officer of the Légion d'honneur in 1903, and Laureate of the Institute of the Academy of Medicine [15–17]. He founded and served as editor-in-chief of the journal *La Presse Médicale* for 30 years, as well as *Revue Générale de Clinique et de Thérapeutique: Journal des Praticiens* beginning in 1887 [18, 19]. His contributions expanded medical knowledge in the fields of neuropathology, hypertension, arteriosclerosis, and arterial cardiopathies (coronary arteries) [20]. As described by F. Santiard regarding Huchard's character:

> Although the faculty recruiting method did not officially award or grant the professor's degree, this remarkable clinician gathered around him a large number of students who were captivated by the clarity of his teaching. They were going to spread around France and abroad the name of the man whom they called Professor Huchard. Those who closely knew him had the opportunity to admire his goodness, charity, and devotion to his patients and pupils, and to see the kind of enthusiasm that aroused him in every noble cause. Endowed with a vibrant, passionate and persuasive word, he also possessed a remarkable talent as a writer, which was superbly affirmed in the *Journal des Praticiens* founded by himself, spreading many truths and supported theses of undeniable utilitarian significance. The theories of Huchard had their admirers as well as fierce adversaries against whom he

> wrestled with an energy and courage for the admiration of all. It is a great and masterful Ligurian that disappears! One can say that Huchard's discoveries have almost completely renewed the therapy of cardiac affections and made this scientist a true benefactor of humanity [15].

In the chapter titled "Traitement de la présclérose" in his book *Consultations Médicales,* Huchard described a finding related to the pulse in patients with hypertension:

> [t]he stability of the pulse, a new sign, consists of the following phenomenon: In the normal state, the number of pulsations decreases from 6 to 8 when passing from the standing to supine position. Graves, who had formerly made this remark, deduced no practical value. Now, numerous observations have taught me that in hypertension, the difference in pulsations in the two positions tends to disappear and may even be reversed. If this difference increases, it is a sign of arterial hypotension. For example, if you have 88 pulses in the vertical station and horizontal decubitus, or even more so 88 in the first attitude and 96 or 100 in the second, you are in a state of arterial hypertension. If you have 88 lying down, and 100 or 110 standing, it's hypotension [21, p. 187].

Current methods for assessing for orthostatic hypotension involves subtracting the difference in blood pressure obtained after standing or sitting from a lying position. Orthostatic hypotension is defined by the presence of a ≥ 20 mmHg drop in systolic or ≥10 mmHg drop in diastolic blood pressure occurring after 3 minutes standing (or sitting). An increase in the pulse of at least 30 beats per minute occurring after 3 minutes of standing suggests hypovolemia independent of whether the patient fulfills the criteria for orthostatic hypotension [22]. Thus, Huchard sign refers to the pulse that does not decrease, and conversely may increase, when changing from the standing to supine position in patients with hypertension (Table 4.1).

Pende Sign

Nicola Pende (1880–1970) was born in Noicattaro (Bari), Italy and received his medical degree from the Faculty of Medicine at the University of Rome in 1903 [23, 24]. After graduation, he worked as medical assistant at the Hospital of Rome followed by an internship at the Institute of General Pathology where he conducted research in endocrinology from 1903 to 1909. In 1907, he taught special medical pathology and in 1908 was promoted Associate Professor of Internal Pathology [23, 25]. He was appointed to the special pathology department of the Royal University of Palermo in 1909 and from 1909 to 1912 served as assistant to Giacinto Viola (1870–1943) at the Institute of Special Medical Pathology, University of Palmero, later serving as Professor of Pathology at this same institution [23]. In 1914, he served at the medical clinics in Berlin and Naples under Friedrich Kraus (1858–1936) and Pietro Castellino (1864–1933) respectively [23]. In 1915, during World War I, he was a medical captain at the military hospitals at Bari, Italy and major and director of the military hospital for disabled men in Rome, and Padua Italy at Vittorio Emanuele Hospital in 1916 [23]. He published the first edition of his treatise titled

Endocrinologia-Patologia e Clinica degli Organi a Secrezione (Clinical Pathology of the Organs of Secretion) in 1916. He was an assistant in medical pathology in 1919 and from 1921 to 1923 served as head of the General Medical and Semiotic Medicine Clinic at the University of Messina, Italy [23]. Here, he was awarded the title of Extraordinary Professor followed by Ordinary Professor of the Clinic and Specialist in Clinical and Special Medical Pathology in 1923 [23]. In 1924, he was the founding rector of the Faculty of Medicine and Surgery at the University of Bari, renamed after Benito Mussolini in 1925 [23].

In 1924, he joined the National Fascist Party and in 1926 founded the first Institute of biotypology and human orthogenesis in Genoa, Italy [23]. The orthogenic clinics were designed to improve the physical, moral, and intellectual aspects of Italians and shape an individual's "orthogenic biotypical profile" to be aligned with principles set forth by the fascist regime [23, 26]. This concept was based on the conceptualization of the study on the relationship between endocrine-vegetative system and biotypical aspects in which hormone secretion is the determinant link between morphology, psychology, and characters of the individual. Hence, through endocrinology, he believed that he was able to identify a biotypological profile or pscyho-physical personality of an individual comprised of the elements consisting of the individual, family and racial inheritances as well as the phenomenal aspects of individuality (morphological, physiological, ethical and affective, and intellective) [23]. Based on these concepts, Pende also conceived of a political and social biology theory in which the classes were the result of a biotypological characteristic that determined social role. Thus, Pende's endocrinology "became the fundamental instrument of the eugenic and demographic policies of the Fascist regime" [27].

He was appointed Senator of the Kingdom for scientific merit of Italy in 1935 and appointed by Mussolini as Chair of Medical Pathology and Clinical Methodology at the University of Rome in 1935 [23]. There he directed the Institute of Medical Pathology and established the biotypological-orthogenetic institute [23]. He directed the medical sciences section of the Italian encyclopedia and in 1937 was appointed head of the eugenic section of the National Research Center [23].

Nicola Pende was believed to be among one of the 42 persons who signed the Manifesto of Race, also referred to as the Charter of Race in 1938, a public declaration regarding racial laws in Fascist Italy. The anti-Semitic laws "stripped the Jews of Italian citizenship and governmental and professional positions." Pende, in his defense, claimed that his signature had been affixed without his approval to the document [28, 29]. Since eponyms are honorific terms, any name associated with war crimes, anti-semitic, or racist connotations should be removed from the literature and discourse [28, 29]. The name Pende has fallen into disfavor because of his proclivities toward anti-semitic and racist ideology. In response, Rome removed the names of Pende as well as other scientist who signed the manifesto from its street [30].

In 1941, he was appointed rector of the Italian Academy of Littorio and in 1956 was the recipient of the first-class gold medal awarded for merit by Giovanni Gronch (1887–1978) President of Italy [23, 31]. He was the recipient of the Bllabli-Valier prize for his work on the organs of internal section, the best medical work published in the preceding year, by the Venice Real Istituto [32, 33]. At the time of this award he served as Professor of Pathology at the University of Palermo.

Pende described in his article titled "Sopra una triade sintomatica dell'ipertiroidismo costuzionale: sua importanza diagnostic nelle forme larvate di tireotoxisi" (Over a triad of symptomatic constitutional hyperthyroidisms: its diagnostic importance in the early form of thyrotoxicosis), a sign which he believed to be useful in diagnosing Basedow's disease (hereditary or endogenous hyperthyroidism):

> Very high variable pressure, i.e. large distance between the systolic blood pressure and the diastolic. I consider this phenomenon besides aortic insufficiency absolutely characteristic of hyperthyroidism. (…) For the most part, when this exists, we find a high systolic pressure of up to 160-190 mm, (RIVA Rocci palpation method) and the diastolic pressure of 50-70 (Korotkov's listening method) [34, p. 311–312].

He acknowledged that other physicians previously identified high variable pressure in this condition but they believed that it was not clinically significant. He reported that this finding was:

> [f]or me one of the cardinal signs of the disease due to the characteristic and permissive action of the thyroid hormone on the heart and arterioles. It is therefore also equally pathognomonic of constitutional hyperthyroidism and in cases where it is absent, I doubt that the patient has hyperthyroidism and therefore suspect the presence of another endocrine abnormality. From research done in my clinic on this sign in Basedow patients subjected with good results to radiotherapy or iodine, there is a relationship between the intensity of the symptom and seriousness of the morbid picture. Treatment of this syndrome with radiotherapy or other treatments causes the systolic and diastolic pressures to approach those found in normal subjects. This confirms that it is a true thyrogenic effect on the arterial pressure [34, p. 312].

Pende found in his series that this sign occurred in 95% of patients with hyperthyroidism and was absent in patients with atherosclerosis, nephrosclerosis, or heart failure in whom the diastolic blood pressure is already elevated [34]. He believed that this sign was useful in determining the severity of the clinical syndrome and response to treatment. Thus, Pende sign refers to the presence of a marked elevation in pulse pressure in patients with thyrotoxicosis (Table 4.1).

Wood and Selzer Sign

Paul Hamilton Wood (1907–1962) was born in Conoor, India and graduated from medical school at Melbourne University in 1931 [35–38]. He completed a resident post at Christchurch General Hospital, New Zealand. In London, England he served as a house physician at Brompton Hospital (Hospital for Consumption and Diseases of the Chest) in 1933 and resident medical outpatient officer at the National Heart Hospital in 1934 [35, 38, 39]. Wood, under the aegis of Sir Francis Richard Fraser (1885–1964), served as one of the first assistants in the department of medicine and joined the staff of the newly established British Postgraduate Medical School at the

University of London at Hammersmith Hospital in 1935 [35–38]. In 1937, he served as a consulting physician for outpatients at the National Heart Hospital followed by a consulting physician position at Hammersmith Hospital and later the British Post-Graduate Medical School in 1941. In the prior year, he was appointed Fellow of the Royal College of Physicians, London [36].

During World War II, he was promoted to the local rank of brigadier in 1945 and recipient of the Officer of the Order of the British Empire award. After World War II, he returned to Hammersmith Hospital as a Physician and Senior Lecturer and in 1947 was appointed first Dean of the Institute of Cardiology. In 1948, he was Physician-in-Charge of the Cardiology Department and Lecturer at Brompton Hospital [36, 39]. He was appointed the first Director of Postgraduate Institute of Cardiology affiliated with the National Heart Hospital in 1949 [36, 38, 39]. The Institute of Cardiology along with the Institute of Diseases of the Chest served as the research arms of the British Postgraduate Medical Foundation (BPMF) of the University of London. These two institutes merged and were renamed the Cardiothoracic Institute in 1972 and The National Heart and Lung Institute in 1988 [40].

In 1950, he published his book *Diseases of the Heart and Circulation* [35]. He was a honorary member of the Swiss Society of Cardiology [36]. As a description of his character:

> His alluring teaching, the colorful style of his writings and lessons, and his tireless eagerness to pursue unresolved problems in the specialty made him an unmatched leader. Responding with constant benevolence to calls from societies or universities to teach, he roamed the world tirelessly. (…) In spite of his health, he was thus one of the most brilliant messengers of contemporary medical science, and a servant worthy of a grand country. (…) A number of young Swiss physicians have had the privilege of attending Brompton Hospital or the National Heart Hospital. They acquired in contact with this extraordinary clinician, Wood ideas and principles that will mark them throughout their career [36, p. 19]. Good physicians who are also good teachers and able research workers are difficult to find. Wood was eminent in all these fields. He was one of those rare people who have an original mind and yet value established views until there is evidence that calls for their revision. (…) He was a superb clinician who liked and understood his patients, and a sound, and sometimes brilliant, diagnosis was only the start for he meant to do everything possible for them. (…) His manner with patients was intense and direct with an appeal to their intelligence, so that the intelligent were captivated and the more simple gladly accepted his clear explanations. His world-wide fame as a consultant grew each year because apart from his ability and his reputation he had a sensitive concern for every patient in his care. (…) As a teacher, he was outstanding and his methods always excited lively comment among his registrars and post-graduate students. A history was more exciting and rational with him as interpreter. His acute observation, his sensitive palpation, and his careful auscultation gave him more signs than most others could detect [38, p. 664].

His life-time achievements can be summarized as one who was a clinical cardiologist and teacher with extraordinary talent and command of the cardiovascular physical examination. He was gifted with the ability to masterfully correlate data found during cardiac catheterization to bedside physical examination findings and diagnosis [38].

Arthur Selzer (1911–1991) was born in Poland and received his medical degree from Uniwersytet Jana kazimierzs Wydzial Lekarski, Lvov, Poland in 1935 [41, 42].

He served with Paul Wood (1907–1962) at the Postgraduate Medical School and at the Hammersmith Hospital from 1936 to 1938 [42]. In 1959, he developed the Division of Cardiology and Cardiology Fellowship Program at Stanford Hospital [43]. That same year he was the founder and served on the Board of Directors for the newly established San Francisco Institute of Medical Science and in 1961 was appointed to the Research Committee at this institute [43]. He published the book *The Heart: Its Function in Health and Disease* in 1966, *Principles of Clinical Cardiology: An Analytical Approach* in 1974, and *Understanding Heart Disease* posthumously in 1992. In 1971, he was Clinical Professor of Medicine at the University of California San Francisco [44]. Selzer served as Governor of the American College of Cardiology Northern California region from 1971 to 1974, Member of the California Academy of Medicine and President from 1972 to 1973, Fellow of the American College of Cardiology in 1983, and Master of the American College of Physicians [44, 45].

Wood and Selzer described a preliminary electrocardiographic finding identified in patients with left ventricular failure secondary to hypertensive heart disease and of aortic insufficiency, "The P wave is widened and of low voltage; it is also usually bifid or flat-topped" [46]. They believed that the wide bifid P wave found in this condition was due to increased stress on the left atrium [46] (Table 4.1).

Salus Sign

Robert Salus (1877–1961) was born in Pizen, Czech Republic and received his medical degree in 1902. In 1909, he habilitated in ophthalmology and beginning in 1916 served as Professor of Ophthalmology at the German Karl Ferdinand University, Prague [47, 48]. Salus described the "nicking sign" or deviation of the retinal vein in cases of atherosclerosis or hypertension:

> Only nicking of the vein or a change of its course in addition to its apparent interruption by the crossing artery is definite proof of an involvement of the vessel wall. In such an event, it is not the obscuring of the vein but the change in the course or the indentation of the vein (frequently a sign present even in early forms of arteriosclerosis and to be discussed later) that permits one to make a positive diagnosis [49, p. 85]. (…) In the nicking sign, the vein is slightly indented by the crossing artery which causes the "nicking" or even a very small arch that just corresponds to the width of the crossing artery. In other instances, the vein deviates in a more or less obtuse angle as in an attempt to shun the crossing artery [49, p. 86].

Thus, Salus sign is a retinal venous finding found in patients with atherosclerosis and hypertension characterized by an indentation or deflection (nicking) of the retinal vein by the crossing of the retinal arteriole (arteriovenous crossing) (Table 4.1, Fig. 4.2).

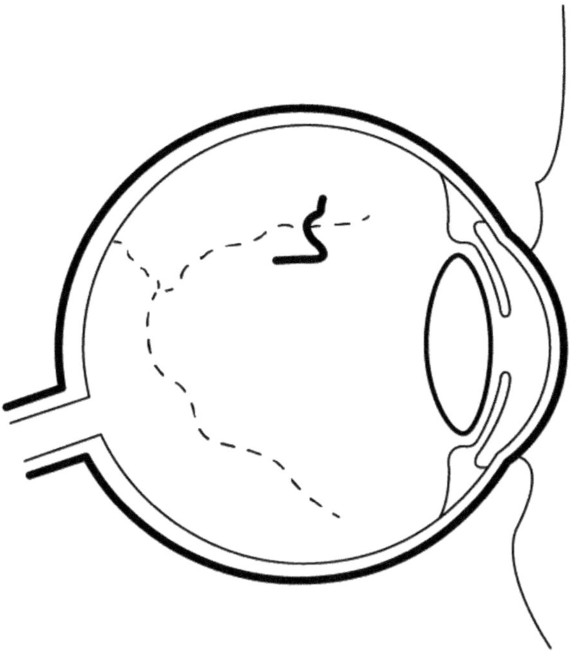

Fig. 4.2 Salus sign (by Ryan Yale)

Cunningham Vasopressor Sign of Potential Hypertension

Robert Sydney Cunningham (1891–1963) was born in Anderson South Carolina and received his medical degree from the Johns Hopkins University School of Medicine in 1915 [50–52]. After graduation, he served as an instructor and in 1922 was appointed Associate Professor of Anatomy at Johns Hopkins Medical Center. He was appointment First Lieutenant Medical Reserve Corps from 1917 to 1919 [53, 54]. He chaired the Department of Anatomy at Vanderbilt University Medical School from 1925 to 1937 and served as Dean of the Albany Medical School, Albany NY, beginning in 1937. At the time of his publication titled "Difference in blood pressure values determined by inflating and deflating the cuff of the sphygmomanometer" in 1946, Cunningham was Captain in the Marine Corps of the United States [55]. Later he received an appointment as visiting Professor of Histology at the University of Virginia, Richmond. Among his other accomplishments, he was a member of the American Association of Anatomists, American

Physiology Society, and Richmond Medical Academy [54]. Cunningham described a method using a sphygmomanometer to determine whether a patient has hypertension. The procedure involved:

> In making measurements of the blood pressure care was observed in placing the sphygmomanometer cuff on the left arm smoothly and in such a way that pressure would not force the lower edge of the cuff against the stethoscope so that noise would not be produced. The cuff was inflated slowly until first sound (diastolic reading) was audible. It was then inflated more rapidly but smoothly, until the sounds disappeared (systolic reading). After raising the mercury column 30 to 40 mm. higher, the pressure was then determined in the usual manner with the mercury falling. Thus, the first sound to appear when the cuff was inflated corresponded to the last sound when it was deflated, and the last sound during inflation corresponded to the first sound on deflation [55, p. 220].

In patients with hypertension he found:

> [t]hat the systolic peak seemed to follow the cuff pressure. That is, the sounds might disappear at a certain level during inflation of the cuff, only to return if the inflation were stopped at that level; the sound might disappear on further inflation and reappear at a higher level until a maximum point was reached beyond which there was no further rise [55, p. 221].

As summarized by Robertson, "If the systolic reading on falling is 20 millimeter or more higher than on rising, the patient is believed to be a candidate for hypertension" Cunningham believed that this, "[a]pparent response is the result of a stimulus from the vascular autonomic system reflexly affecting the cardiac and vascular tone and that the type and degree of response depends upon which fibers are hyperirritable at the time" [55, p. 222] (Table 4.1).

Bonnet Sign

Paul Bonnet (1884–1959) was born in Lyon, France and served as *externe* and *interne* des Hôpitaux Lyon in 1903 and 1906 respectively [56, 57]. He was chief of Professor Mathieu Jaboulay's (1860–1913) clinic in 1910 and was assistant to Professor Léon Tixier (1877–1976) in 1914. For his extraordinary duty during World War I he was the recipient of the Légion d'honneur and Croix de Guerre [56, 57]. He was surgical agrégé in 1920, hospital surgeon from 1924 to 1932, and appointed by the Faculty of Medicine upon the retirement of Professor Étienne Rollet (1862–1937) as Professor of the Ophthalmology Clinic of l'Hôtel-Dieu de Lyon [56, 57]. In 1952 he published his book *Ophtalmologie Clinique* (Clinical Ophthalmology) designed for ophthalmology students [58]. As a description of his character as described by Louis Paufique:

> First, he had the qualities of a first-rate teacher. Being very interested in trainees, he taught them the essentials of the specialty, by quickly drawing on the blackboard the necessary diagrams, as a method to display the answers to each question in clear and precise language [56, p. 78]. (…) But the most extraordinary aspect was to see this surgeon advancing in

> medicine, becoming much more interested in the medical rather than the surgical aspects of Ophthalmology, driven by his curiosity towards general pathology, and captivated by the precision of his examinations with the ophthalmoscope or with the flashlight. Numerous publications made by him or in collaboration with his students showed the interest he brought in these studies, the real erudition he had acquired, and the quality of his observations [56, p. 78–79].

Bonnet described a retinal finding identified on fundoscopic examination:

> [t]he sign of prethrombosis is evidence for adjacent arteriosclerosis. In a hypertensive patient with arteriosclerosis observed over a period of more than 15 years, our attention was one day attracted by a sign observed at a distance from the papilla. A collateral vein when approaching the superior temporal artery was stopped at the crossing of a branch of the superficial temporal artery. We see the vein upstream of the crossing dilated, inflated, and abutting, like the "head of a snake" against the arterial wall… (…) This sign is nonetheless indicative that the artery, in the vicinity of the crossing, is sclerotic. (…) The sign of prethrombosis therefore has a real semiological value. It most properly belongs to a form of slowly evolving arteriosclerosis-related hypertension, which for years and even decades may be observed by ophthalmoscopic observation [59, p. 33–34].

Thus, Bonnet sign refers to the presence of "banking" or dilation of the retinal veins distal to the arteriovenous crossing in patients with atherosclerosis caused by hypertension (Table 4.1, Fig. 4.3).

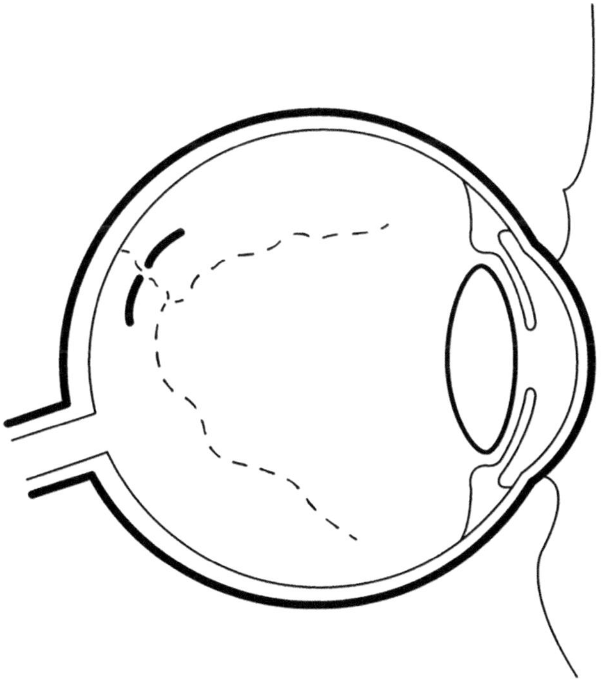

Fig. 4.3 Bonnet sign (by Ryan Yale)

Conclusion

Hypertension is one of several traditional risk factors contributing to the development of cardiovascular and atherosclerotic disease. Early recognition is important in order to prevent cardiovascular complications. The ophthalmoscopic examination provides a fundoscopic image of the retinal vessels in patients with uncontrolled hypertension and atherosclerosis. The bedside clinical diagnosis of hypertension is supported based on the appearance of the retinal arteries and veins, enumerated as signs, along with other key indicators demonstrating evidence of end-organ damage. These bedside signs along with other techniques, including echocardiography and ambulatory blood pressure monitoring, further assist in diagnosis.

References

1. Hales S. Statical Essays Containing Haemastiatics; or, An Account of Some Hydraulic and Hydrostatical Experiments Made on the Blood Vessels of Animals. 2nd ed. London: W. Innts and R. Manby; 1740.
2. Faivre J. Études expérimentales sur les lésions organiques du coeur. Gaz méd de Par. 1856;47:726–9.
3. Marey J. Recherches sur le pouls au moyen d'un appareil enregistreur le sphygmographe présenté à la Société de Biologie. Paris: E. Thunot et Cie; 1860.
4. Von Basch S. Ueber die Messung des Blutdrucks am Menschen. Ztschr f klin Med. 1881;2:79–96.
5. Riva-Rocci S. Un nuovo sfigmomanometro. Gazz med ital, Torino. 1896–97;50:981–1017.
6. Riva-Rocci S. Un nuovo sfigmomanometro. In: Lavori dei congressi di medicina interna, settimo Congresso Tenuto in Roma nell'Ottobre 1896. Roma; 1896. p. 180–1.
7. Rabinowitz LA. Blutdruckbestimmungen an unverletzten Gefässen des Menschen und der Thiere: Dissertation, Königsberg 1881. Jahresb ü d Leistungen in d Ges Med. 1881;16:203–4.
8. Hill H, Barnard H. New sphygmometers for estimating arterial pressure. J Physiol. 1898-1899;23:67–8.
9. Lewis WH. The evolution of clinical sphygmomanometry. Bull N Y Acad Med. 1941;17(11):871–81. Korotkoff NS, translator. On methods of studying blood pressure. Bull. Imperial Mil. Med. Acad. (St. Petersburg), 1905;11:365.
10. J.B.L. Obituary: Robert Marcus Gunn, M.A, M.B. Edin; F.R.C.S. Eng. Br Med J. 1909;2:1719–21.
11. Johnston AW, Johnston A, editors. Robert Marcus Gunn, M.A., M.B., C.M. Edin; F.R.C.S. Eng; senior surgeon, Royal London Ophthalmic Hospital, Moorfields, etc. In: Old-Lore Miscellany of Orkney Shetland Caithness and Sutherland, vol. 4, part 1. London: The Club; 1911. p. 102–5.
12. [No author]. Robert Marcus Gunn M.A.; M.B., C.M. (Edin.), F.R.C.S. (Eng.). Am Jour Ophth. 1910;27–28:49–51.
13. Mahmoudi Nezhad GD, Jalalpour MH, Dalfardi B. Robert Marcus Gunn (1850-1909). J Neurol. 2015;262(11):2599–600.
14. Gunn R. Ophthalmoscopic evidence of (1) arterial changes associated with chronic renal disease, and (2) of increased arterial tension. Trans Ophth Soc UK. 1892;12:124–5.
15. Santiard F. Huchard. In: Augé C, éditeur. Larousse Mensuel Illustré: Revue Encyclopédique Universelle. Tome deuxième. Paris: Librairie Larousse; 1911–1913. p. 37.

16. Ringrose H. Huchard, Dr. Henri. In: The International Who's Who: Who's Who in the World, Incorporated with the International Blue Book. Philadelphia: The Central Newspaper Union; 1910. p. 613–4.
17. [No author]. Foreign news and notes: miscellany. Philadelphia Med J. 1903;11:274.
18. [No author]. Foreign news and notes: in honor of Henri Huchard. Philadelphia Med J. 1903;11:714.
19. [No author]. Foreign news: medical news. JAMA. 1910;55:2165.
20. [No author]. Henri Huchard. Med Rec. 1911;79:448.
21. Huchard H. Traitement de la présclérose. In: Consultations médicales clinique et thérapeutique. Deuxième éd. Paris: Librairie J.-B. Baillière et fils; 1901. p. 186–200.
22. Preventing falls in hospitals. Tool 3F. Orthostatic vital sign measurements. Agency for Healthcare Research and Quality. Rockville. https://www.ahrq.gov/professionals/systems/hospital/fallpxtoolkit/fallpxtk-tool3f.html. Accessed 12 Dec 2019.
23. Betta E. Pende, Nicola. Dizionario Biografico degli Italiani. Treccani. 2015;82. http://www.treccani.it/enciclopedia/nicola-pende_(Dizionario-Biografico)/. Accessed 18 Jan 2020.
24. Nicola Pende's birthplace. Himetop. The history of medicine topographical database. http://himetop.wikidot.com/nicola-pende-s-birthplace. Accessed 22 Dec 2018.
25. [No author]. Medical news: foreign university intelligence. Lancet. 1908;1:824.
26. Nicola Pende, la via italiana al razzismo Quotidiano di Bari. 21 Aprile 2018. https://quotidianodibari.it/nicola-pende-la-via-italiana-al-razzismo/. Accessed 15 Jan 2019.
27. Strategie politiche ed esigenze scientifiche: il ruolo di Nicola Pende nell' istituzione e nell'organizzazione dell'Università di Bari. Annali di Storia delle Universita Italiane 2013;17. http://www.cisui.unibo.it/annali/17/testi/03_Dell_Era_frameset.htm. Accessed 5 Jan 2019.
28. Nicola Pende scienziato razzista. La Repubblica. 14 settembre 2006. https://ricerca.repubblica.it/repubblica/archivio/repubblica/2006/09/14/nicola-pend-scienziato-razzista.html. Accessed 15 Jan 2019.
29. Eliminare dalla toponomastica barese via Nicola Pende. ARCA Centro di iniziativa democratica. http://www.arcabari.it/2013/02/eliminare-dalla-toponomastica-barese-via-nicola-pende/. Accessed 15 Jan 2019.
30. Rome to remove race law signatories. ANSA en Politics. 22 January 2018. http://www.ansa.it/english/news/politics/2018/01/22/rome-to-remove-race-law-signatories_da4c7f1b-1743-47d9-8434-52aac7230c0c.html. Accessed 15 Jan 2019.
31. Bari cancella via Nicola Pende. La Gazetta del Mezzogiorno. 01 Febbraio 2006. https://www.lagazzettadelmezzogiorno.it/news/home/44099/bari-cancella-via-nicola-pende.html?refresh_ce. Accessed 15 Jan 2019.
32. [No author]. Award to Dr. Pende. New York Med Jour. 1920;112:197.
33. [No author]. Prize to Pende. JAMA. 1920;75:115.
34. Pende N. Sopra una triade sintomatica dell iperiroidiso costituzionale; sua importzanza diagnostic nelle ale; sua importanza diagnostic nelle forme larvate di tireotoxicosi. Endocrinol Patol Costit. 1926;1:311–2.
35. Trail RR. Paul Hamilton Wood. Lives of the fellows. Royal College of Physicians. http://munksroll.rcplondon.ac.uk/Biography/Details/4869. Accessed 10 Sep 2019.
36. P.W.D. Paul H. Wood (1907–1962). Cardiologia. 1962;2:18–9.
37. Dimond EG. The meteoric career of Paul Wood. Clin Cardiol. 1987;10:371–2.
38. Campbell M. Paul Wood. Br Heart J. 1962;24:661–5.
39. Bauer G. Wood, Paul Hamilton (1907–1962). Australian Dictionary of Biography. National Centre of Biography, Australian National University. 2002.
40. Our history and alumni. Imperial College of London. National heart and Lung Institute @ 2019 Imperial College London. https://www.imperial.ac.uk/nhli/about-us/our-history-and-alumni/. Accessed 10 Sep 2019.
41. [No author]. Obituary listing. JAMA. 1992;267:1853.
42. [No author]. News of colleagues. Br Heart J. 1993;69:96.
43. CPMCRI history. Sutter Health. https://www.sutterhealth.org/research/cpmcri/history. Accessed 10 Jan 2019.

44. [No author]. Bulletin briefs: Arthur Selzer. UC Synergy: Hospitals and Clinics News. 1971;1(4):7.
45. Arthur Selzer M.D. Distinguished Fellow Award. https://www.acc.org/~/media/Non-Clinical/Files-PDFs-Excel-MS-Word-etc/Membership/Award%20Programs/List%20of%20Distinguished%20Fellowship%20Awardees%201966%202014.pdf?la=en. Accessed 10 Jan 2019.
46. Wood P, Selzer A. A new sign of left ventricular failure. Br Heart J. 1939;49:81–5.
47. Prof. Dr. Robert Salus. Geni. https://www.geni.com/people/Prof-Dr-Robert-Salus/6000000018851778703. Accessed 30 Mar 2019.
48. Saubermann C. Necrologia: Robert Salus. Buchbesprechung. Karger; 1961. https://www.karger.com/Article/PDF/304098. Accessed 30 Mar 2019.
49. Salus R. A contribution to the diagnosis of atherosclerosis and hypertension. Am J Opthlmol. 1958;45:81–92.
50. Robert Sydney Cunningham, Geni. https://www.geni.com/people/Robert-Cunningham-MD/6000000015789306504. Accessed 20 Jun 2019.
51. [No author]. Cunningham, Robert Sydney. American Medical Directory. 1921;7:660.
52. Robert Sydney Cunningham. Medicine in Maryland, 1752–1920. https://mdhistoryonline.net/2018/06/02/md55175/amp/. Accessed 20 Jun 2019.
53. [No author]. Nominations and confirmations. Air-Navy-Air Force Register and Defense Times. 1918;65:83.
54. Robert Sydney Cunningham. Praebook. https://prabook.com/web/robert_sydney.cunningham/1113063. Accessed 20 Jun 2019.
55. Cunningham RS. Difference in blood pressure values determined by inflating and deflating the cuff of the sphygmomanometer. Am Heart J. 1946;31:220–2.
56. Paufique L. Paul Bonnet (1884–1959). Arch Ophtalmol Rev Gen Ophtalmol. 1960;20:77–80.
57. Paufique L. Paul Bonnet (1884–1959). J Med Lyon. 1960;41:1–3.
58. Bonnet P. Ophtalmologie. In: Les sources du travail bibliographique. Genève: Librairie Droz; 1958. p. 481.
59. Bonnet P. Le signe de préthrombose observé sur les vaisseaux de la rétine dans l'hypertension artérielle; sa valeur sémiologique. Arch d'Opth. 1951;11:12–34.

Chapter 5
Aortic Regurgitation Murmurs

Introduction

A multitude of cardiac and peripheral phenomena, eponymously ascribed as signs, have been described in aortic regurgitation (AR) to honor physicians' contributions to medicine. They were identified based on applying the bedside skills of observation, auscultation, palpation, maneuvers, and the sphygmomanometer. These bedside signs have diminished in use since the advent of echocardiographic and other imaging techniques of the heart. With the exception of Corrigan, Duroziez, and Hill signs, they have not been well studied and gaps remain in knowledge regarding evidence of their applicability in clinical practice. In general, for those signs which have been studied, there are a number of limitations with studies such as selection bias, inconsistent case definition and reference standard, and wide ranges of disease severities. Additionally, there is a paucity of data assessing the relationship between a sign and disease severity. Despite these shortcomings, we contend that these signs should be taught since they impart an appreciation for the keen insights applied by physicians in recognizing or eliciting them on physical examination. They also further enhance our understanding about the pathophysiology of disease and provide opportunities for further investigation. Described in this chapter is brief historical information of the person who reported the sign, its original description, and if known, its sensitivity, specificity, and validity in clinical practice. The name for the description of this pathological finding affecting the aortic valve has changed over the years and has encompassed such terms as retroversion of the valves, incompetence, insufficiency, and regurgitation. It is understood that each term is meant to describe the condition by which the aortic valves do not close tightly causing blood to flow back into the left ventricle during diastole.

S. H. Yale et al., *Cardiovascular Eponymic Signs*,
https://doi.org/10.1007/978-3-030-67596-7_5

Historical Background

The history of the aortic valve dates back to Galen of Pergamon (130–c.200 CE), who in the fifth volume of *Opera Omnia* acknowledged the work and described the views regarding the function of the membranes (valves) of the human heart as promulgated by his predecessor Erasistratus (c.304 BC–c.250 BC):

> The use of the membranes, as he thinks, is to perform for the heart contrary functions, alternating at successive intervals. Those attached to the vessels which bring in materials, when pressed from without inward, yield to the influx of the materials, and, falling into the cavities of the heart, throw open its orifices and leave an unobstructed passage for what is drawn into it. For these matters, he says, do not come in of their own impulse, as into a passive receptacle; but the heart itself, expanding like a brazier's bellows, distends itself by its diastole. The membranes attached, on the other hand, to the vessels of exit, act in the contrary way. For, turning from within outward, they yield before the efflux and open the orifices when the heart discharges its contents; while in the whole remaining intervals they exactly close the orifices, preventing any return of what has been discharged [1, p. 251].

Galen believed, unlike Erasistratus, that the valves even in their normal state allow for the backflow of blood, "The valves of the heart are a provision of nature to prevent this otherwise inevitable regurgitation, though even they are not quite efficient" [2, p. xliii–1].

Raymond Vieussens (c.1635–1715) is credited for describing one of the earliest recorded accounts of the pulse in 1695 in the disease later recognized as aortic regurgitation (AR). He published this finding in his book *Traité Nouveau de la Structure et des Causes du Mouvement naturel du Coeur* (New Treatise on the Structure and Causes of the Natural Movement of the Heart) in 1715:

> [I] examined his pulse which appeared to be full, fast, hard, unequal, and so strong that the artery of both arms struck my fingertips, similar to a tense rope when violently shacked. The pulse of this patient, whom I had never seen before, persuaded me that he was laboring from a violent palpation of the heart. I was not deceived, for having questioned him upon the fact, he told me that for a long time he had not slept comfortably because the strong beating of his heart occurred on either side or even on his back if his head were not very high. He added that when he was lying on one side or the other, and particularly on the left, it seemed as though he was being struck on his ribs with a hammer [3, p. 107].

Hence, Vieussens described the pulse in aortic insufficiency although he did not associate this finding with the diseased aortic valve.

It was William Cowper (1666–1709) who described the symptoms and pathological findings of the disease, later recognized as aortic insufficiency, in two patients with aortic valve disease in his paper titled "Of ossifications or petrifications in the coats of arteries, particularly in the valves of the great artery" published in *Philosophical Transactions* in 1705:

> The three semilunar valves of the aorta, which hinder the blood from returning to the heart, after it is expelled thence by its systole or contraction, these valves in this case were somewhat thicker, and not so pliable as naturally, and did not so adequately apply to each other, as is expressed by aaa. Fig. 14. Whence it happened sometimes, that the blood in the great artery (AAA. Fig. 1) would recoil, and interrupt the heart in its systole [4, p. 1971].

In the second case of a 40-year-old man the symptoms:

> [w]ere extraordinary, shortness of breath, especially of any fatigue, with an intermission of one stroke in three of the pulse; his posture of sitting up was more eligible than any other; he complained of great faintness and now and then pain about the heart, the extreme parts often cold, which towards his death increased more and more on him; his legs and arms being gangrened some hours before. (…) Upon opening the chest of the heart, particularly its left ventricule, was found larger than that of an ordinary ox, and filled with coagulated blood [4, p. 1972].

Cowper concluded based on the patient's symptoms and pathologic examination:

> The explication of the symptoms in both these cases is obvious enough, for though the person in the first instance did not die of the same disease with the last mentioned, yet the symptoms in his illness plainly showed what must follow, from the disorders of these valves, as they are rendered more or less useless. For as their office is to prevent the return of the blood into the heart, in its diastole, by exactly shutting up the passage of the aorta, (as the flaps in water engines) so if by any accident they are hindered from doing their duty, as they were by the petrifactions mentioned, the consequences must be, not only a regurgitation of blood into the heart, but they baulk its impulsive force, when the muscular fibres (which are in these valves) cannot contract, to prepare the passage for the blood of the left ventricle when to be expelled into the aorta. (…) In both these cases, the left ventricule of the heart was dilated proportionally to the ill constitution of these valves, which clearly shows these valves give that assistance to the heart in its orifice, that it cannot be without, and that it gradually suffers according to their indisposition [4, p. 1973].

Hence, the term *cor bovinum* is attributed to Cowper's description of the heart in patients with aortic insufficiency as likened to the phrase "larger than of an ordinary ox."

It was René-Joseph-Hyacinthe Bertin (1757–1828) who recognized as early as 1824 the function of the aortic and pulmonary valves, "both are arranged as to oppose a sufficient obstacle to the retrograde flow of the blood in the ventricule" [5, p. xxi]. Thomas Hodgkin (1798–1866), who was made aware of this condition by Charles Aston Key, another physician working at Guy Hospital in London, made the first most accurate description of the disease later referred to as aortic insufficiency. Hodgkin read two letters to the Hunterian Society, written to Dr. Key titled, "On retroversion of the valves of the aorta." The first one was on February 21, 1827, and the second on February 18, 1829. In the first letter he wrote, "My Dear Friend, Thou wilt probably recollect having pointed out to me, a few months ago, a particular state of the valves of the aorta, which, by admitting of their falling back towards the ventricle, unfits them for the performance of their function." [6, p. 433]. Hodgkin coined the term "retroversion of the valves" to describe this condition, "To avoid circumlocution, and in defect of a better name, I shall designate by the term retroversion of the valves that disease state which allows of their dropping in towards the ventricle, instead of effectually closing the vessel against a reflux of blood." [6, p. 433]. In both letters, he described seven patients with this condition and enumerated several important pathologic aspects of retroversion of the valves. In the second letter he described symptoms seen in the case of a 28-year-old physician:

> Besides the general and inordinately violent arterial action, which was very rapid and frequent, though perfectly regular, there was a remarkable thrill in the pulse, and the carotids were seen violently beating on both sides. The contractions of the ventricles were marked by strong impulse, and a constant *bruit de scie*. Which presented this peculiarity, that it as double, attending the systole as well as the diastole, but not exciting the idea of being at all connected with the auricles [6, p. 438].

Austin Flint's contributions in the areas of physical diagnosis and diseases of the heart are considered invaluable to the field of cardiology and study of cardiac murmurs. His other, not widely known but most noteworthy contribution was related to the pitch of the percussion note or respiratory sounds [7, 8]. Flint identified two cases where an auscultatory mitral diastolic murmur was found in association with aortic regurgitant murmur. This finding was eponymously named in his honor as the Austin Flint murmur. He further explained this phenomenon:

> The murmur is often rough than soft. The roughness is often peculiar. It is a blubbering sound, resembling that produced by throwing the lips or the tongue into vibration of the lips or tongue by the breath in expiration. I suppose that the murmur is caused, in these cases, by the vibration of the mitral curtains, and that the vibrations of the lips or tongue by the breath represents the mechanism of the murmur as well as imitates the characteristics of the sound [9, p. 50]. (…) Now in cases of considerable aortic insufficiency, the left ventricle is rapidly filled with blood flowing back from the aorta as well as from the auricle, before the auricular contraction takes place. The distension of the ventricle is such that the mitral curtains are brought into coaptation, and when the auricular contraction takes place the mitral direct current passing between the curtains throws them into vibration and gives rise to the characteristic blubbering murmur. The physical condition is in effect analogous to contraction of the mitral orifice from an adhesion of the curtains at their sides, the latter condition, as clinical observation abundantly proves, giving rise to a mitral direct murmur of a similar character [9, p. 53].

A wide variety of extracardiac phenomena have been eponymously named after physicians who identified findings occurring in association with aortic regurgitation. These physicians applied the physical examination skills of observation, palpation, auscultation, and other maneuvers to identify and describe these signs. The signs are described chronologically based on the year they were reported. In this review, the term aortic regurgitation and aortic insufficiency are used interchangeably.

Signs

Cuming Sign

Thomas Cuming (1798–1887) was born in Armagh, Northern Ireland, United Kingdom, and received his medical degree from the University of Edinburgh in 1819 [10]. He was appointed physician to the Wellesley Fever Hospital, Dublin, Ireland, and also served as assistant physician and lecturer at the Pitt Street Institute for the Diseases of Children [10]. In 1829, he practiced medicine in Armagh where his notoriety became well recognized through his work in treating epidemic fever, cholera, and consumption (tuberculosis) in children [10]. In 1857, he was appointed Fellow of the King and Queen's College of Physicians and bestowed the degree of MD from the University of Dublin [10].

He also served for 37 years as visiting physician to the Armagh District Lunatic Asylum [10]. As described of his character:

> No doubt one so well and widely known and loved will long live in the affections of many whom his skill has relieved and his friendship aided; but even those whom his skills has relieved and his friendship sided; but even those who most loved him, however they may deplore his loss, can scarcely regret his passage into rest after so long and active a career of usefulness and beneficence. Of Thomas Cuming may be said, in the full sense of the words, that he died full of years and honours [10, p. 653].

Thomas Cuming described the clinical and autopsy findings in his paper entitled, "A case of diseased heart with observations" published in the *Dublin Hospital Reports* in 1822, involving an 88-year-old man with incompetency of the aortic valve:

> Although the shriveled and contracted state of the aortic valve prevented them from completely closing the ventriculo-aortic aperture, and they allowed a reflux of blood from the artery into the ventricle, there was no diminution of the aortic aperture itself, and therefore a full stream of blood was thrown into the artery at each stroke of the ventricle; whence arose the full, hard, and vibrating pulse, which, conjoined with the violence of the pulsation in the region of the heart, led me to suspect an active, rather than passive enlargement of the ventricle [11, p. 330].

Cuming sign thus refers to the presence of the full, hard (pounding), and vibratory pulse in patients with aortic insufficiency [12]. Cuming report is noteworthy in his ability to correlate pathologic findings with clinical symptoms and relate these to the proposed pathogenesis of the disease [13] (Table 5.1).

Corrigan Sign (Pulse)

Sir Dominic John Corrigan (1802–1880) was born in Dublin, Ireland, studied medicine in Dublin and Edinburgh, and received his medical degree from the University of Edinburgh in 1825 [14]. He served as a physician at Meath Dispensary, Cork-Street Fever and Charitable Infirmary Hospital (also known as Jervis Street Hospital), Dublin, from 1830 to 1840. He was appointed to the House of Industry Hospitals (The Richmond Hospital, Whitworth Medical Hospital, and Hardwicke Fever Hospital) from 1840 to 1866 [14–16]. In his teaching positions as Professor of Medicine, he taught at Diggs Street School, Peter Street School, and Carmichael College of Medicine (formerly Richmond Hospital) [14, 17]. As commissioner for national education and an elected Member of Parliament for the city of Dublin from 1870 to 1874, he devoted his attention to and was an ardent supporter and voice for Catholic education [15, 18]. In 1871, he was appointed Vice-Chancellor of the Senate of the Queen's University [14]. He was appointed Physician-in-Ordinary to Queen Victoria, Ireland, in 1874 and named Baronet of the Empire in 1866 [15,

Table 5.1 Signs of aortic regurgitation

Name	Year	Description of sign	Method
Cuming [11]	1822	Full, hard (pounding) and vibratory pulse.	Palpation
Corrigan [22]	1832	*Visible* pulsation of the arteries of the neck and superior extremities.	Inspection
Watson [30]	1844	Jerky or shock-like impulse felt at the elbow, femoral, and carotid arteries.	Palpation
Duroziez [36]	1861	There are two ways to produce the double soft blowing sound-with the stethoscope or hand. (1) *Stethoscope*: Gradually press the stethoscope obliterating its surface. There is a moment when the double soft blowing sound occurs. (2) *Hand*: Place the stethoscope on the artery without pressing it. Then press using the hand sequentially, first proximal and second distal to the instrument. Proximal pressure will produce the first soft blowing sound and distal pressure will produce the second soft blowing sound.	Stethoscope Palpation
Traube [41]	1867	Faint double sound auscultated over the femoral artery.	Auscultation
Quincke [51]	1868	At the border between the white and a red nail bed, one observes a forward and backward movement synchronized with the heartbeat. In warm external air, the nails are uniformly reddened. Under these circumstances in order to create a lighter zone on the nail, either apply a naturally uniform pressure or hold the hand in the air.	Inspection
Becker [53]	1872	On ophthalmoscopic examination, fundic retinal vessels show spontaneous arterial pulsation. The degree of visibility of the retinal pulsation is seen more clearly if the patient walks up and down stairs quickly or consumes alcohol.	Inspection
De Musset [55]	1877	With every pulse there is a slight involuntary toss of the head that can be stopped by pressing the nape of the neck with the thumb and forefinger.	Inspection
Rosenbach [61]	1878	Pulsation of the liver during systole.	Palpation
Gerhardt [68]	1882	Pulsation of the spleen during systole.	Palpation
Müller [74]	1889	The red tonsils and anterior and posterior palatal arches move medially, synchronously with each carotid pulse. On the soft palate, a pulsation is seen with the free edge of the uvula moving downwards. Each pulsation causes narrowing of the palate opening caused by the contractions of the palatal arches, tonsils, soft palate, and the uvula. At the same time, a rhythmic increase in the intensity of the redness of the palate is observed.	Inspection
Hill [81]	1909	Marked difference in systolic blood pressure between the arms and legs in the recumbent position.	Sphygmomanometer

Table 5.1 (continued)

Name	Year	Description of sign	Method
Landolfi [84]	1909	Passive rhythmic movement of narrowing and dilatation of the pupil, independent of the ambient light. The changes of the iris are synchronous to the movements of the heart. Narrowing of the pupil corresponds to ventricular systole and dilatation to ventricular diastole. This phenomenon is accentuated by having the subject stand, administering digitalis, or compressing the femoral or abdominal aorta. It is less obvious when the patient is lying down or kept at prolonged rest, consumption of bromides, or inhale nitrite.	Inspection
Minervini [86]	1910	The patient is examined in a sitting position with the head slightly turned back and mouth open. Careful inspection of the oral cavity reveals that there is a movement of the tongue from bottom to top, rhythmic and synchronous to the heartbeat. This movement is best seen when the tongue rests on the floor of the mouth than when it is pulled out of the mouth. With a tongue depressor apply moderate pressure to the tongue. The tongue depressor always lifts upwards by rhythmic jolts.	Inspection
Sailer [88]	1928	Splenic pulsation seen in cases of aortic insufficiency and bacterial endocarditis.	Palpation
Palfrey [92]	1952	The examiner raises the arm vertically above the heart and auscultates over the volar aspect of radial artery. If no arterial tone is heard aortic insufficiency is not severe and may be only mild. If the tone is heard over the elevated wrist, a diastolic blood pressure of about 45 by mercurial manometer. With the arm still elevated, move the stethoscope gradually proximally until at some point the tone suddenly disappears. The lower this point, the less the diastolic pressure. If the tone is present as low as the elbow the diastolic pressure is approximately 30 mmHg.	Maneuver
Mayne [95]	1953	The blood pressure is taken with the arm elevated. In this position in otherwise healthy individuals, the diastolic blood pressure is 10 mmHg lower when the arm is in a vertical compared to horizontal position. In patients with aortic insufficiency the values exceed 15 mmHg.	Sphygmomanometer
Dennison/Shelley [98]	1958	Pulsatility of the cervix.	Inspection
Harvey [103]	1963	Diastolic murmur heard best along the right compared to the left sternal border.	Auscultation
Penny [107]	1988	Pulsating wheal on the cheek containing a blanched center and surround ring of erythema.	Inspection
Morton and Mahon [108]	2002	Facial flushing or "flashing" occurring during the upstroke and downstroke of the arterial wave. Facial flush is most pronounced with the patient in the sitting position at an approximately 45 degree angle.	Inspection
Sherman [111]	2004	Dorsalis pedis pulse associated with a prominent and rapid arterial upstroke.	Palpation
Ashrafian [113]	2008	Subtle rhythmic anterior propulsion of the eyes occurring with systole.	Inspection

18–20]. Among Corrigan's other noteworthy accomplishments, he received the honorary degree of Doctor in Medicine from the University of Dublin in 1849, Honorary Fellowship from the Royal College of Physicians of Ireland in 1856 and served as President to the Royal College of Physician, Ireland for five consecutive terms between 1859 and 1864 [16, 18, 19]. Corrigan was one of the founders of the Dublin Pathological Society in 1838, later served as its President. He was a member of the Royal College of Surgeons, London, in 1843 and in 1849 was the recipient of the honorary degree, Doctor of Medicine, from the University of Dublin [14]. From 1858 to 1863 he served as President of King's and Queen's College of Physicians [21]. In recognition of his contribution to medicine and government he was anointed baronet in 1866 [14]. In 1875, he was elected as the first president of the Pharmaceutical Society of Ireland [14]. His notoriety was well-recognizing and in this capacity he served as President of the Royal Irish Academy and Zoological Society in Ireland, Harverian Society in London, and Academy of Medicine, Paris [20].

His obituary provides a glimpse of the legacy of his life's work, contribution to medicine, and tribute to his accomplishments, "We can scarcely praise too highly a man who could show such discernment, and who could add to such scientific and professional labours work as a public-spirited citizen and statesman which makes his death to be lamented as a national loss." [16, p. 269]. In an address delivered to medical students during distribution of prizes to students at St. Mary's Hospital, Corrigan spoke of his view of the medical profession

> I should tire you were I to enumerate the numerous and vices my kind friends pressed on me as to the best way of getting on. I listened to all, and I must confess that I was at first inclined to grow sad and to regret I had entered a profession which, up to that time, presented to my young dream glorious eminences to be attained by battling forward under the flag "Excelsior." But, as I was beginning to despair, there was a little book published, *The Lives of British Physicians*, extending from Linacre in 1410, to Gooch's death in 1830, a period of about 400 years. If my young friends have not perused the book I would advise those who are ambitious of eminence to read it, and I think they will come to the same conclusion to which I was led from its perusal, that there is but one road to excellence and success in our profession, and that is by steady study and hard labour; and you will at least always have this consolation in your dreariest hour of labour, that "no proud man's contumely," no "insolence of office" nor "spurns that patient merit of the unworthy takes" can bar your way [19, p. 410].

Corrigan described three signs, in his paper entitled "On permanent patency of the mouth of the aorta, or inadequacy of the aortic valves" published in *Edinburgh Medical and Surgical Journal* in 1832, the first of which referred to the *visible* pulsation that bears his namesake (Table 5.1):

> 1st, Visible pulsation of the arteries of the head and superior extremities. 2nd, *Bruit de soufflet* in the ascending aorta, in the carotids, and subclavians. 3rd, *Bruit de soufflet* and *fremissement*, or a peculiar rushing thrill felt by the finger, in the carotids and subclavians. In conjunction with these may be reckoned the pulse, which is invariably full. When a patient affected by the disease is tripped, the arterial trunks of the head, neck and superior extremities immediately catch the eye by their singular pulsation. At each diastole the subclavian, carotid, temporal, brachial, and in some cases even the palmar arteries, are suddenly thrown from their bed, bounding up under the skin. (…) From its singular and striking appearance, the name of visible pulsation is given to this beating of the arteries. It is accompanied with *bruit de soufflet* in the ascending aorta, carotids, and subclavians; and in the carotids and subclavian, where they can be examined by the finger, there is felt *fremissement*, or the peculiar rushing thrill, accompanying with *bruit de soufflet* each diastole of these vessels. These three signs are so intimately connected with the pathological cause of the disease, and arise so directly from the mechanical inadequacy of the valves, that they afford unerring indications of the nature of the disease [22, p. 227–228].

He was the first to account for the pathophysiology of the *visible* pulsation of the arteries in the neck and upper extremity in patients with aortic insufficiency:

> [T]he ascending aorta and arteries arising from it, pouring back a portion of their blood, become, after each contraction of the ventricle, flaccid or lessened in their diameter. While they are in this state, the ventricle again contracts and impels quickly into these vessels a quantity of blood which suddenly and greatly dilates them. The *diastole* of these vessels is thus marked by so sudden and so great an increase of size as to present the visible pulsation which constitutes one of the signs of the disease [22, p. 228].

It is of historic interest that Corrigan also reported the effects related to the appearance of the pulsation caused by change in arm and leg position:

> [i]ncrease the pulsation of the brachial and palmar arteries in a most striking degree by merely elevating his arms to a perpendicular position above his head. He thus enabled the brachial and palmar arteries to empty themselves more easily back upon the aorta. They became more flaccid, and then, on the next contraction of the ventricle, their diastole became comparatively greater, and their visible pulsation of course more marked. The same effect could be produced in the arteries of the lower extremities by lying down and elevating the legs on an inclined plane [22, p. 229].

Armand Trousseau imparted the name *Maladie de Corrigan* (Corrigan's disease) in recognition of Corrigan's description of this disease [16]. It is important to note that it was Thomas Watson of London in 1843 who described the *palpable* "water-hammer" pulse of aortic insufficiency (see Watson sign). What Corrigan observed in 1823 was the *visible* pulsation of the neck and upper extremities in aortic insufficiency.

It is noteworthy that James Hope in his book, *A Treatise on Diseases of the Heart and Great Vessels* published in 1831, most thoroughly described the *palpable* pulse in aortic insufficiency:

> Aortic regurgitation produces a pre-eminently *jerking* pulse, a high degree of the pulse of unfilled arteries as seen in anemia from any cause. The diastole or beat of the artery is short and quick, as if the blood were smartly jerked or shot under the finger, the vessel during the intervals feeling unusually empty. This is the most remarkable, appreciable, and constant pulse produced by the disease of the heart. In the immense majority of cases, the practitioner may conjecture the disease by this sign alone. It differs from the jerking pulse of anemia, in being more marked, and in not necessarily being frequent, as the anaemic pulse is, when its jerk is distinct. It may be absent, or scarcely appreciable, if the regurgitation be very slight; and it may be neutralized by free mitral regurgitation (Payne) or great contraction, in consequence of the enfeebling effect of these legions on the pulse [23].

Hope in his third edition to this book wrote in a footnote regarding Corrigan's writings on the pulse:

> I described this pulse (which had not previously been noticed by a writer on diseases of the heart) in several parts of the first edition of the present work in 1831. Dr. Corrigan, who wrote in 1832 or 1833 on permanent patency of the aortic valves as supposed new disease, has so completely overlooked this pulse as even to state the reverse: "it rises without any jerk under the finger" (Dublin Jour. vol. x. p. 186) [23].

As previously noted, Vieussen in 1715 first described the palpable pulse found in aortic insufficiency although he did not associate it with the diseased aortic valve [3]. Additionally, Cuming in 1822 correlates and attributed the characteristics of the palpable pulse to the symptoms of aortic valve disease.

A systematic review conducted by Babu et al. assessed five studies (1908–2001) that evaluated the Corrigan pulse. Each study included more than 10 adults with chronic AR and variable degrees of disease severity. Based on the case definition used in these studies, the sign was erroneously defined as a "palpable pulse which increases when the wrist is elevated." Despite limitations in study design including case definition, selection bias (lack of controls), inconsistent or non-reported disease severities (mild, moderate, severe) and diagnostic reference standard, a sensitivity of 38–95% was found with a single study reporting a specificity of 16%. These findings suggest that this maneuver, erroneously named Corrigan pulse, lacked sufficient sensitivity and specificity to be useful in clinical practice [24].

Watson Sign

Sir Thomas Watson (1792–1882) was born in Kentisbeare, Devonshire, England, and received his medical training at St. Bartholomew's Hospital and the Universities of Edinburgh and Cambridge, the latter is where he received his medical degree in 1825 [25–28]. He was elected Fellow of the Royal College of Physicians (FRCP) London in 1826, and from 1827 to 1843 served as physician to the Middlesex Hospital [25, 27]. At King's College he was appointed Professor of Forensic Medicine from 1831 to 1836, followed by a Professorship of the Principles and Practice of Medicine. He was appointed Chair of Clinical Medicine at the University of London (University College) for 1 year followed by a transition with this same title to King's Hospital, one which he served from 1836 to 1840 [29]. In 1859, he was appointed Physician Extraordinary to the Queen and Baronet in 1866, and Physician in Ordinary to the Queen in 1870 [27]. In the Royal College of Physicians, he held numerous positions including Censor (1828, 1837, 1838), Council (multiple times between 1833 and 1868), Representative of the College in the General Council of Medical Education (1858), and President (1862–1867) [27, 29]. He received numerous other accolades and honorary titles including doctor of law and civil law from Cambridge and Oxford respectively and fellow at St. John's College and King and Queen's College of Physicians, Ireland [28]. As described of his character:

> His sense of justice, his habitual reference of all questions of detail to unassailable principle, his flexibility of mind, and his quick perception of character, gave him a rare but well-justified ascendancy over even his ablest of his contemporaries; and while Sir Thomas Watson practiced his profession he was, during a long period, recognized without dispute as its leader [25].

As written by Charles West, a colleague at the College of Physicians:

> [H]is moral as well as his intellectual qualities had much to do with the estimate which all formed of his character. His faculties were remarkably well balanced, his mind was eminently fair. He had that gift-the attribute and the reward of truth-the power intuitively to detect all specious error. (…) The courteous consideration with which he treated his juniors, the pains he took in investigating the case, the endeavor to conceal an error without sacrificing the interests of the patient, were qualities which no younger man who met him in combination could ever forget [29, p. 736].

Watson in 1844 likened the pulse of aortic insufficiency to a toy:

> The pulse of aortic regurgitation is very striking and peculiar: sudden, like the blow of a hammer, without any prolonged swell of the artery. It always reminds me of the well-known chemical toy, formed by including a small quantity of liquid in a glass tube, exhausted of air, and hermetically sealed. On reversing the tube, the liquid falls from one end of it to the other with hard short knock, as if it were a mass of lead. The sensation given to the fingers by the pulse, when there is much regurgitation through the aortic valves, is very similar to this. It is as if successive balls of blood were suddenly shot along under the finger [30, p. 603].

He described the location of the "water hammer" pulse in a patient with aortic insufficiency:

> The shock of this man's artery was plainly to be felt, through his clothes, by one's hand laid lightly upon the bend of his arm. His wife told me that, for five years past, this jarring blow had made it uncomfortable for her to take his arm when they were walking together. This same kind of jerking impulse was strikingly perceptible in the femoral arteries and in the carotids [30, p. 603].

Another method for eliciting this sign described by other authors involves the examiner raising the arm at the wrist above the head while the patient is reclined. Using the opposite hand, the examiner grasps the flexor aspect of the forearm, feeling for a tapping impulse or shock over the thenar eminence [31]. Thus, raising the patient's arm above the level of the heart intensifies the radial pulse at the forearm [32] (Table 5.1).

Duroziez Sign

Paul Louis Duroziez (1826–1897) was born in Paris, and received his medical degree from the Faculty of Medicine in Paris in 1853 [33, 34]. Notably, he completed an externship under Jean-Baptiste Bouillaud (1796–1881) from 1849 to 1850 at the Charité, Paris, and from 1856 to 1858 served as Clinical Chief at the Charité in Bouillaud's service [33]. In 1870 during the Franco-Prussian War, he was as an ambulance physician and surgeon major of the 14th Infantry Battalion for the French army [33]. In the First Ward of Paris, he served as member of the Commission of Public Hygiene in 1879 and in 1889 as medical inspector of the schools [35]. He was elected President of the French Society of Medicine in 1882 and in 1895 received the Légion d'honneur, France [34, 35].

He recognized that it was in fact Bouillaud, who in 1841 identified an "intermittent double soft blowing sound in the femoral artery in difficult and complicated cases of aortic insufficiency. It is a pathognomonic sign of this condition" [36, p. 417]. Duroziez noted that the production of the abnormal second murmur (systolic sound) is infrequently seen in the arteries of the lower extremity due to the relative absence of reflux of blood [36] (Table 5.1):

> [n]o one, I believe, has given it the importance that it deserves. Everyone has spoken of the soft blowing sound occurring in arterial diastole, which quite often exists without compression of the artery. Very few authors have spoken of the soft blowing sound during systole. Most often it does not exist by itself as it needs to be sought and brought out. The first soft blowing sound occurs as a result of the powerful force of ventricular contraction while the second soft blowing sound is produced by the systole of the arteries in the legs, a much smaller force which needs help, and this aided by compression of the artery. (…) [w]hat commonly occurs is that when aortic insufficiency is found in association with aortic or mitral stenosis, the arteries are moderately dilated with blood and it is difficult to hear the second heart murmur. Although we pay great attention to this finding, it still does not appear regularly. It will not be found when weak pulsations are present. The murmur appears or disappears depending upon the force of the heartbeat. Sometimes it can be heard in both femoral arteries and other times in only one. To summarize, in order for the distension and recoil to appear, a sufficient systole of the arteries is required. A careful examination is essential [36, p. 426–427].

He described the method by applying upstream (proximal) and downstream (distal) pressure for eliciting the double murmur over the femoral artery:

> There are two ways to produce this double soft blowing sound, with the stethoscope or hand. Gradually press the stethoscope until the artery is obliterate. There is a moment when the double soft blowing sound appears. If the second soft blowing sound easily occurs, we can simply put the stethoscope on the artery without pressure. Then press the hand successively above and below the stethoscope. Pressure above produces the first soft blowing sound, while pressure below produces the second soft blowing sound. This provides clear proof that the second soft blowing sound is produced by the arteries of the leg, which causes the blood to flow backwards and somehow empty the capillaries [36, p. 426–427].

Duroziez therefore found that:

> [c]ompression of the artery with the stethoscope helps to make the second sound more intense. We see that a single or double abnormal murmur constantly takes place in the arter-

> ies. Therefore, it must be an important sign to recognize aortic insufficiency. However, because this sound is common to other diseases its absolute semeiological value has less value. The systolic sound of the arteries is much more difficult to auscultate than the diastolic sound and thus has escaped several observers [36, p. 422].

Duroziez reported that the intermittent double soft blowing sounds in the femoral arteries are found in other conditions including typhoid fever, lead poisoning, and anemia. It is distinguished from aortic insufficiency since it, “lasts only a few days and by decreasing the pressure the sound is now continuous” [36, p. 425]. Hence, although Bouillaud originally identified the sign through auscultation, it was Duroziez who identified the method for unmasking the sound through compression and auscultating the femoral artery.

In a systematic review of five studies (1911–1981) a sensitivity ranging from 33% to 81% and specificity from 35% to 100% was identified for Duroziez sign [24]. Each study enrolled more than 10 adults with chronic AR and variable degrees of disease severity. These studies had methodological limitations such as inconsistency in case definition performance, study selection, and reference standards used, and therefore limits the ability to draw a meaningful conclusion regarding the sign’s utility in clinical practice [24].

Traube Sign

Ludwig Traube (1818–1876) was born in Ratibor, Prussian Silesia, and received his medical degree from the University of Breslau in 1840. He continued his studies under Joseph Škoda (1801–1881) and Carl von Rokitansky (1804–1878) in Vienna, and returned to Berlin in 1842 as a practicing physician [37–39]. The 1848 revolution afforded Jewish physicians the right to practice medicine in the hospital and the ministry of education through a student movement was persuaded to appoint Traube an assistantship in the Charité Hospital [37, 38]. In 1849, he served a civil assistantship at Johann Lukas Schönlein’s (1793–1864) clinic where he was responsible for teaching percussion and auscultation of diseases of the chest, followed by a habilitation as an Adjunct Professor at the University of Berlin in 1851 [37, 38]. He was appointed director of Diseases of the Chest at the Charité Hospital in 1853 and within his department assigned the title of *propaedeutic* (preparatory) clinic in 1855 [38]. In 1862, he was Ordinary Professor at Friedrich Wilhelm Institute (Prussian institution for army surgeons) and in 1866 named Geheimer Medizinal Rath (highest rank for medical advisors), a powerful regimented political title within Prussia affording these individuals the unquestionable authority to establish the type of medical care to be delivered throughout the medical system [39, 40]. It was not until 1872 that Traube finally received an appointment as Ordinary Professor in the Medical Faculty in Berlin, which had been intentionally upheld by his chief Friedrich Theodor von Frerichs (1819–1885) and ministry of education. His other appointments included honorary member of the German Physicians Society in Paris in 1873 and title of Doctor of the University at the University of Leiden, The

Netherlands, in 1875 [38]. He is best recognized in Germany as the father of experimental pathology. He was responsible for the introduction of physiological experimentation in clinical medicine which led to the recognition of medicine as a biologic science. As written by Rudolf Virchow (1821–1902) in memory of Traube's role in transforming the study of medicine:

> Traube's goal was quite clear then. He himself expressed it in the foreword to the "contributions" in the following words: Sharp questions arising out of a thorough knowledge of the facts obtained concerning conditions or perceived phenomena. Definitive answers are the result of a systematic series of precise experiments and indeed the direct implications of these experiments. What he sought were not just facts but explanations. Of course, actual explanations proved by the experiment and not merely speculative interpretations. A very laudable goal, because it clarified the details of the systematic process through which the final result is formulated and accepted [37, p. 209–210].

Dr. Oscar Fraentzel (1838–1894), an assistant and nephew working in Traube's clinic, reported in 1867 the peculiar findings identified by Traube in several patients with aortic insufficiency [41]. Fraentzel described the case of a 28-year-old male where:

> The femoral arteries are not abnormally tense and the pulse wave is very high. You hear two tones, a loud systolic and weak diastolic tone [41, p. 455]. Geh.-Rath Traube has only recently become aware of the occurrence of a double tone in the femoral artery in the case of insufficiency of the aortic valves. In two cases he found post-mortem, unusually large and in one case almost complete insufficiency of the aortic valves. Despite careful examination intra-vitam and post-mortem, these two cases in no way differed from those usually seen [41, p. 456].

Traube provided an explanation for the findings of the "double tone":

> [b]oth the normal and abnormal appearances of the circulatory apparatus sounds occur because the membranes move from a state of low to a state of high tension. Their intensity varies based on the difference in tone produced in rapid succession by the membrane. In this way, three of the most common acoustic signs which we observe in the case of aortic insufficiency are casually explained by: a) the sounds of the femoral artery, b) the rough systolic murmur in the carotids, c) the lack of the systolic sound at the apex of the heart. The femoral artery shows the strongest tension among the superficial arteries accessible to palpation as it is one that is certainly considerably larger than, for example, the carotid. Under ordinary conditions, this tension remains significant even during diastole and the increase in tension during systole is so small that a sound perceptible to our ear does not arise. This is different in aortic valve insufficiency since blood flows not only into the capillaries but also into the left ventricle during diastole. The tension of the arteries at the end of diastole must be far less than under normal conditions. On the other hand, a greater amount of blood is transported into the aortic system during systole than that found in healthy people. Thereby, this increases the difference in tension in the arterial wall at the end of diastole and during systole. Therefore, only now can a sound emerge [41, p. 456].

Furthermore, he accounted for the relationship between the presence of the double sound over the femoral artery and severity of aortic insufficiency recognizing that the double tone sound occurs only in cases of severe aortic insufficiency:

> The connection between the appearance of two sounds over the femoral artery and the size of the insufficiency is, after all, also clear. If it is established that a membrane, such as a string, can be made to sound when it changes rapidly from a state of lower tension to that of a higher tension then conversely sounding vibrations must be able to be caused by the condition of higher tension rapidly followed by a state of lower tension. Apparently, in this as in the other cases, the molecules that are brought out of their equilibrium position must vibrate before they steadily assume the new equilibrium position. In fact, experience teaches that strings that suddenly become slack can be made to sound. In cases of severe insufficiency of the semilunar valves and considerable volume of the left ventricle, the aortic system must during diastole forcibly lose large quantities of blood in a short period of time. This causes the walls of the more distant arteries, such as the femoral artery, to vibrate stronger and faster than in cases of less insufficiency [41, p. 457].

Traube in his 1872 paper titled "Ueber den Doppelton in der Cruralis bei Insuffizienz der Aortenklappe" (About a double tone in the femoral artery in the case of an insufficient aortic valve) reported on five cases of aortic insufficiency where the auscultatory findings of a "double tone" over the femoral artery occurred spontaneously without the requirement for compressing the femoral artery (Table 5.1):

> If the stethoscope is easily applied to the groin as is customary in Germany without any impairment of the arterial lumen then insufficiency of the aortic valves, as is known, is distinctly pronounced in the majority of cases. A ventricular-systole falling tone, which often has the intensity of a heart sound and sometimes appears louder is present. In my experience, this sound is often replaced or accompanied with a murmur. The murmur, and this is a point in which I deviate from Duroziez, never has the character produced by compressing the femoral artery. It is always much softer, and in the majority of cases much weaker than the compression noise. Anyone who is aware of all this must find it almost incomprehensible how one could confuse the results of Duroziez's work, with those contained in a report from my clinic, which was published two and a half years later. I believe that this confusion had already preserved the name I used to describe the phenomenon that I discovered on the femoral artery. In my report there is no discussion of a "double tone in the femoral artery" anywhere, as in Duroziez's case. Since Škoda, however, we are accustomed in Germany to distinguish sharply between a tone and murmur. We speak of a tone only when it occurs with the sound phenomena that more or less resembles normal heart sounds. In fact I have found in only a few cases of insufficiency of the aortic valves, five-up to this moment, the double tone in the femoral artery. This shows such concurrence with the phenomenon of the normal cardiac tone that one, who at the best of intentions, could hardly determine that it is different. In such cases the femoral artery not only leaves a true tone during the period of the ventricular systole, as in the usual case of aortic insufficiency, but also during ventricular diastole when the sound is recognized to be similar to a heart sound [42, p. 573–574].

Traube's finding was indeed a rare occurrence and identified by him in only five cases over 5 years. The sign is found only in cases of severe aortic insufficiency with severe left ventricular dilation [43]. He also reported that the double tone sound was not pathognomonic for aortic insufficiency and is found in patients "who are prostrate from severe feverish disease" [41, 42]. It should be recognized that Bouillaud had recognized this similar finding 30 years prior to Traube's description.

Quincke (Sign) Pulse

Heinrich Irenaeus Quincke (1842–1922) was born in Frankfurt-am-Main, Germany, studied medicine at Berlin, Würzburg, and Heidelberg Universities, and received his medical degree from the University of Berlin in 1863 [44, 45]. He then furthered his studies in Switzerland, Paris, and London [46, 47]. He served as an assistant to Friedrich Theodor von Frerichs (1819–1885) at the Charity Hospital in Berlin from 1867 to 1870. In 1872, he was appointed Professor of Internal Medicine at the University of Berne, Switzerland, and served as Chair of Internal Medicine in 1873 [48]. In 1888, he was Professor of Medicine at the University of Kiel, Germany, a position he held for the next 30 years [45, 46, 48]. In 1900, he served as the rector of Christian-Albrechts-University in Kiel, followed by an appointment at Senckenberg Institute, Frankfurt am Main, in 1908. He was the recipient of an honorary degree of Legum Doctor (Doctor of Laws, LLD) from the University of Glasgow in 1901 [49]. Quincke had a remarkable medical career and as a quintessential internist he contributed in multiple therapeutic areas such as in the fields of allergy (angioedema of anaphylaxis also known as Quincke's edema), cardiology (aortic insufficiency Quincke's pulse), neurology (performed the first lumbar puncture using a cannula for diagnostic and therapeutic purposes and characterized cerebrospinal fluid), pulmonary (Quincke position or a position with the patient lying prone with head down to facilitate drainage of lung abscess, as well as the first to surgically drain a lung abscess), hematology (named poikilocytosis in patient with pernicious anemia and identified its relationship to gastric cancer) [44, 49, 50]. As described of his character:

> By character and by training he was stern with himself in his adherence to his chosen tasks and no less firm in his guidance of others. Behind this was his loyalty and such a plaint interest that it bent itself to the needs of all with whom he worked for their aid or their instruction. His lectures were comprehensive, clear in their unraveling of tangled problems. But above all his clinical work as it chiefly occupied his attention revealed that power of investigation and of instruction which made him the revered teacher and brought his work to the fulfillment which has enriched all branches of internal medicine [47].

He described the location and appearance of the nail bed where the capillary pulse is identified (Table 5.1):

> [t]he border between the more whitish blood-poor area and redder, more intensely injected part of the capillary system of the nail bed. In the majority of the persons examined, one will observe a forward and backward movement at the border of the red and white parts synchronizing with the heartbeat [51, p. 357].

He reported the method used for eliciting the capillary pulse in cases where the nail bed is confluently red:

> But not every fingernail show the mentioned white zone with general blood supply caused by the strong and frequent action of the heart and high arterial pressure. In the warm external air, the nails are uniformly reddened. Under these circumstances in order to create a lighter zone on the nail one can either apply a (naturally uniform) pressure there, or, better yet, hold the hand in the air [51, p. 357].

Quincke found that the capillary pulse was most commonly seen in the index finger and absent in the toes. He believed that transparency of the nail bed, decreased elasticity of the capillaries, lower blood volume and decreased blood flow are local conditions required to visualize the pulse [51]. Systemic factors such as arterial hypertension, elevated ambient temperatures, and tachycardia, which lead to redness of the nail bed, masks the capillary pulse [51]. Quincke also reported the finding of post-systolic pulsation of the veins on the dorsum of the hands, and in one patient on the dorsum of the foot in aortic insufficiency:

> [f]or here, as in the capillary pulse, certain conditions are necessary for the appearance of this phenomenon. The skin must be as thin and limp as possible (no increase in water) with the veins filled to a certain extent. (...) Therefore, both elevation of the arm and severe inhibition of venous blood flow will make the pulse of the vein disappear [51, p. 358].

It is of historic interest that Quincke was the first to describe in a male patient that he:

> [h]ad the opportunity of observing capillary pulse in the living man also in a place other than the fingernails, namely on the retina, indeed in the last case of aortic valve incompetence mentioned still under my care. In addition to an exceptionally strong arterial pulse of retina which is visible far beyond the limits of the papilla, a visible arterial pulse of the retina was also seen in the upright position in both eyes. The uniform systolic blushing and diastolic paling of the optic papilla is presumably due to an alternately strong and weaker filling of the existing capillary network located here. Most striking is the change of color in the middle at the border of the physiological excavation, whereas in the case of the fingernail it fluctuates between red and less red with the pulse. Beyond the limits of the papilla the capillary pulse though probably present is not visible since the change in color nuance does not appear so sharp due to the dark choroidal background. By the way, in neither of the two eyes is another abnormality demonstrable to which the pulsation phenomenon could be accounted [51, p. 358].

It was Otto Becker, who acknowledged and credited Quincke's earlier publication on the retinal pulsation findings in aortic insufficiency. Becker described in a large series of patients with aortic insufficiency pulsation of the retinal arteries (see Becker Sign).

Becker Sign

Otto Becker (1828–1890) was born in Domhof, Mecklenburg, Germany, and received his doctorate from the University of Vienna in 1859 [52]. He served as an assistant to Carl Ferdinand Ritter von Arit (1812–1887) excelling in the field of ophthalmology. He habilitated as an Adjunct Professor in 1867 in Vienna and was appointed first Ordinary Professor of Ophthalmology at Heidelberg Eye Clinic. At the University of Heidelberg, he served as Chairman and hospital administrator. His area of interests involved the lens as well as the location and function of the ciliary body. His other significant contribution was the translation and improved clarity of Donder's original work on refraction and accommodation of the eye [52].

Becker described in details and further elucidated the retinal and optic nerve findings in a large number of patients with heart disease and "in the retina and optic nerve, in the case of aortic insufficiency of the aortic valves, a spontaneously occurring arterial pulse can be detected" [53, p. 206]. As enumerated by Becker, Quincke also noted that:

> The diastolic pulse of the central retinal vein, which is so often present in the normal case, is also exceptionally present in this case. Since the development of this pulsation has not yet been fully elucidated, and indeed it is probably not due to reproduction by the capillaries, it should not be further discussed here [53, p. 207].

Becker was aware that "Quincke had previously published the same consideration in two places" [53, p. 206]. He acknowledged Quincke's findings and credited him for being the first to see the spontaneous retinal arterial pulse in aortic insufficiency [53]. Becker, however, reported a finding which differed from Quincke's original observation:

> From all this, it is almost certain that the spontaneous arterial pulse is invariably found in the eyes of individuals suffering from aortic valve insufficiency. So far, only a single case was investigated by me and it was an individual with severe anemia. My observations on this point are therefore not entirely in agreement with the information provided by Quincke who found the phenomenon at all times in cases of pronounced valvular defect. According to our research, however, the degree of visibility of the pulse also changed with exercise. If we have the patient go up and down stairs quickly or if the heart action had been aroused by the consumption of alcohol we perceived the retinal pulsation much more clearly. (…) It must therefore be left open whether perhaps in such cases the phenomenon can be evoked [53, p. 258].

Becker sign thus refers to the retinal arterial pulse found on an ophthalmoscopic examination in a patient with aortic valve insufficiency and anemia, more pronounced with exercise and tachycardia (Table 5.1).

De Musset Sign

The sign was eponymously named after a French poet and dramatist suffering from AR. Alfred Louis Charles de Musset (1810–1857) described his symptoms in the poem "La nuit de mai" (A May night):

> Why beats my heart so fast? / What is this thrill that terrifies my pulses? / Did I hear / A stranger's knock? / Why does my dying lamp / Blaze into sudden light? / Sweet heaven, help me! I tremble. / Who is this? Who calls? 'Tis no one / And all I hear is the untiring clock / That knells the poorness of my solitude [54, p. 11].

Paul de Musset, in an autobiography about his brother Alfred, wrote about a symptom that he observed and eponymously named after his brother:

> One morning in March, when we were at breakfast, I perceived that my brother, at every pulse-beat, gave a slight involuntary toss of the head. He demanded to know why my mother and I looked at him curiously; and we told him what we had observed. "I did not know," he replied, "that that was visible; but I can set your minds at rest." He pressed the

> nape of his neck in some way with his thumb and forefinger, and his head immediately ceased to mark the pulsations of his heart. "You perceive," he said, "that this terrible disorder can be cured by a very cheap and simple method" [55, p. 235].

Paul de Musset further wrote about his brother's course and diagnosis:

> I had observed in 1842, and which had developed stealthily, made rapid progress during the winter of 1856. I do not know why the physician, who understood the nature of it perfectly, should have thought fit to keep it a secret. It was an affection of the valves of the aorta [55, p. 279].

Thus, de Musset sign refers to head bobbing found in patients with severe aortic insufficiency (Table 5.1).

Rosenbach Sign

Ottomar Ernst Felix Rosenbach (1851–1907) was born in Krappitz (Silesia), Germany (currently Poland), and received his medical degree from the University of Breslau, Germany (currently Poland), in 1874 [56]. At the University of Jena, he served as an assistant to the medical hospital and dispensary from 1874 to 1877 [56, 57]. At Allerheiligen-Hospital in Breslau, he served as Assistant and Adjunct Professor in 1877 and Chief of Medicine from 1877 to 1893 [56]. He was appointed Extraordinary Professor at the University in 1888 and in 1896 continued his medical practice in Berlin [57].

Rosenbach is considered a pioneer leading the concept of functional diseases and functional diagnosis based on a physiological rather than anatomical or structural approach to disease pathogenesis [58]. His earlier work entitled "Der Mechanismus und die Diagnose der Mageninsuffizienz" (The mechanism and the diagnosis of gastric insufficiency) published in 1878, introduced the concept of motor or mechanical insufficiency in various diseased organ systems. Ismar Isidor Boas (1858–1938) acknowledged Rosenbach's groundbreaking work and recognized him "to be considered the founder of the functional diagnosis of gastric diseases" [57–59]. A description of his character:

> There can be no difference of opinion, even among those who do not agree that among the prominent men of our profession and or time, Rosenbach was, more than any other, an original thinker, observer and investigator, who made no concessions to the extravagant fashions in medicine of the present day [60].

Ottomar Rosenbach acknowledged that most cases of hepatic pulsation are caused by tricuspid insufficiency. He also recognized that:

> The earlier view that pulsation of the liver is most commonly directly due to the elevation and lowering of its surface in tricuspid insufficiency, similar to an arterial vessel of the pulsating inferior vena cava, is true in most cases. (…) The observation given at the onset is to show that there are indeed cases that occur in which a pulsation of the liver, which differs no way from that caused by insufficiency of the tricuspid, is observed… [61, p. 498].

Rosenbach mentioned conditions of adjacent organs (hypertrophic heart disease, abdominal aorta aneurysms, and adjacent vessels) which also cause liver pulsation [61]. He also identified in a patient with aortic insufficiency:

> Recently, I have again observed a case of insufficiency of the highest level of the aortic valves in which exquisite systolic liver pulsation existed without signs of tricuspid insufficiency. However, since the section was denied, it was impossible to verify the assumed cardiac findings by autopsy and therefore as much as I am objectively convinced of the correctness of the diagnosis, I must rely on the detailed discussion and without the use of the case for my views [61, p. 523].

Thus, Rosenbach sign refers to the presence of hepatic pulsation in patients with aortic insufficiency (Table 5.1).

Gerhardt Sign

Carl Adolph Christian Jacob Gerhardt (1883–1902) was born in Speyer, Germany, and received his doctorate from University of Würzburg in 1856. He served as an assistant to Wilheim Griesinger (1817–1868) at the Tübingen Clinic and studied under Rudolf Virchow (1821–1902), Franz von Rinecker (1811–1883), and Heinrich von Bamberger (1822–1888) at Würzburg [62, 63]. He spent 2 years at Swabian University, Germany, where he taught auscultation and percussion, pharmacology, and completed his habilitation thesis on the diaphragm [62]. In 1852, he returned to the University of Würzburg where he taught diseases of the larynx, auscultation and percussion, and published the *Handbuch der Kinderkrankheiten* (Handbook of Childhood Diseases).

He was named Adjunct Professor in Würzburg in 1860 and the following year was promoted to Full Professor at the medical clinic in Jena [62, 63]. While at Jena he published his book, *Lehrbuch der Auscultation und Percussion mit besonderer Berücksichtigung der Inspection, Betastung und Messung der Brust und des Unterleibes zu diagnostischen Zwecken* (Textbook of Auscultation and Percussion with Particular Attention to the Inspection, Palpation and Measurement of the Chest and Abdomen for Diagnostic Purposes) in 1866 [62, 64]. He succeeded his teachers Heinrich von Bamberger at Würzburg in 1872 and Friedrich Theodor von Frerichs in Berlin in 1885 [63]. His primary areas of interest involved diseases of the heart, lungs, larynx, and children [63]. Among his other accomplishments, he was the first to describe erythromelalgia in 1892 (Gerhardt's disease). One of Gerhardt's greatest discoveries was that he synthesized acetylsalicylic acid, commonly known as aspirin, in 1853 [65]. He also devised the ferric chloride test for the identification of urinary acetic acid in acetonemia [66]. There are two other signs attributed to his name. First, another "Gerhardt sign" (Change of sound sign) in reference to the change in percussion sound when the patient changes from a standing to supine position in cases of pyo-pneumothorax. Second, adductor paralysis of the larynx in thoracic aortic aneurysm [67]. As described of his character:

> He excelled all of those in one quality which was characteristic. In his writings, as in his speeches, there was never a superfluous expression. Every sentence expressed a fact, a truth. Abridgment is impossible. Every word, as it was heard or read, is to the point, earnest, concise, almost blunt, carefully considered weighty. (…) The simplicity, straightforwardness, and honesty of his spiritual and moral nature at that time, developed later, in the matured scientist and practitioner, that logical and fascinating style which, while not lacing in elegance, appealed directly to the scientific consciousness and thought [63, p. 500].

Gerhardt reported the case of a 27-year-old with chronic aortic insufficiency, presumably caused by previous rheumatic fever, who was found on physical examination to have an enlarged spleen in which:

> [a] surprising phenomenon was the marked pulsation in which the hard mass swelled with each heart systole, expanding on all sides, and shrinking again during diastole. One heard a dull double tone above the mass only at the upper edge of the heart sound. (…) The pulsation of the swollen spleen was so clear in this case that it could be demonstrated to numerous observers. As one could grasp the spleen tip with the fingers it was easy to prove that it was not a displacement of the spleen by the movement of the apex, but a true systolic swelling of the organ [68, p. 449].

He further identified two other patients with well-compensated aortic insufficiency, pericarditis, splenomegaly, and spleen pulsation. Gerhardt recognized that "two factors seem to be of particular importance for the development of the pulsatile spleen described here: the abnormal blood pressure related to aortic insufficiency and rapid relaxation of the vessel walls" [68, p. 450]. He recognized that splenic pulsation was found in conditions other than aortic insufficiency and believed it was caused by an abnormal increases and decreases in blood pressure and rapid relaxation of the blood vessels [69] (Table 5.1).

Müller Sign

Friedrich von Müller (1858–1941) was born in Augsburg, Germany, acquired his medical training in Munich, Tübingen, and Würzburg in Germany, and completed his doctorate from the latter university in 1882 [70, 71]. From 1882 to 1885, he was appointed assistant at Carl Gerhard's (1822–1902) clinic at the University of Würzburg, returning to Berlin with Gerhard as senior assistant at the Charity Hospital in 1885 [71]. From 1877 to 1888, he served as an Adjunct Professor of internal medicine at Friedrich Wilhelm University Berlin, and in 1889 was Chief of the Polyclinic at the University of Bonn, Germany, followed by a position as Chief of the Polyclinic at the University of Breslau, Germany (currently Wroclaw, Poland), in 1896 [70, 72]. From 1892 to 1899, he was director of the polyclinic at the University of Marburg, Germany, where he rose to the rank of dean of the faculty [70]. He served as Chair of the Department of Medicine at the University of Basel, Switzerland, in 1899, appointed chief of the Second Medical Clinic in Munich from 1902 to 1937, and rector of the University of Munich, Germany in 1914 [70, 71].

His other accolades include serving as President of the annual German Congress of Internal Medicine Vienna in 1907 and President of the German Academy of Sciences Leopoldina in 1927 [72, 73].

He observed in a 22-year-old female with aortic insufficiency and intermittent angina:

> [r]hythmic movement of the palate. The inflammatory reddened tonsils and the anterior and posterior palatal arches moved medially, synchronously with each carotid pulse. Also on the soft palate, a pulsation was found when the free edge of the uvula moved downwards. In this way, the contraction of the palatal arches and tonsils as well as the soft palate and the uvula came together with each pulse causing a narrowing of the palate opening. At the same time, a rhythmic strengthening of the redness of the palate was observed [74, p. 251].

He postulated that the cause of these findings:

> As far as the genesis of the phenomenon is concerned it is natural to think that the increased pulsation of the carotids produces a co-vibration of the palatal arches and tonsils, which move medially each time. But this is still not completely sufficient for the explanation, since the free edge of the soft palate and the uvula also pulsate and move downward. The amplification of the pulsation during angina also accounts for the fact that we have to deal with a greater quantity of blood which occurs with each pulse-wave and with this a swelling of its parts [74, p. 252].

Müller believed that palate pulsation was not a rare phenomenon since he identified this in 4 to 7 patients with aortic insufficiency (Table 5.1). We are unaware of any study that assessed the sensitivity or specificity of this sign.

Hill Sign

Sir Leonard Eskrine Hill (1866–1952) was born in Bruce Castle, Tottenham, England, and received his MRCS (Member of the Royal College of Surgeons of England) and LRCP (Licentiate of the Royal College of Physicians) degrees in 1889, and MB (Bachelor of Medicine, Bachelor of Surgery) from the University College London in 1890 [75, 76]. The Sharpey Scholarship at the University College afforded him the opportunity to study physiology under Edward Albert Sharpey-Schäfer (1850–1935) (considered founder of endocrinology in collaboration with George Oliver (1841–1915) who discovered adrenaline and coined the terms endocrine and insulin). Later he worked as an assistant to Sir John Scott Burdon-Sanderson (1828–1905) (discovered the inhibition of bacteria by penicillium) at Oxford, returning to the University College in 1891 as an Assistant Professor to Schäfer [75, 76]. In 1895, he served as Lecturer in Physiology at the London Hospital. He was elected to the Royal Society in 1900 and in 1912 was Professor of Physiology at the London College [75]. From 1914 to 1930, he was appointed Director of Applied Physiology at the National Institute for Medical Research and subsequently served as Director of Research at the St. John Clinic and Institute of Physical Medicine [75]. He was knighted in 1930.

Hill's applied research spanned multiple therapeutic areas and collaborations. His early research focus was on the cerebral circulation, intracranial pressure and vasomotor and abdominal muscle tone in maintaining upright posture. These concepts were included in his 1896 book titled *The Physiology and Pathology of the Cerebral Circulation* [75]. With Harold Barnard (1868–1908), he developed the armlet method for determining arterial blood pressure [75]. In association with John James Rickard Macleod (1876–1935) and Major Greenwood (1880–1949) his work focused on the effects and management of high atmospheric pressure and decompression during diving [76]. In collaboration with Martin Flack (1882–1931), they studied the regulation of breathing [75, 76]. His later work involved studies on environmental conditions (ambient temperature, humidity, and air movement) on human health and work-capacity, a field of medicine later recognized as occupational health [76]. As Director of Research at St. John Clinic and Institute of Physical Medicine, he studies the therapeutic effects of ultraviolet and infrared radiation in the formation of vitamin D.

Hill receives numerous accolades including being elected fellow of the Royal Society and University College of London, Honorary LLD from the University of Aberdeen (1931), and Honorary Associate of the Royal Institute of British Architects (ARIBA) [75]. For his contributions to the study of ventilation and the effects of light and solar radiation, he was the recipient of the Gold Medal of the Institution of Mining and Metallurgy and the Thomas Kay Sidey Medal of the Royal Society of New Zealand, respectively [75]. His avocation involved painting in oil, water-color, and pastel and writing children books.

Martin William Flack (1882–1931) was born in Borden, Kent, England, and received his medical degree from the London Hospital in 1908. His work as a student under the aegis of Sir Arthur Keith (1866–1955) lead to their anatomical discovery of which they named the sino-auricular node in 1906 [77]. During his medical training he also served as an assistant demonstrator of physiology in Sir Leonard Hill's laboratory, resuming this position after working in the Continental Laboratories where he conducted further research confirming that the sino-auricular node was responsible for the heartbeat, as well as investigations on the nerve supply to the thyroid gland [77]. In collaboration with Sir Leonard Hill, they published *A Textbook of Physiology* in 1919 and conducted research on the physiologic effects of oxygen debt and carbon dioxide excess [77]. He was appointed Director of the Department of Medical Research for the Royal Air Force at Mount Vernon Hospital London in 1915 [77]. Here he was involved in research assessing pilots' fitness for airplane flight. He was awarded Central Chancery of the Orders of Knighthood by the Royal Air Force in 1919 in recognition of his work during the War [78]. As a tribute to Martin Flack and a description of his character, Air Vice-Marshal Sir David Munro wrote:

> I have seldom met a man who had so strong a sense of loyalty, and to the Service which he served so well his loss will be almost irreparable. But it is not only for his knowledge and capabilities that he will be missed; he was, in all his relations, one of the most simple, genuine, and good-hearted of men, and I am sure that there are very many who, like myself, will have experienced in his death a real sense of personal loss [77, p. 404].

Wilfred Watkinson Holtzmann (1877–1944) was born in Bradford, West Yorkshire, England, and received his BCh degree in 1903 and MA and MB in 1904 from the University of Cambridge [79, 80]. He was initially involved in medical practice at Clipsley Lodge, Haydock Lancashire. He also served as a medical superintendent at Haydock Cottage Hospital and later appointed surgeon at Hospital St. Helens in the United Kingdom [80]. After World War I, he served as a surgeon at West Herts Hospital, Hemel Hempstead [80]. He was appointed Fellow of the Royal College of Surgeons, England in 1908 [79, 80].

Hill, Flack, and Holtzmann reported in their 1909 paper entitled "The measurement of systolic blood pressure in man" that:

> Holtzmann, acting on the suggestion of one of us (L.H.), made some independent observations of a similar kind and like result, in the London Hospital. He also tried the pressure in two or three cases of aortic regurgitation, and told us that he had found a noticeable difference between arm and leg reading in such. Following up on this interesting observation we have found that in all cases of aortic regurgitation there is this marked difference, which is not abolished by the method of oscillating the pressure up and down near the obliteration pressure. So marked is this difference that we believe we could pick out the cases of aortic regurgitation by it alone [81, p. 76].

They concluded emphasizing the importance of their findings as a sign of aortic insufficiency that: "A difference between arm and leg readings is most marked in all cases of aortic regurgitation, and when such patients are lying quiet in bed this difference is a diagnostic sign of aortic regurgitation" [81, p. 81] (Table 5.1). In a later paper Hill and Rowland confirmed earlier findings:

> In a paper by one of us (L.H.) written in co-operation with Martin Flack and W. Holtzmann, results were published which show that the systolic pressure taken in the arm and leg differ widely in cases of aortic regurgitation; so much so that this difference becomes of diagnostic value [82, p. 220].

They attributed this difference in systolic blood pressure to "greater conductance of the systolic wave by the leg arteries, which are held in a more contracted state in cases of aortic regurgitation" [82, p. 221]. Hill sign is moderately sensitive but is not specific since there are several conditions that result in a false positive (thyrotoxicosis, sepsis, beriberi, pregnancy, and strenuous exertion) or false negative (aortic stenosis, peripheral vascular occlusive disease) result.

Babu et al. in a systematic review of seven studies on Hill sign, whereby each included at least 10 adults with chronic aortic insufficiency and variable degrees of disease severity, found for those which reported these findings a sensitivity and specificity range from 0% to 100% and 71% to 100% respectively. Limitations of these studies were related to selection biases, inconsistent reference standards and in some studies non-specified severities of aortic insufficiency [24]. Frank et al. found a popliteal-brachial index greater than 20 mmHg discriminated between patients with moderate to severe from those with mild AR [83].

Landolfi Sign

Michele Landolfi (1878–1959) was born in Airola, Italy. Being a pupil of Leonard Bianchi (1848–1927), Pietro Francesco Castellino (Castelino) (1864–1933) and Antonio Cardarelli (1831–1927), he graduated from the Medical School in Naples, Italy in 1902. A year later, Landolfi began serving as assistant at the Clinic of Domenico Capozzi (1829–1907) at the *Ospedale degli Incurabili* (Hospital for the Incurables) of Naples. As a Professor of Medical Semiotics at the University of Naples in later years, he was the founder and first President of Association of Italian Blood Volunteers (AVIS), and also served as the editor-in-chief of two medical journals, *Riforma Medica* and *Folia Medica*. He received accolades such as the Commander of the Crown of Italy and the Knight of the Mauritian Order [84].

Landolfi examined the eyes in a series of 24 patients with pure or complicated aortic insufficiency. In one patient he identified (Table 5.1):

> [a] rhythmic movement of narrowing and dilatation of the pupil independent of the will of the patient and the ambient lighting. (…) [b]ecause the changes of the iris were synchronous to the movements of the heart, narrowing of the pupil corresponded to ventricular systole and dilatation to diastole [84].

He described the methods that accentuated the findings within the iris and in three additional patients, the effect of foxglove (*Digitalis*):

> This phenomenon was accentuated by keeping the subject standing, administering foxglove, running, or compressing the femoral or abdominal aorta. In contrast, it became less obvious when the patient was lying down, kept at prolonged rest, or when he took bromides or inhaled nitrite [84].

He accounted for the pathogenesis of this finding:

> It is due to the fact that during ventricular systole the energetic impulse of the blood causes hyperemia of the iris and consequently miosis. During diastole, the rapid return of blood causes anemia of the iris and hence mydriasis. In other words, the repletion of the iris vessels dilates the iris and diminishes the diameter of the pupil. The opposite occurs when the amount of blood in the iris vessels decrease. We find therefore, that circulatory hippus of aortic insufficiency is constituted by the succession of these alternative movements. Research previous conducted by M. Mosso demonstrated that there is a constant correlation between the state of the peripheral vessels and the state of the pupil. The circulatory hippus, therefore, is only an exaggeration of the physiological cardiovascular hippus [84].

Landolfi stated that the sign is seen in patients with left ventricular hypertrophy and a Corrigan pulse:

> The pathological cardiovascular hippus, i.e., the rhythmic hippus that is synchronous with movements of the heart and very accentuated manifest during systole only in pure well-compensated aortic insufficiency. The sign when it exists is therefore pathognomonic of this affection, but its absence has no meaning [84].

We are unaware of any study that assessed the sensitivity or specificity of this sign.

Minervini Sign

There is limited historical information on Leone Minervini (?–1924). At the time of the publication of his paper, he was an assistant at the *Ospedale degli Incurabili* (Hospital for the Incurables) of Naples, Italy. He served as Associate Professor of Medical Pathology of Revista Università beginning in 1912 [85]. In his paper entitled "Le pouls de la langue dans l'insuffisance aortique" (The pulse of the tongue in aortic insufficiency), Minervini identified with the use of a tongue depressor:

> [t]hat the underlying tongue communicated with the jerks of the instrument from bottom to top, rhythmic and synchronous to the arterial pulsations. It was a real pulse of the tongue due to the rhythmic jerks of the lingual artery caused by the energetic impulse of the tongue. (…) [I]n fact, not only is the tongue pulsating but the entire floor of the mouth presents a rhythmic uplift and lowering synchronous with the cardiosystole-arteriodiastole and the cardiodiastole-arteriosystole. The pulse of the tongue is accompanied, moreover, by a state of turgescent of this organ and with slight swelling of the floor of the mouth lifted upwards. During the heart diastole, the pulse naturally falls back abruptly and at the same time the tongue becomes less swollen and lowers to resume the same position as before with the new systole of the heart [86, p. 481].

He further described the method for examining the patient to distinguish tongue movements, which may naturally occur to the sides or back and forth, from those seen in aortic insufficiency:

> In order to detect the phenomenon in question, the patient is examined in a sitting position with his head slightly turned back and mouth open. By carefully inspecting the oral cavity in positive cases there is tongue movement from the bottom to top, rhythmic and synchronous to the heartbeat. This movement is better seen when the tongue rests on the floor of the mouth than when it is drawn out of the mouth. In this last position, the instinctive and inevitable contractions of the lingual muscles causes a hardening of the organ obscuring the arterial jerks. (…) [I]t is possible to use a metallic or glass tongue depressor. It is then sufficient to apply with this instrument moderate pressure to see the pulse of the tongue occurring in all its clarity. The tongue depressor always lifts upwards by rhythmic jolts analogous to rhythmic jerks of the head or abrupt movement of a laryngo-tracheal jerk [86, p. 481].

Minervini further identified during which stages the tongue pulsation is best seen in aortic insufficiency:

> The intensity of the phenomenon in question, moreover, parallels the state of the arterial pressure and the pulse of the tongue and is best visible when there is hypertrophy of the left ventricle. It decreases in intensity and even disappears completely during periods when the blood pressure falls and at the same time as the decrease in ventricular capacity and systolic impulse begins to appear. It reappears, on the contrary, in advanced stages of the disease [86, p. 481].

Thus, Minervini sign refers to the presence of tongue pulsations in patients with aortic insufficiency (Table 5.1). We are unaware of any study that assessed the sensitivity or specificity of this sign.

Sailer Sign

Joseph Sailer (1867–1928) was born in Philadelphia, Pennsylvania, and received his medical degree from the University of Pennsylvania in 1891 [87]. He completed an internship at Presbyterian and Philadelphia General Hospitals followed by additional training in neurology and pathology in Zurich, Paris, and Vienna. Upon his return to the United States, he served as demonstrator of morbid anatomy in the department of Pathology under the aegis of Simon Flexner (1863–1946) at the University of Pennsylvania [87]. This was followed by a transition to clinical medicine where he was appointed initially as instructor and subsequently first Associate, Assistant, and Professor at the Philadelphia General Hospital in 1912. He served as first Chair of the newly formed Department of Gastroenterology in the Philadelphia Polyclinic. He was a member of the American Gastro-Enterological Association beginning in 1907, chief promoter of Philadelphia's Children's Heart Hospital, and one of the original founders of the American Heart Association in 1924 [87]. In a memorial address about Joseph Sailer, David Rieseman, a friend and colleague of Sailer wrote, "In Joseph Sailer the American Gastro-Enterological Association has lost more than a mere member, it has lost an influence for progress and an inspiration to higher ideals. His name will live in our annals and in the annals of American medicine." [87, p. 578]. Sailer described the case of a 27-year-old male with aortic insufficiency who developed *streptococcal viridians* endocarditis and fever. He stated that, "If one can draw conclusion from four cases described in detail, the condition necessary to cause the pulsation of the spleen are a severe type of aortic regurgitation and an infectious process." [88, p. 452]. He believed that splenic pulsation was caused by "the enlargement and softening of the spleen that occurs in the infection, however, must contribute to the occurrence, the chief cause of which is the excessive pulse pressure that occurs in aortic regurgitation" [88]. Thus, Sailer is credited for describing splenic pulsation in patients with aortic insufficiency in bacterial endocarditis (Table 5.1). We are unaware of any study that assessed the sensitivity or specificity of this sign.

Palfrey Sign

Francis Winslow Palfrey (1876–1953) received his medical degree from the Harvard Medical School in 1902 [89, 90]. He completed his medical training at Massachusetts General Hospital and Children's Hospital in Boston [89]. During World War I, he was commissioned major and medical chief of the bases hospital in Charlotte North Carolina [91]. He taught clinical medicine at Harvard Medical School from 1905 to 1939 and served as secretary of the faculty of medicine until 1917 [89, 90]. In 1906, he was appointed assistant, in 1917 instructor and in 1929 Assistant Professor of Medicine at Harvard Medical School [91]. With his colleague Simeon Burt Wolbach (1880–1954) and John Lancelot Todd (1876–1949) they were successful in identifying the causal relationship and pathogenesis between rickettssial organism and typhus [89].

Francis W. Palfrey reasoned that the auscultatory pistol shot sound heard in patients with severe aortic insufficiency represents the palpatory "shock" felt by the examining finger. Thus, by changing the position of the arm from a horizontal to vertical position while feeling for the shock and listening for the short and loud snapping or pistol-shot sounds, he identified a bedside maneuver to assist in determining the severity of aortic insufficiency (Fig. 5.1). The maneuver as described by Palfrey involves the following:

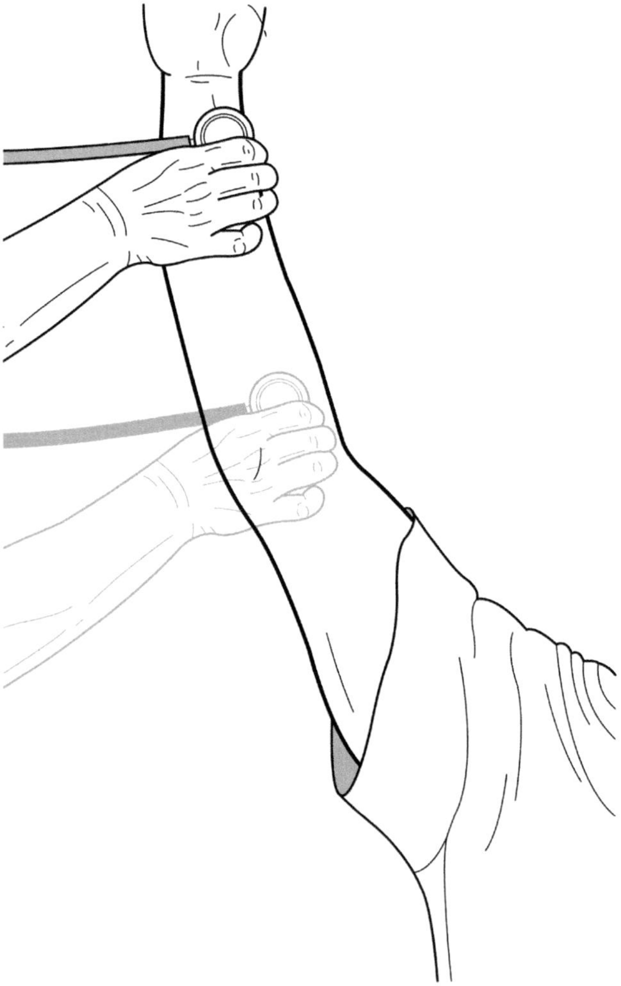

Fig. 5.1 Palfrey sign (by Ryan Yale)

> [r]aise the arm vertically above the heart and listen to the front of the wrist. If no arterial tone is heard it may be concluded that the insufficiency is not marked and may be slight. If the tone is heard over the elevated wrist but not lower it means a diastolic blood pressure of about 45 by mercurial manometer. (…) Next, with the arm still elevated, it is well to move the stethoscope gradually downward until at some point the tone suddenly disappears. The lower this point, the less the diastolic pressure; if the tone is present as low as the elbow it means a diastolic pressure of about 30 [92, p. 772].

These principles were based on Palfrey's understanding of the pressure changes occurring in a vertical column of blood when moved from a horizontal to upright position. In the normal state the diastolic pressure remains greater than the reduction in the column of blood and no signs are heard. However, in patients with less severe forms of aortic insufficiency the pistol-shot sounds may be heard only when the wrist is held vertically such that in these patients the diastolic pressure is lowered below the column of arterial blood. Thus, Palfrey identified an auscultatory method which by changing the position of the patient's arm, the severity of aortic insufficiency could be determined (Table 5.1). We are unaware of any study that assessed the sensitivity or specificity of this sign.

Mayne Sign

There is limited historical information available on Brian Mayne. He served as a physician at the Meath Hospital in Dublin, Ireland, in 1947. He became a Fellow of the Royal College of Physicians of Ireland (FRCPI) in the same year and was elected secretary/treasurer at the first inaugural meeting and later President of the Irish Cardiac Society from 1959 to 1960 [93]. Although officially retired in 1981, he continued to serve at the Meath Hospital until 1983 [94]. Mayne described a new physical sign that he believed might be helpful in cases of aortic insufficiency not detected by other methods. The maneuver is performed by (Table 5.1):

> Taking the blood pressure with the arm elevated, as it is held in the position in which Corrigan's pulse is elicited. It seems rational to suppose that in this position, the reflux of blood from the arm is accelerated, and that the regurgitation of blood from the aorta is probably also accelerated, by increasing the hydrostatic head of pressure in the aortic arch [95, p. 80].

He found that in otherwise healthy patients the diastolic blood pressure is 10 mmHg lower when the arm is in a vertical compared to the horizontal position. In patients with aortic insufficiency the value exceeds 15 mmHg. Happes et al. studied Mayne sign in 40 patients with aortic regurgitation of different severities ranging from mild to severe and 30 controls without aortic regurgitation using Doppler echocardiography. There was no correlation between the presence and severity of aortic regurgitation and Mayne sign. They did however identify an inverse relationship between age and change in diastolic blood pressure. Results from this study suggest that Mayne sign is an unreliable clinical finding in patients with aortic regurgitation and is found in otherwise healthy younger people [96]. Abbas and Sapira identified the sign in 65% of otherwise healthy persons [97]. We are unaware of any study that assessed the sensitivity or specificity of this sign.

Dennison Sign

Alfred Dudley Dennison, Jr. (1914–1988) was born in Johnstown, New York. He received his doctor of medicine degree from Cornell University in 1939. An Associate in Medicine at the Indiana University Medical School, presented a sign at the Michigan Academy of General Practice Fall Postgraduate Clinic on November 12, 1958 and published it in *The Journal of the Indiana State Medical Association* in 1959 [98].

Dennison wrote about the finding of a pulsating cervix seen in a patient with aortic insufficiency:

> We have hoped to make a young aspirant in the field of obstetrics and gynecology quite famous by placing his name in the historical stream of eponyms. Dr. Richard Shelley, our outgoing resident in obstetrics and gynecology, was surprised and perplexed to note a vigorously pulsating cervix as he peered at this organ through the speculum. He summoned the resident in medicine for consultation, demonstrated the pulsating cervix, and after the astute resident in medicine had listened to the precordium and noted free aortic insufficiency; it became quite apparent that the vigorous pulsation was isochronous with the heat beat. Such comments may not bring fame and fortune to this young man, but the ensuring jocularity has made the game of medicine more fun [98, p. 1284].

Thus, although Dennison's name has been ascribed to this attribution, it was in fact Richard Shelley, a resident at the Indiana University Medical School who was the first to observe this finding. Thus, it is also referred to as Shelley sign (Table 5.1). We are unaware of any study that assessed the sensitivity or specificity of this sign.

Harvey Sign

Watkins Proctor Harvey (1918–2007) was born in Lynchburg, Virginia, and received his medical degree from Duke University School of Medicine in 1943 [99]. He served under Samuel A. Levine (1891–1966) as the first cardiology fellow at Peter Bent Brigham Hospital at Harvard [99, 100]. He was appointed first Chair, established the Division of Cardiology and cardiology fellowship at Georgetown University. His expertise was related to the art of physical diagnosis and clinical auscultation for cardiovascular disease and master teacher of cardiology. As an inventor, he designed the Harvey Welch Allyn Tycos stethoscope series and the triple-header and elite stethoscopes which further enhanced acoustic sounds [101]. He passed on his knowledge of the clinical examination, publishing or co-authoring several books including Samuel Levine's second edition *Clinical Auscultation of the Heart, Clinical Auscultation of the Heart and Cardiac Pearls, Clinical Auscultation of the Cardiovascular System* and *Clinical Recognition and Treatment of the Common Arrhythmias.* As a tribute to his accomplishments as a gifted teacher, an amphitheater was built at Georgetown and dedicated to his namesake in 2015. It was designed specifically to teach diagnostic skills and heart sounds, a task that Dr. Proctor Harvey deemed so very important in the art of medicine [102]. He served as

President of the American Heart Association from 1969 to 1970 and honored by receiving the James B. Herrick Award in 1978 for his contribution to the teaching of cardiology [100]. As described by Dr. Stephen Ray Mitchell, Dean for Medical Education at Georgetown University School of Medicine, "most would agree he became the father of bedside auscultation across this country and around the world" [101].

Harvey, Michael A. Corrado, and Joseph K. Perloff reported that the murmur of severe aortic insufficiency was located along the right sternal border compared to the more common left sternal border in approximately 20% of patients:

> In some, however, transmission has been atypical in that the murmurs were louder along the *right* sternal border rather than the *left*. This finding of a "right-sided" aortic diastolic murmur has served as an immediate clue that these patients generally represent categories of aortic insufficiency not rheumatic, but of more unusual etiology, and generally associated with dilation and rightward displacement of the aortic root. (…) In addition, "right-sided" aortic diastolic murmurs may also result from deformity limited to the aortic valve itself and without any apparent dilation and rightward displacement of the aortic root [103, p. 29].

They found that the right-sided murmur was more commonly present in patients with an aneurysm and/or dissection of the first portion of the aorta and an aneurysm involving the sinus of Valsalva, syphilis, Marfans's syndrome, hypertension, arteriosclerosis, rheumatoid spondylitis, trauma, and osteogenesis imperfecta, that affect the aortic root and cause dilation and rightward displacement of the aorta. Additionally, a right-sided murmur is found in conditions which affect the aortic valve including bacterial endocarditis, syphilis, trauma, sclerosis, and interventricular septal defects with aortic insufficiency [103] (Table 5.1). Thus, Harvey sign refers to the presence of a right-sided heart murmur in patients with severe aortic insufficiency.

Penny Sign

William J. Penny graduated from medical school at the University College of Cork, Ireland, in 1976 [104]. He was elected Fellow of the Royal College of Physicians (FRCP), Ireland. He serves in the Department of Cardiology at the University of Wales College of Medicine in Cardiff, UK, and has an appointment at Spire Cardiff Hospital [105]. He is an honorary clinical teacher of cardiology at Cardiff University and former President of the Welsh Cardiovascular Society. He previously served on the *Postgraduate Medical Journal* editorial board [106].

Penny described the finding of a pulsating wheal, containing a blanched center and surrounding ring of erythema that was seen on the cheek of a 55-year-old woman with severe aortic insufficiency after an aortogram. He reported this as the "flashing wheal" sign and attributed this finding to the presence of visible dilation of the dermal capillary, a result of the urticarial reaction to contrast [107, p. 1158–1159] (Table 5.1). We are unaware of any study that evaluated the sensitivity or specificity of this sign.

Morton and Mahon Sign

There is limited historical information on G. Morton, a previous trainee of Dr. Mahon. At the time of their publication, they served on staff at the Morriston Hospital, Swansea, Wales, United Kingdom [108]. Simon Mahon received his MB, ChB, in Medicine in 1989 and served as a Clinical Lecturer in Cardiothoracic Anesthesia at the University of Liverpool from 1995 to 1997 [109]. He was a Consultant in Cardiothoracic Anaesthesia and Intensive Care Medicine from 1997 to 2002 at Swansea NHS Trust and at Carmarthenshire NHS Trust from 2002 to 2008 [109]. He was Associate Medical Director of NHS Wales from 2008 to 2009 followed by serving as Executive Medical Director at Hywel Dda Health Board, Wales from 2009 to 2012 [109]. He currently serves as Consultant Anaesthetist at Carmarthen, Carmarthenshire, United Kingdom [109]. They identified in a 79-year-old man with chronic aortic insufficiency, "[f]acial flushing or 'flashing' was continuous and correlated to the upstroke of the arterial waveform and pulse oximeter; it would also blanch with the down stroke of the arterial waveform" [108, p. 501]. They conjectured that "this facial flash may be more pronounced with the patient sitting at approximately 45 degrees head up on the trolley (as on that morning)" [108, p. 502]. Thus, Morton and Mahon sign refers to facial flushing seen in patients with chronic aortic insufficiency (Table 5.1). We are unaware of any study that evaluated the sensitivity or specificity of this sign.

Sherman Sign

Fredrick T. Sherman received his medical degree from Temple University in 1972. He was Clinical Professor of Geriatrics, Palliative Medicine, and Medicine at Mount Sinai Hospital until 2009 [110]. He served as Chief Medical Officer for Community, Managed Care Services from 2009 to 2014 and currently is the founding member and secretary for "Literacy is a Family Experience (LIFE), Inc."[111].

Sherman identified what he referred to as a "geriatric physical sign." He described the distinct findings on physical examination of the dorsalis pedis pulse in elderly patients:

> Any adult age >75, whose dorsalis pedis pulse is quickly located and is unexpectedly prominent, has chronic aortic regurgitation or insufficiency until proven otherwise. The key descriptors are: 1) "quickly" located, i.e., appreciated within 1 to 2 seconds of palpating the dorsum of the foot; and 2) "unexpectedly" prominent with a rapid arterial upstroke [112].

We are unaware of any study that evaluated the sensitivity or specificity of this sign (Table 5.1).

Ashrafian Sign

Hutan Ashrafian received his MBBS degree from the University College of London, Masters of Business Administration from the University of Warwick's Business School, and Doctor of Philosophy from the Imperial College of London [113]. He is a member of the Royal College of Surgeons of England. Since 2017, he has served as honorary senior clinical fellow in surgery at the Imperial College Healthcare NHS trust and Chief Scientific Advisor at the Institute of Global Health Innovation Surgeon for Digital Medical Research, Industry, and Policy at the Imperial College of London [113].

He described the case of a 67-year-old man with chronic aortic insufficiency with "subtle rhythmical anterior propulsion of both eyes that followed the pattern of systole" [114, p. 421]. Although the exact distance measured from the apex of the cornea to a point on the lateral orbital rim using an exopthalmometer was not provided, values greater than 21 mm in Caucasians signifies proptosis [115]. Since this patient did not meet this criterion, the author applied the term "pulsatile pseudoproptosis" to describe the clinical finding [114, p. 421.] He believed that the finding was caused by "increased ocular pulse amplitude" [114, p. 423]. We are unaware of any study that evaluated the sensitivity or specificity of this sign (Table 5.1).

Conclusion

Twenty-three signs have been identified in persons with aortic insufficiency and eponymously ascribed to honor physicians' findings or in the case of de Musset, his brother's observation. For the majority of these eponyms, their sensitivity and specificity have not been studied and thus the utility of these signs in clinical practice is largely unknown. Even among Corrigan, Duroziez, and Hill signs, which have been further assessed, weaknesses in study design and methodology (e.g., selection bias, diagnostic standards used) limits the ability to draw meaningful conclusions regarding their accuracy and validity as bedside tools in clinical practice. Moreover, only two studies assessed the severity of aortic insufficiency for Corrigan and Hill sign using echocardiography and aortography respectively. Only for Hill sign was a correlation found between increasing severity of AR and widening of the popliteal-brachial plexus gradient [24]. Despite these limitations, we believe that it is important that these signs be taught to students and physicians as they reinforce the importance of applying the fundamental aspects of examination in diagnosis, enhance understanding of the pathophysiology of disease, and provide opportunities for further investigation in order to determine their accuracy and validity in clinical practice.

References

1. Dalton C. Chapter 4: Galen. In: Doctrines of the Circulation: A History of Physiological Opinion and Discovery in Regard to the Circulation of the Blood. Philadelphia: Henry C. Leas's Son & Co; 1884. p. 250–1.
2. Galen. Synopsis of chapters. In: Galen on the Natural Facilities. Brock AJ, translator. London: William Heinemann; 1916. p. xliii–1.
3. Vieussens R. De la structure de la surface interne de ventricule gauche du coeur. In: Traité nouveau de la structure et des causes du mouvement naturel du coeur. Toulouse: Jean Guillemette; 1715. p. 101–20.
4. Cowper W. Of ossifications or petrifications in the coats of arteries, particularly in the valves of the great artery. Phil Trans. 1702–1705;23–24:1970–7.
5. Bertin RJH. Introduction. In: Traité des maladies du coeur et des gros vaisseaux. Paris: J.-B. Baillière; 1824. p. xvii–xlviii.
6. Hodgkin T. On retroversion of the valves of the aorta. Lond M Gaz. 1828–1829;3:433–43.
7. Willius FA, Keys TE. Austin Flint (1812–1886). In: Classics of Cardiology, vol 2. New York: Dover Publications; 1941. p. 499–501.
8. Flint A. On the distinctive characters of the pulmonary signs obtained by percussion and auscultation. Am J M Sc. 1862;43–4:305–20.
9. Flint A. On cardiac murmurs. Am J M Sc. 1862;43-4:29–54.
10. [No author]. Obituary: Thomas Cuming. Br Med J. 1887;2:653.
11. Cuming T. A case of diseased heart with observations. Dublin Hosp Rep. 1822;3:319–34.
12. Zacek P. Eponyms linked with aortic regurgitation. In: Vojacek J, Zacek P, Domiik J, editors. Aortic Regurgitation. Cham: Springer International Publishing; 2016. p. 41–2.
13. Kligfield P. An annotation of the pulse in aortic regurgitation: Thomas Cuming, 1822. Am J Card. 1979;44:370–1.
14. Willius FA, Keys TE. Sir Dominic John Corrigan (1802–1880). In: Classics of Cardiology, vol. 2. New York: Dover Publications; 1941. p. 419–22.
15. O'Brien ET. The man behind the eponym: Sir Dominic John Corrigan (1802–1880). N Engl J Med. 1981;304:365–6.
16. [No author]. Obituary: Sir Dominic J Corrigan, Bart M.D. Edin. Lancet. 1880;118:268–9.
17. [No author]. Obituary: Sir Dominic John Corrigan, Bart M.D. Br Med J. 1880;1:227.
18. Major RH. Dominic John Corrigan (1802–1880). In: Classic Descriptions of Disease with Biographical Sketches of the Authors. 3rd ed. Illinois: Charles C. Thomas; 1932. p. 352–6.
19. Corrigan D. Address delivered on the occasion of the distribution of prizes in St. Mary's hospital medical school. Lancet. 1873;2:409–13.
20. Agnew RA. The achievement of Dominic John Corrigan. Med Hist. 1965;9:230–40.
21. Stone J. Sir Dominic John Corrigan. In: Profiles in Cardiology. New Jersey: The Foundation for Advances in Medicine and Science; 2003. p. 64–7.
22. Corrigan DJ. On permanent patency of the mouth of the aorta, or inadequacy of the aortic valves. Edinb Med Surg J. 1832;37:225–45.
23. Hope J. Signs, diagnosis, prognosis, and terminations of disease of the valves: pulses in regurgitation through the aortic valves. In: A Treatise of the Diseases of the Heart and Great Vessels and on the Affections which may be Mistaken for Them. Philadelphia: Lea and Blanchard; 1846. p. 362.
24. Babu AN, Kymes SM, Carpenter-Fryer SM. Eponyms and the diagnosis of aortic regurgitation: what says the evidence? Ann Intern Med. 2004;138:736–42.
25. [No author]. Sir Thomas Watson. Br Med J. 1882;2:1282.
26. [No author]. Obituary: Sir Thomas Watson. Lancet. 1882;2:1131.
27. [No author]. Obituary: Sir Thomas Watson, MD FRS. Med Rec. 1822;22:723.
28. Munk W. Thomas (Sir) Watson Lives of the fellows. Heritage Centre: Royal College of Physicians. London; 2009. http://munksroll.rcplondon.ac.uk/Biography/Details/4657. Accessed 9 Mar 2019.

29. [No author]. Obituary: Sir Thomas Watson. Med Times Gaz. 1882;2:735–7.
30. Watson T. Disease of the heart. In: Lectures on the Principles and Practice of Physic. Philadelphia: Lea and Blanchard; 1844. p. 585–607.
31. Suvarna JCD. Watson's hammer pulse. J Postgrad Med. 2008;54:163–5.
32. Mackenzie J. Valvular defects. In: Diseases of the Heart. London: Oxford Medical Publications; 1918. p. 329–35.
33. Major RH. Paul-Louis Duroziez: diseases of the circulatory system. In: Classic Description of Disease. Illinois: Charles C. Thomas; 1945. p. 363–4.
34. Berry D. History of cardiology: Paul Louis Duroziez, MD. Circulation. 2006;114(22):188.
35. Wilius FE, Keys TE. Paul Louis Duroziez (1826–1897). In: Classic of Cardiology, vol. 2. New York: Dover Publications; 1941. p. 492–6.
36. Duroziez P. Du double souffle intermittent crural, comme signe de l'insuffisance aortique. Arch Gén de Méd. 1861;17:417–43.
37. Virchow R. Zur Erinnerung an L. Traube. Berl klin Wchnschr. 1876;13:209–10.
38. Morrison H. Ludwig Traube. Boston Med Surg J. 1927;196:1097–101.
39. Singer I. Traube, Ludwig. In: The Jewish Encyclopedia, vol. 12. New York: Funk and Wagnalls Company; 1907. p. 235.
40. Brog HW. Flashback on evidence-based medicine: the Prussian *Geheim Rath*. JPANDS. 2015;20:92–4.
41. Fraentzel [O]. Ueber zwei eigentümliche Phänomene bei Insuffizienz der Aortenklappen. Berl klin Wchnschr. 1867;4:355–457.
42. Traube L. Ueber den Doppelton in der Cruralis bei Insuffizienz der Aortenklappen. Berl klin Wchnshr. 1872;9:573–4.
43. Sapira JD. The heart. In: The Art & Science of Bedside Diagnosis. Baltimore: Williams & Wilken; 2012. p. 283–330.
44. Minagar A, Lowis GW. Dr Heinrich Irenaeus Quincke (1842–1922): clinical neurologist of Kiel. J Med Biogr. 2001;9:12–5.
45. [No author]. Obituary: Heinrich Irenaeus Quincke. J Nerv Ment Dis. 1922;56:547–8.
46. Cozanitis DA. Heinrich Irenaeus Quincke (1842–1922): the Nobel Prize but for the problem of age. Presse Med. 2013;42:464–79.
47. [No author]. Obituary: Heinrich Quincke. Lancet. 1922;202:1259.
48. [No author]. Clinical of Kiel: Heinrich Irenaeus Quincke (1842–1922). JAMA. 1966;196:1152–3.
49. Heinrich Quincke. The University of Glasgow Story. University of Glasgow. https://www.universitystory.gla.ac.uk/biography/?id=WH27240&type=P. Accessed 2 May 2019.
50. Pearce JMS. Walter Essex Wynter, Quincke, and lumbar puncture. J Neurol Neurosurg Psychiatry. 1994;57:179.
51. Quincke H. Beobachtungen über capillar- und venenpuls. Berl klin Wchnschr. 1868;5:357–9.
52. Czerny V. Otto Becker gedächtnisrede gehalten im Auftrage der medizinischen Fakultät in der Aula der Universität. Heidelberg: Gustav Koester; 1890. p. 3–12.
53. Becker O. Ueber die sichtbaren Erscheinungen der Blutbewegung in der menschlichen Netzhaut. Arch f Opth. 1872;18:206–96.
54. De Musset A. May night. In: The Poet and the Muse. London: Richard Bentley and Son; 1880. p. 10–17.
55. De Musset P. The Biography of Alfred de Musset. Preston HW, translator. Boston: Roberts Brothers; 1877.
56. Singer I. Haneman FT. Ottomar Ernst Felix. Jewish Encyclopedia. Rosenbach; 1906. http://www.jewishencyclopedia.com/articles/12837-rosenbach-ottomar-ernst-felix. Accessed 10 Mar 2019.
57. Guttman W. Zum andenken an Ottomar Rosenbach. Leipzig: Verlag von J.A. Barth; 1908. p. 5–16.
58. Faber K. Nosography in modern internal medicine. Ann Med Hist. 1922;4:1–63.
59. Morrison H. Ottomar Rosenbach, pioneer in the development of the concept of functional disease and functional diagnosis in internal medicine. Ann Intern Med. 1937;11:527–36.

60. [No author]. Ottomar Rosenbach. Med Brief. 1907;35:367.
61. Rosenbach O. Ueber arterielle Leberpulsation. Deutsche med Wchnschr. 1878;6:498–500, 519–23.
62. Heubner O. Carl Gerhardt. Jahrb f Kinderh. 1902;56:250–2.
63. Jacobi A. In memoriam Carl Gerhardt, birth May 5, 1833, died July 21, 1902. In: Robinson WJ, editor. Miscellaneous Addresses and Writings, vol. 7. New York: The Critic and Guide Company; 1909. p. 499–500.
64. Gerhardt C. Metallklang. In: Lehrbuch der Auscultation und Percussion: mit besonderer Berücksichtigung der Besichtigung, Betastung und Messung der Brust und des Unterleibes zu diagnostischen Zwecken. Tübingen: Verlag der H. Laupp'schen Buchhandlung; 1833. p. 184–7.
65. Hall CW. Gerhardt, Karl Jakob Christian Adolph. In: A Biographical Dictionary of People in Engineering: From the Earliest Records to 2000. Indiana: Purdue University Press; 2008. p. 81.
66. Medvei VC. The story of insulin. In: The History of Clinical Endocrinology. Carnforth, Lancs: The Parthenon Publishing Group; 1993. p. 249–57.
67. White FA. Gerhardt's sign. In: Physical Signs in Medicine and Surgery: Rare, Lost and Forgotten Physical Signs. Ocala: Museum Press Books; 2009. p. 106.
68. Gerhardt C. Pulsierender milztumor. Ztschr f klin Med. 1882;4:449–50.
69. Gerhardt C. Aorteninsuffizienz und milz pulsationen. Centralbl f klin Med. 1888;9:1–4.
70. Wormer EJ. Müller, Friedrich von. Neue deutsche Biographie. 1997;18:379–81.
71. [No author]. Friedrich von Muller. Br Med J. 1951;2:340.
72. Biografie, Friedrich von Muller. Wissenschaftliche sammlungen. Teil-Katalog der wissenschaftlichen sammlungen. Humbolot-Universitat zu Berlin. https://www.sammlungen.hu-berlin.de/objekte/-/17224/. Accessed 15 May 2019.
73. [No author]. Friedrich von Müller and William Osler. N Engl J Med. 1955;252(2):76–7.
74. Mueller F. Pulsation des Gaumens bei Aorteninsuffizienz. In: Zur Pathologie des weichen Gaumens. Berlin: Charité-Annalen; 1889. p. 251–2.
75. Douglas CG. Leonard Erskine Hill, 1866–1952. Biographical memoirs of fellows of the Royal Society: The Royal Society Publishing; 1953. https://royalsocietypublishing.org/doi/abs/10.1098/rsbm.1953.0009. Accessed 10 May 2019.
76. Hill AB, Hill B. The life of Sir Leonard Erskine Hill FRS (1866–1952). Proc Roy Soc Med. 1968;61(3):307–16.
77. [No author]. Group Captain Martin Flack, C.B.E. Br Med J. 1931;2(3686):402–4.
78. [No author]. Major (Hon. Lt.-Col) Martin William Flack, M.B., Central Chancery of the Orders of Knighthood, Royal Air Force. Lond M Gaz. 1918;31098:92.
79. Dr. Wilfred Watkinson Holtzmann BS MB FRCS. The West Dorset Hanns. 2019. https://www.hannfamily.org.uk/Hannfamily-o/p79.htm. Accessed 2 Jun 2019.
80. Watkinson, Wilfred (1877–1944). Royal College of Surgeons. Plarr's Lives of the Fellows. The Royal College of Surgeons of England. 2013. https://livesonline.rcseng.ac.uk/client/en_GB/lives/search/detailnonmodal/ent:$002f$002fSD_ASSET$002f0$002f376931/one?qu=%22rcs%3A+E004748%22&rt=false%7C%7C%7CIDENTIFIER%7C%7C%7Cresource+Identifier. Accessed 6 May 2019.
81. Hill L, Flack M, Holtzman W. The measurement of systolic blood pressure in man. Heart. 1909;1:73–82.
82. Hill L, Rowlands RA. Systolic blood pressure: (1) in change of posture, (2) in cases of aortic regurgitation. Heart. 1911-1912;3:219–22.
83. Frank MJ, Casanegra P, Migliori AJ, Levinson GE. The clinical evaluation of aortic regurgitation. Arch Intern Med. 1965;116:219–23.
84. Landolfi M. Un nouveau signe de l'insuffisance aortique: l'hippus circulatoire. Semaine méd. 1909;29:349.
85. Minervini L. L'universita italiana. Rivista dell'istruzione superiore. 1924;20:152.
86. Minervini L. Le pouls de la langue dans l'insuffisance aortique. Semaine méd. 1910;30:481–90.

87. [No author]. Joseph Sailer RD. Am J Surg. 1929;7:576–8.
88. Sailer J. Pulsating spleen in aortic insufficiency. Am Heart J. 1928;3:447–53.
89. [No author]. Francis Winslow Palfrey, 1876–1953. N Engl J Med. 1953;9:383–4.
90. [No author]. Corporation records. The Harvard Graduates' Magazine. 1917;26:103–300.
91. Francis Winslow Palfrey, Clinical Medicine. [Internet]. Assistants. Quinquennial Catalogue of the Officers and Graduates of Harvard University. 1636–1910. Cambridge Massachusetts. Published by the University 1910. https://books.google.com/books?id=J3MqAAAAYAAJ&pg=PA105&lpg=PA105&dq=Francis+Winslow+Palfrey&source=bl&ots=omHzd6Voki&sig=FlvffU8Fg-qiV3Vi1AtF8lghmBE&hl=en&sa=X&ved=2ahUKEwiD4oGAxb7fAhUBba0KHUyHDcwQ6AewD3oECAMQAQ#v=onepage&q=Francis%20Winslow%20Palfrey&f=false. Accessed 20 Mar 2019.
92. Palfrey FW. Auscultation of the Corrigan or water-hammer pulse. N Engl J Med. 1952;247:771–2.
93. Irish Cardiac Society. Annual Scientific Meeting & AGM. 6–8 October 2016 Newpark Hotel, Kilkenny, Ireland. http://www.irishcardiacsociety.com/documents/ICS_AGM_Prog_2016_SCREEN.pd. Accessed 10 May 2019.
94. Meath Hospital, Dublin: annual report for the year ended 31st December 1979. Lenus The Irish Health Repository. https://www.lenus.ie/bitstream/handle/10147/45526/8189.pdf?sequence=1&isAllowed=y. Accessed 5 May 2019.
95. Mayne B. On aortic regurgitation: a new physical sign. Ir J Med Sci. 1953;6:80–1.
96. Happes M, Kamran H, Salciccioli L, Ko EH, Lazar JM. Mayne's sign is mainly related to younger age and not to aortic regurgitation. Blood Press Monit. 2010;15:305–7.
97. Abbas F, Sapira JD. Mayne's sign is not pathognomonic of aortic insufficiency. South Med J. 1987;80:1051–2.
98. Dennison AD Jr. Aortic regurgitation multiple eponyms, physical signs and etiologies. J Indiana State Med Assoc. 1958;52:1283–9.
99. Leonard JJ. Profiles in cardiology: W. Proctor Harvey. Clin Cardiol. 1991;14:180–2.
100. Biography of W. Proctor Harvey. Georgetown University School of Medicine. https://som.georgetown.edu/harveysociety/harveyfounderbio. Accessed 12 Apr 2019.
101. Robertson E. Watkins Proctor Harvey, cardiologist, dies at 89. Richmond Times Dispatch. 7 Oct 2007.
102. W. Proctor Harvey Amphitheater. Notes from Neil. Sunday, October 25, 2015. http://medstarresearch.blogspot.com/2015/10/w-proctor-harvey-amphitheater.html. Accessed 10 May 2019.
103. Harvey WP, Corrado MA, Perloff JK. Right-sided murmurs of aortic insufficiency (diastolic murmurs better heard to the right of the sternum rather than the left). Am J Med Sci. 1963;245:29–43.
104. Dr. William Penny. British Cardiovascular Society. http://www.bcs.com/programmesessions/biog.asp?bcsid=805. Accessed 14 May 2019.
105. Dr. William J Penny, Consultant Cardiologist MD, FRCP. Spire Cardiff Hospital. https://www.spirehealthcare.com/spire-cardiff-hospital/consultants/dr-w-j-penny-c1390182/. Accessed 10 Jan 2019.
106. William J Penny (Cardiff, UK) editorial board Postgrad Med J. The journal of continuing professional development. 2006. https://pmj.bmj.com/content/postgradmedj/82/964.toc.pdf. Accessed 12 May 2019.
107. Penny WJ. The sign of the flashing wheal in aortic regurgitation. Am J Cardiol. 1988;6:1158–9.
108. Morton G, Mahon S. The facial flushing or aortic regurgitation. Anaesthesia. 2002;57:501–2.
109. Dr. Simon Mahon. Linkedin. https://www.linkedin.com/in/dr-simon-mahon-22816a43/?originalSubdomain=uk. Accessed 4 Mar 2020.
110. Fredrick T Sherman. Mount Sinai. Ichan School of Medicine at Mount Sinai. https://www.mountsinai.org/profiles/fredrick-t-sherman. Accessed 10 May 2019.
111. Fredrick T. Sherman MD, MSc. Linkedin. https://www.linkedin.com/in/fredrick-t-sherman-md-msc-a25a1823. Accessed 10 May 2019.

112. Sherman FT. Sherman sign predicts aortic regurgitation: from foot fetish to clinical pearl. Geriatrics. 2004;59:7.
113. Hutain Ashrafian. Likedin. https://www.likedin.com/in/hutan-ashrafian-2a8993169/. Accessed 10 May 2019.
114. Ashrafian H. Pulsatile pseudo-proptosis, aortic regurgitation and 31 eponyms. Int J Cardiol. 2008;107:421–3.
115. Henkind P, Priest RS, Schiller G. Prolapse of iris, surgical proptosis. In: Compendium of Ophthalmology. Philadelphia: J.B. Lippincott Company; 1983. p. 242.

Chapter 6
Tricuspid Insufficiency Murmurs

Introduction

The word "tricuspid" is derived from the Latin, *tri* (three) and *cuspis* (cuspidis, a projection or point). Thus, the tricuspid valve is the anatomical structure in the heart with three valve leaflets (cusps) which separates the right atrium and ventricle. A variety of bedside signs have been discovered during the physical examination in patients with tricuspid insufficiency (TI) as a means to differentiate and diagnose this disease. These signs were elicited by examiners who applied one or more key fundamental physical examination skills including observation, palpation, auscultation, and passive maneuvers to identify or unmasked underlying TI. These signs have been eponymously named to honor those physicians' contributions to medicine. With the exception of Pasteur (abdominojugular test) and Carvallo signs, the majority have not been well studied and thus their utility in clinical practice remains unknown. Despite the lack of consistent performance, technique, and case definition; the presence of a positive abdominojugular test increases the probability for diagnosing conditions that cause elevated right atrial or ventricular filling pressure and thus represents an accurate indirect method for determining whether the left atrial pressure is increased or pulmonary capillary wedge pressures ≥15 mmHg on cardiac catheterization. An understanding of the historical significance of these signs as originally described provides an appreciation for these findings and reinforces the importance of applying bedside techniques during the physical examination. Knowledge of these signs may also enhance one's understanding of the pathophysiology of disease and provide opportunities for further investigation.

The history of the tricuspid valve dates back to Erasistratus (c. 304 BC – c. 250 BC) who is believed to be the first to identify and describe this membrane (valve) [1]. Since his original writings were lost in antiquity, they were described later by Galen of Pergamon:

S. H. Yale et al., *Cardiovascular Eponymic Signs*,
https://doi.org/10.1007/978-3-030-67596-7_6

> Erasistratus, in his treatise on fevers, has described how membranes are attached to the mouths of the vessels which serve the heart in the alternate reception and expulsion of materials. Some have ventured to deny the existence of these membranes, implying that they were made up by Erasistratus for the purpose of supporting his doctrine; but they have now come to be so well known to physicians generally, that one would seem very ill informed not to be acquainted with them. At the mouth of the vena cava there are three, shaped very much like spear points; whence, I suppose, they were called "tricuspids" by some of the Erasistrateans [2, p. 250].

Hombert described in 1704 in his paper "Observation sur un battement de veines semblable au battement des artères" (Observation of the beat of the veins like the beat of the arteries), the finding of a pulsation within the cervical (jugular) vein:

> [t]hese violent contractions are joined to the heart's normal contractions, compressing the blood contained in its cavities more violently than by its normal contractions. These violent contractions mixes the blood in the veins causing repulsion of the valves such that they are pried open by the violent effort forced upon them by the heart. The blood repulses by jerks, causing the veins to swelling at intervals and giving the impression that they can be measured. This is similar to the pulsation normally felt in the arteries closest to the heart. These pulsations were caused by the forceful contractions of the heart and exactly follow each contractions. They are different from pulsations within the arteries, which have always seemed to me to have a single contraction independent of the heart. It is possible to compare this unusual reflux of blood in the veins with the swelling and repulsion of the flowing waters of the rivers by the high tides. The extraordinary swelling of the veins, which is always observed in this patient caused by the clogged arteries, gives us an opportunity to easily explain all the symptoms with which he was afflicted [3, p. 161].

Since the eighteenth century, a variety of signs have been identified on physical examination through observation, or elicited through palpation of the abdomen or other maneuvers, to confirm the diagnosis of TI. These signs have been named eponymously to honor the person's discovery. Our goal in this chapter is to provide a brief historical background of the person and sign as originally reported, and if known, its sensitivity, specificity, and utility in clinical practice. The signs are described chronologically from the date they were first reported.

Signs

Lancisi Sign

Joannis (Giovanni) Maria Lancisi (1654–1720) was born in Rome, Italy, and received his doctor of medicine and philosophy degrees from the Collegio di Sapienza in 1672 [4, 5]. He served as assistant physician at San Spirito Hospital in Sassia, Rome in 1676, appointed professor of anatomy in 1684, and professor of theory and medical practice at Collegio di Sapienza in 1697 [4]. As papal physician to Pope Innocent XI in 1688 and later Innocent XII and his successor Clement XI, he was bestowed the illustrious title "Physician to the Pontiff" [5, 6]. In his first book *De Subitaneis Mortibus* (On Sudden Death) published in 1707, Lancisi recognized that heart disease and recurrent syncope are causes of sudden death [7]. In the second part of his treatise, *De Motu Cordis et Aneurysmatibus* (On the Motion of the Heart and on Aneurysms) published in 1728, he wrote about the causes (hereditary, intra- and extra-mechanical obstruction, syphilis, and emotions) and signs of right cardiac enlargement (pulsation of jugular veins) [8]. Lancisi's contributions and influences in medicine spanned multiple different areas including anatomy, pathology, epidemiology, and clinical practice. His work can best be described as applied anatomy and clinicopathologic correlate to disease [9]. In the field of epidemiology, he recognized the role and habitat of the mosquito in causing malaria and thus provided some of the earliest evidence of zoonotic disease, its transmission, and prevention. His work is significant in that it provided the foundation for the pathological description of heart disease [9].

Lancisi described in the second part of his two-part treatise published posthumously in 1728 titled *De Motu Cordis et Aneurysmatibus*, his observation and cause for dilation of the jugular vein:

> From the dilation of the right auricle and ventricle there are two especially important results that are worth most careful consideration, for it I they above all that bring about the alternating dilation of the jugulars. In the first place, when thee cavities are extremely dilated and enlarged, a far too large amount of blood is collected in them; next, the orifice of the stem of the vena cava also becomes too large for it to be completely closed by the valves attached to it. Thus, it comes to pass that, when the heart contracts, the blood from the right ventricle is not only propelled to the lungs through the pulmonary artery, but both because of its excessive amount and on account of the incompletely closed valve at the mouth of vena cava, it is driven back again through the gaping chink of the valves and forced back along the whole path of the superior vena cava; then from that path it flows straight on into the jugulars more violently than into the other branches of the cava, because the jugulars are situated directly in line with this motion of the blood. (…) This dilation is more apparent in the neck, because there, bedside the ordinary integuments, there occur neither muscle nor anything else that can compress or conceal it. But when systole of the heart cease, the blood without delay flows back downward from the jugulars into the vena cava; hence the jugulars cease to swell and in their turn collapse [10, p. 309].

Morgagni believed that dilation of the right ventricle did not account for all cases of jugular venous distension:

> Lancisi proposed this venous pulsation as a diagnostic of dilation in the right cavities of the heart; but it sometimes arises where no such enlargement had taken place. If, for instance, either of the tricuspid valves become contracted or inflexible, it will consequently be incapacitated to perform its functions; or if any of the chordae tendineae are ulcerated, ruptured, or relaxed, and thus rendered inadequate to retain the valve in its situation, so as to close the orifice, some blood will return into the veins when the ventricle contracts. Certainly this symptom often indicates dilation of the right cavities of the heart; but occasionally it denotes some other affection which either exists in those cavities, or, at least, maintains such a relation to them as to interfere with the transmission of blood through the right side of this organ [11, p. 340].

Thus, Lancisi sign refers to dilation of the jugular veins in the neck occurring during systole and their collapse during diastole due to right ventricle enlargement (Table 6.1).

Table 6.1 Tricuspid insufficiency (TI) signs

Name	Year	Description of sign	Method
Lancisi [10]	1745	Dilation of the jugular veins in the neck occurring during systole and their collapse during diastole caused by right ventricle enlargement.	Observation
Pasteur [17]	1885	Distension, with or without pulsation, of the superficial veins of the neck occurring when firm pressure is exerted over the liver in the direction of the spinal column.	Observation Palpation
Carvallo [32]	1946	The murmur is produced by asking the patient to take a deep breath or to hold his/her breath after a deep inspiration. In some patients the murmur may occur during normal inspiration. The greater intensity of the murmur may be with changes in pitch. The maximum intensity is found at the tricuspid area, but the site may be located either to the right or to the left of the sternum. Furthermore, an increased murmur may also be heard close to the apex.	Auscultation
Terry [35]	1959	In TI, a ventricular extrasystole does not result in either an arterial pulsation or a second heart sound. It does however cause substantial pulsation in the jugular veins. Furthermore, if the normal ventricular systoles are causing expansile hepatic pulsation, the ventricular extrasystoles will usually create an easily perceptible hepatic pulsation. If hepatic pulsation occurs in the absence of TI, the pulsations are transmitted from the abdominal aorta. In this instance, an extrasystole that fails to produce an arterial pulsation will also fail to produce a hepatic pulsation.	Observation
Luisada [39]	1967	Movement of the head to the right occurring during the period of collapse of the distended jugular vein and diastolic rumble murmur on the right side of heart.	Observation
Vitums [41]	1969	Passive elevation of the legs increases the intensity of the TI murmur.	Maneuver
Byrd [44]	1984	Lateral pulsation of the earlobe in patients with TI.	Observation
Chow [45]	1990	Pulsatile varicose veins with a prominent systolic wave. The pulsations persist despite elevation of the legs.	Observation Maneuver

Pasteur Sign

William Pasteur (1885–1943) was born in Geneva, Switzerland, and received his medical degree from the University College Hospital, London in 1880 [12]. He was an assistant followed by honorary staff physician to the Middlesex Hospital and Queen's Hospital for Children in Bethnal Green, eventually assuming the title of consulting physician [13, 14]. In 1891, he was elected Fellow of the Royal College of Physicians (FRCP), London, and served as dean of Middlesex Medical School from 1896 to 1902 [13, 15]. He served on the Cancer Investigation Committee of the Middlesex Hospital from 1908 to 1909 [16].

As a description of his character as written in his obituary:

> A man of inborn dignity, with a straightforward and kindly manner which reflected his true nature, Dr. William Pasteur was looked up to by all. Here one felt, is a physician who will give his whole mind to the case and treat it with wisdom and understanding. Such clinical teachers leave the mark of their personality on a receptive student when he passes into practice [13].

W. Pasteur described a sign of TI (Fig. 6.1) which, "[c]onsists in a distension, with or without pulsation of the superficial veins of the neck, occurring when firm pressure is exerted over the liver in the direction of the spinal column, and independent of the movements of respiration." [17]. He believed that the sign is useful in "cases where the usual signs of tricuspid regurgitation are ill-developed or in abeyance, and that it may prove a valuable factor in the difficult general problem of prognosis in cases of cardiac disease" [17]. Pasteur was only able to elicit this sign in cases of liver enlargement caused by chronic passive congestion [17] (Table 6.1).

It should be recognized that it was Rondot who coined the term "hepatojugular reflux":

> In a certain number of morbid conditions accompanied by dilation of the right heart with more or less marked insufficiency of the myocardium, the compression of the liver causes a sudden swelling of the superficial jugular veins, to which may be called the hepato-jugular reflux, for distension occurs from bottom to top, beginning at the superior border of the clavicle, in the opposite direction of the normal course of blood in these vessels [18, p. 567].

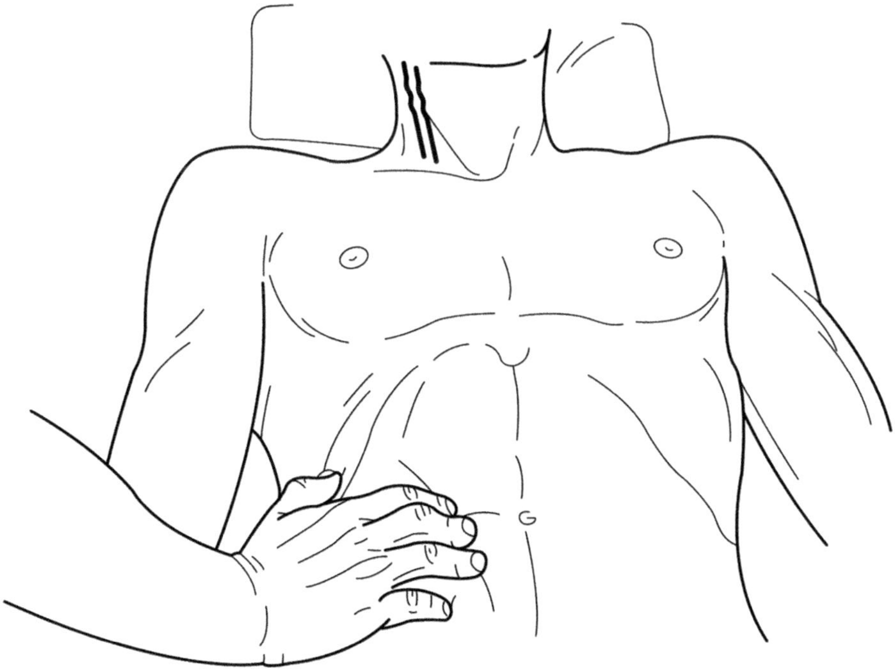

Fig. 6.1 Pasteur sign (by Ryan Yale)

He used bimanual compression of the liver since he was unable to elicit the sign when compressing the posterior part as described by Pasteur. Rondot identified factors which limits the performance of this test including obesity, ascites, and marked abdominal distention. When performing the maneuver he reported:

> But a very important point of the technique consists in making sure that the patient does not make a respiratory effort and does not stop breathing. If the patient resists the compression, ask him to breathe normally and gently succeed in obtaining the reflux by increasing the degree of inward pressure. (…) In order to elicit the phenomenon in question, it is preferable to place the subject horizontally with the lower limbs flexed. Compression is performed backwards, by supporting and preventing the inward movement of the hypochondrium by the left hand, and by depressing the abdominal wall backwards and forwards sufficiently vigorously below the right false ribs. This bi-manual palpation is generally well tolerated if care is taken to gradually increase the compression in cases where the liver is painful. (…) After drawing the dullness of the heart, one frequently can recognize where the reflux occurs. The area of dullness to the right of the sternum below the second intercostal space widens almost instantaneously. In 7 cases, this amplification oscillated between 2 and 8 centimeters, disappeared with the decompression of the liver, and reoccurred each time it was applied. (…) The auscultation of the heart performed while a helper exercised the compression of the liver, allowed me to identify other changes including a very faint and low tone of the first tricuspid sound, and in a single case the very clear attenuation of a xiphoidal murmur which in some cases occurred in a less obvious manner [18, p. 568].

Hepatojugular reflex or more aptly referred to as abdominojugular test is used to assess central venous pressure in patients with left or right ventricular failure. Physicians have modified the definition of the Pasteur sign by quantifying the significance of a positive test result. Hence a positive test is a sustained elevation of the jugular venous pulse greater than 3–4 cm above the sternal notch for 10–15 seconds [19–22]. A fall of the jugular venous pulse more than 4 cm upon release of the abdominal pressure has also been proposed as a positive test [22]. Another method described by Burch is to press firmly over the periumbilical area for 30 seconds. The height or the fall from baseline of 4 cm in the jugular venous pulsation is a positive test [23]. To the best of our knowledge, there are no studies that directly compared these techniques. Nevertheless as articulated by Brostoff, it is important that abdominal pressure be maintained for 30 seconds, confirm that the elevated JVP is sustained and not transient, and avoid pressing directly over the liver since it may be painful for the patient [24]. Burch developed an ingenious device in an attempt to standardize and quantitate the amount of pressure applied over the hepatic area when performing abdominojugular reflux test [23].

The interobserver agreement while assessing the abdominojugular test in patients with heart failure ranged from 92% to 97% confirming good reproducibility among different examiners [25, 26]. The presence of this sign has been found to enhance the probability of identifying patients with congestive heart failure and an elevated left atrial pressure or pulmonary capillary wedge pressure (PCWP) >15 mmHg on cardiac catheterization [25, 27, 28]. Thus, a positive result increases and its absence decreases the probability of heart failure.

In The Evaluation Study of Congestive Heart Failure and Pulmonary Artery Catheterization Effectiveness (ESCAPE) study among 186 patients with a PCWP >22 mmHg identified during cardiac catheterization, 147 (65%) were found on examination to have a positive and 39 (51%) negative hepatojugular reflux. Neither the method of performing the test or cutoff used for a positive test was specified. Overall, a sensitivity of 65%, specificity of 64%, positive likelihood ratio (LR) 1.79, and negative LR 1.82 were reported [29]. The lack of standardization for performing and defining a positive test may have contributed to the reduced accuracy of the abdominojugular test in identifying elevated left atrial pressure compared to earlier studies [29]. A positive test is attributed to a variety of causes that leads to the inability of right heart to handle additional increases in venous return. These include such condition as right ventricular failure, tricuspid regurgitation (TR) and stenosis, constrictive pericarditis, cardiac tamponade, and left ventricular failure with elevated left atrial pressure.

Variations in LRs may be due to differences in techniques and definition of a positive test result used when performing the test. As originally described by Pasteur, firm pressure is applied using a single hand exerted over the liver in the direction of the spinal column independent of respiratory movements. Rondot described a bimanual technique with the patients in the supine position with knee flexed. Pressure is applied with the left hand in the left hypochondrium right hand over the right false ribs posteriorly and cephald. He specified that the test should not be performed during deep inspiration.

Although the pathogenesis of the test is unknown, two prevailing theories include (1) increased systemic venous pressure in the setting of increased venous tone and/or (2) dilation of the inferior vena caused by the increased systemic venous pressures [23, 24]. In both cases, increased blood volume in these vessels is shifted from the smaller (e.g., splanchnic) to larger central veins (e.g., jugular veins, and inferior vena cava) which are unable to adjust to changes in volume when compressed due to their high venous tone.

Carvallo Sign

José Manuel Rivero Carvallo (1905–1993) was born in Tehuacán, Puebla, Mexico and received his medical training at his home country, then the University of Sorbonne, Paris, graduating from the latter in 1932 [30]. After graduation, he served as a member of the cardiology clinic at the Hôpital de la Pitié, Paris [30]. He returned to Mexico in 1934 and was appointed to Pavilion 21 of the General Hospital in Mexico City [31]. From 1944 to 1970, he served as head of clinical services and clinical researcher, as well as Professor of Medical Clinic in the Faculty of Medicine at the Universidad Nacional Autónoma de México (UNAM) [31].

Carvallo described a method for eliciting or increasing the intensity of the tricuspid murmur:

> The murmur is produced by ordering the patient to make deep inspirations or to hold his breath after a deep inspiration; a very small period of inspiratory apnea as seen during the examination when children cry, may be enough to make the acoustic change noticeable. In some patients the characteristic murmur can be noticed during normal inspiration. The greater intensity of the murmur may be associated or not with changes in pitch; the increase of intensity is almost always absolute. (…) The maximum intensity belong

> to the tricuspidal focus, but the site may be changed either to the right or to the left of the sternal bone; there were cases recorded where increase of the murmur was heard close to the apex [32, p. 539].

Carvallo found that this sign was present in 50 patients (90%) with TI. Validation studies reported a sensitivity ranging from 61% to 100%. Cha et al., using intracardiac phonocardiography in 35 patients with valvular heart disease, confirmed on right ventriculography and intracardiac phonocardiography Carvallo sign in 19 (54%) of the patients. In 16 patients with a Carvallo sign, TI was confirmed as being absent in five patients. Findings from this study suggest that this sign, if present, is useful for confirming TI but its absence does not exclude the diagnosis [33] (Table 6.1).

There is another sign named eponymously for Carvallo which he reported in 1962 in his paper titled "El signo de doble choque apexiano" (Sign of the double apical thrust) as a method to differentiate true (mitral) from apparent (tricuspid) apex of the heart. He recognized that in some patients with disease involving the tricuspid valve, the right heart becomes hypertrophied and dilates causing it to rotate clockwise along its longitudinal axis and counterclockwise around its transverse axis. This causes the right ventricle to occupy the position previously assumed by the left (anterior and lateral aspect) of the heart while the left ventricle shifts backward:

> [t]he patient is placed on his back and the apex area is found. The palm of the hand is placed over this area while the tips of the fingers are placed from the 4th to the 7th left intercostal spaces at the level of the left axillary line. Without separating the hand the patient is asked to turn to his left at which time, a new apical thrust appears under the tips of the explorer's fingers which is the true apex. The other thrust was actually the apparent apex [34, p. 397].

The double apical thrust sign was used to identify TI in patients with concomitant mitral insufficiency.

Terry Sign

There is limited historical information on R. Barratt Terry. At the time of the publication of his paper describing his sign, he was a member of the departments of medicine at Passavant Memorial Hospital, Northwestern University Medical School, and Cook County Hospital, Chicago, Illinois. He described a bedside method to differentiate hepatic pulsation due to TI murmur from those transmitted by the abdominal aorta in cases of ventricular extrasystole(s):

> In tricuspid incompetence, such a ventricular extrasystole also fails to create an arterial pulsation or a second heart sound, but it does cause substantial pulsation in the jugular veins; and, if the normal ventricular systoles are causing expansile hepatic pulsation, the ventricular extrasystoles will usually create an easily perceptible hepatic pulsation. If there is hepatic pulsation in the absence of tricuspid incompetence, it is transmitted from the abdominal aorta. In this instance, an extrasystole that fails to produce an arterial pulsation will also fail to produce hepatic pulsation [35, p. 158].

Terry identified in a patient with TI and ventricular bigeminy caused by digitalis intoxication:

> [e]ach normal systole results in simultaneous palpable carotid pulsation, visible jugular pulsation, and palpable hepatic pulsation; each ventricular extrasystole results in simultaneous jugular and hepatic pulsation, but no arterial pulsation occurs and no second heart sound is produced. The persistent occurrence of two hepatic pulsation for each single arterial pulsation is a striking clinical phenomenon as well as a useful physical sign [35, p. 158].

Thus, Terry sign refers to the presence of jugular venous distention and hepatic pulsation, without either a palpable arterial pulsation or second heart sound, heard during auscultation in patients with TI and premature ventricular contractions. It also serves as a method to differentiate hepatic pulsation caused by TI from abdominal aortic aneurysms (Table 6.1).

Luisada Sign

Aldo Augusto Luisada (1901–1987) was born in Florence, Italy, and received his medical degree in 1924, graduating cum laude from Royal University, Florence, Italy [36]. Prior to immigrating to the United States in 1939, he served at the Royal University in Naples (1931 to 1935) and in Sassari, Italy (1935 to 1936) as faculty and professor of medicine respectively [36]. From 1943 to 1949, he was appointed to the faculty at Tufts College School of Medicine, Boston, Professor of Medicine, and from 1949 to 1971 was Chief of Cardiovascular Research at the Chicago Medical School and Chairman of Cardiovascular Medicine at Mt. Sinai Hospital, Chicago. This was followed by an appointment as Chairman of the Department of Cardiology, Oak Forest Hospital, Illinois from 1971 to 1983 [36, 37]. He authored 5 textbooks, 11 monographs, and over 400 publications [37]. Even after retirement, he remained active in medicine volunteering at the Downey Veterans Administration and Michael Reese Hospital and Medical Center [37]. As a description of his character:

> [A]ldo Luisada embodies qualities of greatness that elude enumeration; he has been more than a teacher. Countless cardiologist are indebted to him for his years of dedication in his chosen field and for his training of young physicians. His presence on the cardiologic scene has been and continues to be a stimulus and inspiration [38].

Aldo Luisada, Stanley Wissner, and Parkash D. Gupta observed the finding of core pulmonale secondary to primary pulmonary hypertension in a 51-year-old male with, “[a] rhythmic motion of the head toward the right at each heart beat.” [39, p. 141]. A recording of the head movement, “showed that the largest movement occurred during the systolic collapse of the jugular vein (which was larger on the right side) in coincidence with the functional diastolic rumble (tricuspid flow murmur).” [39, p. 142].

Thus, Luisada sign refers to the movement of the head to the right occurring during the period of collapse of the distended jugular vein and diastolic rumble murmur in the right side of heart in patients with TI (Table 6.1).

Vitums Sign

Vitolds C. Vitums graduated from George Washington School of Medicine in 1968 [40]. At the time of his publication he was an intern in Medicine at George Washington University Division, Veterans Administration Hospital. Vitums, Gooch, and Evans assessed the effectiveness of three maneuvers that increased the intensity of the TI murmur: (1) Carvallo sign or increased in the intensity of the systolic murmur following deep inspiration, (2) gentle compression by the palm of the examiner's hand beneath the right costal margin or the lower liver edge for approximately 5 second, (3) passive elevation of the patient's legs by an additional person (…) [41, p. 533].

They found that liver squeeze (pressure) or leg raising was most effective method to increase the intensity of the TI murmur:

> When inspiration fails to cause transient hemodynamic alterations to a degree which causes changes in the physical signs emanating from the right heart. (…) The aim is to further augment systemic venous return and thereby exaggerate the flow differentials to the right and left heat chambers [41, p. 535].

Thus, Vitums sign refers to passive elevation of the legs as a method to augment blood volume to the right side of the heart and thereby increasing the intensity of the TI murmur (Table 6.1, Fig. 6.2).

Byrd Sign

Milton Daniel Byrd (1939–) was born in Atlanta, Georgia, and graduated from Emory University School of Medicine in 1964. He completed his internship and internal medicine residency at Georgia Baptist Hospital, Atlanta, Georgia (currently WellStar Atlanta Medical Center) [42]. He received his cardiology training under Joseph Gordon Barrow, Gerald Fletcher, and Henry Joseph Llewellyn Marriott among others. Byrd was Clinical Professor of Medicine and Cardiology at Emory University School of Medicine. He is currently in private practice at the WellStar Atlanta Medical Center [43]. He served on the executive committee and was appointed Chief of Staff at Georgia Baptist Hospital and is a member of the American College of Physicians, American Society of Internal Medicine, American College of Cardiology, and American Heart Association [42].

Byrd described his experience with the possible pathognomonic sign of lateral pulsation of the earlobe in patients with TI. He noted that earlobe pulsation may occur "even if the typical deep jugular V waves are not prominent." Furthermore, "this earlobe pulsation may occur when the TR is not severe enough to produce the more easily recognized deep jugular vein systolic V wave" [44].

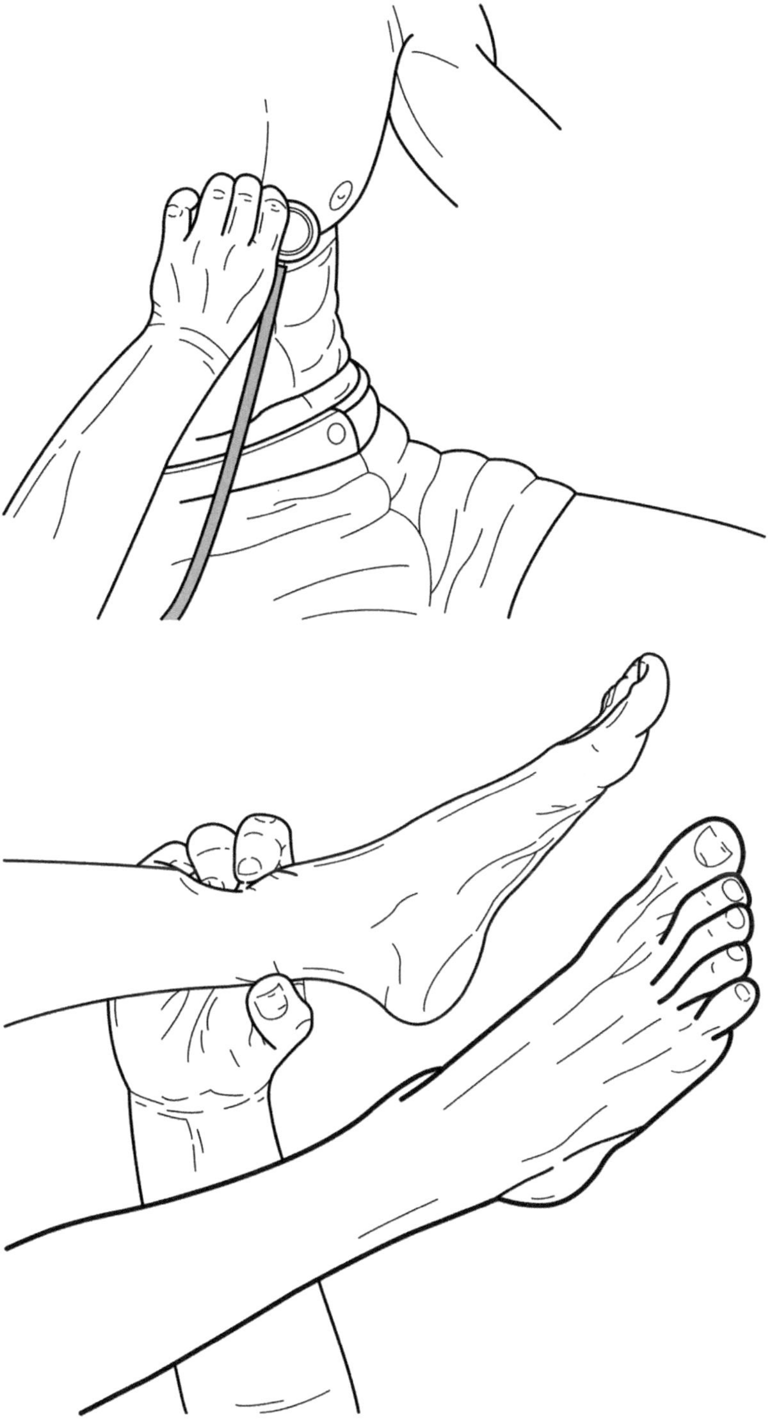

Fig. 6.2 Vitums sign (by Ryan Yale)

He also recognized that this phenomenon is also present in patients with diastolic dysfunction, pulmonary hypertension, cardiac cirrhosis, and TR, and resolves with treatment of the underlying disease [43]. Thus, the presence of this sign in other diseases suggests that it lacks sufficient specificity to be used in the clinical diagnosis of TI (Table 6.1).

Chow Sign

There is limited historical information on W.H. Chow. At the time of his publication with K.L. Cheung, he served in the Department of Medicine at the Graham Hospital in Aberdeen, Hong Kong. W.H. Chow and K.L. Cheung observed the finding in a 51-year-old female with mitral stenosis TI caused by rheumatic heart disease and serve saphenous venous varicosities, "[t]he varicose veins pulsated with a prominent systolic wave. (…) The pulsation persisted despite the elevation of her legs, indicating that her TI was severe" [45]. Thus, Chow sign refers to the presence of pulsation of the saphenous vein during systolic ventricular contraction (Table 6.1).

Conclusion

Signs of TI involve using the physical examination skills of observation, palpation, auscultation, and passive elevation of the extremities. Luisada, Chow, and Vitums signs are examples where although other physicians' names were listed on the publication, only one name is associated with the eponymic sign. In these cases it may have been due to that he was either the first or most senior author at the time of the publication. Despite these contentions regarding the use of eponymous signs, they are for the most part ingrained in the medical literature. Most signs have not been studied and thus their utility as a bedside diagnostic tool remains unknown. The hepatojugular reflux or more correctly referred to as abdominojugular test is a notable exception identified in this review. This test has been so modified since its initial description by Pasteur in 1888 in an attempt to quantitate, and thereby, standardize the meaning of a positive test. However, the lack of a consistent standard case definition limits the ability to compare different studies. As emphasized by one author, it is important that the test be performed exactly as described in the study in order to obtain similar results [20, 21]. Despite the fact that many of these signs have not been further studied, we content that they are important and be taught to students as they are valuable in emphasizing the importance of observation and palpation during the physical examination. The use of maneuver to enhance these signs also provides insights into the pathophysiologic mechanism of disease. Furthermore, knowledge of these signs provides opportunities for further investigation and comparison of different techniques.

References

1. Skinner HA. The Origin of Medical Terms. Baltimore: The Williams & Wilkins Company; 1949.
2. Dalton C. Chapter IV: Galen. In: Doctrines of the Circulation: A History of Physiological Opinion and Discovery, in regard to the Circulation of the Blood. Philadelphia: Henry C. Leas's Son & Co; 1884. p. 229–84.
3. Hombert M. Observation sur un battement de veines semblables au battement des artères. Hist Acad Roy d Sc. 1722;2:159–63.
4. Bett WR. Giovanni Maria Lancisi (1654–1720). Nature. 1954;174:781.
5. Fye WB. Giovanni Maria Lancisi, 1654–1720. Clin Cardiol. 1990;13:670–1.
6. Major RM. Giovanni Maria Lancisi. In: Clinical Description of Disease with Biographical Sketches of the Authors. 3rd ed. Illinois: Charles C. Thomas; 1945. p. 448–50.
7. Lancisi GM. De Subitaneis Mortibus. Rome: Francisci Buagni; 1707.
8. Lancisi GM. De Motu Cordis et Aneurysmatibus. Roma: Giovanni Maria Salvioni; 1728.
9. [No author]. Giovanni Maria Lancisi (1654–1720): cardiologist, forensic physician, epidemiologist. JAMA. 1964;189:375–6.
10. Lancisi G. Pulsation of the jugular vein, a pathognomonic sign. In: Aneurysms – The Latin Text of De Aneurysmatibus, Rome 1745. Wright WC, translator. New York: The Macmillan Company; 1952. p. 309–12.
11. Morgagni JP. Case 5: dilation of the right auricle and ventricle, from contraction of the aorta. In: The Seat and Causes of Diseases, Investigated by Anatomy, vol. 1. Cooke W, translator. Boston: Wells and Lilly and HC Carey and I Lea Philadelphia; 1824. p. 339–43.
12. Lee JA. The other Pasteur: changing views on the postoperative chest. Anaesthesia. 1978;33:362–6.
13. [No author]. William Pasteur CB, CMG MD, FRCP. Br Med J. 1943;2:376.
14. Brown GH. William Pasteur. Lives of the fellows. 2009. http://munksroll.rcplondon.ac.uk/Biography/Details/3470. Accessed 28 May 2019.
15. Thomson HC. The Story of the Middlesex Hospital Medical School, 1835–1935. London: John Murray; 1935.
16. Pasteur W. Cancer investigation committee (1908–1909). In: Lazarus-Barlow WS, editor. Archives of the Middlesex Hospital, vol. 13, Seventh Report from the Cancer Research Laboratory. London: MacMillan and Co; 1908.
17. Pasteur W. Note on a new physical sign of tricuspid regurgitation. Lancet. 1885;2:524.
18. Rondot E. Le reflux hepato-jugulaire. Gazette Hebd Sc Méd Bordeaux. 1898;19:567–71.
19. Wiese J. The abdominojugular reflux sign. Am J Med. 2000;109:59–61.
20. Simel DL, Cook D. Update: central venous pressure. In: Simel DL, Rennie D, editors. The Rational Clinical Examination: Evidence-Based Clinical Diagnosis. New York: McGraw Medical; 2009. p. 133–5.
21. Cook DJ, Simel DL. Does this patient have abnormal central venous pressure? In: Simel DL, Rennie D, editors. The Rational Clinical Examination: Evidence-Based Clinical Diagnosis. New York: McGraw Medical; 2009. p. 125–31.
22. McGee S. Abdominojugular test: inspection of the neck veins. In: Evidence-Based Physical Diagnosis. 3rd ed. Pennsylvania: Elsevier; 2012. p. 301.
23. Burch GE, Ray CT. Mechanism of the hepatojugular reflux in congestive heart failure. Am Heart J. 1954;48:373–82.
24. Brostoff JM. Re-examining examination: misconceptions in clinical medicine. J R Soc Med. 2009;102:11–5.
25. Butman S, Ewy GA, Standen JR, Kern KB, Hahn E. Bedside cardiovascular examination in patients with severe chronic heart failure: importance of rest or inducible jugular venous distention. J Am Coll Cardiol. 1993;22:968–74.
26. Omar HR, Guglin M. Clinical and prognostic significance of positive hepatojugular reflux on discharge in acute heart failure: insights from the ESCAPE trial. Biomed Res Int. 2017; article ID: 5734749.

27. Shabetai R, Fowler NV, Gunteroth W. The hemodynamics of cardiac tamponade and constrictive pericarditis. Am J Cardiol. 1970;26:480–9.
28. Ewy GA. The abdominojugular test: technique and hemodynamic correlates. Ann Intern Med. 1988;109:456–60.
29. Drazner MH, Hellkamp AS, Leier CV, Shah MR, Miller LW, Russell SD, et al. Value of clinician assessment of hemodynamics in advanced heart failure: the ESCAPE trial. Cir Heart Fail. 2008;1:170–7.
30. Fresquet JL. Jose Manuel Rivero Carvallo (1905–1993). Historia de la Medicina. https://www.historiadelamedicina.org/rivero.html. Accessed 3 Mar 2019.
31. De Micheli A. Centenario del natalicio de un distinguido cardiólogo mexixano, Dr. José Rivero Carvello. Arch Cardiol Méx. 2005;75:118–20.
32. Rivero-Carvallo JM. Signo para el diagnóstico de las insuficiencias tricuspídeas. Arch Inst Cardiol Mex. 1946;16:531–40.
33. Cha SD, Gooch AS, Maranhao V, Koehler E. Intracardiac phonocardiography in tricuspid regurgitation: relation to clinical and angiographic findings. Am J Card. 1981;48:578–83.
34. Rivero-Carvallo JM. El signo de doble choque apexiano. Arch Inst Cardiol Mex. 1962;32:387–99.
35. Terry RB. Coupled hepatic pulsations in tricuspid incompetence; a new physical sign. Am Heart J. 1959;57:158–9.
36. Aldo A. Luisada cardiologist, educator. Prabook. https://prabook.com/web/aldo_a.luisada/122523. Accessed 15 Apr 2019.
37. Heart Researcher, Teacher Dr. Aldo Luisada, 86. Chicago Tribune. December 27, 1987. https://www.chicagotribune.com/news/ct-xpm-1987-11-27-8703290301-story.html. Accessed 8 Apr 2019.
38. Kaplan MA, Sarnoff SJ, Liu CK. Aldo A. Luisada MD, FACC: Physician, scientist, teacher. Am J Cardiol. 1971;28:236.
39. Luisada AA, Wissner S, Gupta PD. Lateral head movements as a sign of tricuspid insufficiency. Cardiologia. 1967;50:140–6.
40. The New Alumni. GW Medicine Summer. 1968. https://hsrc.himmelfarb.gwu.edu/cgi/viewcontent.cgi?article=1024&context=gwmed. Accessed 9 May 2019.
41. Vitums VC, Gooch AS, Evans JM. Bedside maneuvers to augment the murmur of tricuspid regurgitation. Med Ann Dist Columbia. 1969;38:533–5.
42. Milton Daniel Byrd. Doximetry. https://www.doximity.com/pub/milton-byrd-md. Accessed 3 Feb 2019.
43. [No author]. Personal Communication. Milton Daniel Byrd. Accessed 28 Dec 2018.
44. Byrd MD. Lateral systolic pulsation of the earlobe: a sign of tricuspid regurgitation. Am J Cardiol. 1984;54:244.
45. Chow WH, Cheung CL. Pulsatile varicose veins: a sign of tricuspid regurgitation. Br J Clin Pract. 1990;44:669.

Chapter 7
Miscellaneous Murmurs and Findings

Introduction

Signs of aortic and tricuspid insufficiency murmurs are covered in Chapters "Aortic Regurgitation Murmurs" and "Tricuspid Insufficiency Murmurs." Herein are reviewed those remaining signs detected through auscultation, maneuvers, sphygmomanometer, or radiographic techniques. Auscultatory signs include murmurs caused by a ventricular septal defect (Roger) or sounds identified in mitral stenosis (Fraentzel). Other findings include methods used to differentiate radiating aortic murmur from those arising in carotid stenosis (Riesman), distinguishing functional from organic aortic insufficiency murmurs (Loewenberg), and determining which phase of the cardiac cycle a murmur is present (Farfel). Suzman described a maneuver to accentuate the superficial collateral veins in patients with coarctation of aorta. Goetz, through an intravenous contrast technique, radiographically visualized a patent ductus arteriosus. Some of these findings remain clinically relevant as bedside techniques. Recognized are physicians and their honorary signs as told through historical information regarding their character, contributions, and accomplishments to medicine and beyond. The signs are reported sequentially based on the date of their original publication.

Signs

Roger Murmur Sign

Sir Georges Eugène Henri Roger (1860–1946) was born in Paris and received his Doctor of Medicine degree from the Medical Faculty of Paris in 1887 [1–3]. He was agrégé of the Faculty of Medicine in 1892, hospital physician at the Contagious Hospital at Porte d'Aubervilliers from 1895 to 1903, and a physician in the

S. H. Yale et al., *Cardiovascular Eponymic Signs*,
https://doi.org/10.1007/978-3-030-67596-7_7

Charity Hospital in 1903 [3]. Roger was Professor of Experimental and Comparative Pathology, Paris, in 1904, Professor of the Institute of Colonial Medicine in 1905, and Dean of the Faculty of Medicine at the University of Paris in 1917 [2, 3]. He was elected foreign correspondent in 1924 and honorary foreign member in 1926.

Roger was a member of the Societies of Biology and Medical and Natural Science in Brussels, Pathological and Anatomy Section of the National Academy of Medicine in Paris from 1910 to 1946, as well as the Academies of Milan, Warsaw, Turin, Madrid, and Buenos Aires [1, 2]. He was Knighted in 1908, Officer in 1917 and Commander of the Légion d'honneur in 1923, Officer of the Order of Leopold, Commander of the Crown of Italy, and Crown of Romania and Polish Renaissance [2, 3]. Roger identified auscultatory findings in patients with a ventricular septal defect (VSD):

> This cardiac anomaly has no objective symptom that makes it recognizable; it was almost exclusively found by auscultation. After having examined thousands of children for forty years it was thanks to the stethoscope examinations, which were constantly repeated, that I correlated the sounds with pathological anatomy in order to separate this anomaly of the heart from other malformations or diseases, established their distinct clinical existence, and confirm its characteristics as a pathognomonic sign [4, p. 1075].

He described the auscultatory findings in patients with a VSD (Table 7.1):

> This cardiac anomaly, of which I have just completed the first clinical study, is important from a practical point of view in order to distinguish it from other malformations or especially from other heart diseases. It is revealed only by auscultation. It announces itself by a physical sign, the characters of which are quite special. It is loud and extends in a wide area. It is unique, begins and extends so as to encompass systole. It has its maximum intensity not at the tip (as in the alterations of atrioventricular orifices), the base on the right (as in the narrowing of the aorta), or at the left pulmonary area (as in the stenosis of the artery), but at the upper third of the precordial region. In the middle of the precordium it divides itself so it decreases in intensity as one gradually moves away from this central point. It is fixed, not transmitted within the arteries, and does not coincide with any signs other than the purring thrill. An anomalous noise which unites this set of characters is the pathognomonic sign of non-occlusion of the ventricle septum. The cause of this malformation or whether it is confused with other congenital or acquired lesions is currently unknown. This diagnosis is made easily by carefully evaluating the physical signs which vary in number, location, and character in this heart disease [4, p. 1091].

Roger recognized that the reason why some patients with interventricular septal defects were cyanotic was due to concomitant pulmonary artery stenosis [4]. The murmur of VSD has also been described as a loud, rough, systolic sound audible at the left third to fifth intercostal space and in some cases is heard over the entire precordium. It radiates transversely to the right of the precordium and is heard throughout both normal heart sounds (pansystolic or holosystolic), often obscuring these sounds and may be associated with a thrill [5]. His name is also eponymously attributed to the esophagosalivary or "Roger" reflex, which is the occurrence of salivation after stimulation of the lower portion of the esophagus [6].

Table 7.1 Miscellaneous murmur signs

Name	Year	Description of sign	Method
Roger [4]	1879	Loud murmur which extends in a wide area encompassing systole. It has its maximum intensity at the upper third of the precordial region. In the middle of the precordium it divides so it decreases in intensity as one gradually moves away from this central point. It is fixed, not transmitted within arteries, and does not coincide with any sign other than the purring thrill.	Auscultation
Fraentzel [12]	1889	Presytolic (modified interrupted diastolic) murmur in patients with mild-moderate mitral stenosis.	Auscultation
Herring, HE [19]	1911	Faint murmur heard at the distal aspect of the sternum that continues for a short time after death.	Auscultation
Riesman [22]	1922	The diaphragm of the stethoscope is placed over the clavicle. If the murmur radiates it is heard along the bone.	Auscultation
Farfel [26]	1939	The blood pressure is taken and then re-inflated such that the mercury column is set midway between systolic and diastolic blood pressure readings. If one listens to the normal heart, it will be found that the upward excursion of the mercury column coincides with the second heart sound. In this way one has already established a point at which systole ends. Knowing that the second heart and the impulse at the mercury column occur concurrently, one should note whether the murmur in question immediately precedes this phenomenon, as would be true of a systolic murmur, or follows it, which would be the case with a diastolic murmur.	Sphygmomanometer
Loewenberg [32]	1940	Normally, the systolic pressure in the arm and in the thigh are about equal. When both an aortic diastolic murmur and a low diastolic blood pressure are present, one may make the diagnosis of functional aortic insufficiency if the levels of the systolic blood pressure in the arm and in the thigh are in about the same proportion as normal. In organic aortic insufficiency, the systolic blood pressure is between 50 and 100 mm of mercury higher in the thigh than in the arm. In functional aortic insufficiency, no such variation occurs. The systolic pressure in the thigh is about the same or only slightly higher than the arm.	Sphygmomanometer
Suzman [33]	1947	Ask the patient to stoop or bend forward and with the arms hanging down vertically or to lie prone on a couch with a pillow under the chest and the arms hanging down over the edge.	Observation
Goetz [37]	1951	Defect in the outline of the main pulmonary artery seen at the time when the contrast medium is passing through the pulmonary artery—2 to 3 seconds after the injection of the diodone. As the blood from the aorta does not contain any diodone at that time, the admixture of blood from the aorta via the patient ductus with the blood in the pulmonary artery containing the diodone shows up on the film as a filling defect.	Radiography

Fraentzel Sign

Oscar Maximilian Victor Fraentzel (1838–1894) was born in Meseritz (Miedzyrzecz), Poland, and received his medical degree from the Friedrich Wilhelm Institute for Military Medical Education (Kaiser Wilhelm Academy), Berlin, in 1860 [7–9]. Here he received his medical training under such eminent physicians, including Johannes Peter Müller (1801–1858), Friedrich Schlemm (1795–1858), Rudolph Virchow (1821–1902), Bernard von Langenbeck (1810–1887), Johann Christian Jüngken (1794–1875), Friedrich Theodor von Frerichs (1819–1885), Moritz Heinrich Romberg (1795–1873), and Johann Ludwig Casper (1796–1864) [7]. His medical career spanned services in the military and the university. In 1861, he was appointed subordinate physician in the Guards Pioneer Battalion and that same year assigned to the Westfälische Füsilier-Regiment No. 37, promoted to Assistant Physician, and assigned to the third Lower Silesian Infantry Regiment No. 50 in 1863 (Russian-Polish Border) [8, 9]. In 1865, he was appointed senior physician at the Friedrich-Wilhelm Institute and that same year promoted to medical officer and commanded the battle of Langensalza (war between French forces and allied Prussian and Hanoverian forces) in 1866 [8, 9].

From 1867 to 1869 he served as assistant at the propaedeutic medical clinic at Charité Universitätsmedizin, Berlin, led by Ludwig Traube [8, 9]. In 1868, he habilitated as an associate professor at Friedrich Wilhelm University, Berlin, resigned his position with Traube at Charité, and transferred as staff and department physician to the first Foot Division of the Guards Field Artillery Regiment in 1869 [8, 9]. From 1869 to 1873, he was appointed director of the Augusta Hospital, Berlin, and Director of the Internal Division at Charité [8–10]. During the Franco-Prussian War (1870–1871), he was chief physician of the third Field Hospital of the Guards Corps [8]. In 1873, he served as chief physician of the Cholera Field Hospital and was senior staff physician second class and physician of the second Guards Field Artillery Regiment [8, 9]. He was appointed Associate Professor in 1875 and extraordinary member of the Reich Health Office and Privy Medical Council in 1883 and 1889, respectively. He was discharged from military service as general physician second class in 1893 [8, 9].

Fraentzel was elected Chairman in the Association of Internal Medicine and served as a member of the Medical Examination Commission from 1874 to 1875 [8, 9]. He received numerous military awards throughout his career including the Rothen-Adler Order fourth Class sword for his leadership during the Schleswig-Holstein war from 1863 to 1864, Iron Cross second Class aw. B. in 1872 for his valent medical and military leadership, batch of a first-grade surgeon in 1882, patent for this batch in 1883, the third Order Crown Order, and the third Order Rothe Eagle Order with the bow and swords on the ring added in peace [8, 9]. His character as described in his obituary:

> Fraentzel's importance as a clinician lies in the vigor with which he developed from Traube's teachings including his exactness at the patient's bed, his instruction directed always to the art of healing, and the applied practice of medicine. (...) For the medical

> Corps, his dual appointment as medical officer and excellent university teacher was particularly gratifying and advantageous because he never ceased to regard his military position, whose duties he always advocated in all his numerous other voluntary obligations, as the starting point and center of his collective activity. (…) Precisely because of the value which he himself attached to his military position, he greatly contributed to fortifying and increasing the appraise of the Corps of Medical Officers in the circles of the university teachers and of the teaching administration. Moreover, a large number of medical officers owes him an appreciation for further education in the scientific disciplines and a wealth of practical advice of creative experience in his writings, which served as a source of continued education [8, p. 560].

Traube described four types of murmurs and sounds heard during diastole in mitral stenosis:

> (a) As a prolonged murmur increasing in intensity toward the end of diastole and lasting until the next systole.
> (b) In the form of two diastolic sounds which often resemble tones. In the more common cases, the first sound is similar to a tone while the second sound represents a murmur lasting until the beginning of the next systole.
> (c) In the form of a short presystolic sound.
> (d) As an unmodified murmur that is separated by a pause from the next systole [11, p. 251].

He classified the different varieties of the diastolic murmur into the following categories:

1. Separated from the next systole by a pause.
   (a) A loud prolonged murmur which increases toward the end of diastole and lasts until the following systole.
   (b) A short murmur, occurring only at the end of diastole, the so-called presystolic noise.
   (c) A murmur formed from two different sounds of which the second lasts until the following systole.

2. Not separated from the next systole by a pause.
   (a) A diastolic murmur which is distinctly separated by the following systole, that is, similar to the diastolic murmur of insufficiency of the aortic valves.
   (b) Two different diastolic sounds, the second of which is also distinguished by a distinct pause from the next systole. These diastolic sounds can be either tones or short murmurs [11, p. 251–252].

Fraentzel, nephew and at one time assistant of Traube, acknowledged Traube's prior description of the diastolic double tone in mitral stenosis:

> According to his experience he explains that the diastolic double-tone occurs comparatively infrequently in individuals who show no signs of a valvular defect, whereas in cases of definite mitral stenosis a comparatively rare pure diastolic double-tone is encountered. One must say that Traube placed importance on the pure diastolic double tone in contrast to a similar phenomenon which occurs rather frequently in mitral stenosis. That is, during diastole 2 very short noises or first a tone and then a short noise is identified [12, p. 58].

Fraentzel explained the different length of the pauses:

> On closer examination of the latter, one is convinced that two sounds that form the double tone and the first heart sound are not separated by equal pauses. The pause between the second diastolic sound and the next systolic tone is shorter than that separating the first

> diastolic sound, but also shorter than the pause which separates the systolic tone from the first heart sound. Thus, the second sound of the diastolic double tone forms, as it were, a sign for the next systolic tone. Now, if it can be established that the systolic tone audible over the ventricles is caused by vibrations by which the mitral and tricuspid valves are displaced by their rapidly increasing tension during ventricular systole, than it may be assumed that audible vibrations may be present and arise when they are tense under the influence of atrial contraction. Under normal conditions the tension is too low to produce a sound, but if the energy of the atrial contraction grows for any reason, then the latter will also be able to produce a sound which precedes systolic so that one identifies a diastolic double tone. Traube expressly calls this double tone "a kind of gallop rhythm," which means that in his view the gallop rhythm usually has to occur by a different mechanism [12, p. 58].

Thus, Fraentzel recognized another type of sound in patients with mild-moderate mitral stenosis occurring during diastolic which can be referred to as a presystolic murmur or an "interrupted modified diastolic murmur" (Table 7.1). The murmur is loudest and caused by increased velocity of blood flow at the beginning and end of diastole, the latter due to atrial contraction [13].

Hering (HE) Sign

Heinrich Ewald (HE) Hering (1866–1948) was born in Vienna, Austria [14]. He served as adjunct professor in physiology at the University of Prague in 1895, extraordinary professor in 1900, and professor of general and experimental pathology in 1902 [14, 15]. He was appointed rector of the German University in Prague in 1913, followed by a position as Director of Pathologic Physiology at the University of Cologne, Germany [14, 16].

HE Hering primary area of study involved understanding the role of the carotid sinus in regulating pulse (negative chronotropic) and blood pressure (vasodepressor) in response to electrical stimulation or pressure (carotid sinus reflex) and pulsus irregularis perpetrus currently named atrial fibrillation [14–18]. HE Hering described in his paper "Ueber ein Postmortales Auskultations Phänomen beim Menschen" (About a postmortem auscultation phenomenon in man) a postmortem auscultatory continuous murmur:

> Recently I came to the bedside of a patient when she passed away. I saw the last breaths and some pulsations in the supraclavicular fossa. When the latter were no longer visible, I auscultated the heart in the area of the apex. I could no longer hear heart sounds but did notice a continuous low murmur. I then placed the stethoscope over the lower end of the sternum where the sound was clearly audible. To insure it was not a subjective sound I put the stethoscope on my forehead; it was not heard here. I again auscultated at the same places previously described. I immediately let my two assistants, Drs. Rihl and Eibegger, auscultate in all three places and both confirmed my observation [19, p. 4].

He identified this sound *intra vitam* and found that:

> You will also perceive that noise if you place, for example, the stethoscope so that it rests on the back of the hand on the second and third metacarpal bones and do not compress the

> intermetacarpal space. You make your hand completely limp on the table so as not to contract the muscles. (…) [i]t is of course necessary that it be as quiet as possible in the room [19, p. 5].

Hering accounted for what he believed to be the origin of the sound, "On the basis of all these empirical facts it is most likely that the postmortem noise I perceive is a vascular noise. I have called it postmorbid since the individual was dead according to the usual criteria as there was no evidence of either respiration or cardiac activity." [19, p. 5]. He recognized the limitations as well as potential medical–legal benefits of his findings in determining the time of death:

> It is possible that one does not always hear these sound postmortem as they last for a variable duration, usually not more than one or two minutes. For example, they cannot be heard, or only heard for a short time post-mortem, when the heart rate is slow. We know from animal experiments that under certain circumstances the heart still beats weakly even without a blood supply. In these cases the flow of blood from the arteries into the veins sometimes occurs before the heart stops. However, under certain circumstances, one may still hear sounds even if the heart is quiet weak, that is too weak to pump blood to trigger even a detectable auscultation phenomena. In these cases, the postmortem noise should be the last auscultatory finding pointing to a persisting stream of blood. (…) Finally, it should be mentioned that under certain circumstances the sound has great importance from a judicial-medical purpose [19, p. 5].

Thus, Hering sign refers to a faint murmur heard at the distal aspect of the sternum continuing for a short time after death (Table 7.1).

Riesman Sign

David Riesman (1867–1940) was born in Saxe-Weimar, Germany, and received his medical degree from the University of Pennsylvania in 1892 [20, 21]. He served as Adjunct Professor of Clinical Medicine at the Philadelphia Polyclinic from 1900 to 1918, and Assistant Professor from 1908 to 1912 followed by Professor of Medicine at the University of Pennsylvania from 1912 to 1933. In 1933, he was appointed Emeritus Professor of the History of Medicine at the University of Pennsylvania [20, 21]. Throughout his career, he served as a consultant physician at the Women's, Chestnut Hill, Jewish, and Kensington hospitals [21]. He served as President of the Medical Board of the Philadelphia General Hospital and member of the tuberculosis and cardiovascular boards. He was a Fellow of the American College of Physicians and American Association for the Advancement of Science [21].

Riesman described an auscultatory method to distinguish whether a murmur heard in the neck is due to an aortic murmur or arises from areas of carotid stenosis (Table 7.1):

> To avoid this source of error the stethoscope, which must be either a Bowles or some other form of diaphragm stethoscope, should be placed over the clavicle. If the murmur is a transmissible one it will be well heard all along the bone, where no artery can possibly be pressed upon [22, p. 5].

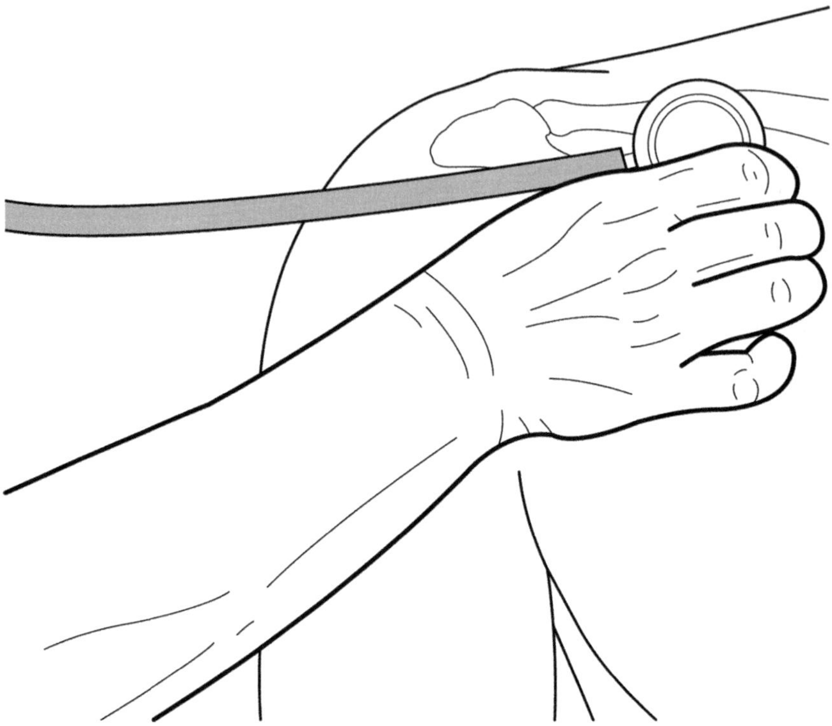

Fig. 7.1 Riesman sign (by Ryan Yale)

Likewise, in cases such as hypertension where the aortic second sound is unexpectedly found not to be loud, the sound was accentuated when the stethoscope was placed over the clavicles [22] (Fig. 7.1). He proposed that "some extrinsic mechanical factor interferes with the transmission of the intensified second sound to the usual place of auscultating, in the second right interspace. The same factors do not interfere with the audibility of the sound over the clavicles" [22, p. 6].

Farfel's Heart Murmur Timing Sign

Bernard Baruch Farfel (1911–2004) was born in New York City, NY, and received his medical degree from New York University [23]. He served as Associate Professor of Clinical Medicine at Baylor College of Medicine, Houston. He was a founding member of the Jewish Institute for Medical Research in Houston in 1963 and served as President of the Houston Society of Internal Medicine, Founding Chairman of the Board of the Jewish Institute for Medical Research, President of the Jewish Family Services (1966–1968), as well as a member of other councils and services

[23, 24]. He was the recipient of numerous honors and awards for recognition of his service including the American Jewish Committee's Max H. Nathan Award, the National Conference of Christians and Jews' Brotherhood Award, and the B'nai B'rith Women of Houston's first Good Heart Award [23, 25]. As a description of his character:

> A man of exquisite kindness, compassion, and spirit, Dr. Farfel was a true healer, who enriched the lives of all who knew him. (…) Dr. Farfel had a great deal of compassion for his patients, family and friends. He was known for his sense of humor, sweet disposition, and commitment to his family [23].

He described an observational and auscultatory bedside method using a sphygmomanometer for determining whether a murmur is present during the systolic or diastolic phase of the cardiac cycle:

> After I have taken the patient's blood pressure, I leave the cuff in place and set the mercury column at about midway between the systolic and diastolic blood pressure readings. This is done so as to obtain good excursions of the column with each beat. If one listens to the normal heart, it will be found that the upward excursion of the mercury column is coincident with the second heart sound. In this way one has already established a point at which systole ends. Knowing that the second heart and the impulse given to the mercury are coincidental, one should note whether the murmur in question immediately precedes this phenomenon, as would be true of a systolic murmur, or follows it, which would be the case with a diastolic murmur [26, p. 1642].

Thus, Farfel sign is a method for timing when a murmur occurs during the cardiac cycle. The visual upward excursion of the column of a mercury sphygmomanometer coincides with the auscultatory second heart sound (Table 7.1).

Loewenberg Sign

Samuel Aaron Loewenberg (1881–1958) was born in Libau, Latvia, and received his medical degree, graduating with honors from the Medico Chirurgical College (current University of Pennsylvania Medical School), Philadelphia, in 1903 [27, 28]. He was an Instructor in Medicine at the Medico-Chirurgical College and Hospital, Philadelphia in 1904 [29]. From 1908 to 1937, he was a visiting physician at the Eagleville Sanatorium for Consumptives. He served at the Liberties Hospital (later incorporated into the Albert Einstein Medical College) from 1921 to 1951 [27]. He had the privilege of working with such eminent physicians as Ferdinand Widal (Paris) (1862–1929), Karl Frederik Wenckebach (1864–1940), Hans Eppinger (1879–1946) and Jakob Erdheim (Vienna) (1874–1937), Sir James Mackenzie (1853–1925) and Thomas Lewis (London) (1881–1945), and Anthon Gohn (Prague) (1866–1936). He was a visiting physician at Philadelphia General Hospital in the medical department from 1927 to 1948, followed by an appointment as consulting physician [27]. He was Consulting Physician to the Philadelphia Hospital for

Contagious Diseases and the Philadelphia Psychiatric Hospital in 1940 [27, 30]. Loewenberg was appointed Assistant Professor of Medicine in 1910 and demonstrator of physical diagnosis when the Medical Chirurgical College joined to become the University of Pennsylvania in 1914. During World War I, he was a contract surgeon, captain, commanding officer, and Chief of the Heart and Lung Examining Demobilization Board in 1919 [27].

During his career he authored four textbooks including *Diagnostic Methods and Interpretations in Internal Medicine* (1928), *Medical Diagnosis and Symptomatology* (1929), *Medical and Physical Diagnosis: Interpretation of Findings* (1929), and *Clinical Endocrinology* (1937). He was a member of a number of societies including the American Heart Association, American College of Physicians, and the National Tuberculosis Association to name a few [31].

Loewenberg reported a method for differentiating functional from organic aortic insufficiency:

> Normally the systolic pressure in the arm and in the thigh are about equal. When both an aortic diastolic murmur and a low diastolic blood pressure are present, one may make the diagnosis of functional aortic insufficiency if the levels of the systolic blood pressure in the arm and in the thigh are in about the same proportion as in the normal. In organic aortic insufficiency the systolic blood pressure is between 50 and 100 mm. of mercury higher in the thigh than in the arm. In functional aortic insufficiency no such variation occurs; the systolic pressure in the thigh is about the same or only slightly higher than the arm [32, p. 991–992].

Thus, Loewenberg sign refers to the presence of systolic blood pressure which is equal to or slightly higher in the thigh than in the arm in functional aortic insufficiency (Table 7.1).

Suzman Sign

There is limited historical information on S. Suzman. At the time of his publication when he described his sign he was serving at Guy's Hospital and National Heart Hospital Cardiac Department and the Thoracic Surgical Unit, London, England.

Suzman described a method to emphasize the superficial collateral veins of the back and sides of the chest in patients with suspected coarctation of the aorta. The maneuver consists of (Table 7.1), "Causing the patient to stoop or bend forward and with the arms hanging down vertically. An equally good method is for the patient to lie prone on a couch with a pillow under the chest and the arms hanging down over the edge of the couch." [33, p. 310]. He believed that this finding was caused by "partial compression and obstruction (in cases where the sign is positive) of the subclavian artery in the costo-clavicular space, and any change of posture that widens this space will thus release pressure on the subclavian artery and so cause a sudden filling up of superficial arteries" [33] (Fig. 7.2).

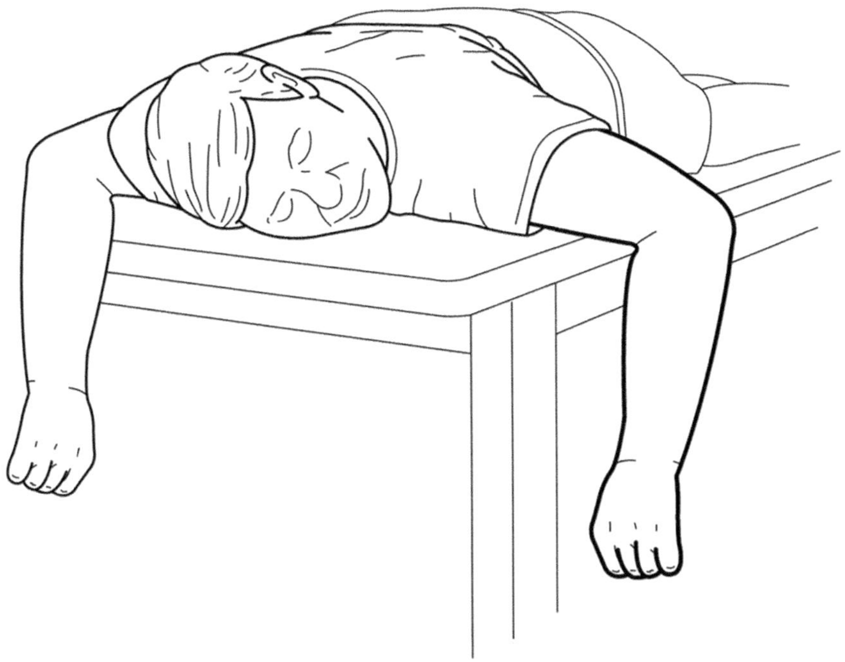

Fig. 7.2 Suzman sign (by Ryan Yale)

Goetz Sign

Robert Hans Goetz (1910–2000) was born in Frankfurt, Germany, and graduated from the University of Frankfurt in 1934. He left Germany because of his anti-Nazi views during the National Socialist Party regime and continued his training in Bern, Switzerland, where he earned his medical degree from the University of Bern in 1936. This was followed by a brief appointment, because of a 1 year visa, in the Department of Physiology in Edinburgh University in 1937 [34]. That same year he accepted a research fellowship as a research scientist at the J.S. Marais Surgical Research Laboratory in the Department of Surgery at the University of Cape Town, South Africa [35]. He subsequently established a vascular laboratory at Groote Schuur Hospital and was appointed Associate Professor of Surgical Research at the University of Cape Town Medical School [34]. He left South Africa due to his views of the apartheid movement and emigrated to the United States. He earned the Vesalius Medal for his field work in understanding the physiology and blood pressure of the giraffe. In 1957, he became Associate Professor of Surgery at Albert Einstein College of Medicine of Yeshiva University and in 1961, Professor and Attending surgeon at Bronx Municipal

Hospital [34]. He was credited for performing the first successful coronary artery bypass operation in 1960 and received a patent for the intra-aortic balloon pump [36].

R.H. Goetz described a radiographic sign for the detection of a patent ductus arteriosus (Table 7.1):

> The sign consists of a defect in the outline of the main pulmonary artery and is seen at a time when the contrast medium is passing through the pulmonary artery, that is, two to three seconds after the injection of the diodone. As the blood from the aorta does not contain any diodone at that time, the admixture of blood from the aorta via the patient ductus with the blood in the pulmonary artery containing the diodone shows up on the film as a filling defect [37, p. 242].

He believed that identification of the filling defect is an important finding in cases where "the opening is rather small and where consequently, both the dilation of the pulmonary artery and the re-opacification of the pulmonary artery are absent." [37, p. 246].

Conclusion

A variety of auscultatory findings such as VSD and presystolic murmur or interrupted modified diastolic murmur in mitral stenosis were determined through meticulous use of the stethoscope. The sphygmomanometer assisted in identifying the timing of the murmur during the cardiac cycle and to distinguish functional from organic aortic valvular insufficiency. Through the use of a sphygmomanometer, Loewenberg used a technique, originally described by Hill, Flank, and Holtzman in 1909, to diagnose aortic insufficiency and differentiated it from functional aortic insufficiency. These findings reported as eponymous signs should reinforce to physicians that the bedside cardiac examination, using relatively simple instruments, may be helpful in diagnosing and differentiating disease. The sensitivity and specificity of these signs have not been further studied providing the opportunity for further investigation.

References

1. Rouvillois H, Trémolières F. Roger Georges Eugène Henri. Comité des travaux historiques et scientifiques. Insitut rattaché à l'École nationale des chartes. Dernière mise à jour le 26 oct. 2019. https://cths.fr/an/savant.php?id=4637. Accessed 28 Mar 2020.
2. Henri Roger L. Académie royale de Médecine de Belgique. Fédération Wallonie-Bruxelles. http://www.armb.be/index.php?id=4500. Accessed 20 Jul 2019.
3. Leonore. Roger, George Eugène Henri. http://www2.culture.gouv.fr/public/mistral/leonore_fr?ACTION=CHERCHER&FIELD_1=COTE&VALUE_1=19800035%2F238%2F31573. Accessed 21 Jul 2019.
4. Roger H. Recherches cliniques sur la communication congénitale des deux coeurs, par inocclusion du septum interventriculaire. Bull Acad de Méd. 1879;8:1074–94,1189–91.

5. Barker F. Congenital diseases of the heart. In: The Clinical Diagnosis of Internal Diseases: General Diagnosis, Infections, Respiratory and Circulatory Systems, vol. 2. New York: Appleton and Company; 1916. p. 895–7.
6. Rogers, Georges Henri. The Free Dictionary by Farlex. 2003–1019. https://medical-dictionary.thefreedictionary.com/Georges+Henri+Roger. Accessed 10 Feb 2019.
7. [No author]. Biographische Mittheilungen. Leopoldina 1894;30:207–8.
8. [No author]. Fraentzel O. Deutsche mil ärztl Zeitschr. 1894;23:558–60.
9. Historischen Commission bei der Königlichen Akademie der Wissenschaften. Allgemeine Deutsche Biographie. Leipzig: Verlag von Dunder & Humblot; 1904.
10. [No author]. Obituary: Dr. Oscar Fraentzel. Lancet. 1894;2:765.
11. Traube L. Ueber das diastolische Geräusch bei Stenose des Ostium venosum sinistrum. Ges Beitr z Path u Physiol. 1871;3:251–2.
12. Fraentzel O. Vierte Vorlesung. In: Vorlesungen über die Krankheiten des Herzens: Die ideiopathischen Herzvergrösserungen. Berlin: Verlag von August Hirschwald; 1889. p. 56–73.
13. Kelly AOJ. Diseases of the endocardium. In: The Practice of Medicine: A Guide to the Nature, Discrimination and Management of Disease. Philadelphia: Lea & Febiger; 1910. p. 445–77.
14. Major RH. Auricular fibrillation, Heinrich Ewald Hering. In: Classic Description of Disease. Illinois: Charles C. Thomas; 1932. p. 390–2.
15. Zimmer HG. Heinrich Ewald Hering and the carotid sinus reflex. Clin Cardiol. 2004;27:485–6.
16. [No author]. Heinrich Hering, Jr. (1866–1948): pathologic physiologist. JAMA 1965;193:185–6.
17. Hering HE. Die Karotissinusreflexe auf Herz und Gefässe, vom Normal-Physiologischen, Pathologisch-Physiologischen und Klinischen Standpunkt. Steinkopff: Dresden; 1927.
18. Hering HE. Pulsus Irregularis Perpetuus. Prag med Wchnschr. 1903;28:377–81.
19. Herring HE. Ueber ein postmortales Auskultations-Phänomen beim Menschen. Deutsche med Wchnschr. 1911;37:4–5.
20. David Riesman (physician) 2017. https://en.wikipedia.org/wiki/David_Riesman_(physician). Accessed 12 Jul 2019.
21. Riesman D. Prabook. 2019. https://prabook.com/web/david.riesman/1111886. Accessed 10 Jul 2019.
22. Riesman D. Some points in physical diagnosis. Trans Assoc Am Physicians. 1922;37:4–6.
23. Houston Chronicle. Obituaries. Bernard Farfel MD. 2019. https://www.legacy.com/obituaries/houstonchronicle/obituary.aspx?n=bernard-farfel&pid=2280895. Accessed 10 Sep 2019.
24. Mishpacha. A Publication of Jewish Family Services. 100 Years A bridge to the future. JFS Jewish Family Services. Houston, Texas. 2013. http://www.jfshouston.org/pdfs/Mishpacha_Spring_2013.pdf. Accessed 10 Sep 2019.
25. Levy VS. If You Build It, They Will Heal. JHV Jewish Herald Voice. Greater Houston's Jewish News Media since 1908. http://jhvonline.com/if-you-build-it-they-will-heal-p16054-89.htm. Accessed 11 Sep 2019.
26. Farfel B. A method of timing heart murmurs. JAMA. 1939;113:1642–3.
27. Samuel A. Loewenberg, M.D. Jefferson Alumni Bulletin. 1959;11:17.
28. [No author]. General Magazine and Historical Chronicle, vol. 44. New Jersey: University of Pennsylvania and General Alumni Society; 1941.
29. Henry FP, Shoemaker JV, editors. Founders' Week Memorial Volume: Containing an Account of the Two Hundred and Twenty-fifth Anniversary of the Founding of the City of Philadelphia, and Histories of its Principal Scientific Institutions, Medical Colleges, Hospital, etc. Philadelphia; 1909.
30. [No author]. Book reviews: Medical diagnosis and symptomatology, Samuel A. Loewenberg MD, FACP. AJCP. 1942;12(4):239.
31. Loewenberg S. Geographic list of members. In: National Tuberculosis Association - Transactions of the Sixteenth Annual Meeting. St. Louis, MO; 1920. p. 601.
32. Loewenberg SA. Valuable sign in diagnosis of functional aortic insufficiency. Ann Intern Med. 1940;14:991–2.

33. Suzman SA. New sign in coarctation of the aorta. Br Heart J. 1947;9:310.
34. Konstantinov IE, Robert H. Goetz: the surgeon who performed the first successful clinical coronary artery bypass operation. Ann Thorac Surg. 2000;69:1966–72.
35. Mitchell G. Robert Goetz: a pioneer of the study of the physiology of animals in the wild. Trans R Soc S Afr. 2008;63:182–5.
36. Saxon W. Robert Goetz, 90, Innovator In Coronary Bypass Surgery. NY Times. https://www.nytimes.com/2000/12/20/us/robert-goetz-90-innovator-in-coronary-bypass-surgery.html. Accessed 20 Jul 2019.
37. Goetz RH. A new angiocardiographic sign of ductus arteriosus. Br Heart J. 1951;13:242–6.

Chapter 8
Physical Signs and Medical Eponyms of Pericarditis: Inspection

Introduction

Inspection is derived from the Old French *inspeccion*, Latin *inspectionem* (a looking into) and *pie* root spek (to observe) [1]. Inspection is the first of the four basic tenets of the physical examination along with palpation, percussion, and auscultation and involves looking or observing. The word pericardium was first named by Galen of Pergamon (c.130 CE–c.200 CE) and is derived from the Greek preposition *peri* (about or around) and the word *kardia* (heart) [2]. Pericarditis originated from the Greek suffix *-itis,* a simple adjectival ending and later the genitive form of the adjective to mean inflammation of the named organ [2].

Pericarditis is the term used to describe the spectrum of diseases that includes acute and chronic types. Acute pericarditis consists of effusive and fibrinous forms while chronic pericarditis consists of effusive, adhesive, mixed (effusive-adhesive) and constrictive forms and its combinations. The terminology used by physicians prior to the advent of imaging techniques is less specific even when postmortem studies were performed. For example, the term adherent pericarditis is currently referred to chronic adhesive or adhesive-constrictive pericarditis with the latter implying constrictive physiological changes.

Reprinted, in part, from Erciyes Medical Journal, vol 41, Ye F, Tekiner H, Yale ES, Mazza JJ, Yale S, Physical signs of inspection and medical eponyms in Pericarditis Part I: 1761 to 1852. pages 223–229, 2019, with permission from Erciyes University Faculty of Medicine.
Reprinted, in part, from Erciyes Medical Journal, vol 41, Ye F, Tekiner H, Yale ES, Mazza JJ, Yale S. Physical signs of inspection and medical eponyms of Pericarditis Part II: 1864 to 1895, pages 230–234, 2019, with permission from Erciyes University Faculty of Medicine.
Reprinted, in part, from Erciyes Medical Journal, vol 41, Ye F, Tekiner H, Yale ES, Mazza JJ, Yale S. Physical signs of inspection and medical eponyms in Pericarditis Part III: 1900 to 1964, pages 41–43, 2019, with permission from Erciyes University Faculty of Medicine.

S. H. Yale et al., *Cardiovascular Eponymic Signs*,
https://doi.org/10.1007/978-3-030-67596-7_8

Physicians during this time period, if they were to excel in the art of clinical medicine, were required to develop proficiency in diagnosis using the senses of sight, touch, and hearing which respectively involved the application of inspection, palpation, percussion, and auscultation. From these investigations, they identified and reported signs for which thereafter have been eponymously ascribed to their namesake.

Inspection, the first basic tenet routinely taught during the physical examination is often overlooked, underappreciated, and discarded as being unimportant and insignificant, and thus only given cursory significance. It is the method for identifying physical signs by observation and may provide clues about the condition of the patient and the underlying disease process [2]. As emphasized by DeGowin and DeGowin in their book *Bedside Diagnostic Examination,* "More diagnoses are probably made by inspection than by all other methods combined. The method is the most difficult to learn because no systematic approach can encompass the variety of signs" [3, p. 34]. Although observation seems like a "simple" technique, it in fact requires training, patience, perceptibility, and practice. The medical term inspection, although technically used in reference to the physical examination, is applied in this chapter when "observing" a sign detected through a radiograph or electrocardiogram.

Covered in this review are eponymic signs of inspection of the precordium seen in patients with acute effusive and fibrinous pericarditis and chronic adhesive-constrictive pericarditis. Findings observed during the physical examination include such things as observing the arterial and jugular venous pulse and shape, as well as the strength and contour of chest and abdominal wall for bulging or retraction of the precordium and epigastrium. These signs were often detected, described, and reported in patients with advanced disease and have not been well studied; therefore, it is unknown how useful they are in current clinical practice. Knowledge of these signs enhances understanding of the pathophysiology of disease and provides a window into the world of the bedside physical examination required prior to the advent of sophisticated diagnostic tests. These findings, depicted as medical eponyms, may impart important clues for diagnosticians to identify the underlying condition and explain the pathophysiological mechanism of the disease process.

Our goals in this chapter is to provide the reader with a unique and novel perspective and appreciation of the signs of pericarditis by first providing a synopsis of the physician who observed the sign, its original description, and if available the sensitivity, specificity, and predictive value of the sign and its application in more modern-day clinical practice. The signs are presented chronologically based on the year that they were first reported (Table 8.1).

Table 8.1 Pericardial inspection eponyms signs

Name	Year	Description of sign	Significance
Auenbrugger [5]	1761	Swelling or bulging of the epigastrium.	Pericardial effusion
Heim-Kreysig [18]	1816	Systolic elevation of the thorax and depression of the left ribs.	Adhesive-constrictive pericarditis
Sander [22]	1823	During systole the cardiac apex rise forward toward the fifth rib and a depression forms in the epigastrium under the left ribs. During inspiration the depression is deeper but the shock weaker, the converse occurs during expiration.	Adhesive-constrictive pericarditis
Hope [32]	1839	Systolic forward protrusion and retraction of the left precordial region.	Adhesive-constrictive pericarditis
Williams [37]	1840	Protrusion of the chest wall involving the cartilage of the middle ribs along with a retraction or depression of the epigastrium.	Adhesive-constrictive pericarditis
Bouillaud [48]	1846	Depression of the precordial region.	Adhesive-constrictive pericarditis
Škoda [52]	1852	Systolic retraction and diastolic elevation occurring at the lower half of the sternum.	Adhesive-constrictive pericarditis
Friedreich [57]	1864	During diastole there is a rapid and brief jerking and venous collapse seen best at the anterior jugular vein. During systole the veins become gradually dilated and filled.	Adhesive-constrictive pericarditis
Duchenne [63]	1883	During inspiration the epigastric and hypochondriac regions are depressed and the chest dilates. During expiration these movements are reversed. When the diaphragm is weak these signs are seen only during forced respiration.	Pericardial effusion
Broadbent [72]	1895	Retraction synchronous with the cardiac systole occurring posteriorly in the region of the left and right eleventh and twelfth ribs. This is most marked on the left compared to the right side.	Adhesive-constrictive pericarditis
Ogle [77]	1900	Distension of the external jugular veins unaltered during inspiration and without visible pulsation.	Acute purulent pericarditis
Keith [84]	1904	Expansion of the walls of his chest and body in a lateral direction during inspiration.	Adhesive-constrictive pericarditis
Wenckebach [87]	1907	Limited upward movement of the chest that and inspiratory retraction of the lower sternum and ribs.	Adhesive-constrictive pericarditis
Hirtz [92]	1911	Patient in the bed on his/her knees, body bent forward, and supported by the elbows.	Acute effusive pericarditis

(continued)

Table 8.1 (continued)

Name	Year	Description of sign	Significance
Wynter [98]	1911	Depression of the abdominal wall in the epigastrium during inspiration.	Acute fibrinous pericarditis
Volhard [106]	1923	Retraction of the heart and chest wall during systole and its return during diastole. Described fluoroscopically as a “see-saw” pattern.	Adhesive-constrictive pericarditis
Schmieden [111]	1926	Radiographic and operative finding of systolic elevation of the diaphragm.	Adhesive-constrictive pericarditis
Rabin [117]	1952	With the neck in a neutral position, elevation of the aortic arch on swallowing.	Adhesive-constrictive pericarditis
Spodick [120]	1974	The predominant P-R segment depression across the pericardium document the posterior component. Because of these P-R segment deviations, it is of practical importance in acute pericarditis to consider the T-P segment to be the electrocardiographic base line to avoid mistaking P-R segment depression for S-T segment elevation.	Acute pericarditis

Signs

Auenbrugger Sign

Joseph Leopold Edler von Auenbrugger (1722–1809) was born at Graz in Styria, Austria, and studied medicine at the University of Vienna [4]. He served at the Spanish Military Hospital in Vienna in 1751, initially as an assistant and subsequently as a physician [4]. It was in 1754 that Auenbrugger noted differences in sounds by striking the chest wall [4]. He published his observation, methods, and results of percussion in his book titled *Inventum Novum Ex Percussione Thoracis Humani, Ut Signo Abstrusos Interni Pectoris Morbos Detegendi* (A New Discovery that Enables the Physician using Percussion of the Human Thorax to Detect Diseases Hidden within the Chest) in1761 [5]. His finding was initially dismissed and later revived by Jean-Nicolas Corvisart (1755–1821), a French physician who embraced this technique [4].

Auenbrugger described in his aforementioned book under the 12 observation of dropsy of the chest, subheading XLVI, Dropsy of the Pericardium, his observation of two signs which bears his namesake, "A swelling is perceived in the praecordia, which can readily be distinguished by its superior resistance, from the stomach distended by flatus." [5, p. 401]. Thus, this sign refers to significant protuberation of the epigastrium in massive pericardial effusion [6]. He also described his observation of a flat percussion sound on the chest in cases of pericardial effusion, "The sound in the cardiac region, which I have already stated (III. 2.3.) to be naturally more obscure than in the other parts of the chest; is now as completely deadened as if the percussion were applied to a fleshy limb." [5, p. 401]. This eponym also named Auenbrugger sign, refers to the presence of dullness in Traube's space, a crescent shape region bounded by the lower edge of the left lung, anterior border of the spleen, left costal margin and inferior margin of the left lobe of the liver, due to a large pericardial effusion displaced by descent of the left lobe of the liver [7] (Table 8.1). We are not aware of any study which evaluated the sensitivity or specificity of this sign.

Heim-Kreysig Sign

Ernst Ludwig Heim (1747–1834) was born in Solz, Thuringia, received his doctorate at Halle in 1776, and conducted his medical studies at Jena, Thuringia, and Leipzig, Saxony [8–10]. He served at Spandau as a government physician of the Havel district in 1776 and for the region Osthavelland in 1778 [9, 11]. In 1780, he moved to Berlin achieving the rank of professor at the university and in 1806 served as senior physician to the Armendirektorium (Executive Director for the poor) [9]. He was recognized for his service by the city of Berlin being named honorary citizen in 1822 [9]. Heim was the recipient of the Knight of the Red Eagle Order of the Third Class by the King of Prussia and of the Nordstern Order by the King of Sweden [12]. In addition to his advocacy in promoting public health, he was also a botanist with a special interest in mosses [8].

Friedrich Ludwig Kreysig (1770–1839) was born in Eilenburg, Saxony and received his habilitation (medical doctorate) at the University of Leipzig in 1795 [13, 14]. He was appointed professor of anatomy and botany in Wittenberg in 1801 and professor of special pathology and therapy at Medical-Surgical Academy and Director of the Medical Clinic in 1815 [14–16]. He served as a foreign member of the Royal Swedish Academy of Sciences in 1828 [14]. His interests were in the areas of botany and diseases of the heart. As such, he was a founding member of the Society for Nature and Medicine and member of the Society of German Scientists and Physicians, Dresden [17]. In addition to the sign which he described with Heim, Kreysig was influential in describing the inflammatory process in endocarditis [14].

In 1816, Friedrich Ludwig Kreysig reported in his paper entitled "Die Krankheiten des Herzens" (The diseases of the heart), a visible and palpatory finding in cases of pericardial adhesions:

> For there is a violent pounding in the chest which is generally periodic and persistent. Instead of what other authors call palpitations, this knock is visible outwards, often audible, not infrequently associated with a whistling sound occurring during systole. (…) [b]ut is also distinguished by visible changes in the thorax. One can identify it by placing the palm of the hand on the lowest portion of the chest in the region of the corresponding diaphragm. In fact, in this latter position especially if the patient is allowed to walk back and forth around the room a few times, the hand receives a violent shock or feeling as if it were torn violently from the corresponding diaphragm. If one looks at the thorax, one sees that it is not only violently shaken and raised upwards by every cardiac systole, but at the same time one always notices a deepening of the left ribs as if there was a depression. The discovery of this latter circumstance and sign I owe to the keen insight of the experienced Privy Councilor, Dr. Heim in Berlin [18, p. 623].

Thus, Heim-Kreysig sign refers to elevation of the thorax and concavity or depression of the left ribs occurring during cardiac systole in patients with presumed adhesive-constrictive pericarditis (Table 8.1). They may also have been the first to describe what is referred to as the audible "pericardial knock." We are unaware of any studies that evaluated the sensitivity and specificity of this sign.

Sander Sign

James Sander (1777–1843), father of another well-known physician, William Rutherford Sander, was an English physician who practiced in Edinburgh, Scotland. James Sander was involved in the early study of digitalis [19]. He was a member of the Medical Society of Edinburgh and served as a President of the Royal Society of Medicine and Royal Physical Society of Edinburgh [20, 21]. Sander reported that in the adherent pericardium:

> During ventricular contraction the heart is shorter, rounder, and narrows in order to expel blood. The apex moves forward towards the fifth rib causing the lower portion of the pericardium and all that is adherent to it to rise with the diaphragm. At the same time, a depression occurs under the left ribs in the epigastrium. Next, the two atrium simultaneously contract and the ventricles relax and dilate to receive blood. The apex of the heart suddenly attempts to move downwards, and unable to do so transmits a shock to the adherent pericardium, diaphragm, and other parts. A small elevation is visible on the chest where the depression previously occurred, but now extends slightly lower. Strictly speaking, the depression precedes the shock since the contraction of the atrium represents the beginning of the cardiac cycle. It is a perpetual strong undulating movement, lower than that which is normally felt in the region of the heart. Thus, during inspiration and expiration the two phenomena are separated by contractions of the atrium and ventricles and unite by a single pulsation in the radial artery. The collapse and pulsation of the radial artery is isochronous with the pulsation and depression under the ribs respectively. During inspiration the hollow is deeper and a greater portion of the diaphragm is lowered, since the heart needs to generate more force to overcome the resistance caused by adhesions. Consequently, since the adhering parts have now moved further away from the chest wall during the heart's descent, the shock is weakly transmitted to the chest. The opposite occurs during expiration [22, p. 156–157].

Sander believed that he identified a "[m]echanical sign, always produced by the same unique cause. It is a sign which never deceives and allows us to easily recognize adhesions of the pericardium even when it is complicated by other diseases of the heart or chest." [22, p. 157]. Laënnec wrote in his book *Traité de l'auscultation médiate et des maladies des poumons et du cœur* (Treatise of the Diseases of the Chest and of Mediate Auscultation), "I have understood than an English physician, Dr. Sander, has announced as an infallible sign of the adhesion of the pericardium to the heart, the existence of a hollow, during each systole of the organ, in the epigastrium, immediately below the left false ribs." [23, p. 677–678]. Thus, Sander sign refers to the presence of a hollow or depression occurring under the left ribs in the epigastrium occurring during systole in patients with presumed adhesive-constrictive pericarditis (Table 8.1). We are unaware of any study which evaluated the sensitivity or specificity of this sign.

Hope Sign

James Hope (1801–1841) was born at Stockport, England, and received his medical degree from Edinburgh University in 1825 [24]. In 1828, he obtained the College of Physician degree as a licentiate and served as physician to the Marylebone Infirmary in 1831 [24]. He published the first (English) edition of his critically acclaimed book *A Treatise on the Diseases of the Heart and Great Vessels* in 1831 which described his work on heart sounds and murmurs [25–27]. That same year, he was elected fellow of the Royal Society of Medicine [28]. He published another influential book in 1833 entitled *Principles and Illustrations of Morbid Anatomy adapted to the Elements of M Andral and to the Cyclopaedia of Practical Medicine Being a Complete Series of Lithographic Drawings, from Originals by the Author: with Description and Summary Allusions to Cases, Symptoms, Treatment, & c* [29, 30]. He was appointed full physician at St. George's Hospital in 1839 and fellow of the London College of Physicians in 1840.

James's father, Thomas Hope, provided him with the following words of wisdom which was forever beholden to him, "First, never keep a patient ill longer than you can possibly help. Secondly, never take a fee to which you do not feel yourself to be justly entitled. And thirdly, always *pray* for your patients." A short time before his death, Dr. Hope said that these maxims had been the rule of his conduct, and that he could testify to their success [31, p. 51].

James Hope in his book entitled *A Treatise on the Diseases of the Heart and Great Vessels* described two signs which he believed to be important to support the diagnosis of adherent pericardium caused by rheumatic heart disease:

1. [t]he heart, though enlarged, and when, therefore, it ought to beat preternaturally low down in the chest, beats as high up as natural, and sometimes occasions a prominence of the cartilages of the left precordial ribs. (…) We should, indeed, naturally expect that the adhesion would brace up the organ, and that, when enlarged and not able to descend, it must, being bounded behind by the spine, force the walls of the precordial region forward.
2. [a]brupt, jogging, or tumbling motion of the heart, very perceptible in the precordial region with the cylinder. It is more distinct when the heart is hypertrophous and dilated; and, under these circumstances, I have found the jogs correspond with the ventricular systole and diastole respectively, that of the diastole being sometimes nearly as strong as the other, and having the character of a receding motion suddenly arrested. (…) This jogging motion is distinguished from the undulatory movement of fluid in the pericardium, both by its nature, by the exact synchronism of the jogs with the sounds, and by the feeling that the heart, at each systole, comes in immediate contact with the thoracic walls. I suppose the double jog to be occasioned by the heart being bound down to the spine by the adhesion, whence it is tilted forwards as often as the rounded swell of the ventricles, both during their systole and their diastole, meets the resistance of the spinal column. (…) The jogs would, of course, be increased by hypertrophy, and also by aortic regurgitation, which imparts abruptness to the heart's action [32, p. 194].

Thus, Hope sign refers to the systolic protrusion of the chest wall in left precordial region in patients with presumed adhesive-constrictive pericarditis [33] (Table 8.1). We are unaware of any studies which evaluated the sensitivity or specificity of this sign.

Williams Sign

Charles James Blasius Williams (1805–1889) was born in the Hungerford Almshouse, Wiltshire, and received his medical degree from the University of Edinburgh, Scotland in 1824 [34]. He practiced medicine at St. George's University, London in 1830, elected fellow of the Royal Society of Medicine in 1835, and

Fellow of the Royal College of Physicians, Edinburgh in 1840 [35]. In the Royal College, he also served other eminent titles including Goulstonian Lecturer in 1841, Censor in 1846, and Lumleian Lecturer in 1862 [34]. In 1839, he was appointed Professor of Medicine and physician to the University College, London [34, 35]. He served as Presidents to numerous societies including the Harveian and Westminster Medical Societies, Pathological Society of London in 1846, New Sydenham in 1858, and Royal Medical and Chirurgical Society from 1873 to 1875 [34, 35]. He also served as Physician Extraordinary to the Queen in 1874 and Consulting Physician for the Hospital of Consumption, Brompton, for which he took an active role in its founding in 1841 [34, 36].

Williams in his book entitled *The Pathology and Diagnosis of Disease of the Chest Compromising a Rational Exposition of their Physical Signs* published in 1840, described the visible and palpatory findings identified in patients with adherent pericarditis:

> But it often happens in case of close adhesions, that prior to their formation the pericardial sac has adhered in its distended state to the walls of the chest at the left of the sternum, so that when the heart also adheres to the sac, it constantly pulsates in close contact with their walls. This combination of circumstances gives us very appreciable signs. In the first place, the motions of the heart may be seen and felt much more plainly and widely than usual, drawing in the intercostal spaces at each systole. Then these motions, instead of being, as usual intercepted by the expansion of the lung in a full inspiration, are always close to the walls of the chest; for these walls, instead of, as usual rising from the heart upwards and outward at each inspiration, carry the heart with them in all their movements. Under these circumstances, therefore, there will be proportioned to the adhesion and the size of the heart, a space in which the pulsation are felt, and the sound on percussion is always dull in every stage of respiration, and in every posture of the body. (…) When the heart is thus generally adherent to the pericardium, and this to the diaphragm and walls of the chest, the enlargement of the organ, which very commonly ensues, cannot readily take place as usual, downwards, and to the left; but it proceeds upwards and downwards, carrying with it the wall of the chest, to which it gives a remarkable projection about the ends and cartilages of the middle ribs. I have seen this accompanied by a retraction or hollow at the epigastrium [37, p. 240].

Thus, Williams sign refers to the systolic protrusion of the precordium and retraction of the epigastrium in patients with presumed adhesive-constrictive pericarditis (Table 8.1). We are unaware of any studies that evaluated the sensitivity or specificity of this sign.

Bouillaud Sign

Jean-Baptiste Bouillaud (1796–1881) was born at Bragette, France, and received his medical doctorate in 1823 with the thesis entitled *Essai sur le diagnostic des anevrismes de l'aorte et specialement sur les signes que fournit l'auscultation dans cette maladie* (Test on the diagnosis of aneurysms of the aorta and especially on the signs that the auscultation provides in this disease) [38].

He was elected to the French Academy of Medicine in 1826. He served as Professor of Clinical Medicine at Hôpital de la Charité and physician at Hôpital de la Pitie, Paris, in 1831, and Dean of the Paris Faculty of Medicine in 1848 [38, 39]. He was elected President of the French Academy of Medicine in 1862, President of the First International Congress of Medicine in Paris in 1867, Commander of the Légion d'honneur and member of the Institut de France in the section of medicine of the Académie des Sciences in 1868 [40].

Bouillaud made a number of significant contributions to medicine particularly in the field of cardiovascular and neurological diseases. He performed detailed analysis weighing and measuring hearts, differentiated different types of valvular heart diseases through auscultation, identified the *bruit de diable* (venous hum heard over the right internal jugular vein and *bruit de rappel* (false reduplication) of the second heart sound (open-snap) heard over the apex in patients with mitral stenosis, gallop rhythm, *faux pas du coeur* (weak heart beat and absent peripheral pulse), congenital heart disease, neurologic disease (identified that the speech center is localized to the anterior lobe of the brain and that the cerebellum is involved in coordinate movements), and tympanic sound heard on percussing the chest above the level of a pleural effusion (later reported by and eponymously named Škoda's sign) [38, 39].

In addition to the signs which bear his namesake, included and discussed are other discoveries in the field of cardiovascular medicine for which Bouillaud is credited. We included this information not only because of its historical importance but also to provide the reader with an appreciation of the extent and depth of his overall contribution to medicine, one which may not be well recognized. In the preface to his book, *Traité clinique des maladies du coeur* (Clinical Treatise of Heart Diseases) published in 1835, he described and assigned the terms "endocardium" and "endocarditis" to the heart which has also been termed in honor of Bouillaud's discovery, the *Maladie de Bouillard*, by Armand Trousseau (1801–1867), or "Bouillaud's cardiac sign" [41]. Bouillaud assigned a "law of coincidence" which involved establishing an association between articular disease and inflammatory involvement of all layers of the heart (pancarditis) in patients with acute generalized articular rheumatism (rheumatic fever) [42]. He reported in a paper entitled "De l'oblitération des veines et de son influence sur la formation des hydropisies partielles: Considérations sur les hydropisies passives et générales" (Obliteration of the veins and its influence on the formation of partial dropsy: Considerations on the passive and general dropsy) the presence of dropsy (later termed edema) occurring in the lower extremities of seven patient caused by obliteration of the vein by a fibrinous clot. In three of these patients, there was a tumor identified at autopsy [43]. It is recognized that this report was published over 30 years prior to Virchow description and coining of the terms thrombosis and embolism in 1856 and 1860 respectively, and 50 years prior to Trousseau's paper on cancer and thrombosis published in 1873 [44–46]. Bouillaud also described a metallic sound heard over the heart in patients with cardiac hypertrophy, acknowledging Laënnec's prior discovery [47]. In 1846, he reported a method for diagnosing adhesive pericardium:

> [i]t is only by means of certain physical signs, so far neglected, that for some years now we have been able to establish the diagnosis in several individuals- a diagnosis still rather obscure for us when we published the first edition of the Clinical Treatise on the Diseased Heart. In six or seven subjects, we identified the relationship between general adhesion of the pericardium and the following signs: (i) obvious depression of the precordial region analogous to that observed in a side of the chest caused by pleurisy with adhesion. This finding in the precordial region is a sign of great importance. If the hand and ear are applied to the precordial region, one recognizes that the heart does not move as freely as it does in the normal state; its beats are somewhat impeded and the apex of the heart does not strike the chest wall with a sharp and distinctive force as usual [48, p. 415–416].

Thus, Bouillaud sign refers to the presence of persistent retraction of the precordium caused by presumed adhesive-constrictive pericarditis [6] (Table 8.1). We are unaware of any studies which evaluated the sensitivity or specificity of this sign.

Škoda Sign

Josef Škoda (1805–1881) was born in Pilsen, Bohemia (currently Czechia), and received his medical degree from the University of Vienna in 1831. In Vienna, he worked at Karl von Rokitansky's Pathology-Anatomy Institute followed by an appointment as an assistant physician in 1831, full physician in 1841, and Professor of Clinical Medicine in the Internal Department of the K.K. Allgemeines Krankenhaus (General Infirmary) in 1846 [49]. Both he and Carl von Rokitansky (1804–1878) were considered the founders of the new Vienna School of Medicine [49]. His primary research interest and studies were centered around the effects of percussion and auscultation on physical acoustics which cumulated with the publication of these finding in the book entitled *Abhandlung über Perkussion und Auskultation* (Treatise on Percussion and Auscultation) in 1839 [50]. In this text, he described the better known percussion tympanic sound heard above a pleural effusion. He was appointed Professor and Chair of Internal Diseases in 1846 and Vice-Dean of the medical faculty, Vienna Faculty of Medicine in 1849 [51]. A description of his character as enumerated in his obituary:

> Recognising morbid anatomy as the sole basis for an accurate diagnosis he endeavoured to unravel the complex phenomena of disease, to reduce them to their simple elements, and *per viam exclusion* to arrive at an exact diagnosis. None of his old pupils can ever forget his singular accuracy in this, any more than they can forget the remarkable lesson in rational scepticism daily exemplified in his wards [49, p. 286] (…) [t]he careful manner in which he investigated or ran over the points of a case, the logical accuracy with which he made his deductions, and the pathological knowledge with which he clenched them, fascinated though they did not charm, and left an impression of mental power that quite counterbalanced his somewhat insignificant and ungainly figure and boyish appearance forty years ago [49, p. 287].

Josef Škoda described three patients with an adherent pericardium associated with systolic depression and diastolic elevation at the intercostal spaces to the left of the apical heart beat:

> [t]he diagnosis of this disease is based on the finding that during systole the heart does not move down and to the left, but rather the apex of the heart is pulled upward to the right. (...) The apex of the heart does not produce a systolic shock; one either does not feel at all or it seems to impart a pulsation during diastole *). At the interscapular space corresponding to the apex of the heart, as well as one or two intercostal spaces higher, depressions become visible with each systole. Both the heart and pericardium as well as the pericardial and costal pleural are adherent. Without the latter adhesion, a retraction of the left intercostal spaces does not take place, and in such cases one must try to recognize the systolic retraction of the apex by the sense of touch. (...) The investigation must also be based on the fact that the apex of the heart is now driven against the chest wall the same time that systolic retraction of one or more intercostal spaces is occurring. The systolic retraction of the lower half of the sternum is a sure sign that fusion of the heart with the pericardium and fixation of the heart on the spine is present [52, p. 314].

Thus, Škoda sign refers to an indentation or depression at the apex or to the left of the heart with systole, and elevation occurring at the same site during diastole, in patients with presumed adhesive-constrictive pericarditis (Table 8.1). We are unaware of any study which evaluated the sensitivity or specificity of this sign.

Friedreich Sign

Nikolaus Friedreich (1825–1882) was born in Würzburg, Germany, studied medicine in Würzburg in 1844 and Heidelberg in 1847, and received his doctorate in 1850 [53, 54]. He habilitated as Privatdozent (adjunct professor) for Special Pathology and Therapeutics in 1853 and appointed Professor extraordinarius of Pathologic Anatomy in Würzburg (a position formerly held by Rudolf Virchow) in 1857 [54, 55]. In 1858, Friedreich was appointed Director of the Medical Clinic, Professor and Chair of Pathology and Therapeutics, and Professor Ordinarius at the University of Heidelberg [54]. As a student of Rudolf Virchow (1821–1902) in Würzberg, he was profoundly influenced by his approach to medicine that was founded on the principles of cellular pathology and pathological process. His area of special interest was in clinical diagnostics. In collaboration with Friedrich August Kekulé (1829–1896) they determined that amyloid [term coined by Rudolph Virchow (1821–1902)] was a proteinaceous substance [54]. His name is perhaps best recognized and associated with his work on hereditary spinal ataxia (Friedreich's Ataxia) as described in his paper entitled "Ueber Ataxie mit besonderer Berücksichtigung der hereditären Formen" (About ataxia with special consideration of the hereditary forms) published in *Virchow's Archives* in 1877. As a description of Friedreich's scientific approach:

> All the works of Friedreich, however the smallest as well as the most extensive, have a common character and characteristic built on a firm foundation of pathological anatomy. They are distinguished by a universal historical and literary knowledge, an all-encompassing

> comprehension and command of the subject, thoroughness, and clarity of representation [53, p. 973].

A description of his character as formulated by Adolf Kussmual (1822–1902):

> Seeing the young clinician in his hospital was both valuable and gratifying. For him, the endeavor was not duty and work but pleasure and enjoyment. The clinic was not merely a scientific workshop, but also a matter of affection. You could not find a gentler, more humane person with the sick than Friedreich. His mild, quiet dignity, and welfare for others brought comfort and confidence to all, and for some it was a cure. There was no greater master in the technique of the physical examination as no one came close to him in the art of percussion. One could find no better percussion hammers or plethimeters than Friedreich's fingers. Even on the most corpulent person, he lured the notes far and wide [54, p. 203–204].

Friedreich reported initially in his chapter "Die Krankheiten des Herzens" (The diseases of the heart) in *Virchow's Handbuch der speciellen Pathologie und Therapie* (Virchow's Handbook of Special Pathology and Therapy) in 1861, a "peculiar phenomenon of the cervical veins which he interpreted as a new sign for the diagnosis of cardiac adhesions." [56]. In his paper entitled "Zur Diagnose der Herzbeutelverwachsungen" (For the diagnosis of pericardial adhesions) published in 1864, Friedreich stated:

> Since then, I confirmed the diagnosis of pericardial adhesions in a case at autopsy as well as in patients who presented with the same symptoms. I now consider the previous finding with a high level of certainty as being sufficiently well-founded, and I believe that I can assign a new and essential sign to the somewhat uncertain diagnosis of the pericardial adhesions. At the same time, the two cases described appear to me to be suitable for clarifying and modifying some other points concerning the diagnosis of pericardial adhesions [57, p. 296–297]. (...) The two cases presented here, which in many respects agree with each other, seem so instructive in the diagnosis of pericardial adhesion, that their specific description, as well as a closer examination of the phenomena observed during the course of the disease may well be justified [57, p. 304].

He explained and proposed a pathogenesis for systolic retraction and diastolic recoil of the chest and later its effects on the jugular vein reasoning in both cases:

> There seems to me to be no doubt that such widespread systolic retraction must occur particularly when the longitudinal axis of the heart shortens during systole. This shortening pulls the diaphragm strongly upwards and its points of insertion on the chest inward. This motion also affects the adjacent higher portions of the thoracic wall which are required to follow to a certain extent. The occurrence of this phenomenon seems to be caused by more intimate adhesions of the lower surface of the heart with the diaphragm, which were unusually strong in the second case described. It seems plausible that the latter phenomenon occurs only in cases when there are fixed adhesions to the diaphragm even in the absence of obliteration of the entire pericardial cavity. This prevents the downward sliding motion of the heart on the diaphragm, allowing the diaphragm to be pulled upward by the systolic shortening of the heart. In contrast, if there are no diaphragmatic adhesions despite existing pericardial adhesions in the upper parts of the heart, the above phenomenon may well be missed because a space becomes available due to systolic shortening and elevation of the heart caused by either the expansion of the lung or even by a slight upward movement of the diaphragm. Shortening of the apex of the heart is marked by a circumscribed depression, occurring during systole in the intercostal space in question, due to pressure caused by intestinal gas. The remarkable fact is that systolic retraction of the chest wall was particu-

> larly pronounced during inspiration. This may be used to support the view that the tighter, flattened, and shortened diaphragm had to be pushed higher especially with deep inspirations. This finding is more noticeable in inspiration than during expiration when the diaphragm is in a flaccid and curved position. (...) Apart from the diaphragmatic adhesions, another findings is the extensive systolic retraction of the chest wall. That is, a complete and sufficiently strong energy of cardiac contractions is required to overcome the elastic resistance of the thorax [57, p. 307–309].

Friedreich described the appearance of the jugular veins during systole and diastole:

> A clear visible sudden swelling alternating with the carotid pulse was seen simultaneously with the diastolic recoil of the chest wall followed by a rapid and brief jerking diastolic venous collapse. In one case, the entire right and left supraclavicular regions were in a quick short movement, recessed, and pulled inwards. In both cases the diastolic collapse was best seen in the right supraclavicular regions extending downwards just below the clavicle and externally at the external jugular vein, most marked at the anterior jugular vein. During systolic retraction of the thoracic wall the veins were again gradually dilated and filled to a not insignificant degree (in the second case with a double motion corresponding to the contraction of the atrium and ventricle), and during diastole collapsed and complete disappeared. The phenomena of the veins described were so peculiar and striking that they could not be confused with any of the more common conditions of the jugular veins. [57, p. 310–311].

Furthermore, he accounted for the occurrence of this finding in adhesive pericarditis:

> To a certain extent the sudden decrease in pressure on the lungs produced by the inward movement of the chest wall must be conducive to a rapid outflow of blood from the jugular veins. The finding of blood flowing from the jugular veins during diastole is due to the rapid recoil of the chest wall, rapid and deep inspiration, and previous systolic retraction. Moreover, the reason for the above appearance seemed to be attributed to a change of position of the diaphragm caused by the recoil of the chest wall. With the return of the ribs and the lower part of the sternum into a deeper and flatter position, the heart contrary to the conditions prevailing under normal conditions, also moves during diastole because it is adherent to the diaphragm [57, p. 311].

He acknowledged the work by other authors in this field of study:

> The phenomenon described here of a rapid diastolic collapse of the cervical veins and gradually swelling in systole has already been mentioned by other observers. Skoda regards this rare symptom as a sign of paralysis of the right atrium, though it is difficult to see how it should arise in the latter state. As a sign of pericardial obliteration, I found the phenomenon neither described nor written by any authors known to me [57, p. 312].

Thus, Friedreich sign refers to diastolic collapse of the jugular veins in patients with adhesive- constrictive pericarditis (Table 8.1). In a study of 15 cases of constrictive pericarditis and 17 normal controls, diastolic venous collapse was identified in 8 of 15 cases [58]. Lang et al. identified Friedreich sign in 15 of 16 patients with constrictive pericarditis. It is generally absent in cases of cardiac tamponade, as it is more often associated with a restrictive and heavily calcified pericardial disease [59].

Duchenne Sign

Guillaume-Benjamin-Amand Duchenne (1806–1875) was born at Boulogne-sur-Mer (Boulogne), France, studied medicine in Paris, where he was taught by such eminent physicians as Jean Cruveilhier (1791–1874), Alfred-Armand-Louis-Marie Velpeau (1795–1867), Baron Guillaume Dupuytren (1777–1835) and René Laënnec (1781–1826), and graduated in 1831 [60, 61]. Subsequently, he practiced in Boulogne and returned to Paris as a private practitioner in 1842, where he encountered Pierre-François Olive Rayer (1793–1867), Armand Trousseau (1801–1867) and Jean-Martin Charcot (1825–1893) at Charité, Hôtel-Dieu, and Salpêtrière hospitals respectively [60, 61]. Both Trousseau and Charcot were influential in that they encouraged Duchenne to publish his discoveries [60]. Despite not having an appointment or position at the University, he remained committed to conducting clinical neurology research. He described his position related to this matter in his book entitled *De l'électrisation localisée et de son application à la pathologie et à la thérapeutique* (From localized electrization and its application to pathology and therapeutics) in response to criticism he received related to his failure to address the study of pathological anatomy during his clinical studies of glosso-labial-laryngeal paralysis:

> I must answer these reproaches that I do not think I deserved. Those who said it probably did not know that I was only allowed to glean, so to speak, from our hospitals. If I were able to exist scientifically it was because I was fortunate enough to browse through the many services of the hospital, collecting clinical facts which have, I will not say, disdainfully escaped the observation of all. Those who criticized me should know that when I discovered a new finding, I was not allowed to talk about people I made them on during my lifetime clinical research. If I had been a hospital doctor, I would have had the freedom to complete these cases by anatomical-pathological research. But then I could not have fulfilled the task of researcher which I imposed on myself. I am convinced that my principal work on progressive muscular atrophy, atrophic paralysis of childhood, progressive locomotor ataxia, glosso-labio-laryngeal paralysis and pseudo-hypertrophic paralysis among other, would never have seen the light of day. To accomplish this required a wider field of observation spanning all hospitals in Paris. If I renounce and still renounce the honors of an official position, it is because of my duty to give myself entirely and freely to my irresistible taste for physiological and pathological research. Should I be a subject of reproach for the disinterestedness of having made science solely out of love for it? [62, p. 601].

Duchenne noted that there are different causes of diaphragmatic paralysis including "palsies due to the inflammation of adjacent organs" [63, p. 329]. He further described that the symptoms occurring in these condition are:

> [n]oticeable during respiration and are as follows: At the moment of inspiration, the epigastric and hypochondriac regions are depressed and the chest dilates, during expiration these movements are reversed. When the diaphragm is weak these signs are only seen during forced respiration, but during tranquil breathing as well as in healthy persons the bulging of the belly and the expansion of the chest occurs together [63, p. 330].

Thus, Duchenne sign refers to depression of the epigastric and hypochondriac regions in patients with diaphragmatic paralysis and pericardial effusion. We were unable to confirm the publication where he described this relationship in pericardial effusion [64] (Table 8.1). Duchenne made numerous discoveries and contributions to the medical literature with eponymous conditions and disease that bears his namesake including Duchenne attitude, Duchenne Disease (Tabes dorsalis, progressive bulbar palsy), Duchenne paralysis, Duchenne-Aran Disease, Duchenne Erb-Palsy Paralysis, and Duchenne-Griesinger Disease (Duchenne Muscular Atrophy or Dystrophy) [60, 65]. We are unaware of any study that evaluated the sensitivity or specificity of this sign.

Broadbent Sign

William Henry Broadbent (1835–1907) was born at Longwood, near Huddersfield, England, passed the qualifying examination by the College of Physicians, London in 1857, and received his medical degree from the University of London in 1860 [66, 67]. He served at St. Mary's Hospital in 1858, London Fever Hospital in 1860, and Western General Dispensary as an outpatient, full, and later consulting physician respectively [68]. He was a member of the Royal College of Physicians in 1861, fellow in 1869, censor 1888–1890, and senior censor from 1895 to1896 [67, 69]. He was appointed President of the Harveian Society in 1863, Medical Society of London in 1881, Clinical Society from 1887 to 1888, and Neurological Society from 1895 to 1896 [68, 69]. In 1897, he was elected fellow of the Royal Society and received honorary titles of LLD from the Universities of Edinburgh in 1896, St. Andrew in 1897, and Toronto in 1906, and Doctor of Science (D.Sc.) from the University of Leed in 1904 [67, 69–71]. He is the recipient of a number of distinguished honors including Knight Commander of the Victorian Order in 1901, Grand Cross and Insignia of the Légion d'honneur in 1904, and physician extraordinary to Queen Victoria and physician-in-ordinary to King Edward [67, 69, 70]. His work spanned the fields of cardiology and neurology and areas of cancer and typhoid [71].

In a tribute to Broadbent's character, a former student wrote in an obituary the following description:

> Those who kept in touch with him could always be sure of kindly and wise counsel for the asking, whether the matter were one as to a career, a perplexing case, or personal or domestic illness. In the first two of these contingencies I have myself repeatedly experienced his unfailing kindness; in the last I have known of instances where all the engagements of a busy life have been put aside to make time to give freely his aid in consultation at the bedside of some former pupil, not only in or near London, but at distances involving a railway journey of many hours each day [69, p. 71].

William Broadbent described in 1895 in his paper entitled "An unpublished physical sign" the finding identified in four patients of a:

> [v]isible retraction, synchronous with the cardiac systole, of the left back in the region of the eleventh and twelfth ribs, and in three of which there is also systolic retraction of less degree in the same region of the right back. In all the cases there is a definite history of pericarditis, and in three of them there are other conditions strongly suggesting an adherent pericardium [72, p. 200].

Furthermore, he discussed the findings of adherent pericardium at the Medical Society's Transaction in 1898:

> A systolic tug of the left false ribs posteriorly communicated by the diaphragm may be conspicuous. The recoil from the drag may be so distinct as to look and feel to the hand like pulsation, and in the first case in which I observed it, now more than 20 years since-a case of left empyema-it was taken for pulsation, and it was supposed that a pulsating tumour of some kind underlay the empyema. A post-mortem examination showed that the cause was adherent pericardium . I have often seen this tugging since, and in some cases it can be made to affect the right false ribs by causing the patient in the sitting posture to lean over to the left so as to throw the drag of the heart upon the right half of the diaphragm. It must be added that this indication is not infallible, as the tugging has been observed when the heart was hypertrophied without adhesions [73, p. 25].

He accounted for the proposed pathogenesis of this occurrence due to the:

> Diaphragm, which, if pulled upon, would have more effect on the floating eleventh and twelfth ribs than on the other more fixed ones. In cases of large heart with adherent pericardium there is a considerable area of the ventricles closely adherent to the central tendon of the diaphragm, and the powerful contraction of the hypertrophied heart must give a decided tug to this structure. That it should affect the ribs more often on the left side would be expected from the adhesion being manly to the left of the middle line; the liver also, which is often large in these cases, may restrain the movement to the right [74, p. 200].

He believed that "systolic retraction of the lower ribs on the lateral or posterior aspect of the thorax is of the greatest importance, and can scarcely be due to anything else than pericardial disease" [74, p. 56]. Broadbent sign thus refers to the systolic retraction of the chest wall near the eleventh and twelfth rib posteriorly due to pericardial adhesion in patients with adhesive-constrictive pericarditis (Table 8.1). We are unaware of any study that evaluated the sensitivity or specificity of this sign.

Ogle Sign

Cyril Ogle (1861–1931) was born near Sheffield, UK, attended medical school at St. George's Hospital, London beginning in 1883, qualified in 1888, appointed assistant in 1897, physician in 1904, and consulting physician in 1926. He was elected member of the Royal College of Physicians, London in 1891 and fellow in 1899 [75]. He was active in the chapter serving as an examiner in pharmacy, medicine, councilor, censor and from 1922–1927 Vice-President of the Clinical Section [76]. As a tribute to his character H.R. wrote: "His exceptional abilities were fully recognized by his colleagues and pupils, who paid him the well-deserved tribute of making him the doctors' doctor. A more willing and unselfish friend cannot be imagined, and it is certain that he spent his life in the service of others" [76, p. 426].

Cyril Ogle and Herbert Allingham described in a patient with purulent pericarditis that: "[b]oth external jugular veins were very distended, not altering during inspiration, and without visible pulsation or even flicker, but they contained liquid blood" [77, p. 693]. Thus, Ogle sign refers to the presence of distension of the external jugular veins without pulsation in patients with purulent pericarditis (Table 8.1).

Nonpulsatile distended jugular veins are found in cases of obstruction (e.g., constrictive pericarditis, mediastinitis, thrombosis of the upper thoracic veins) or by unilateral or bilateral compression (e.g., enlarged mediastinal or cervical lymph nodes, aortic aneurysm) resulting in impaired venous return to the right heart [78]. The height of distension of nonpulsatile jugular veins, unlike pulsatile jugular veins, is neither affected by changes in upper body position nor during respiration [78]. Thus, this is a useful method for distinguishing possible causes. The finding of distended neck veins in a wide variety of diseases suggests that it is a nonspecific sign in the diagnosis of constrictive pericarditis.

Keith Sign

Sir Arthur Keith (1866–1955) was born at Old Machar, Aberdeen, Scotland, began his medical training at Marischal College, Aberdeen, Scotland, in 1884 and graduated with an MB in 1888 [79, 80]. The following year he accepted a position as a medical officer in Siam, Thailand where he also developed his interest in botany collecting over 500 flora specimens [81]. He returned to London in 1891, pursuing his primary interest in comparative anatomy and paleontology and in 1894 received his medical degree at Aberdeen University and fellowship from the Royal College of Surgeons, England. He lectured on Anatomy at the London Hospital Medical School in 1895 where he was involved in the study on the anatomical bases of the mechanisms of respiration and cardiac function including cardiac arrhythmias with Sir James Mackenzie (1853–1925) and Martin Flack (1882–1932) [80, 81]. In collaboration with Flack, they identified the sino-auricular (sino-artial) node [80, 81]. In 1908, he was appointed Hunterian Professor and Conservator of the Hunterian Museum at the Royal College of Surgeons England, between 1914 and 1918 was elected President to the Royal Anthropological Institute, and from 1916 to 1933 was acting editor of the *Journal of Anatomy* [80–83]. His other accolades included being appointed Fullerian Professor of Physiology of the Royal Institute of Great Britain from 1918 to 1923, elected Rector of Aberdeen University in 1930, and knighted in 1923 [81, 82]. Keith's life work and career can be summarized into three facets:

> He was, of course, primarily a human anatomist and his knowledge of human anatomy (particularly in relation to its clinical applications) was quite profound. Secondly he was a comparative anatomist having an unrivalled personal acquaintance with the morphology of the higher Primates. Thirdly, he was a physical anthropologist who allowed his interests to stray far beyond the narrow field represented by measuring tape and calipers [81, p. 155].

He was the recipient of six honorary degrees including the LLD from University of Aberdeen, Doctor of Law from Birmingham and Leeds, and Doctor of Science from Durham, Manchester and Oxford [80]. He described the phenomenon of lateral thoracic respiratory expansion in cases of pericardial adhesions (Table 8.1):

> When the pericardium becomes fixed by adhesions to the lungs and chest wall a number of obscure symptoms follow owing to the arrest of the normal respiratory movement of

> the heart. The type of respiration may change; the patient, instead of gaining his inspiratory space by a forward heave of his abdominal wall, due to the descent of the diaphragm, inspires by expanding the walls of his chest and body in a lateral direction [84, p. 558]. (…) In that movement the central part of the diaphragm and its crura take no part [84, p. 559].

We are unaware of any studies which evaluated the sensitivity or specificity of this sign.

Wenckebach Sign

Karel Frederik (Karl Friedrich) Wenckebach (1864–1940) was born at The Hague, Netherlands, and received his medical degree from the University of Utrecht in 1888 [85]. That same year, he had an initial appointment as an assistant at the Institute of Zoology and subsequently in the Departments of Pathology and Normal Anatomy [85]. He served at the University of Groningen, the Netherlands, as Professor of Pathology and Therapeutics and Clinic, and Director of Pathology Laboratories from 1901 to 1911 [85, 86]. He was appointed Chair of Medicine at the University of Strasbourg from 1911 to 1914 and University of Vienna from 1914 to 1929. In the Royal College of Physicians of London and Edinburgh and Royal Society of Medicine, he was an honorary fellow and a foreign corresponding member of the British Medical Association [85]. Sir Thomas Lewis amply described the extent of Wenckebach's studies in the field of cardiovascular disease:

> When as a young man I first met Wenckebach it was at Groningen, where he then held the chair of medicine. He had already reached fame by his independent analysis of cardiac irregularities, using the radial pulse only; this work, published as whole in his first book, *Die Arrhythmie*, in 1903, was a brilliant achievement and the foundation of much that followed. (…) In later years, by publishing an instance in which quinine stopped attacks of auricular fibrillation, he made a first observation that led quickly to the successful use of quinidine for chronic fibrillation. His work upon beriberi heart, undertaken in post-war years in the Dutch East Indies, again broke fresh ground and must be regarded as of high importance [85].

Wenckebach showed by taking photographs during respiration in a patient with adherent pericardium, instead of the lateral expansion of the chest as described by Keith, there is during inspiration:

> [o]nly an upward movement of the chest and that is very limited. There is no forward movement of the chest wall whatever. Looking at the patient, we see an inspiratory retraction of the lower part of the sternum and ribs. (…) So we find in this disease a paradoxical respiratory movement of the chest, a pendant to the so-called paradoxical pulse [87, p. 66].

He accounted for this finding that adhesions cause the diaphragm to:

> [n]ot only pull at the heart, but pulls at the chest wall in front. (...) The absence of a marked descent of the diaphragm in inspiration is proved by the ascent of the vaulting of the abdominal wall. Even we see an inward movement probably due to the fact that the chest with the adherent diaphragm is strongly heaved off from the abdominal contents [87, p. 66].

Wenckebach thought that:

> [i]t is a very valuable sign for the diagnosis of adherent pericardium [87, p. 65]. (...) So every new symptoms has to be welcomed, and I venture to think that the arrest or even retraction of the lower part of the sternum with its cartilage in inspiration *must* be found in every case whether there are adhesions between diaphragm, heart, and chest wall [87, p. 67].

It is of historical interest that Francis Sibson described in 1881 the finding of limited anterior chest well expansion in his chapter on adherent pericardium:

> When, however, the heart is, as usual, enlarged, being often affected with valvular disease, the adhesions may be short, fibrous, and binding; and the front of the organ maybe fixed to the two lower thirds of the sternum and the adjoining cartilages by pleuro-pericardial adhesions, so that the automatic and respiratory movements of the heart, and the inspiratory expansion of the lungs, are restrained; thus the discovery of the adhesions during life may generally in such cases be made by a careful study of the physical signs; its diagnosis being the more certain and easy in proportion as the heart is more enlarged, and more firmly fixed to the anterior walls of the chest [88, p. 203].

Thus, Wenckebach sign refers to the absence of anterior movement of the chest during inspiration in patients with adhesive-constrictive pericarditis (Table 8.1). We are unaware of any studies which evaluated the sensitivity or specificity of this sign.

Hirtz Sign

Edgard Hirtz (1849–1916) was born in Winzenheim, Haut-Rhin, Alsace and received his medical training at Old Faculty of Strasbourg and Paris. He continued his training under Louis-Alexandre Saint-Germain (1835–1897), Noël Guéneau de Mussy (1813–1885), and Paul Camille Hippolyte Brouardel (1837–1906) in Paris. He was appointed physician at the Paris Hospital in 1887, head of the Department at Necker Hospital, Paris, and officer of the Légion d'honneur in 1910 [89–91]. Edgard Hirtz described in his paper entitled "Knee chest position as a sign of pericarditis" the findings in a patient with acute generalized articular rheumatism and dyspnea:

> He was obliged to sit up, leaning forward for a few minutes at a time, but even this position did not give him the desired relief. The patient was relieved of his dyspnea only when he assumed the knee-chest position, which he instinctively took himself. It is this singular position which attracted my attention when I first saw the patient. He was upon his knees on the bed, his body bent forward, and supported by his elbows. The first sight of this individual in a condition of intense anxiety, cyanosis and very short of breath, bent forward in the knee-chest position made me think of the possibility of pericarditis with marked effusion, even without proceeding with the examination [92, p. 122].

Based on his observations and the improvement of dyspnea with thoracentesis:

> I believe, in fact, that the knee-chest position necessitated by an intense dyspnea is a characteristic sign of pericarditis with large effusions. While this sign is rare, it seems to have a definite value; for in my experience it always indicates the presence of a large pericardial effusion [92, p. 123].

Thus, Hirtz sign refers to the improvement in the symptom of dyspnea when the patient assumes the "knee chest posture" in patients with marked pericardial effusion (Table 8.1, Fig. 8.1). This sign has also been found to be helpful in patients with

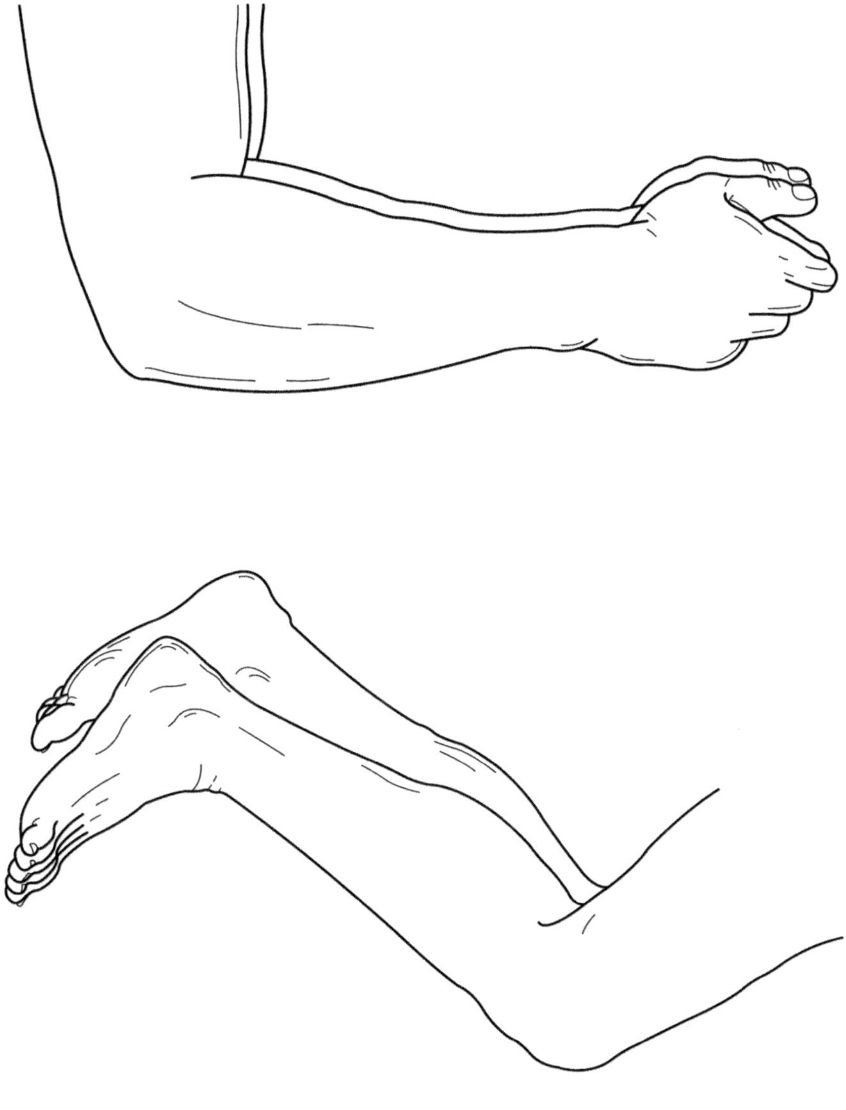

Fig. 8.1 Hirtz sign (by Ryan Yale)

"rheumatic, tuberculous, scarlet fever, and nephritic pericardial effusions." [93, p. 49]. Hirtz acknowledged in his manuscript that Franz Zehetmayer (1813–1846) in 1845 and Pierre Merklen (1852–1906) in 1892 each reported a case where a patient with large pericardial effusion assumed the knee-chest position [92].

Wynter Sign

Walter Essex Wynter (1860–1945) was born in Brompton, London, England, received his medical training at Middlesex and St. Bartholomew Hospital, London, and medical degree in 1888 [94]. He served as assistant in 1891, full physician in 1901, and consulting physician in 1925, at the Middlesex Hospital [94]. He was elected Fellow of the Royal College of Physicians, London in 1897 [95]. In addition to the sign which bears his namesake, it is of historical interest that he reported in 1891 a lumbar puncture technique, the same year, but 1 month after Heinrich Irenaeus Quincke (1844–1922) performed the first lumbar puncture. His technique differed from Quincke in that it involved an incision in the dura followed by insertion of a Southey's tube with rubber drainage at L2 intervertebral space, rather than a very fine cannula between the third and fourth lumbar vertebral arch [96, 97]. Wynter described a sign that he identified in patients with acute fibrinous pericarditis secondary to rheumatic heart disease with predominantly polyarthritis:

> The sign suggested in this communication is inhibition of the action of the diaphragm, indicated by suppression of normal abdominal respiratory movement. (…) [t]he cessation of phrenic action is bilateral, and consequently absence of abdominal movement is as obvious as in abdominal disorders, albeit other abdominal manifestations, such as muscular rigidity and general tenderness are lacking [98, p. 40].

He recognized that, "[i]nflammation of the pericardium, possibly commencing in some other part than that immediately in contact with the chest wall, indicated by its presence by reflex inhibition of the diaphragm some days before the appearance of ordinary sign." [98, p. 42]. Thus, "Loss of abdominal movement, as a sign of pericarditis is the more valuable, in that it may precede and outlast the other indications, and so afford grounds for anticipatory or retrospective diagnosis." [98, p. 45]. He acknowledged and referred to the work in Sibson's textbook *Collected Works of Francis Sibson* published in 1901 where this finding was described:

> The respiratory play of the upper ribs was more than doubled in extent in three-fourths of the cases observed (5 of 7), so that respiratory was as a rule high. This was due to the arrest or restraint of the action of the diaphragm caused by extensive inflammation of the central tendon of the diaphragm, where it forms the floor of the pericardium [99, p. 141].

Furthermore, Sibson accounted for the proposed pathogenesis of this finding.

> The inspiratory movement of the abdomen below the ensiform cartilage was either reversed (in 12), arrested (in 1), or restrained (in 6) in every case of pericarditis in which that sign was observed. This is at once accounted for by the inflammation, in that disease, of the central tendon of the diaphragm where it forms the floor of the pericardium, which leads to the virtual paralysis of the central portion of the diaphragm. This fact, that the anterior wall

> of the epigastric space, instead of advancing, recedes during inspiration, gives us a physical sign of great value in the diagnosis of pericarditis, and of the advance and decline of that disease [99, p. 142].

Thus, Wynter sign refers to the depression of abdominal wall in the epigastrium during inspiration in patients with acute fibrinous pericarditis (Table 8.1). We are unaware of any studies that evaluated the sensitivity or specificity of this sign.

Volhard Sign

Franz Volhard (1872–1950) was born in Munich, Germany, and received his medical education at the Universities of Bonn, Strasbourg, and Halle, Germany, completing his state examination from the University of Halle in 1897 [100, 101]. In Berlin, he worked as a morbid anatomist followed by a position as a lecturer at the University Gieβen in 1898 [100, 102, 103]. He served as Director of the Clinic of Internal Medicine at the Dortmund Municipal Hospital in 1905 (102, 104). He was the Director of the Municipal Hospital in Mannheim in 1908, chief of internal medicine from 1910 to 1918, and appointed Professor and Director of the Clinic of Internal Medicine at the University of Halle in 1918 [102, 103]. He accepted the position of Professor of Medicine at Frankfurt am Main, Germany in 1928, and was President of the German Society of Internal Medicine in 1930 [101, 103].

He received an honorary doctorate from the Sorbonne (University of Paris) in 1933 and was the co-editor of *Zentralblatt für innere Medizin* and chief editor of the *Neue medizinische Welt* [104, 105]. His research involved multiple therapeutic areas including nephrology (hypertension, low-protein diet in uremia, clinical aspects of uremia and isosthenuria marker of chronic renal disease), pulmonary (positive pressure respirator and method to assess peak flows at the bedside in bronchospastic and emphysematous lung disease), cardiovascular (increased venous pressure in pericarditis and retinal vasospasms in severe hypertension with proteinuria), infectious diseases, neurology, and gastroenterology (identified and characterized gastric lipase) [102–104]. He is perhaps best recognized for his work on diseases of the kidney. Volhard with his colleague Karl Theodor Fahr (1877–1945) in their monograph *Die Brightsche Nierenkrankheit: Klinik, Pathologie und Atlas* (Bright's Kidney Disease: Clinic, Pathology and Atlas) published in 1914 revolutionized the field of nephrology by classifying renal disease (Bright's disease) into three main groups: inflammatory diseases which involved the glomeruli or glomerulonephritis (nephritis), degenerative disease or nephrosis, and arteriosclerotic (sclerotic) renal disease [102, 103, 105]. Their work was influential in distinguishing benign from malignant nephrosclerosis forms of hypertension. In regard to the extent of his contribution to nephrology:

> It remains true, however, that no one since Bright has done more than Franz Volhard to advance knowledge in this important branch of medicine. For more than a generation his clinic at Frankfurt was a Mecca for those interested in renal disease, and his teaching and methods for long prevailed throughout the civilized world [105].

With his colleague Viktor Schmieden, they reported their observation of the motion of the chest wall in a patient with calcific pericarditis with adhesions:

> It is possible to distinguish two types of callous pericarditis depending on whether external adhesion of the pericardium to the chest wall or shrinkage of the callous thickened pericardium dominates the clinical picture. The difference is that in the one case, mediastinal factors are more important than the fusion of the heart to the chest wall. In this latter circumstance the heart becomes overtaxed during systole because during each contraction it must overcome the resistance of the relatively rigid chest wall by increasing its pull inward to the left. In the other case, in which the callous grip on the heart predominates, diastole is primarily affected. In the first case we see the picture of a more or less profound weakness of the heart muscle and the entire pulmonary margins and heart during respiration on the fluoroscopic plate, and most importantly, the characteristic retraction of the heart and chest wall during systole and its return in diastole [106, p. 5].

Volhard's name is only ascribed to this physical finding. By convention since both names appeared in the publication, it would be more commonplace to refer to this sign as the Volhard-Schmieden sign in recognition of the contributions by both authors. Thus, the Volhard sign has been referred to as the "see-saw" movement of the chest. That is, the systolic displacement of the thorax to the left with an opposite (rightward) movement in diastole [107] (Table 8.1). They recognized that this sign is not pathognomonic and identified it in cases of severe mitral stenosis:

> Yes, even here we often find systolic constriction of the heart in the region of the right ventricle lying adjacent to the chest wall, and a swinging movement of the chest wall, reminiscent of the spinning of the chest wall in mediastinopericarditis. Instead of quietness over the heart, we feel a moderately lifting action of the right ventricle in the region of the cardiac dullness and below the left costal arch, and hear the characteristic mitral rhythm and the diastolic sound above the tapping apex beat [106, p. 6].

This suggests that the sign presumably lacks sufficient specificity when used alone in the diagnosis of adhesive pericarditis.

Schmieden Sign

Victor (Viktor) Gottfried Otto Schmieden (1874–1945) was born in Berlin, Germany, and received his medical training at the Universities of Freiburg, Munich, Berlin, and Bonn and medical doctorate from the University of Bonn. He was a trainee assistant at the Pathological Institute of the University of Göttingen from 1898 to 1900. He habilitated for surgery in Bonn in 1903, and was a Privatdozent (adjunct professor) in 1907 [108]. Between 1908 and 1913, he was appointed Professor of Surgery at Friedrich-Wilhelms-Universität, Berlin, was a Professor and Chair of surgery at the University of Halle from 1913 to 1919, and served as second Professor of ordinary for Surgery at Frankfurt University in 1919 [108, 109]. He was also a member of the German Academy of Sciences Leopoldina in 1916 [108].

He made a number of contributions to medicine including laparotomy for management of abdominal gunshot wounds, pericardiectomy for calcific pericarditis (Schmieden Operation) and recognized the sequence from adenomatous polyps to colorectal cancer (dysplasia-carcinoma) recommending total colectomy for patients with polyposis coli [110, 111]. In addition to the sign which he reported with Volhard, he also described the fluoroscopic appearance of the diaphragm in cases of constrictive pericarditis caused by adhesion between the pericardium, mediastinum and pleura. In this case, there is systolic elevation of the diaphragm due to attachments between the diaphragm and cardiac apex [112]. Interestingly, he also described this phenomenon intraoperatively:

> After the lateral and posterior surface of the left ventricle is free, the diaphragmatic surface and the apex are separated with sharp and blunt dissection. The result of this is very impressive. The diaphragmatic portion of the callus, surrounds this section of the heart like petals. The apex, bounded to the diaphragm, cannot produce the normal systolic retraction. On the contrary it becomes elongated during systole and ends sharply. After this section has been freed, the apex regains its normal systolic retraction [111, p. 91].

Thus, Schmieden sign is a radiographic finding in patients with adhesive-constrictive pericarditis where there is systolic elevation of the diaphragm during inspiration [107] (Table 8.1).

Rabin Sign

Coleman Berley Rabin (1900–1991) was born in New York City and received his medical degree from Columbia University College of Physicians and Surgeons in 1922 [113]. He was an intern at Mount Sinai Hospital in 1922 where he completed training in the Pathology laboratory from 1927 to 1938 [114]. He was Clinical Assistant Professor of Medicine at Mount Sinai School of Medicine, elected President of the American College of Chest Physician, and recognized for his professional achievements in medicine by receiving the Townsend Harris Medal by the Associated Alumni of the College of the City of New York [114, 115].

As described by Benjamin Felson in chapter 24 entitled "Some special signs in roentgenology" in Rabin's book *Roentgenology of the Chest* published in 1958, "With the neck in a neutral position, elevation of the aortic arch on swallowing indicates an abnormal adherence of the arch to the trachea. Rabin has called this the *aortic swallowing sign*." [116, p. 259–260]. Faber noted that this finding may be found in patients with pulmonary emphysema, luetic aortitis and aneurysm, mediastinal tumor, adhesive pericarditis and typically as a sign in constrictive pericarditis. As to the pathogenesis of this sign, it is believed to be caused by increased tension of the paratracheal connective tissue in the case of severe pulmonary emphysema when the heart and aorta assume a downward displacement and when elongation of the aortic arch results in the connective tissue between the aorta and trachea to tighten [116]. Thus, Rabin sign or "aortic swallowing sign" refers to the presence of elevation of the cardiopericardial silhouette detected fluoroscopically on swallowing due to external pericardial adhesion, as originally reported in Rabin's book *Radiology of the Chest: Diagnostic Roentgenology* in 1952 [117] (Table 8.1). The presence of this sign in other diseases suggests that it lacks sufficient specificity for the diagnosis of adhesive pericarditis.

Spodick Sign

David H. Spodick (1927–2019) was born in Hartford Connecticut and graduated from New York Medical College in 1950 [118]. He completed an internship at St. Francis Hospital, Hartford Connecticut and residency at Beth Israel Hospital and New England Medical Center [118]. After completing advanced fellowship training in cardiology he served at Lemuel Shattuck Hospital for 19 years followed by a position of Chief of Cardiology at St. Vincent Hospital, Worcester Massachusetts. He was Director Emeritus of the Cardiovascular Medicine Fellowship Program at St. Vincent Hospital and Professor of Medicine Emeritus at the University of Massachusetts Medical School [119]. Spodick published extensively and is the recipient of numerous accolades including the Melvin L. Marcus Memorial Award by the International Academy of Cardiology at the third World Congress of Heart Disease for his distinguished contribution as a gifted teacher in cardiology [119]. As a testimony to his character Gordon Saperia wrote, "David Spodick has reminded us all that we should not be too certain of what we know and the open mindedness may be our greatest intellectual asset." [118].

Spodick retrospectively studied electrocardiograms of 50 clinically diagnosed cases of acute pericarditis. In this study "The T-P interval was the base line for P-R and S-T changes [120, p. 471]." He noted that:

> The predominant P-R segment depression across the pericardium document the posterior component. Because of these P-R segment deviations, it is of practical importance in acute pericarditis to consider the T-P segment to be the electrocardiographic base line to avoid mistaking P-R segment depression for S-T segment elevation [120, p. 474].

Thus, Spodick sign refers to the presence of S-T segment elevation and P-R depression above or below the isoelectric T-P segment in acute pericarditis (Table 8.1).

Based on this point of reference, S-T segment elevation was found in 48 (96%) of patients and P-R segment depression in 41 of 50 patients (82%) with acute pericarditis [120]. In patients with acute pericarditis and absence of the typical findings of ST segment deviation, P-R segment deviation were found in 14 of 19 (74%) of patients [121]. Kranin emphasized the importance of the physical examination in patients with acute pericarditis. In their study of 31 patients with a pericardial friction rub, diagnostic electrocardiographic changes was identified in only one patient [122].

Conclusion

Through inspection, physicians observed depressions and bulging of the chest and abdominal walls, changes in height of the jugular veins, and electrocardiographic and radiographic findings as methods to detect acute and chronic pericarditis. There are few studies which evaluated the sensitivity or specificity of these signs. Thus, their usefulness and applicability in modern day clinical practice are unknown. Furthermore, detection of these signs is less likely since patients more commonly present earlier in the course of this disease resulting in fewer cases of advanced disease. Nevertheless, they are important to appreciate, as they provide an explanation of the pathogenesis and pathophysiology of the disease, reemphasize to clinicians the skill of inspection or observation as a crucial skill to master during the initial part of the physical examination, and provide a greater appreciation for the importance of this aspect of the physical examination in diagnosis. They represent the window to better learn and diagnose disease and provide a more profound appreciation of clinical medicine.

References

1. Inspection (n.) Online etymology dictionary. 2001–2012. https://www.etymonline.com/word/inspection. Accessed 26 Nov 2018.
2. Skinner HA. The Origin of Medical Terms. Baltimore: Williams & Wilkins Company; 1949.
3. DeGowin EK, DeGowin RL. Bedside Diagnostic Examination. New York: Macmillan Publishing Co; 1981.
4. Willius FA, Keys TE. Joseph Leopold Auenbrugger. In: Classics of Cardiology, vol. 1. New York: Henry Schuman; 1941. p. 191–2.
5. Auenbrugger L. On percussion of the chest being a translation of Auerbrugger's original treatise entitled "Inventum novum ex percussione thoracis humani, ut singo abstrsos interni perctoris morbos detegendi [Vienna, 1761]. Forbes J, translator. London: The Johns Hopkins Press; 1824. p. 73–403.
6. Birrer RB, Birrer CD. Medical Diagnostic Signs: A Reference Collection of Eponymic Bedside Signs. Springfield: Charles C. Thomas Publisher; 1982.
7. Spodick DH. Acute Pericarditis. New York: Grune & Stratton; 1959.
8. Wagner R. Grundriss der Encyklopädie und Methodologie der medizinischen Wissenschaften nach geschichtlicher Ansicht. Erlangen: JJ Palm and Ernst Enke; 1838.
9. Heim EL. Epoche Napoleon von der Bastille bis Waterloo. 2003–2018. http://www.epoche-napoleon.net/de/bio/h/heim.html. Accessed 1 Dec 2018.
10. Heim EL. Stiftung Historische Kirchhöfe und Friedhöfe in Berlin-Brandenburg. http://stiftung-historische-friedhoefe.de/ernst-ludwig-heim/. Accessed 1 Dec 2018.
11. Bauer J. Life of Alexander von Humboldt. Bauer J, translator. London: Ingram, Cooke, & Co; 1851.
12. Heim EL. Neuer Nekrolog der deutschen zwölfter Jahrgang, 1834. Zweiter Teil. Weimar: Druck und Verlag von Bernh; 1836. p. 705–36.
13. Heidel C, Kreysign LM, Ludwig F. Die Professoren der Medizinischen Fakultät Carl Gustav Carus Dresden und ihrer Vorgängereinrichtungen 1814–2004, vol. 20. München: KG Saur; 2005.
14. Friedrich Ludwig Kreysig: German physician. https://upclosed.com/people/friedrich-ludwig-kreysig/. Accessed 1 Dec 2018.

15. Pierer HA. Kreysig. In: Pierer's Universal-Lexikon der Vergangenheit und Gegenwartt, vol. 9. Altenburg: Verlagsbuchhandlung; 1860. p. 810–1.
16. Callisen ACP. Kreysig (Friedr. Ludw.). In: ACP C, editor. Medicinisches Schriftsteller-Lexikon der Jetzt Lebenden Verfasser, 29. Band. Copenhagen: Taubstummen-Institute zu Schleswig; 1841. p. 346.
17. Friedrich Ludwig Kreyssig. Stadtwiki Dresden. 2016. http://www.stadtwikidd.de/wiki/Friedrich_Ludwig_Kreyssig. Accessed 2 Dec 2018.
18. Kreysig FL. Ueber die Unterscheidungsmerkmale der Verwachsung des Herzbeutels mit dem Herzen. In: Die Krankheiten des Herzens Systematisch Bearbeitet und Durch Eigne Beobachtungen Erläutert. Zweiter Teil. Berlin: Maurerschen Buchhandlung; 1816. p. 616–28.
19. [No author]. Obituary: William Rutherford Sanders. Edinb Obst Soc. 1881:939–49.
20. Sanders J. General List of the Members of the Royal Medical Society of Edinburgh. Edinburgh: A. & D. Padon; 1806. p. 28.
21. Sanders JA. Treatise on pulmonary consumption, in which a new view of the principles of its treatment is supported by original observations on every period of the disease. Crit Rev. 1808;13:309–15.
22. Sanders J. Remarques sur le diagnostic de l'adhérence du péricarde au coeur. Arc Gén de Méd. 1823;1:153–7.
23. Laennec RTH. Traité de l'auscultation médiate et des maladies des poumons et du coeur. Forbes J, translator. New York: Samuel Wood & Sons; 1830.
24. Lee S, James H. Dictionary of National Biography, vol. 27. New York: Macmillan and Co.; 1891. p. 316–7.
25. Hope JA. Treatise on the Diseases of the Heart and Great Vessels. Philadelphia: Lea & Blanchard; 1842.
26. Fye B. Profiles in cardiology: James Hope. Clin Cardiol. 1989;12:358–9.
27. Willius FA, Keys TE. James Hope. In: Classics of Cardiology, vol. 2. New York: Henry Schuman, Inc.; 1941. p. 403–18.
28. James Hope. Lives of the fellows. Royal College of Physicians. 2009. http://munksroll.rcplondon.ac.uk/Biography/Details/2262. Accessed 1 Dec 2018.
29. [No author]. Dr. James Hope. Nature. 1941;147:605–6.
30. Hope J. Principles and Illustrations of Morbid Anatomy Adapted to the Elements of M. Andral and to the Cyclopaedia of Practical Medicine. Cincinnati: DeSilver and Burr; 1844.
31. Grant K. Professional education. In: Memoir of the late James Hope, M.D., Physician to St. George's Hospital. London: J. Hatchard & Sons; 1842. p. 20–51.
32. Hope J. Adhesions of the pericardium. In: A Treatise of the Disease of Heart and Great Vessels. 3rd ed. London: John Churchill; 1839. p. 191–5.
33. Spodick DH. Chronic and Constrictive Pericarditis. New York: Grune and Stratton; 1964.
34. Lee S. Williams, Charles James Blasius (1805–1899). In: Dictionary of National Biography, vol. 21. New York: The Macmillan Company; 1909. p. 383–4.
35. [No author]. Obituary: Williams CJB, physician extraordinary to the queen. Br Med J. 1889;1(1474):745–6.
36. Williams CJB. Analytical and classified catalogue of the library of the parliament of Queensland. In: O'Donovan D, editor. Volume III: Q-Z and Supplement. Brisbane: E. Gregory, Government Printer; 1900. p. 2670.
37. CJB W. Inflammatory diseases: pericarditis. In: The Pathology and Diagnosis of Diseases of the Chest Compromising a Rational Exposition of Their Physical Signs. 4th ed. London: John Churchill; 1840. p. 233–46.
38. Rolleston JD. Jean Bapiste Bouillaud (1796–1881): a pioneer in cardiology and neurology. Pro R Soc Med. 1931;24:1253–62.
39. Silverman BD. Jean Bapiste Bouillaud. Clin Card. 1996;19:836–7.
40. Eling P, Brunia K. Who was the red dean? J Hist Neurosci. 2017;26:111–8.
41. Bouillaud J. Traité clinique des maladies du coeur: Précéde de recherches nouvelles sur l'anatomie et la physiologie de cet organe. Paris: J.-B. Baillière; 1835.

42. Bouillaud J. Traité clinique du rhumatisme articulaire et de la loi de coïncidence des inflammations du coeur avec cette maladie. Paris: J-B. Baillière; 1840.
43. Bouillaud J. De l'oblitération des veines et de son influence sur la formation des hydropisies partielles: considérations sur les hydropisies passives et generals. Archives Gén de Méd.1823;2:188–204.
44. Virchow R. Phlogose und Thrombose in Gefäßsystem. In: Gesammelte Abhandlungen zur wissenschaftlichen Medicin. Berlin: von Meiniger; 1856. p. 458-635.
45. Virchow R. Purulent cysts in the heart. In: Cellular Pathology as based upon Physiological and Pathological Histology. Chance F, translator. London: John Churchill; 1860. p. 196–219.
46. Trousseau A. Phlegmasia Alba Dolens. In: Lecture on Clinical Medicine: Delivered at the Hotel-Dieu, Paris, vol. 5. Cormack JR, Bazire PV, translators. Philadelphia: Lindsay & Blakiston; 1873. p. 281–332.
47. Bouillaud J. Des bruits anormaux produits par la percussion du coeur contre les parois pectorals. In: Traité clinique des maladies du coeur, précéde de recherches nouvelles surl'anatomie et la physiologie de cet organe. Paris: J.-B. Baillière; 1835. p. 193–5.
48. Bouillaud JB. De la péricardite ou de l'inflammation du péricarde, et de ses suites: caractères anatomiques. In: Traité de nosographie médicale. Paris: J.-B. Baillière; 1846. p. 405–17.
49. [No author]. Obituary: Skoda J. Edinb M J. 1881;27:286–7.
50. Skoda J. Abhandlung über Perkussion und Auskultation. Vienna: J.G. Ritter von Mösel and Braumuller; 1839.
51. Sakula A. Joseph Skoda, 1805–81: a centenary tribute to a pioneer of thoracic medicine. Thorax. 1981;36:404–11.
52. Skoda J. Ueber die Erscheinungen, aus denen sich die Verwachsung des Herzens mit dem Herzbeutel an lebenden Menschen erkennen lässt. Zeitschr der Gesellschaft der Aerzte zu Wien. 1852;1:306–15.
53. [No author]. Nikolaus Friedreich. Wien med Presse. 1882;23:971–4.
54. Kussmaul A. Nikolaus Friedreich. Deutsches Arch f klin Med. 1883;32:191–208.
55. Miller JW. Friedreich's ataxia. Med Rev. 1916;22:192–5.
56. Friedreich N. Krankheiten des Herzens. In: Virchow's Handbuch der speciellen Pathologie und Therapie, vol. 5. Erlangen: Verlag von Ferdinand Enke; 1861. p. 385–530.
57. Friedreich N. Zur Diagnose der Herzbeutelverwachsungen. Archiv f path Anat. 1864;29:296–312.
58. Morand P, Gaudeau B, Wiart JP. The jugular pulse in constrictive pericarditis: correlations between hemodynamics and external recordings. Arch Mal Coeur Vaiss. 1975;68:65–75.
59. Lange RL, Botticelli JT, Tsagarsi TJ, Walker JA, Gani M, Bustamante RA. Diagnostic signs in compressive cardiac disorders. Circulation. 1966;33:763–77.
60. Broussolle E, Poirier J, Clarac F, Barbara JG. Figures and institutions of the neurological sciences in Paris from 1800 to 1950, part III. Rev Neurol. 2012;168:301–20.
61. Poore GV. A short sketch of the life and work of Duchenne (de Boulogne). In: Selections from the Clinical Works of Dr. Duchenne (de Boulogne). Poore GV, translator. London: The New Sydenham Society; 1883. p. ix–xx.
62. Duchenne GB. De l'électrisation localisée et de son application à la pathologie et à la thérapeutique. Troisième éd. Paris: J.-B. Baillière; 1872.
63. Duchenne GB. Paralysis and contracture of the diaphragm. In: Selections from the Clinical Works of Dr. Duchenne (de Boulogne). Poore GV, translator. London: The New Sydenham Society; 1883. p. 325–33.
64. Birrer RD, Birrer CD. Medical Diagnostic Signs: A Reference Collection of Eponymic Bedside Signs. Springfield: Charles C. Thomas Publisher; 1982.
65. Firkin BG, Whitworth JA. Dictionary of Medical Eponyms. Boca Raton: A CRC Press Company; 2002.
66. [No author]. Profiles in cardiology: William Henry Broadbent. Clin Cardiol. 1990;13:62–4.
67. [No author]. Obituary: W. Broadbent, M.D., F.R.C.P. Br Med J. 1907;2:177.

68. Death of Sir William Broadbent, the King's physician. The Register, Abelaide, South Australia, July 12, 1907. https://trove.nla.gov.au/newspaper/article/56531453. Accessed 12 Dec 2018.
69. [No author]. Obituary: Sir William Broadbent Bart. St. Louis Med Rev. 1907;56:71–2.
70. Sir William Henry Broadbent, Bart; K.C.V.O; 1835–1907. vii-x. http://rspb.royalsocietypublishing.org/content/royprsb/80/544/0.full.pdf. Accessed 15 Dec 2018.
71. William Henry (Sir) Broadbent. Lives of the fellows. Royal College of Physicians. http://munksroll.rcplondon.ac.uk/Biography/Details/561. Accessed 15 Dec 2018.
72. Broadbent W. An unpublished physical sign. Lancet. 1895;2:200–1.
73. Broadbent W. Adherent pericardium. In: Selections from the Writings, Medical and Neurological of Sir William Broadbent. London: Oxford University Press; 1908. p. 21–6.
74. Broadbent JFH. Adherent Pericardium. New York: William Wood & Company; 1896.
75. Cyril Ogle. Lives of the fellows. Royal College of Physicians. Munks Roll: Volume IV. http://munksroll.rcplondon.ac.uk/Biography/Details/3363. Accessed 22 Dec 2018.
76. [No author]. Obituary: Cyril Ogle D.M., F.R.C.P. Br Med J. 1931;1(3661):426–7.
77. Ogle C, Allingham H. A suggestion for a method of opening the pericardial sac, founded upon a case of purulent pericarditis. Lancet. 1900;1:693–5.
78. Verhave JH. Distended neck veins: their diagnostic and clinical significance. Rocky Mt Med J. 1963;60:34–6.
79. Campbell M. Sir Arthur Keith. Br Heart J. 1955;17:409–10.
80. [No author]. Sir Arthur Keith (1865–1955), Keith-flack node. JAMA. 1967;200:164–5.
81. Clark WE. Le Gros Arthur Keith, 1866–1955. Biogr Mems Fell R Soc. 1955;1:145–61.
82. Arthur Keith (1866–1955) Biography of Arthur Keith. The Royal Institution Science Lives Here. http://www.rigb.org/our-history/people/k/arthur-keith. Accessed 2 Jan 2019.
83. Fleure HJ. Sir Arthur Keith, F.R.S., 1866–1955. Man. 1956;56:123–4.
84. Keith A. Abstract of The Hunterian Lecture on the evolution and action of certain muscular structure of the heart. Lancet. 1904;1:556–9.
85. [No author]. Obituary: Prof. K. F. Wenckebach, MD Hon. FRCP. Br Med J. 1941;1:219.
86. Stephenson HH, editor. Wenckebach, Karl Frederick. In: Who's Who in Science. London: J. & A. Churchill; 1913. p. 510.
87. Wenckebach KF. Some points in the pathology and treatment of adherent pericardium. Br Med J. 1907;1:63–8.
88. Sibson F. Adherent pericardium. In: Collected Works of Francis Sibson M.D., vol. 4. London: Macmillian & Co.; 1881. p. 202–30.
89. [No author]. Obituary: Dr. Edgard Hirtz. Br Med J. 1917;1:247.
90. Edgard Hirtz (1849–1916). Bibliothèque nationale de France. Data.bnf.fr. https://data.bnf.fr/16236054/edgard_hirtz/. Accessed 10 Jan 2018.
91. Hirtz, Edgard. Biographic base. Paris. http://www.biusante.parisdescartes.fr/histoire/biographies/?refbiogr=8049. Accessed 10 Jan 2018.
92. Hirtz E. La position genu-pectorale, signe pathognomonique des péricardites à gros épanchement. La Tribune médicale 1911;7:122–5.
93. [No author]. Knee chest position as a sign of pericarditis. Buffalo Med J. 1912;67:49.
94. Walter Essex Wynter. Lives of the fellows. Royal College of Physicians. http://munksroll.rcplondon.ac.uk/Biography/Details/4927. Accessed 10 Jan 2019.
95. Walter Essex Wynter (1860–1945) M.D. (Lond.), F.R.C.S. (Eng.). The fight against tuberculosis. Wynter, Walter Essex-Epsom College Archive Website. https://www.yumpu.com/en/document/read/43186077/wynter-walter-essex-epsom-college-archive-website. Accessed 2 Jan 2019.
96. Wynter WE. Four cases of tubercular meningitis in which paracentesis of the theca vertebralis was performed for the relief of fluid pressure. Lancet. 1891;1(3531):981–2.
97. Quincke H. Ueber Hydrocephalus. In: Verhandlungen des Congresses für Innere Medizin, vol. 10. Wiesbaden; 1891. p. 321–39.

98. Wynter WE. Absence of abdominal respiratory movement as an indication of pericarditis. Proc R Soc Med. 1911;4:40–50.
99. Ord WM, editor. Collected Works of Francis Sibson, vol. 4. London: Macmillan and Co.; 1881.
100. Pickering G. The first Volhard lecture Franz Volhard, 1872–1972. Clin Sci Mol Med Suppl. 1973;45:1–10.
101. Wolf G. Franz Volhard and his students' tortuous road to renovascular hypertension. Kidney Int. 2000;57:2156–66.
102. Heidland A, Gerabek W, Sebekova K. Franz Volhard and Theodor Fahr: achievements and controversies in their research in renal disease and hypertension. J Hum Hypertens. 2001;15:5–16.
103. [No author]. Obituary: Franz Volhard. Angiology. 1951;2:81–3.
104. Luft FC, Dietz R. Franz Volhard in historical perspective. Hypertension. 1993;22:253–6.
105. [No author]. Obituary: Franz Volhard, MD. Br Med J. 1950;1(4666):1376.
106. Vollhard F, Schmieden V. Ueber Erkennung und Behandlung der Umklammerung des Herzens durch schwielige Parikarditis. Klin Wchschr. 1923;2:5–9.
107. Spodick DB. Chronic and Constrictive Pericarditis. New York: Grune & Stratton; 1964.
108. Biografie, Viktor Schmieden. Wisssenschaftliche Sammlungen. Teil-Katalog der wissenschaftlichen Sammlungen. Humbold-Universistät zu Berlin. http://www.sammlungen.hu-berlin.de/dokumente/16672/. Accessed 3 Jan 2019.
109. Victor Schmieden. Martin-Luther-Universitat Halle-Wittenberg. 2017. http://www.catalogus-professorum-halensis.de/schmiedenvictor.html. Accessed 4 Jan 2019.
110. Sachs M, Encke A. Victor Schmieden (1874–1945) and his contribution to the development of modern surgery. Zentralbl Chir. 1997;122:597–609.
111. Schmieden V. The technic of cardiolysis. Surg Gynec Obst. 1926;43:80–93.
112. Schwedel JB. Acquired diseases of the heart. In: Rabin CB, editor. Roentgenology of the Chest. Illinois: Charles C. Thomas; 1959. p. 418–33.
113. Rabin CB. Obituary listing. JAMA. 1992;267:2260–1.
114. Eve 18. Associated Alumni of The Mount Sinai Medical Center. Scientific Session April 11, 1970. http://dspace.mssm.edu/bitstream/handle/123456789/440/oh%20EVE%2018%20Alumni%20Day%201970.pdf?sequence=1&isAllowed=y. Accessed 20 Dec 2018.
115. Coleman Berley Rabin. Archives and Special Collections at the Augustus C. Long Health Sciences Library of Columbia University. P&S 12 (Fall 1992). p. 46. https://library-archives.cumc.columbia.edu/obit/coleman-berley-rabin. Accessed 2 Jan 2019.
116. Felson B. Some special signs in chest roentgenology. In: Rabin CB, editor. Roentgenology of the Chest. Illinois: Charles C. Thomas; 1959. p. 248–64.
117. Rabin CB. Radiology of the chest. In: Golden R, editor. Diagnostic Roentgenology. Baltimore: Williams & Wilkins; 1952. p. 147–8.
118. Saperia GM, Bishop RL. David H. Spodick. Clin Cardiol. 2004;27:533–4.
119. David H. Spodick. SafeBeat 2018. https://safebeat.org/endorsements/david_h_spodick_md/. Accessed 5 Dec 2018.
120. Spodick DH. Electrocardiogram in acute pericarditis: distributions of morphologic and axial changes by stages. Am J Cardiol. 1974;33:470–4.
121. Bruce MA, Spodick DH. Atypical electrocardiogram in acute pericarditis: characteristics and prevalence. J Electrocardiol. 1980;13:61–6.
122. Krainin FM, Flessas AP, Spodick DH. Infarction-associated pericarditis: rarity of diagnostic electrocardiogram. N Engl J Med. 1984;311:1211–4.

Chapter 9
Physical Signs and Medical Eponyms of Pericarditis: Palpitation

Introduction

Palpation is derived from the Latin word *palpare*, meaning to feel or touch [1]. The history of palpation of the precordium dates back to ancient Egyptian writings of the Ebers papyrus (c. 1550 BC) in which physicians were able to detect the pulsation of heart beat: "[I]f (…) any physician put his hands (or) his fingers [upon the head, upon the back of the] head, upon the two hands, upon the pulse, upon the two feet" [2, p. 41]. Furthermore, as translated by Breasted, the papyrus:

> [p]ictures the physician as placing his hands or fingers at various points along the body of the patient and discerning the pulsation of the heart from one extremity to the other, the question inevitably arises whether he is not discussing the counting of the pulse in making these references. (…) If so it is the earliest such reference in the history of medicine, for the counting of the pulse was unknown to early Greek medicine and is not mentioned until Democritus and the Hippocratic treatises [2, p. 105].

It was William Harvey (1578–1657) who in 1638 published his observations on the motion of the heart against the chest wall in Chapter II on "Of the motions of the heart, as seen in the dissection of living animals" in the book entitled *Exercitatio Anatomica de Motu Cordis et Sanguinis in Animalibus* (Anatomical Treatise on the Movement of the Heart and Blood in Animals).

> In the first place, when the chest of a living animal opened and the capsule surrounding the heart is cut away, one may see that the heart alternates in movement and rest. There is a time when it moves, and a time when it is quiet. (…) The heart is lifted, and rises up to the apex, so that it strikes the chest at that moment, and the beat may be felt on the outside [3, p. 28–29].

It was René Laënnec (1781–1826) who described in his book *Traité de l'Auscultation Médiate et des Maladies des Poumons et du Coeur* (Treatise on Mediate Auscultation and Lung and Heart Diseases) in 1819, the location of the pulse, movement, and transmission of the left and right ventricular impulses against the chest wall:

S. H. Yale et al., *Cardiovascular Eponymic Signs*,
https://doi.org/10.1007/978-3-030-67596-7_9

> In a healthy person, moderately stout, and whose heart is well-proportioned, the pulsation of this organ is only felt in the cardiac region, that is, in the space comprised between the cartilages of the fourth and seventh ribs, and under the lower end of the sternum. The motions of the left cavities are chiefly perceptible in the former position, those of the right cavities in the latter. This is so much the case that, in disease of one side of the heart only, the pulsation in these two situations give quite different results. When the sternum is short, the pulsations extend to the epigastrium [4, p. 548].

Palpation of the precordium is a relevant part of the physical examination since all significant cardiac movements transmitted by the heart are felt on the chest wall. Palpation or "laying on one's hands" involves tactile sensations detected by the palmar aspects of the fingers and thenar eminence identifying pulsations, size, contour, texture, boundaries, and tenderness. Palpation typically follows observation although this sequence may need to be repeated as necessary to reconfirm impressions. Examination of the patient should occur supine, with the trunk elevated 30 degree, followed by positioning the patient in the partial left lateral decubitus position. The examiner uses the palmar aspect of the hand, in particular, the fingertips and distal metacarpals or thenar eminence (heel) of the hand, varying the amount of pressure based on the precordial site and intensity of underlying sensation. The fingertips are used to detect the precise location of the movements of the heart by applying firm pressure using the thenar surface to detect diffuse systolic movements [5].

Palpation of the chest in patients with more severe pericarditis may produce a palpable thrill. This high-frequency perception, similar to ejection sounds and prominent first and second heart sounds, is best detected by applying firm pressure over the distal metacarpals [5]. There are several palpatory physical signs that may be found on physical examination as described in patients with acute and chronic pericarditis. These signs reported as eponyms provide clinicians with a method to diagnose diseases of the pericardium using bedside physical examination techniques. Our goal in this chapter on palpatory eponymic signs of pericarditis is to provide a brief description of the person who identified and reported the sign as originally described, as well as its sensitivity, specificity, and application in modern day clinical practice. The signs are described chronologically based on the date that they were first published (Table 9.1).

Signs

Griesinger Sign

Wilhelm Griesinger (1817–1868) was born in Stuttgart, Germany, and received his medical training and doctorate at the University of Zürich, Switzerland [6]. After receiving additional training in Paris, he returned to practice in Friedrichshafen at Lake Constance, Germany in 1839, followed by an appointment as a medical assistant at Winnenthal Hospital, Zeller, Germany [6]. He served as Assistant and

Table 9.1 Pericardial palpation eponyms signs

Name	Year	Description of method for eliciting sign	Significance
Griesinger [7]	1856	The pulse is faint or disappears during inspiration and reappears again in expiration.	Fibropurulent mediastinal-pericarditis
Oppolzer [15]	1861	Patient in the supine position with heartbeat weaker at the fourth and fifth intercostal space. With change in position the weakness of the heartbeat extends from the second to sixth intercostal spaces. The attenuated heartbeat involves a triangle area bounded by the left sixth rib, sternal border, and clavicle.	Adhesive pericarditis
Kussmaul [20, 21]	1873	1. Very small or disappearances of the arterial pulses during inspiration with its return during expiration "Paradox" represents the discrepancy between the constant cardiac impulse and reduced or absent arterial pulse. 2. During inspiration there is dilation rather than collapse of the jugular veins.	Fibrous mediastinal-pericarditis
Riegel [44]	1876	Decreased amplitude or volume and increase rate of the pulse during inspiration.	Chronic pericarditis
Jaccoud [48]	1877	At the cardiac apex, depression and rise of the intercostal space occurring during systole and diastole, respectively. Referred to as an "undulating movement" of the chest wall.	Adhesive pericarditis
Oliver [53]	1878	Patient in the erect position, and direct to close his mouth and elevate his chin to the fullest extent. The cricoid cartilage is grasped between the finger and thumb, and gentle upward pressure is applied.	Adhesive pericarditis
Paul [58]	1884	Strong impulse of the heart against the chest wall with a weak impulse at the apex.	Adhesive pericarditis
Graves [62]	1884	Strong impulse of the heart at the precordium with a weaker and thready radial pulse.	Acute pericarditis

Privatdozent (Adjunct Professor) in a medical clinic in Tübingen, Germany, in 1843, Associate Professor at the University of Tübingen in 1847, and Professor of Pathology and Therapy at the University of Kiel, Germany, in 1849 [6]. From 1850 to 1852, he was appointed Director of the Medical School, President of the Medical System in Egypt, and personal physician to the viceroy Abbas Pasha in Cairo, Egypt [6]. He returned to the University of Tübingen in 1854 as full Professor of Medicine and Head of the Clinic. By 1859, he served at the Institute for Mentally Ill Children in Mariaberg, Germany, subsequently accepting a position as Chair of the Clinic in Zürich, Switzerland, where he was instrumental in designing a psychiatry hospital. In his final position, he managed the Polyclinic in Berlin beginning in 1865 [6].

He was editor of the *Archiv für physiologische Heilkunde* and *Archive for Psychiatry and Nervous Disease* in 1867, which was aligned with his interest in psychiatric disorders [6]. He was recognized for his achievement by being named honorary doctor of the medical faculty at the 500th anniversary celebration of the University of Vienna, Austria [6]. Carl Reinhold August Wunderlich (1815–1877) summarized Griesinger's accomplishments as follows:

> [h]e took an active part in the reform of German medicine, which began a little over a quarter of a century ago, and by promoting discourse contributed to the defeat of obsolete prejudices. He made outstanding contributions to the reconstruction of medical science. Through meticulous thorough work, he clarified the behavior of several of the most important forms of disease. He discovered and uncovered new knowledge of disease. Through his astute research and the wealth of groundbreaking new ideas, he became the first authority of our time on the pathology of the brain, nervous diseases and psychiatry. Griesinger's achievements in science have not only been enduring and everlasting, but they are of a special kind which guarantees new knowledge for future generations [6, p. 40].

Adolph Franz Widenmann (1885–1918), a student of Griesinger, wrote in the forward to his inaugural dissertation entitled *Beitrag zur Diagnose der Mediastinitis* (Contribution to the Diagnosis of Mediastinitis):

> One of the most instructive cases, which was discussed in the summer of 1854 at the local medical clinic was a case of pericarditis and mediastinitis, which I as a practitioner had the opportunity to observe more closely. (…) The details of the case were kept in the cabinet of the local clinic. Professor Vierordt gave graphic representations of the remarkable pulse phenomenon in his work "The Teaching of the Arterial Pulse." With great kindness and willingness, my distinguished teacher, Professor Griesinger, supported me in drafting these lines, not only giving me all the literary resources, but also communicating his own experiences on the subject with the utmost care. I am glad to find here the opportunity to express my warmest gratitude to him for this and other evidence of his goodwill [7, p. iv].

Widenmann described the pulse in a 21-year-old journeyman subsequently diagnosed with extensive fibro-purulent pericarditis and mediastinitis after a traumatic puncture wound in the leg as being; "[v]ery noticeable; it is small, trembling, frequent, and very often intermittent, and therefore it cannot be counted" [7, p. 7]. During the course of the patient's illness he noted:

> [t]hat the pulse does not stop at indeterminate intervals and always coincides with inspiration. Throughout the course of inspiration, the pulses become faint or disappear and reappear again during expiration [7, p. 14]. (…) Those indistinct weaker waves always coincide with inspiration while the fuller and stronger waves return during expiration [7, p. 18].

Widenmann concluded based on pulse findings and appearance of the aorta at autopsy that:

> [t]he considerable narrowing in the ascending portion and arch as well as the bending and partial axial rotation of rigid cord-shaped exudates at these points are described above. The uncommon weakness of the pulse explained by these conditions sometimes fades to the point of disappearance during inspiration while cardiac contractions persist [7, p. 31].

Thus, Griesinger sign refers to the diminution or disappearance of the pulse during inspiration in patients with fibropurulent pericarditis and mediastinitis [8] (Table 9.1). The sensitivity and specificity of this sign is discussed under Kussmaul sign. There are two other conditions which he described where his name has been ascribed as "Griesinger sign." The first involves the presence of swelling posterior to the mastoid process in patients with transverse sinus thrombosis [9]. The second, Griesinger Hookworm sign also known as *cachexia aquosa,* which refers to the findings of anemia and malnutrition caused by the parasite *Ancylostoma duodenale* [10].

Oppolzer Sign

Johann Ritter von Oppolzer (1808–1871) was born in Gratzen, Nové Hrady (modern-day Czechia), and received his medical doctorate from the University of Prague in 1835. He was Professor at the Medical Clinic and primary physician in the general hospital in Prague beginning 1841, St. Jacobs Hospital in Leipzig in 1848, and Vienna in 1850 [11]. In Vienna, he served as head of the newly founded Second Medical Clinic and rector from 1860 through 1861 [12]. He was elected foreign member of the Royal Swedish Academy of Sciences in 1863 and awarded the Knight's Cross of the Order of Leopold in 1869 [11, 13]. He supported the concept of a physiological approach to disease prevention, early treatment, symptom relief, and stabilization of the patient based on dietary measures, electrotherapy and balneology, the prevailing treatments available during this time period [14].

Niemeyer published and edited a version of Oppolzer's lecture entitled *Ueber Exsudat in dem Herzbeutel und Verwachsung des letztern; nach Oppolzer* (About exudate in the pericardium and adhesion of the latter, after Oppolzer) in which Oppolzer described a patient with exudative pericarditis where:

> [t]he heartbeat while in the supine position at the 4th and 5th intercostal spaces was weaker than that occurring in the normal state. Furthermore, the heartbeat at the 5th intercostal space was weaker than at the 4th intercostal space. When the patient changes his/her position, the location where the heartbeat was felt also differed. The attenuation now extends from the 2nd to the 6th ribs. The attenuation formed a truncated triangle bounded by the lower edge of the 6th rib to the left of the apex, right sternal border, and a line that begins at the clavicle [15, p. 181].

Thus, Oppolzer sign refers to the weak heartbeat at the fourth and fifth intercostal spaces in the supine position extending from the second to sixth rib in a truncated triangular region border by the left sixth rib, right sternal border, and clavicle when the body position is changed (not-specified) (Table 9.1).

Kussmaul Sign

Adolf Kussmaul (1822–1902) was born in Graben, Germany, and completed his medical studies at Heidelberg University, Germany, followed by additional postgraduate training in Prague and Vienna under Johann Ritter von Oppolzer (1808–1871) and Carl von Rokitansky (1804–1878), respectively [16, 17]. He practiced in Kandern, Switzerland, for 4 years and then pursued additional training in pathological anatomy in Würzberg, Germany, who among his teachers included Rudolf Ludwig Carl Virchow (1821–1902), Rudolf Albert von Kölliker (1817–1905), and Wilhelm Scherer (1841–1886) [18]. Kussmaul received his medical degree from the University of Würzburg, Germany, in 1855 [17]. He was a Privatdozent (Adjunct Professor) in 1856, Professor Extraordinary at the University of Heidelberg, Germany, in 1857, and Professor Ordinary at the University of Erlangen, Germany, from 1859 to 1863 [16]. He practiced at the University of Freiburg, Germany, from 1863 to 1876 and was appointed Chair of Clinical Medicine succeeding Ernst Viktor von Leyden (1832–1910) at the University of Strasbourg, France, from 1876 to 1888. He was honored by the municipality of Heidelberg by receiving the freedom of the city and title of real privy by the Grand Duck of Baden [17].

Kussmaul was a pioneer and the first to describe among others, mesenteric embolism, periarteritis nodosa, osteomyelitis, progressive bulbar paralysis, and the deep, labored respiratory pattern of breathing in patients with diabetic coma and acetemia (diabetic ketoacidosis). His other noteworthy accomplishments included that he was the first to perform esophagoscopy and gastroscopy, use bismuth for peptic ulcer disease, and insert a gastric tube for treatment of gastric dilation [19]. As a tribute to Kussmaul's character, Samuel J. Meltzer (1851–1920) wrote in 1905:

> All of his assistant and pupils could not praise enough his kindness and devotion to his patient. While he was an enthusiastic investigator, he never permitted the study of a case in a manner which could bring harm or discomfort to the patient. The patient was always first and science second, a high principle which should be burned into the minds of our generation of overproductive specialist. Kussmaul told his students he wished them to pass through a serious disease, it would help them to become good physician; they would then understand what care, kindness and tenderness meant to a suffering patient. (…) Above all he laid great stress upon the moral and mental influence of the physician upon his patient. He believed in making the patient at least hopeful and cheerful even if he could not be made well [16, p. 162].

Kussmaul published in a series of three papers entitled "Ueber schwielige Mediastino-Pericarditis und den Paradoxen Puls" (About callous mediastino-pericarditis and the paradox pulse), a unique phenomenon of the arterial pulse and jugular veins (Table 9.1):

> Clinically our attention is directed towards the symptoms of chronic inflammation of the pericardium and its obliteration, to which a peculiar arterial pulse phenomenon and sometimes a peculiar phenomenon involving the jugular veins serves as a criterion for fibrinous mediastinitis. Fibrous mediastinal adhesions cause the sternum during each inspiration, to exert a sweeping pull in front of and along the aortic arch. All arterial pulses become very small or disappear despite a constant heart rate during periods of normal inspiration, only to return immediately upon expiration. I propose to call this pulse a paradox, partly because of the striking mismatch between heart's action and arterial pulse and partly because the pulse, in spite of its inexplicable nature, is in reality a recurring or diminishing one. At the jugular veins, especially the bulb of the jugular vein, the narrow course of the adhesive bands causes a noticeable and considerable swelling, rather than the usual swelling seen during normal inspiration. These events make it possible to diagnosis a moderate mediastinitis associated pericarditis with an approximate degree of certainty in cases where the history, the onset and course of the illness, the physical examination of the heart, and circulatory disturbances, indicate pericarditis and obliteration of the heart but its presence do not permit a definite diagnosis [20, p. 433].

Kussmaul described the palpable pulse in three patients with mediastinopericarditis and correlated his finding using a Marey sphygmograph:

> The most interesting phenomenon found in three patients with mediastinal-pericarditis was the pulse. It was rapid in almost all always exceeding 100, the waves were small, the tension low, and rhythm paradoxical in two respects: (i) despite steady cardiac contractions, the

> pulse disappeared at the palpable finger one or two beats completely or almost completely for short intervals, and then immediately return for two or more beats; (ii) this apparent irregularity was in fact only caused by inequality linked to the phases of respiration. The diminution or disappearance of the pulse was reduced with the greatest regularity with every inspiration, while with each expiration the pulse went back to its former height. These peculiarities were present in all available arteries palpated. From these graphs it is evident that the pulse never quite disappeared, even if it no longer seemed palpable, but was still present although in a dampened form [21, p. 462].

Kussmaul acknowledged the previously observed finding of this phenomenon by Griesinger in 1854 and the publication of Griesinger's observations by A. Widenmann in 1856 from the inaugural dissertation entitled *Beitrag zur Diagnose der Mediastinitis* (Contribution to the Diagnosis of Mediastinitis). Where they differed was in regards to the pathophysiology of the disease:

> Griesinger (op. cit., p. 31) suggested that diminished pulse during inspiration was in his case mainly due to the rigid union of the aortic trunk with the sternum. As the thorax expands the sternum is raised as far as possible causing the aortic trunk, which has grown together with the sternum, to be displaced forward. The adhesions which extend from the aorta to the left sternal region are stretched and strained and accordingly during inspiration, the already narrowed aorta at that point further bends and is now completely constricted. (…) The essential anatomical conditions for the formation of the paradoxical pulse thus appear to be the adherence of the pericardium with the sternum and adhesions from the pericardium to the aorta, before and on the arch, in the form of constricting bands which are always found in this triangular area in adults. It is not absolutely necessary to have a direct union of the vessels with parts of the sternum in front of them. Whether a complete or incomplete union of adhesions from pericardium also give rise to the later observations is unknown, it probably does not [21, p. 462]. (…) As far as the mediastinal fibrosis is concerned, they were not easily overlooked when they occurred with such great abundance as in Griesinger's case. However, in my case there are more strongly developed thickening fibrous cords and thickened strands of connective tissue extending further upwards in the mediastinum identified by careful dissection [21, p. 464].

Thus, the "paradox" that Kussmaul referred to was the sudden and unexpected drop in the pulse with inspiration while the heart rate and rhythm remain unchanged (Table 9.1). Kussmaul also observed in the jugular veins during inspiration, the finding in a case of adhesive pericarditis:

> It was probably due to the fact that the same increased tension occurring in the aorta during inspiration also involves the inferior vena cava or right innominate vein. During each inspiration the already distended jugular veins on the right side became even more distinctly swelled. On the left side, this swelling was not easily recognized. At the same time, a subcutaneous vein, which ran in the direction of the right omohyoid muscle, clearly showed one or two faint retrograde waves with each inspiration. It was not possible to record this phenomenon graphically [21, p. 462].

Kussmaul referenced, based on the communication in *Schmidt's Yearbook*, but was unable to completely access Thomas Fox's 1869 paper published in the *Saint Louis Medical and Surgical Journal*, entitled "Intermittent pulse caused by a dilated bronchus pressing the aorta." Fox described in a 48-year-old male with chronic tuberculosis: "What was interesting as well as perplexing, in this case, was an intermission in every sixth, and sometimes seventh beat of the pulse in the radial arteries, while there was neither intermission nor irregularity in the sounds or beats of the heart" [22, p. 218]. Autopsy revealed the cause for this clinical finding:

> [r]ight bronchus dilated so as almost to admit the hand, while the left was but large enough to admit the index finger. The cause of the intermittent pulse was now apparent, and the manner of its action demonstrated by closing the mouth and one of the nostrils, and inflating the lungs through a tube inserted in the other, when the right bronchus became so dilated as to almost obliterate the aorta. In this way, at each act of inspiration, the attenuated and dilated bronchus was distended, and, pressing upon the ascending aorta, obliterated the pulse. I present this as an interesting case, as I can find none such mentioned by authors, nor is the probability of such a case mentioned in our lectures [22, p. 218].

Kussmaul also acknowledged the findings from other physicians who also observed that the radial pulse was small and almost imperceptible in cases of mediastinal tumors. He believed that:

> Thus, this finding occurs here rarely if at all. The reason for this may lie in the fact that tumors in the mediastinum do not often occupy the position between the aortic arch and sternum or aortic arch and pericardium and if so when they do, they fill this space in a different way than fibrous strands [21, p. 462–463].

For Kussmaul, these report provided further evidence that:

> In any case it is clear from this observation that the paradoxical pulse may also occur without pericarditis. This symptom is always the result of mediastinal disease and we may refer to mediastino-pericarditis only if there is evidence from the history and onset of the disease to assign the diagnosis of pericarditis [21, p. 464].

The "paradoxical pulse" may also be found in patients with underlying pulmonary disease such as bronchial asthma or exacerbation of chronic obstructive pulmonary disease (COPD) where there are wide fluctuation in pleural pressure and right ventricular dilation due to decreased compliance of the lungs or more commonly in cardiac conditions such as pericardial effusions [5, 23]. It is important to recognize that the term "paradoxical" is a misnomer since during normal inspiration in otherwise healthy adults, there is a 3–4 mmHg decline in systolic pressure. Furthermore, with voluntary deep inspiration there may be up to a 10 mmHg drop in systolic pressure [5]. Inspiratory increase in jugular venous distension is also referred to as Kussmaul sign [24].

The paradoxical pulse can be detected through palpation of the brachial artery or through a sphygmomanometer. Using the brachial artery, the patient is seated and positioned to a level that minimizes respiratory excursions. While the patient breathes regularly and is as comfortable as possible, the artery is compressed using the examiner's thumb until the maximum systolic impact is detected. The pressure is gradually released while the examiner simultaneously observes the patient's chest. The point where the pulse diminishes or is extinguished during inspiration while the heart continues to beat is the "paradox," which Kussmaul referenced. He referred to this phenomenon coining the term "paradoxical pulse" in recognition of this diagnostic sign.

Sphygmomanometer, pulse oximetry, and respiratory and arterial waveform analysis are quantitative methods for detecting the paradoxical pulse [25, 26]. In sphygmomanometer-based measurement, the patient is positioned as previously described while the blood pressure cuff is inflated 20 mmHg above the systolic pressure. While the cuff is deflated at a rate of 2–3 mmHg per heartbeat, the brachial artery is auscultated until the first Korotkoff sound is carefully heard and reconfirmed to be occurring only during expiration. The maneuver should then continue until the Korotkoff sounds are heard during both inspiration and expiration. Thus, pulsus paradoxus is present if the difference between peak systolic pressure heard during expiration and both inspiration and expiration exceeds 10 mmHg [23]. The "paradox" is thus an exaggeration of the normal decline of the systolic pressure in patients with underlying cardiac and pulmonary conditions previously enumerated. A sphygmomanometer is useful in the clinical setting where the paradox is not detected using the palpatory technique, particularly in cases where the peak systolic pressure differences are less than 15–20 mmHg [27, 28]. Limitation of this technique includes that it requires meticulous attention to the phase of respiration and difficulty in measuring in patients with low blood pressure, tachycardia, and tachypnea [25, 29].

It is of historic interest that Richard Lower (1631–1691) in his book entitled *Tractatus de Corde* (Treatise on the Heart), published in 1669, wrote about the case of a 30-year-old woman with adhesive pericarditis. He described the characteristic of the pulse during inspiration:

> Besides since the diaphragm is always attached to the pericardium in man, where the heart itself also happens to be united, it cannot be that the heart in every inspiration is drawn down with it, and so much so that the movements of it are so much slowed, and of necessity are suppressed; when the intermission itself of the pulse followed by so constantly every inspiration [30, p. 406].

Giovanni Maria Lancisi's (Johannis Mariae Lancisii, 1654–1720) posthumous 1728 book *De Motu Cordis et Aneurymatibus* (On the Motion of the Heart and Aneurysm), Propositio XXIII, section, "Mire adhesionis Pericardii cum Corde" (Surprising adherence of the pericardium with the heart) described the symptoms and autopsy findings in Joannes Baptista Tomi, a 24-year-old male with adherent pericardium and symptoms of dyspnea, faint and small irregular pulse and distended jugular veins and abdomen. He recognized that the adhesion were responsible for the restrictive movement of the heart [31].

A peak systolic pressure difference greater than 12 mmHg, discriminated patients with from those without pericardial tamponade with a sensitivity of 98%, specificity 83%, and positive and negative likelihood of 5.9 and 0.03 [32]. The low negative likelihood ratio suggests that there is a low probability for not having cardiac tamponade in patients with a peak systolic pressure difference less than 12 mmHg. In a study of 21 consecutive patients with suspected pericardial tamponade, pulsus paradoxus was found to have a sensitivity of 79%, specificity 40% with a positive and negative predictive value of 81% and 40%. In a systematic review on studies for the diagnosis of cardiac tamponade from 1966 to 2006, a sensitivity of 76% (95% confidence interval of 62–92%) was reported. A pulsus paradoxus > or < 10 mmHg with pericardial effusion was associated with a likelihood ratio of 3.3 (CI 1.8–6.3) and 0.03 (CI 0.01–0.24), respectively [33]. A lower sensitivity and specificity of pulsus paradoxus found in some studies for the diagnosis of pericardial tamponade may be explained by the presence of concomitant conditions including atrial septal defect, severe left ventricular dysfunction, severe hypotension, regional tamponade, aortic insufficiency, and aortic stenosis, which eliminates the pressure difference threshold for defining pulsus paradoxus [27, 34, 35]. Furthermore, comorbid conditions that increase peak systolic pressure differences due to pathophysiologic mechanisms include decreasing preload, increasing diastolic left atrial filling, or shift in the ventricular septum are also contributing factors [27, 34–37]. Thus, the presence of pulsus paradoxus in cases of suspected cardiac tamponade increases the likelihood for the presence of this disease. Its absence, however, is not sufficiently specific in excluding the diagnosis.

Studies evaluating elevation of jugular venous pressure with inspiration (Kussmaul sign) have shown a low sensitivity but high specificity in diagnosis. In patients with right ventricular infarction a sensitivity of 17.3% and specificity of 96.8% was identified for Kussmaul sign [38]. In 23 patients with constrictive pericarditis, Kussmaul sign was found in 43% of patients with cardiac tamponade, while in another study in 25 patients with cardiac tamponade, a sensitivity of 26% was reported [39, 40]. These findings suggest that Kussmaul sign is useful in excluding patients who do not have underlying disease.

Riegel Sign

Franz Riegel (1843–1904) was born in Brückenau, Germany, and received his medical degree from the University of Würzburg, Germany. He traveled to Vienna and studied under Johann Ritter von Oppolzer (1808–1871) and Salmon Stricker (1834–1898), returning to Würzburg as an assistant to Heinrich von Bamberger (1822–1888) and Friedrich Wilhelm Scanzoni von Lichtenfels (1821–1891) followed by Carl Jakob Adolf Christian Gerhardt (1833–1902) at the Julius Hospital [41, 42]. He was *privatdozent* (Adjunct Professor) at the University of Würzburg in 1871 and appointed director of the City Hospital in Cologne, Germany, in 1879 [43].

He was selected based on the recommendations of Rudolf Ludwig Carl Virchow (1821–1902) and Heinrich von Bamberger (1822–1888) to lead the Bürger Hospital in Cologne, Germany, and served as Chair and Professor of Medicine at the University of Giessen, Germany, in 1879 [41]. His interest extended into multiple therapeutic areas including gastroenterology (gastric ulcers and diseases of the stomach), cardiovascular diseases (pulse and pathophysiology of the heart), pulmonary (bronchial asthma), nephrology (acute nephritis), and otolaryngology (laryngeal innervation) [41]. In a description of Riegel's approach to science:

> Differing from most of the distinguished clinicians of his time for whom pathological anatomy was the essential factor of their scientific productivity, all of Riegel's works bear a physiological stamp, his interest centered in the functional problems of life, and many of his clinical observations were supplemented by thorough experimental studies [43].

Riegel while assessing the height and rate of pulse curves in patients with rheumatic pericarditis showed:

> [i]t became clear that the small pulses always coincide with a deep inspiration, while the larger ones occurring during expiration. On closer inspection it further appears that individual pulses always gradually decrease in size and then several larger pulses follow and then gradually decrease in size again. Furthermore, it can be seen that each time the impulse becomes less during inspiration, the rapidity of the individual pulse increases, while during expiration the speed decreases as the size of the individual pulse increases. Finally it can be seen that the smaller inspiratory pulses are characterized by a much faster decay and in particular by a very significant recoil wave, while the larger slower expiratory burst are characterized by a considerable decrease recoil wave with significant elevations [44, p. 370].

He accounted for these changes as caused by "changes in the pressure within the thorax during the various stages of respiration" [44, p. 372]. Based on his evaluation of more than 700 pulse curves including healthy individuals performing prolonged inspiration and expiration he concluded:

> From the observations reported here it may be stated that the inspiratory reduction of the pulse as such does not yet justify the conclusion of fibrosing mediastinal pericarditis. On the contrary it is clear that this phenomenon, even if only occurring during deep and slow respirations, can be observed in healthy young individuals. It may, therefore, be desirable to consider in future cases of mediastinal-pericarditis whether the condition in question occurs during deep and/or superficial respiration. Finally, further observations may determine whether in all cases of pathological pulsus paradoxus, if I may call it so in comparison with the physiological pulsus paradoxus just described, whether further inward and expiratory changes of the curvature mentioned above always occur. No mention has been made of the special characteristic of the pulses occurring during inspiration and expiration in a few previous observations of pulsus paradoxus. These relations are not seen from the curves in a few pulse images communicated thus far. From the foregoing investigations, the significance of the pulsus paradoxus is in no way diminished, but it seems desirable in further investigations to give special consideration to the last mentioned points. Of course, very pronounced degrees of the pulsus paradoxus with almost complete disappearance of the pulse at inspiration will never lead to any confusion with these physiological occurrences [44, p. 372].

Thus, Riegel sign refers to the decreased pulse volume and amplitude and increased heart rate occurring during inspiration and increased pulse volume and amplitude but decreased heart rate occurring during expiration in patients with chronic rheumatic pericarditis (Table 9.1). We are unaware of any study that evaluated the sensitivity or specificity of this sign.

Jaccoud Sign

François Sigismond Jaccoud (1830–1913) was born in Geneva, Switzerland, and earned his medical degree in 1860 at the Faculty of Medicine, Paris. He was appointed physician to the hospital of Paris in 1862, Associate Professor in 1863, and Full Professor and Chair of Internal pathology, Medical Clinic at La Pitié,

Paris in 1876 [45, 46]. He was elected to the French Academy of Medicine in 1877 and appointed its permanent Secretary in 1901 [45–47]. He was Knight of the Légion d'honneur, then officer, before being appointed Professor at the Faculty of Medicine. He received the Commander's Cross from the Academy of Medicine [46]. Jaccoud published several books including *Traité de pathologie interne* (*Treatise of Internal Pathology*) in 1871 and *Nouveau dictionnaire de médecine et de chirurgie pratiques* (New Dictionary of Practical Medicine and Surgery), colloquially known as *Jaccoud's Dictionary* from 1864 to 1886 [45]. As a description of his character:

> He was very benevolent, affectionate, and sincerely interested in his students, encouraging them in their works and trying to help them. He had the opportunity of treating some of them with touching solicitude. He was also good and deeply devoted to his entire family [46, p. 28].

Jaccoud described a palpatory finding in patients with chronic pericarditis with adhesions:

> Functional symptoms, as well as physical signs of adhesion, may be absent, but in some cases when present are clear enough to allow diagnosis. The most important of these signs are systolic depression and diastolic uplift of the chest wall at the apex of the heart. The sign known as the systolic depression consists of a sudden depression of the intercostal space corresponding to systole. This depression replaces the raising occurring in the normal state [48, p. 649].

He accounted for the presumed role of adhesions at a point on the chest wall during cardiac contraction:

> The interpretation of this phenomenon is as follows: because of adhesion the point of the heart, fixed in systole, can no longer move down to the left. As the organ is shortened in mass as a result of its contraction, there is a tendency towards an absent pulsation at the apex. At this time the predominant external pressure depresses the chest wall. When the outer surface of the pericardium is itself united to the thorax by short and solid adhesions, the depression is simply due to the traction exerted by these adhesions at the time of the systolic shortening of the heart. These signs are helpful, but their value is not always the same. If the depression is strictly limited to a point, it does not prove the presence of general adhesions. It is easy to conceive, according to the mechanism which has just been exposed, that it is sufficient for a simple adhesion which governs the movement of the point to produce this limit phenomenon; the fact was proved by Traube. On the one hand, the recent observations by Bahr, Friedreich and Galvagni that the peak-bound systolic depression may exist in the absence of any adherence is not certain. On the other hand, extensive systolic depression at several left intercostal spaces, with involvement of the false ribs and the lower end of the sternum, is a pathognomonic symptom. It requires not only general adhesion of the heart, but also to the pericardium, sternum and perhaps the spine. Now as these conditions are not always maintained, the existence of the symptom is probative, but its absence has no precise meaning [48, p. 649–650].

Thus, Jaccoud sign refers to the presence of a systolic lift and diastolic depression (undulating movement) of the intercostal space and costal cartilages of the chest wall [49] (Table 9.1). We are unaware of any study that evaluated the sensitivity or specificity of this sign.

Oliver Sign

William Silver Oliver (1836–1908) was born in Kilfinane, Limerick, Ireland, and received his medical degree from Halfax, Nova Scotia. He entered the army as an Assistant Surgeon in 1857, promoted to staff surgeon in 1872, Surgeon Major in 1873, Brigade Surgeon in 1882, and Honorary Deputy Surgeon-General in 1883 [50, 51]. He designed and patented the accouterments worn by the Canadian military during the Boer War and up to the beginning of the First World War with the goal to redistribute the load to avoid back strain [52]. Oliver described the diagnostic method for detecting a thoracic aneurysm as follows:

> [p]lace the patient in the erect position, and direct him to close his mouth and elevate his chin to the fullest extent, then grasp the cricoid cartilage between the finger and thumb, and use gentle upward pressure on it, when, if dilation or aneurism exist, the pulsation of the aorta will be distinctively felt transmitted through the trachea to the hand. The act of examination will increase laryngeal distress should this accompany the disease [53].

In addition to aortic aneurysm, the "tracheal tug" has also been reported to be found in "certain cases of indurative mediastinitis where the trachea and aorta are firmly bound together" [54, p. 143]. This is a departure from Oliver's first description. Thus, the term Oliver sign has also been used to refer to the presence of tracheal or laryngeal tug occurring with systole caused by mediastinal-pericardial adhesions [49] (Table 9.1).We are unaware of any study, which evaluated the sensitivity or specificity of this sign.

Paul Sign

Constantin Charles Théodore Paul (1833–1896) served as Associate Professor at the Paris Faculty of Medicine in 1866, and physician at St. Antoine, Lariboisière, and Charité Hospitals, Paris [55, 56]. He was a member of the Academy of Medicine in 1880, and recipient of the Grand Cross of the Légion d'honneur in 1876 [55–57]. He published a book on diseases of the heart entitled *Diagnostic et traitement des maladies du coeur* (Diagnosis and Treatment of Heart Diseases) in 1883. He had a special interest in general therapeutics, collaborating with Armand Trousseau (1801–1867) on the 1876 edition of *Traité de thérapeutique et de matière médicale* (Treatise on Therapeutics and Medical Materials) [56].

Costantin Paul in his first book reported that in the diagnosis of pericardial adhesion:

> If cardiac hypertrophy is present, with a violent impulse of the heart as a whole but a feeble impulse of the apex, we are justified in suspecting pericardial adhesions. Under all circumstances, however it must be admitted that the diagnosis remains hypothetical unless the patient is markedly thin [58, p. 73].

Thus, Paul sign refers to the presence of a strong impulse of the heart with a weak impulse at the apex in patients with adhesive pericarditis (Table 9.1). We are unaware of any study that evaluated the sensitivity or specificity of this sign.

Graves Sign

Robert James Graves (1796–1853) was born in Dublin, Ireland, and graduated from Dublin University in 1823 [59]. He served as Chief physician at Meath and later at St. Patrick Dun's Hospital, Dublin. At Meath, he was involved in medical education and research, and instrumental in establishing a bedside teaching program [59, 60]. Beginning in 1827, he served as Professor of the Institutes of Medicine to the King and Queen's College of Ireland [59]. He was editor of the *Dublin Journal of Medical and Chemical Science,* which subsequently became known as the *Dublin Quarterly Journal* (currently *Irish Journal of Medicine*) [59]. He was elected fellow of the Royal Society of the Royal Irish Academy, Honorary Member of several other societies including of the Royal Medical Society of Berlin, and Imperial Medical Society of Vienna [59]. As a description of his character:

> Eminently gifted as he was by nature, endowed with excellent abilities, remarkable powers of observation, and animated with high and noble views, these influences must have had much weight in the formation and determination of his medical character, and, as the sequel of his career fully proved, he was not un worthy to follow in the footsteps of such noble pioneers of science, and to carry out the good work they had commenced [61, p. 201]. (…) As a lecturer, Dr. Graves was distinguished by a force and clearness of language, and an earnestness of manner, which irresistibly commanded attention while his fine person and noble features won the admiration of his hearers. His style as a writer was at once simple yet nervous, and full of graphic power; and his delineations of disease are among the most successful of modern medical compositions [61, p. 204–205]. (…) He was a firm supporter of the dignity and honour of his profession, and during many years enjoyed a large and lucrative practice [61, p. 205].

Although he is best known for his work on hyperthyroidism (Graves disease), he also described angioneurotic edema, scleroderma, erythromelalgia, pin point pupil in pontine hemorrhage, and cough-induced fracture [60]. Robert James Graves found that:

> In some cases of pericarditis the heart's action becomes increased in strength for many hours before any physical sign of pericarditis can be detected, and before any pain is felt in the region of the heart. In such cases, when the usually acknowledged symptoms of pericarditis are added to this already existing augmented action of the heart, the latter goes on increasing, and finally becomes excessively violent, and does not begin to decrease notably for several days after the peculiar symptoms of pericarditis have disappeared. (…) The heart's action may not only precede the physical, but the constitutional symptoms of inflammation of that organ or its membranes, and consequently may be the only beacon to forewarn us of a danger still beyond the visible horizon, and undiscoverable by any other means. Connected with the motions of the heart is the remarkable disparity that exists between the energy of the heart's action and the strength of the pulse; for it often happens

> that the pulsations in the cardiac region are violent, while the pulse is weak and thready at the wrist [62, p. 184–185].

Thus, Graves sign refers to the early presence of increased heart rate in patients with acute pericarditis (Table 9.1). We are unaware of any study that evaluated the sensitivity or specificity of this sign.

Conclusion

Physicians used the tactile sensation of palpation or touch to detect abnormalities involving the chest, arterial pulse, and venous pressure in patients with pericarditis. Using these techniques, later recognized as eponymous sign, assisted clinicians to recognize pericarditis and distinguish it from other cardiac diseases during the era where there were no advanced imaging techniques. It is of interest that these eponymous names have been assigned to some individuals even though the same phenomenon was described at an earlier time. The sensitivity and specificity of most signs have not been studied and thus their applicability and reliability in clinical practice remain unknown. The techniques should be taught to physicians so that they can learn to appreciate subtle aspects and findings found on physical examination, as well as to gain further insight into the pathophysiology mechanisms of disease.

References

1. Skinner HA. The Origin of Medical Terms. Baltimore: Williams & Wilkins Company; 1949.
2. Breasted JH. The Edwin Smith Surgical Papyrus, vol. 1. Chicago, IL: The University of Chicago Press; 1930.
3. Harvey W. The motions of the heart as observed in animals experiments. In: Exercitatio Anatomica De Motus Cordis et Sanguinis in Animalibus. Leake CD, translator. Springfield: Charles C. Thomas; 1928. p. 28–29.
4. Laennec RTH. A Treatise on the Diseases of the Chest and on Mediate Auscultation. Forbes J, translator. New York: Samuel Wood & Sons; 1830.
5. Perloff JK. Physical Examination of the Heart and Circulation. 2nd ed. Philadelphia: W.B. Saunders Company; 1990.
6. Wunderlich CA. Wilhelm Griesinger. In: Biographische Skizze. Leipzig: Verlag von Otto Wigand; 1869. p. 3–40.
7. Griesinger W, Widenmann A. Beitrag zur Diagnose der Mediastinitis. Tübingen: Druck von L. Fr. Fues; 1856.
8. Spodick DH. Acute Pericarditis. New York: Grune & Stratton; 1959.
9. Birrer RB, Birrer CD. Medical Diagnostic Signs: A Reference Collection of Eponymic Bedside Signs. Springfield: Charles C. Thomas Publisher; 1982.
10. White FA. Physical Signs in Medicine and Surgery: An Atlas of Rare, Lost and Forgotten Physical Signs. Ocala: Museum Press Books; 2009.
11. Hirsch A. Oppolzer, Johann Ritter von. In: Allgemeine Deutsche Biographie, vol. 24. Leipzig: Verlag Duncker & Humblot; 1887. p. 405–7.

12. Maisei T. Scholars in Stone and Bronze: The Monuments in the Archaded Courtyard of the University of Vienna. Niewlsen CR, translator. Vienna: Böhlau Verlag; 2008.
13. Johann Ritter von Oppolzer. Wikipedia, The Free Encyclopedia. https://en.wikipedia.org/wiki/Johann_Ritter_von_Oppolzer. Accessed 22 Nov 2018.
14. Spitta A. Der Balneologe und Stoffwechselforscher Josef Seegen (1822–1904). Wien: Angestrebter akademischer Grad Magistra der Philosophie (Mag. Phil.); 2013.
15. Niemeyer P. Ueber Exsudat in dem Herzbeutel und Verwachsung des letztern; nach Oppolzer. Schmidt's Jahrb. 1861;112:181–2.
16. Meltzer SJ. Addresses: the men we lost. Med News Phila. 1905;87:161–3.
17. [No author]. Obituary: Professor Adolf Kussmaul. Lancet. 1902;2:53.
18. [No author]. Foreign news and notes: death of Professor Kussmaul. Phila M J. 1902;9:999.
19. Garrison FH. An Introduction to the History of Medicine with Medical Chronology. 2nd ed. Philadelphia: W.B. Saunders Company; 1917.
20. Kussmaul A. Ueber schwielige Mediastino-Pericarditis und den Paradoxen Puls. Berl klin Wochenschr. 1873;10:433–5.
21. Kussmaul A. Ueber schwielige Mediastino-Pericarditis und den Paradoxen Puls. Berl klin Wochenschr. 1873;10:461–4.
22. Fox T. Intermittent pulse, caused by dilated bronchus pressing upon the aorta. St Louis M & S J. 1869;6:217–81.
23. Bilchick KC, Wise RA. Paradoxical physical findings described by Kussmaul: pulsus paradoxus and Kussmaul's sign. Lancet. 2002;359:1940–2.
24. Reed RM, Ramani GV, Hashmi S. Unraveling the paradox of cardiac tamponade: case presentation and discussion of physiology. BMJ Case Reports. 2012;23:2012.
25. Sarkar M, Bhardwaj R, Madabhavi I, Gowda S, Dogra K. Pulsus paradoxus. Clin Resp J. 2018;12(8):2321–31.
26. Stone MK, Bauch TD, Rubal BJ. Respiratory changes in pulse-oximetry waveform associated with pericardial tamponade. Clin Cardiol. 2006;29(9):411–4.
27. Bandinelli G, Lagi A, Modesti PA. Pulsus paradoxus: an underused tool. Intern Emerg Med. 2007;2:33–5.
28. Fowler NO. Pulsus paradoxus. Heart Dis Stroke. 1994;3:68–9.
29. Jay GD, Onuma K, Davis R, Chen MH, Mansell A, Steele D. Analysis of physician ability in the measurement of pulsus paradoxus by sphygmomanometry. Chest. 2000;1888:348–52.
30. Major RH. Richard Lower (1631–1691), Treatise of the Heart. In: Classic Descriptions of Diseases with Biographical Sketches of the Authors. 3rd ed. Springfield: Charles C. Thomas Publishers; 1945. p. [404–6].
31. Lancisii JM. Propositio XXIII. In: De Motus Cordis et Aneurysmatibus. Romae: Apud Joannem Mariam Salvioni; 1728. p. 38.
32. Guberman BA, Fowler NO, Engel PJ, Gueron M, Allen JM. Cardiac tamponade in medical patients. Circulation. 1981;64:633–40.
33. Roy CL, Minor M, Brookhart A. Does this patient with pericardial effusion have cardiac tamponade. JAMA. 2007;297:1810–8.
34. Argulian E, Messerli F. Misconception and facts about pericardial effusion and cardiac tamponade. Am J Med. 2013;126:858–61.
35. Singh S, Wann LS, Klopfenstein HS, Hartz A, Brooks HL. Usefulness of right ventricular diastolic collapse in diagnosing cardiac tamponade and comparison to pulsus paradoxus. Am J Cardiol. 1986;57(8):652–6.
36. Johnson SK, Naidu RK, Ostopowicz RV, Kumar DR, Bhupathi S, Mazza JJ, Yale SH. Adolf Kussmaul: distinguished clinician and medical practice. Clin Med & Res. 2009;7:107–12.
37. Lee JC, Atwood JE, Lee HJ, Cassimatis DC, Devine PJ, Taylor AJ. Association of pulsus with obesity in normal volunteers. J Am Coll Cardiol. 2006;47:1907–9.
38. Mittal SR, Garg S, Lafgarhia M. Jugular venous pressure and pulse wave form in the diagnosis of right ventricular infarction. Int J Cardiol. 1996;53:253–6.

39. Rey C, Blanchi C, Kauffmann R, Meruane J, Goich J, Godov D. Constrictive pericarditis: diagnostic aspects and surgical results in 23 cases. Rev Med Chil. 1989;117:34–9.
40. Cooper JP, Oliver RM, Currie P, Walker JM, Swanton RH. How do the clinical findings in patients with pericardial effusion influence the success of aspiration. Br Heart J. 1995;73:351–4.
41. Clemm WN. Obituary: Franz Riegel, M.D. N York M J. 1904;80:554–5.
42. [No author]. Franz Riegel. Wien klin Rundschau. 1904;19:734–5.
43. [No author]. Obituary: Meltzer, the men we have lost. Med News. 1905;87:163.
44. Riegel F. Ueber die respiratorischen Aenderungen des Pulses und den Pulsus paradoxus. Berl klin Wchnschr. 1876;26:369–72.
45. [No author]. Paris letter: death of Sigmond Jaccoud. JAMA. 1930;60:1630.
46. Siredy A. Jaccoud et Hérard. Bull méd. 1914;3:25–8.
47. Colby FM, Churchill AL, Krans HS, editors. Necrology: Jaccoud, François Sigismond. In: The New International Year Book: A Compendium of the World's Progress for the Year 1913. New York: Dodd Mead and Company; 1913. p. 481.
48. Jaccoud S. Traité de pathologie interne. 5e éd. Paris: V. Adrien Delahave et Cie; 1877.
49. Spodick DH. Chronic and Constrictive Pericarditis. New York: Grune & Stratton; 1964.
50. [No author]. Medical news: military appointments. Med Times & Gaz. 1872;1:179.
51. [No author]. Obituary: Surgeon-General William Silver Oliver. Br Med J. 1908;1:1337.
52. Patent no. 45782. Filing year 1894. "Army Accoutrement," William Silver Oliver. Made in Canada Patents of Invention and the Story of Canadian Innovation. Library and Archives Canada. Bibliotheque of Archives Canada. http://www.collectionscanada.gc.ca/innovations/023020-2220-e.html. Accessed 4 Dec 2018.
53. Oliver WS. Physical diagnosis of thoracic aneurysm. Lancet. 1878;2:406.
54. Howard CP. The diagnosis of mediastinitis. John Hopkins Hosp Bull. 1915;26:140–4.
55. [No author]. Recent deaths: M. Constantin Paul. Boston M & S J. 1896;134:476.
56. [No author]. Death of Dr. Constantin Paul. Lancet. 1896;1:1101.
57. [No author]. Obituary: Dr. Constantin Paul. Med Rec NY. 1896;49:704.
58. Paul C. Complications of pericarditis: various forms of the disease-pericardial adhesions-course-termination. In: Diagnosis and Treatment of Diseases of the Heart. New York: William Wood & Company; 1884. p. 68–73.
59. [No author]. Necrology. Virginia M & S J. 1853;1:256.
60. Firkin BJ, Whitworth JA. Graves disease. In: Dictionary of Medical Eponyms. 2nd ed. New York: Parthenon Publishing; 1996. p. 156–7.
61. [No author]. Obituary: Robert James Graves, M.D. The Gentleman's Magazine. 1853;15:202–5.
62. Graves RJ. Diseases of the heart lecture: pericarditis. In: Clinical Lectures on the Practice of Medicine. London: The New Sydenham Society; 1884. p. 170–91.

Chapter 10 Physical Signs and Medical Eponyms of Pericarditis: Percussion

Introduction

The word percussion is derived from the Latin *percussio,* meaning beating or striking from one (*percuterre*) who strikes or thrusts [1]. It was Leopold Auenbrugger (1722–1809) who first used this technique in examination of the heart as described in *Inventum Novum Ex Percussione Thoracis Humani Ut Signo Abstrusos Interni Pectoris Morbos Detegendi* (New Invention to Detect the Diseases Hidden Deep Inside the Chest) in 1761 [2]. In John Forbes's 1824 English translation of Auenbrugger's 1761 original treatise in Latin, Auenbrugger wrote in the preface:

> I here present the reader with a new sign which I have discovered for detecting disease of the chest. This consists in the percussion of the human thorax, whereby, according to the character of the particular sound thence elicited, an opinion is formed of the internal state of the cavity [2, p. 379].

He described the findings identified on examination of the precordium, "[o]ver the space occupied by the heart, the sound loses part of its usual clearness, and becomes dull. The whole sternum yields as distinct a sound as the sides of the chest except in the cardiac region where it is somewhat duller." [2, p. 380]. Auenbrugger described under his "Second observation, on the method of percussion" that the direct method of percussion involves striking the thorax "[s]lowly and gently, with the points of the fingers, brought close together and at the same time extended" [3, p. 381]. Furthermore, "during percussion the shirt is to be drawn tight over the chest, or the hand of the operator covered with a glove made of unpolished leather" [2, p. 382]. It was Pierre Adolphe Piorry (1794–1879) who used a pleximeter, an ivory plate device to elicit different tones. Regarding the use of this device he wrote:

> Several English or American physicians, who have done me the honor of attending my lessons, simplify the process I employ by using their finger as a plessimeter. It is the left finger that can fill this office, but it does it imperfectly: it gives less that the ivory plate, the skin which covers it, dampens the impulse; it has a rounded surface which it is not easy to strike perpendicularly; the shock it receives, communicated to the underlying parts, can be painful

S. H. Yale et al., *Cardiovascular Eponymic Signs*,
https://doi.org/10.1007/978-3-030-67596-7_10

> or dangerous because of the narrow surface with which it is related. In addition, the ordinary plessimeter is itself of extreme simplicity; and, in default of such instrument, a coin may be put into use [3, p. 17].

Percussion involves using either a single finger (direct) or more commonly either of the middle two fingers (indirect) methods. Using the indirect technique the palmar aspect of the middle finger of either the right or left hand is affixed firmly to the chest (pleximeter) while this finger is tapped using the middle, rigid, but partially flexed of the other hand (plexor) and wrist as a fulcrum. One or two blows are delivered sequentially with the plexor quickly removed after each strike.

Percussion is a physical skill often neglected during the assessment of patients with acute and chronic pericarditis with or without pericardial effusion. Percussion of the precordium during the physical examination provides information about the extent of a pericardial effusion and for identifying the location of the apex beat when its pulsations cannot be palpably identified in cases of a large pericardial effusion or dilated left and right atria. During percussion the transition from tympani to dullness detected on the precordium moving lateral to medially, respectively, identifies the cardiac apex and extent of pericardial effusion.

Physicians during this time period identified other findings on physical examination ascribed as sign and eponymously defined in honor of their discovery. These signs have not been well studied and thus there is limited information of their application in clinical practice. With the advent of new technological advanced techniques such as echocardiogram for evaluation of the heart, bedside examination and evaluation for signs of the precordium using percussion has for the most part been, unfortunately, abandoned. Nevertheless, these signs are important to appreciate and understand as they were identified and applied at a time when the use of bedside diagnostic techniques and maneuvers were required for diagnosis. Understanding these signs provides clinician a more thorough appreciation of the bedside technique of percussion, insights into anatomical landmarks, and pathophysiology of disease.

Our goal in this chapter on eponymous signs of percussion in pericarditis is to provide the reader an appreciation of bedside physical examination techniques identified at a time when there were limited ways and interventions available to evaluate pathologic symptoms. Reviewed are the person who reported the sign as originally described, and if available, the sensitivity, specificity and predictive value, and its application and usefulness in modern day clinical practice. The signs are described chronologically from the date that they were first reported in the literature.

Signs

Čejka Sign

Josef Rodomil Čejka (Čegka) (1812–1862) was born in Rokycany, Czechoslovakia, and received his medical degree in 1837 from Charles University in Prague [4]. He studied autopsy and physical diagnostics with Carl von Rokitansky (1804–1878) and Josef Škoda (1805–1881), recognizable leaders in Vienna Medicine [5]. He habilitated at the University of Prague lecturing on diseases of the skin in 1847 and served as a member of the German Parliament in 1848 [4]. He was extraordinary Professor and physician at the K.K. Allgemeinen Krankenhause (General Hospital) in 1857 and served as the Dean of the Medical College from 1859 to 1860 [4, 6]. Čejka was a literary prow of Bohemian literature, author of Czech musical terminology, and translator of Shakespearean drama [4].

Čejka described four cases of adherent pericardium (three of which were described in detail) at the Sessional Reports of the Class of Mathematical and Natural Sciences of the Imperial Academy of Sciences in 1851, involving the inward movement of the lower sternum and third to sixth intercostal spaces during systole, its rebound during diastole, and absent apical impulse. He confirmed Škoda's observation regarding disease pathogenesis, that "a firm attachment to the thoracic wall was invariably present, and I have hitherto considered it to be essential" [7, p. 255]. The second case was a percussion finding in a 30-year-old female where:

> The percussion sound was dull on the left side throughout a space extending vertically from the third to sixth rib, and horizontally from the middle of the sternum to the midclavicular line. The upper boundary of this space was almost as broad as the lower boundary. There was no change in the percussion sound with either inspiration and expiration [7, p. 252].

Thus, Čejka sign refers to the presence of left sided thoracic dullness extending vertically in the midclavicular line from the third to sixth ribs and horizontally from the mid-sternum to midclavicular line which remains unchanged during respiration [8] (Table 10.1). We are unaware of any studies which evaluated the sensitivity or specificity of this sign.

Bamberger Sign

Heinrich von Bamberger (1822–1888) was born in Prague and received his medical degree from the University of Prague in 1847 [9]. He was trained by such eminent physicians including Josef Škoda (1805–1881), Carl von Rokitansky (1804–1878), Josef Hyrtl (1810–1894), and Johann Ritter von Oppolzer (1808–1871) [10, 11]. He served as Ordinary Professor of Special Pathology and Therapeutics (Clinical Medicine), and primarius physician at Julius Hospital, Wurzburg in 1854 [10–12]. At that time his colleagues included Johann Lukas Schönlein (1793–1864), Rudolf Ludwig Carl Virchow (1821–1902), and Friedrich Wilhelm Scanzoni von Lichtenfels (1821–1891) [10]. It was at Wurzburg that he published his books *Lehrbuch der Krankheiten des Herzens* (Textbook of Diseases of the Heart) in 1857 and *Die Krankheiten des chylopoetischen Systems* (On the Diseases of the Chylopoietic System) in 1864 [10, 11]. He was appointed medical director at Clinics of the General Hospital, Vienna, in 1872 and Rector at the University of Vienna in 1885 [10]. With Ernst Fuchs (1851–1930), he found *Wiener Klinische Wochenschrift* (Viennese Clinical Weekly), a publication which remains currently in press. He served as Austrian and Bavarian "Hofrath," Knight of the Leopold Order, and a member of the Imperial Royal Society of Physicians in Vienna for which he was President [10]. As described in his obituary, "Bamberger belonged to those happily

Table 10.1 Pericardial percussion eponymous signs

Name	Year	Description of method for eliciting sign	Significance
Cejka [7]	1856	Dullness over the left chest wall extending vertically from the third to sixth ribs and horizontally from the mid-sternum to mid-clavicular line. This area has a fixed sound which does not changed during respiration.	Adherent pericardium
Bamberger [13]	1856	Dullness in the posterior lower region of the left thorax from the lower angle of the scapula downward caused by compression of the left lower lung lobe.	Pericardial effusion
Sansom [15]	1876	Percussion dullness extending above the third rib (in some cases extends from the costal-cartilage of the first or second ribs) to the sixth rib and intercostal space. The line between pulmonary resonance and precordial dullness is well-defined by increased percussion resistance and decreased vibration.	Pericardial effusion
Rotch [21]	1878	Percussion dullness 2–3 cm lateral to the right sternal edge in the fifth intercostal space.	Pericardial effusion
Sibson [28]	1881	Pear-shaped outline of dullness. The upper region of pericardial dullness extends 2 inches in width over the great arteries. This area is much narrower than the great region of dullness over the heart itself, which at its upper portion is about 4 inches wide. The greater width of the cardiac portion of the region of dullness extends mainly to the left. This sudden widening of the area of pericardial dullness from pericardial distension gives that area peaked form above and an indented outline along its left upper border.	Pericardial effusion
Pins [16]	1889	Dullness extending in the shape of a truncated cone with the upper limit (apex), one and half fingerbreadth on the third costal cartilage to the left of the midclavicular line and lower limit (base) at the seventh intercostal space extending from left of the sternal border to one and a half fingerbreadth to the left of the midclavicular line Lateral decubitus or knee-bend position, there is resolution of the previous dull sound and dyspnea.	Pericardial effusion
Ebstein [36]	1892	Dullness due to a pericardial effusion located at the fifth intercostal space at the right border of the sternum (right heart angle). During inspiration resistance and dullness to palpatory percussion is now located in the lower right corner of the pericardium as the liver is displaced downward.	Pericardial effusion
Ewart [40]	1896	An area of dullness extending horizontally from the left of the spine to the scapular (angle) line and vertically below the ninth or tenth ribs. Its shape is that of a square. The extension of the patch in the right chest may become nearly completely dull in cases of large pericardial effusion.	Pericardial effusion
Germe [42]	1897	The dorsal vertebrae are counted by first drawing a cross on the spinous process of the seventh cervical vertebrae (area corresponds to the level of the left atrium). Its upper limit is found by striking the spine from top to bottom until a clearly truncated resistance is felt on the finger. To determine the lower limit, proceed in the opposite direction.	Pericardial effusion

Potain [50]	1901	Percuss beginning from the periphery, moving toward the heart in a serial perpendicular direction. Percussion should not begin over the heart and extending outwards. As long as percussion is on the part of the lung situated outside the heart, the sound is full and equal everywhere, if there is no pulmonary lesion. When one reaches the lung border, the tone of the percussion sound rises suddenly since the depth of the lung vibration becomes less. This point is marked with a pencil line.	Pericardial effusion
Teissier [53]	1911	An area located to the right of the vertebral column above the line of transverse sound (corresponding to the tenth dorsal vertebra) and regarded as the lower limit of the thoracic sound. This area of dullness is in the form of a right triangle whose base corresponds to this lower tone; small side corresponds to the line of the spinous processes, and whose long side, that is, the hypotenuse, marks the line of demarcation between the normal pulmonary sound and the zone of the paravertebral diminished sound. The summit of this triangle exceeds the fourth intercostal spaces. Conventionally referred to as Grocco triangle.	Pericardial effusion
Calvert [58]	1914	In pericardial effusion the right lobe of the liver is low, varying in its position from the fifth interspace to the sixth rib. In contrast, in dilatation of the heart the right lobe of the liver is high varying in position from the fourth to the fifth rib. In each condition, a narrow area of relative lung liver dullness is present.	Pericardial effusion
Conner [63]	1926	Region of dullness to percussion assumes bilaterally the shape of a right-angle triangle, whose apex is in the interscapular region well above the scapular angle, the base corresponding to the base of the thorax, and oblique side extending downward and outward about to the posterior axillary line with the right side potentially appearing smaller compared to the left side.	Pericardial effusion
Moschowitz [67]	1933	Abrupt transition from pulmonary resonance to cardiac dullness extending to the right of the sternum.	Pericardial effusion
Dressler [69]	1960	Flat percussion note elicited over the lower half of the sternum. The larger the effusion, the more likely is it that the flat percussion sound extends as high as the level of the second costal cartilage.	Pericardial effusion

constituted natures in which both endowments are represented. His special power as a clinician and as a consultant may be briefly summarized in this - that he thought as a *savant* and practiced as an artist." [12, p. 1048]. Regarding his skills as a clinician and teacher, the following attributes were described:

> His diagnostic skill was extraordinary, and astonished all who had the opportunity of observing him in his clinical work. Bamberger was not only an earnest investigator and practitioner of great experience and resource, but an eminent teacher. His lectures were remarkable for their clearness and accuracy, and equally attracted students and practitioners [10, p. 1137].

Bamberger in his paper entitled "Über Pericarditis" (On pericarditis) described the signs and symptoms of pericarditis in 57 patients:

> Of the other physical phenomena of pericarditis, the following were most frequent and important in the cases observed: Significant dullness of prolonged duration in the posterior lower region of the left thorax due to compression of the left lower lobe of the lung. It is often confused with left-sided pleuritic exudate, from which it differs, however, in the distinct feeling of vocal fremitus. Rarely is compression of the lungs so strong that there is clear signs of resonance [13, p. 374].

He further stated in his book *Lehrbuch der Krankheiten des Herzens* (Textbook of Diseases of the Heart) in 1857:

> The left lung is compressed by every large pericardial exudate. On the upper lobe, this is usually insignificant and manifests by a tympanitic full sound under the left clavicle (Graves once observed an extensive protrusion of the left lung apex above the clavicle), while the lower lobe is sometimes evacuated to the point of being compressed. Therefore, in almost in every case, the sound on percussion of the dorsal surface of the left thorax is dull and sometime completely absent over the lower angle of the scapula. The respiratory sound there is indeterminate, barely audible, or rarely bronchial. One must not confuse this condition with the not uncommon finding of a simultaneous pleuritic exudate, where palpation from vocal fremitus does not disappear unlike that found in the pericardium. This is one of the most important differential signs [14, p. 121].

Sansom in 1892 described Bamberger's findings in patients with pericardial effusion:

> An important diagnostic sign of pericardial effusion, when this is in considerable amount, first described by Bamberger, is afforded by percussion at the back. With the patient in the sitting position, an area of dulness of about the size of a crown-piece, bounded by resonant lung, can be delimited about the angle of the left scapula. Over this area the signs are increased vocal fremitus, bronchial breathing, and bronchophony. If the patient bends well forward or assumes the knee-elbow position for a short time, the dullness disappears, and in its place a tympanitic sound is elicited; in like manner the former auscultatory signs of lung consolidation vanish, or only slight crepitant rales are heard, which also may soon become inaudible. The former signs return when the vertical position of the body is resumed [15, p. 159].

As confirmed by Pins in 1889, we also were also unable to identify that Bamberger discussed the disappearance of this finding by leaning forward [16]. Hence, we suspect that Sansom was referring to both Bamberger (1856) and Pins (1889) signs in the description of this finding in his text published in 1892 [13, 15, 16]. Bamberger believed that this was a useful sign particularly in children and young adults. In terms of duration of the sign, Sansom found that "It is only present in the early periods of pericardial effusion, and may last from 3 to 6 days. In the later period, however, the signs of local consolidation of the lung may become long persistent" [15, p. 159]. It is of historical interest that Bamberger, Pins, and Ewart all described this same sign and thus it has been referred to as the Bamberger-Pins-Ewart Sign [17] (Table 10.1). As stated, Bamberger sign has been incorrectly referred to the presence of percussion dullness located at the angle of the scapula that becomes resonant with the patient leans forward [8]. We are unaware of any study which evaluated the sensitivity or specificity of this sign.

Sansom Sign

Arthur Ernest Sansom (1838–1907) was born in Wiltshire, UK, received his Doctor of Medicine degree in 1866 and was elected fellow of Royal College of Physicians of London in 1878. He served as physician at several hospitals including the London Hospital, North-Eastern Hospital for Children, Royal Albert Orphan Asylum, and Royal Hospital for Diseases of the Chest, City Road [18]. He pioneered the use of antisepsis in practice and contributed to enhance the understanding of diseases of the heart. His book *Diagnosis of Disease of the Heart and Thoracic Aorta* published in 1876 contained precise illustrations of the physical signs. As described in his obituary:

> His former house physicians or those students who accompanied him in his visits to the wards of the London Hospital will remember the enthusiasm and perseverance with which he obtained such tracings and the pains which he took to explain to those around him the significance and importance which he attached to them [18, p. 844–845].

Arthur Ernest Sansom described an:

> [a]brupt outline of praecordial dullness of pyramidal or pyriform shape in patients with pericardial effusions. When this is observed, there is a great probability of effusion in the pericardial sac. In this case the relative cardiac dulness does not exist; the transition from the resonance of the lung to a very marked dulness is abrupt; moreover, the dulness may extend above the usual limit. Whenever marked dulness extends above the third rib, there is a strong probability of pericardial effusion. If there be much distension of the pericardium with fluid, the area of dulness may extend from the articulation of the first or second costal cartilage above to the sixth rib or sixth intercostal space below. The pericardial sac being filled with fluid, the edge of the lung which overlaps the cardiac area is pushed aside, and the area of deficient resonance, as opposed to dulness, is abolished. The line, therefore, between pulmonary resonance and praecordial dulness is well defined, and the sense of resistance to the fingers on percussion is increased, the vibrations being lessened [15, p. 157].

Thus, Sansom sign refers to the presence of percussion dullness extending from the first and second costal cartilage to the sixth rib or sixth intercostal spaces in patients with a large pericardial effusion [8] (Table 10.1). We are unaware of any studies which evaluated the sensitivity or specificity of this sign.

Rotch Sign

Thomas Morgan Rotch (1849–1914) was born in Philadelphia, Pennsylvania, and graduated from Harvard Medical School in 1874 [19]. From 1874 to 1876 he traveled to Berlin, Vienna, and Heidelberg to further his medical training returning to serve on staff at the Boston Dispensary and Boston City Hospitals and subsequently Infants' and Children's Hospital in Boston (currently Children's Hospital), eventually assuming the rank of Medical Director [19]. He founded the American Pediatric Society, serving as its third President in 1891 and first president of the New England Pediatric Society in 1908. He assumed Presidency of other societies including Suffolk District Medical and Boylston Medical Societies [19]. At Harvard, he served as Full Professor and Chair of Pediatrics in 1893, the first of its kind and model for other departments of pediatrics in the United States [19]. He is best recognized for his work in infant nutrition, establishing the first research milk laboratory that modified the fat, carbohydrate, and protein content of cow's milk so that it resembled breast milk. Thus, he is considered the "founder of modern scientific infant feeding" [19, 20]. His other areas of interest were in radiographic studies on bone development and diseases of infants and children [19]. He published the textbook *Pediatrics* in 1895, the standard work in this field at that time [19].

Rotch identified an area of flatness in the right fifth intercostal space suggestive of a pericardial effusion. He recognized that:

> It probably also appears, at the same time, to the left of the sternum. But the physiological flatness of the heart here obscures it. For diagnosis, then, flatness, at from two to three centimeters from the right edge of the sternum in the fifth intercostal space, would be almost absolutely sufficient to mark the presence of an effusion, unless the opinions of authorities on enlarged heart are proved to be incorrect [21, p. 427].

Thus, Rotch sign refers to the presence of dullness to the right of the sternum at the fifth intercostal space in patients with pericardial effusion (Table 10.1). The sign is similar to both Ewart and Conner signs [22]. We are unaware of any study which evaluated the sensitivity or specificity of this sign.

Sibson Sign

Francis Sibson (1814–1876) was born at Crosscanonby, Cumberland, England [23]. He began his medical education in Edinburgh, received a diploma from the Royal College of Surgeons in 1831, followed by additional professional training at Guy's and Thomas Hospital in London, obtaining his M.B. and Doctor of Medicine degree (gold medal distinction) from the University of London in 1848 [24, 25]. He was actively involved in the Provincial Medical and Surgical Association (British Medical Association), and Metropolitan Counties Branch beginning in 1843 serving as its representative and President of the Council from 1866 to 1869 [24, 25]. He was elected member of the Royal College of Physicians, London, in 1849 and fellow in 1853 [25, 26]. Sibson was an active member of the college as an examiner in medicine, Secretary to the Committee on Classification of Disease, and editor of *The Nomenclature of Disease* [24]. He served as a physician at St. Mary's Hospital in 1851, achieving the rank of Consulting Physician in 1871, and was appointed resident surgeon at the Nottingham General Hospital in 1853 [26]. His publication on *Medical Anatomy or the Illustrations of the Relative Position and Movements of the Internal Organs: Anatomy* (1855–1869) is considered one of his most distinguished and enduring work [24, 27].

Sibson was a member and served on the Councils of the Royal Medical and Chirurgical Society of London from 1863 to 1864 and the Royal Society of Medicine serving on the Council from 1872 to 1874 and Joint Treasure [24]. He received Honorary degrees of MD in 1867 and LLD in 1876 from the Universities of Dublin and Durham, respectively [24, 25]. As a description of his character as described in an obituary:

> Few men were better known in professional circles than Dr. Sibson, and still fewer were more highly respected. His goodness of heart, integrity of character, and personal worth endeared him to a wide circle of professional brethren, as also to numerous private friends and patients, by all whom his sudden death is felt as a great and irreparable loss [24].

In addition to the pericardial sign which bears his name, he also described the subpleural dense fascia which extends and attaches anteriorly to the first rib and costal cartilage, posteriorly to the C7 transverse process and medially to the mediastinal pleura (Sibson's fascia).

Sibson described in his textbook the specific finding of anterior dullness in patients with pericardial effusion:

> This upper region of pericardial dulness, over the great arteries, which is two inches wide, is much narrower than the great region of dulness over the heart itself, which at its upper portion is above four inches wide, the greater width of the cardiac portion of the region of dulness being gained chiefly to the left. This sudden widening of the area of pericardial dulness from distension of the sac gives that area peaked form above, and an indented outline along its left upper border, that distinguish it from the equally high and extensive area of cardiac dulness due to adherent pericardium and valvular disease, when the heart is enlarged in all directions and especially upwards and to the left, and when the upper left border of the region of cardiac dulness presents a very gradual inclination downwards and to the left without a break. (…) This pear-shaped outline of the region of dulness over the pericardium is quite characteristic, and indicates with certainty the presence of extensive effusion into the sac [28, p. 16, 32].

Thus, Sibson sign refers to the presence of a curve extending inward from the upper left border of cardiac dullness in patients with pericardial effusion [17] (Table 10.1). We are unaware of any study which evaluated the sensitivity or specificity of this sign.

Pins Sign

Emil (Elias) Pins (1845–1913) was born in Lemberg, Ukraine, and received his medical degree from the University of Vienna in 1873 [29]. He served as an assistant to Adam Politzer (1835–1920), an otologist at the Allgemeines Krankenhaus (General Hospital) followed by medical practice in Vienna. He recognized that the Friedlander bacillus travels through the Eustachian tube causing middle ear infections in children in 1877 [30].

Pins presented and reported *Ein neues Symptom der Pericarditis* (A new symptoms of pericarditis) at the Wiener Medizinisches Doctoren Collegium meeting on January 21, 1899, and in *Wiener medizinische Wochenschrift* that same year. In his paper, he provided detailed daily descriptions of the same pulmonary finding recognizing in six patients (three in articular rheumatism, two in tuberculosis, and one in Bright's disease) [16, 31]. In the second case, patient P.B. a 17-year-old, he found on day 2 during the examination:

> [t]he cardiac dullness is considerably increased in the shape of a truncated cone. The base is located at the 7th intercostal space and extends from the left sternal border 2 cm to the left midclavicular line with its upper limit on the 3rd costal cartilage being 3 cm in width. When examined in a sitting position, a clear rattling noise can be heard in the area of the base of the heart, but disappears in the horizontal position [16, p. 249].

Physical findings identified the following findings the following day:

> Examination of the lungs on the anterior chest wall as well as on the right back does not reveal anything abnormal. There is indeterminate breathing at the left back and angle of the left scapula where the percussion sound becoming quieter and absent. The damping corresponds to the entire lower left lung lobe. In the middle of the quiet part there is a deep bronchial breathing, in the periphery the respiratory sound is vague. Fremitus is preserved everywhere, and even in the middle of the damping it is somewhat amplified. The patient if he is able, is placed and examined in the knee-bend position. Immediately the findings change. In place of the dullness is a tympanitic sound, instead of the bronchial one can hear indeterminate breathing, the earlier weak bronchophonie has completely disappeared. The heartbeat is clearer and, moreover, in the 3rd and 4th intercostal space tactile fremitus can also be felt. After the patient has again taken the supine position and rested again, he is examined in a sitting position, whereby exactly the former findings are found [16, p. 249].

Pins accounted for the pathogenesis:

> It is obvious that this symptom is not found in all cases of pericarditis. A small amount of pericardial exudate does not cause compression and in a large effusion the exudate is fixed. Too little exudation does not lead to any compression, and movement of the heart and the fluid is not well possible if the exudates are too copious. In the former case there is absolutely no dullness or resonance. In the latter case, resonance may be present but is not affected by changes in position. Furthermore, this symptom will be absent in those cases of pericarditis in which there are adhesions between the heart and parietal pericardium, because the fixed heart may not fall as far backward to compress the lung. However in all other cases it should be found if patients are examined in a different position. The fact that atelectasis, which persists for several days, does not always result in lasting induration in the left lower lobe of the lung is explained by the fact that the patients are forced by their existing breathing difficulties to change their position from time to time and to sit up temporarily, whereby each time the lungs and its compression is improved [16, p. 251].

He acknowledged the previous findings of Bamberger and reported on these limitations:

> Only Bamberger, in his textbook of heart disease, mentions that in large pericardial exudates the left lower lobe of the lung may be so compressed as to cause bronchial respiration, a finding resembling pleurisy. But even Bamberger does not say under what circumstances these compression phenomena are to be found and under which they are not to be found. In particular, no mention is made of the findings caused by changes in position [16, p. 251].

Thus, Pins sign refers to the relief of dyspnea in patients with acute pericarditis when the knees are drawn to the chest, the lateral decubitus position, or leaning forward [8] (Table 10.1). It is often referred to as the Bamberger-Pins-Ewart sign in recognition of the three persons who reported this finding. We are unaware of any study which evaluated the sensitivity or specificity of this sign.

Ebstein Sign

Wilhelm Ebstein (1836–1912) was born in Jauer, Prussia (Silesia, Poland), pursued his medical training in Breslau and Berlin and received his medical degree from the University of Berlin in 1859 [32]. He received his medical training under the auspices of Mortiz Heinrich Romberg (1795–1873), Rudolf Ludwig Virchow (1821–1902), Friedrich Theodor von Frerichs (1819–1885), and Emil du Bois-Reymond (1818–1896) [32, 33]. He qualified as privatdozent (Adjunct Professor) in 1869 and was subsequently appointed Professor and Director of the Medical Polyclinic at the University of Breslau [34]. He served as Professor of Internal Medicine at Göttingen from 1877 to 1906 [35].

He was a prolific writer publishing 237 articles in multiple therapeutic areas, including metabolic, gastrointestinal, infectious, orthopedics, nephrology, hematology, heart disease, as well as medical history [33]. He is best known for his work in the areas of gout, diabetes, and weight loss by a low-carbohydrate diet [33]. His name, in addition to the cardiac sign which bears his namesake, is associated with other eponyms including Pel-Ebstein fever as seen in Hodgkin's lymphoma and other neoplasms, Ebstein anomaly, a rare congenital heart malformation were the tricuspid valve is displaced downward in the right ventricle in conjunction with a patent foramen ovale, and Ebstein's disease or hyaline degeneration of the epithelial cell involving the renal tubules as may be found in patients with diabetes mellitus [35]. Ebstein discussed the limitations of identifying a left sided pericardial effusion:

> At this point I would like to remark that determining the presence of fluid in the lower left corner of the pericardium by percussion causes particular difficulties in cases where the lungs and not the heart is against the chest wall and the nearby tympanitic resounding crescent-shaped space is present. The last-mentioned circumstance is, in my opinion, primarily an hindrance to identify dullness developing in the lower left pericardial angle. (…) In most cases, determining early fluid accumulation in the lower left corner of the pericardium by percussion may not be accurate. The finding of fluid in the lower right corner of the

> pericardium is simpler and more easily accessible to examine unless, in the lower part of the right half of the thorax, other findings are completely deadening the sound, for example, when a right-sided pleural exudate is present [36, p. 430].

He proposed a method for identifying a pericardial effusion on the right side of the chest based on an anatomical approach:

> It is known in healthy people above absolute liver dullness there is a narrow zone of incomplete dullness, so-called relative liver attenuation. It begins in the 4th intercostal space or at the upper margin of the 5th rib, essentially coinciding with the zone which I call liver resistance. I usually find it a little higher than the relative liver attenuation. It can be explained by the fact that liver resistance is determined by the sense of touch alone without the aid of percussion and is probably more subtly developed in the examiner's hands than the ear. Both the usual percussion, as well as palpation or palpatory percussion, in which the sense of hearing and the sense of touch are used, shows that relative liver attenuation prevails. Liver resistance under normal conditions extends medially in the right half of the thorax to the border of the sternum. Now, if a liquid-effusion develops in the cavity of the pericardium, the first part were relative liver-dullness occurs is located most medially. In the liver, there is a dullness arising from the fluid accumulated in the lower right corner of the heart which is clearer and more intense than otherwise present in the area of relative liver dullness. It is completely or almost completely dull. The dullness is more complete the greater the portion of the lung covered by the pericardium expanding and dilating as a result of accumulating exudative fluid. The lower right corner of the fluid-filled pericardium is applied to the thorax wall. As a rule, fluid accumulating in the pericardial cavity can first be detected by the dullness occurring in the 5th intercostal space at the right border of the sternum. The range of the relative liver attenuation is located on the right sternal margin. Liver resistance, an intense, absolute or almost absolute attenuation, can be detected under the circumstances mentioned called heart angle [36, p. 432–433].

He further described what he referred to as the heart angle:

> Schematically reproduced for our purpose this heart angle is nothing more than an acute angle located on the anterior surface of the thorax, the apex turned medianward, forming the projection of the right lower pericardial effusion. The name Herzleberwinkel has occasionally been used in other places where the heart and liver come into contact. The place where the lateral margin of the left lobe of the liver borders the dullness of the heart, forms a more or less obtuse angle. I chose it for this purpose, because it was concise, purposeful, and appropriate and unlikely to cause confusion. If this were the case that one would be able to prevent any misunderstanding by applying the term "right-sided heart angle". For now we want to keep the shorter name… [36, p. 433].

He described the method for identifying the heart angle using percussion:

> The method of examination of the heart angle is moderately simple. We use short and narrow plethimeters which should not be wider and longer than the dimensions of the normal heart angle. We use a glass plessimeter because this has the advantage of being inexpensive and easy to disinfect. In lieu of the plesthimeter, percussion can be performed on the dorsal surface of the third phalanx, while the other phalanges are held in the extended position between the second and third phalanxes. As for the method of percussion, as we have already learned and from what has been said, we use and recommend ordinary percussion. (…) Ordinary percussion should not be too strong for obvious reasons. If percussion is strong enough to detect the so-called relative attenuation of the liver, the difference in the intensity of both is immediately apparent by comparing the dullness occurring in its lateral parts with the attenuation occurring in the ventral angle of the heart. When fluid accumulates in the lower right corner of the pericardium, palpatory percussion gives the examining

> finger nearly the same feeling of increased resistance as that part of the liver directly adjacent to the costal arch and significantly greater resistance than in the area of liver resistance or the so-called relative liver dullness. If one examines the patient while they are being slowly turned and exhales, one finds that during inspiration the liver resistance shifts downward with its dullness and resistance changing. Dullness corresponding to the fluid effusion is now located in the lower right corner of the pericardium. Resistance increases at the heart angle, although it is less severe than when it occurs either during expiration or in middle diaphragm position. Admittedly the practice of this method of investigation is one of the finer percutorial tasks, but it is by no means more difficult than a large number of other methods of investigation [36, p. 435].

He believed that this method was useful for distinguishing cardiac dilation from pericardial effusion and recognized the limitation of this maneuver:

> There is no infallible diagnostic sign here as well answers for the vast majority of disease diagnoses [36, p. 436]. In order to decide whether it is hydropericardium, hemopericardium or pericarditis, be it a fibrinous or purulent, etc., we not only need the findings from percussion, but the aggregates of all methods of examination of the heart including those which are not directly related to the function of the heart. We need to examine the entire body, assess the history, the beginning and the course of the illness, and subjective complaints in order to clarify the nature and quality of the fluid in the pericardium [36, p. 439].

Thus, Ebstein cardiac sign refers to the presence of percussion dullness at the cardiohepatic angle located at the fifth intercostal space [8] (Table 10.1). We are unaware of any study which evaluated the sensitivity or specificity of this sign.

Ewart Sign

William Ewart (1848–1929) was born in London and began his medical training at St. George's Hospital, London, in 1869, qualifying from the Royal College of Surgeons of England in 1871 and received his licensure from the Royal College of Physicians of London in 1872 [37–39]. He served as house physicians at Addenbrooke's Hospital, Cambridge, while attending Gonville and Caius College from 1875 to 1876 [38, 39]. He earned his M.B. degree in 1871, was a member of the Royal College of Physician in 1874, and served as lecturer in physiology and curator of the museum, performing all postmortem examinations at St. George's Hospital and Medical School [38, 39]. He was elected fellow of the Royal College of Physician and appointed assistant physician and pathologist at the Hospital for Consumption and Disease of the Chest, Brompton, in 1881 [38]. He received his M.D. from Cambridge University in 1882 and was appointed assistant physician at St. George's hospital requiring him to resign at Brompton Hospital [38, 39]. He was a full physician in 1887 and consulting physician in 1907 at St. George's Hospital [37]. In the Royal College of Physician, his other appointments included serving as examiner in medicine from 1894 to 1897 and councilor from 1901 to 1903 [38]. He served as chairman of the British Medical Association, Westminster Division, from 1908 to 1909 [38]. As a description of his character in his obituary:

> Indefatigable in his work, he was an enthusiastic teacher, sparing neither time nor trouble in conveying the essence of his knowledge and experience to those who were ready to learn. An afternoon spent with him in the wards afforded a liberal education in intensive clinical investigation and diagnosis. The obvious, however clear was not sufficient for him; he was always searching for something beyond with a persistence and attention to detail which, those unaccustomed to his methods, seemed remarkable. Not content with methods of treatment and diagnosis as he found them, he was unending in his efforts to find something better with an eagerness which was irresistible. By nature an optimist, he approached every problem with a cheery confidence which was as stimulating as it was helpful [38, p. 370].

William Ewart in his paper entitled "Practical aid in the diagnosis of pericardial effusion in connection with the question as to surgical treatment" described 12 signs two of which bear his name. The first is "The first rib sign" in which he was able to, "[f]eel with the finger the upper edge of the first rib as far as its sternal attachment. This points to a raising of the clavicle not only in its outer but also in its inner portion; and to a relaxation of the ligament between it and the first rib." [40, p. 720]. He attributed this finding as "connected with the immobility and with the elevation of the lower ribs, coupled with the greater activity of the superior respiratory region of the chest" [40, p. 720]. The second sign as described by Ewart was one he referred to as the posterior pericardial patch of dullness (Table 10.1):

> A patch of marked dullness is found at the left inner base, extending from the spine for varying distances outwards, usually not quite so far as the scapular (angle) line, and ceasing abruptly with a vertical outer boundary. Above its extension is also variable, according to the size of the effusion; commonly it does not extend higher than the level of the ninth or tenth rib, and here again its horizontal boundary is abrupt. Its shape than is that of a square and it is quite unlike that of any dullness arising from pleuritic effusion. (…) When, however, the effusion is considerable, the extension of the patch in the right chest may become almost absolutely dull [40, p. 720].

Additionally, Ewart also described an area "Immediately below or slightly to the left of the tip of the left scapula a patch about 2 inches in diameter presents well-marked tubular breathing and aegophony" [40, p. 721]. We are unaware of any studies which evaluated the sensitivity or specificity of this sign.

Germe Sign

There is limited historical information on Léon Germe (1837–1898). In 1867, he was appointed Deputy Professor and the Chair of medicine at the Preparatory School of Medicine and Pharmacy, Arras, Northern France [41]. At the time of his publication of his paper "Recherches sur les causes des mouvements du coeur, sur son innervation et son indépendance motrice" (Research on the causes of the movements of the heart, on its innervation and motor independence) in 1897, he was a Professor of Childbirth, Diseases of Women and Children, Preparatory School of Medicine and Pharmacy [42]. He was a corresponding member of the Paris Society of Medicine [43]. His other areas of investigation included respiration and pulmonary circulation (specifically asphyxia and mountain sickness) [44].

In his aforementioned paper, Germe described a percussion method for detecting enlargement of the left atrium or pericardial effusion:

> The limits of the left atrium are traced by dorsal percussion. We first make a cross on the spinous process of the 7th cervical vertebrae, which corresponds to the level of the auricle, and count the dorsal vertebrae starting below this level. Its upper limit is found by striking the spine from top to bottom. As soon as the heel of the plessimeter or the sound from finger pleximeter arrives on this cavity, a clearly truncated resistance is felt on the finger. For the lower limit, proceed in the opposite direction. The height of the left atrium is an average of 5 cm. It can be as high as 8 and even 9 cm. and as low to 3 1/2 cm. Changes in volume are observed at its upper part [42].

Thus, Germe sign refers to the zone of dullness identified when percussing the vertebral column between the fifth and tenth dorsal vertebrae in patients with atrial hypertrophy, atrial dilation, or pericardial effusion [45, 46] (Table 10.1). We are unaware of any study which evaluated the sensitivity or specificity of this sign.

Potain Sign

Pierre Carl Édouard Potain (1825–1901) was born in Paris, France, and received his medical degree from the University of Paris in 1853 with the doctorate thesis entitled *Les soufflés vesiculaires qui suivent les hémorrhagies* (The vesicular blisters that follow bleeding). At the University of Paris, he was Adjunct Professor in 1859, physician to Menages Infirmary in 1860, St. Antoine Hospital in 1865, and Necker Hospital in 1866. He was appointed Professor of Medical Pathology in 1876 and subsequently Professor of Clinical Medicine in the faculty of medicine serving as a teacher at Necker and Charity Hospitals [47, 48]. His textbook entitled *Leçons cliniques de la Charité* (Clinical Lessons at the Charity), published in 1894, remained the standard for disease of the heart during this time period [47]. He was Honorary Professor of the Faculty of Medicine, Paris, member of the Institute of France and Academy of Medicine in 1882, and honored by the French government as Commander of the Légion d'honneur [47, 49]. In his obituary, his personal characteristics were described:

> His kindness to the pupils, his gentleness to his poor patients, his justice in the examination of students, which was always tempered with kindness, made him one of the most beloved of all the teachers in the faculty of medicine. (…) He deserved the administration and veneration which were recently manifested anew when he resigned his position as clinical teacher last year and was made honorary professor, and his pupils from all over the world united to present him with a gold medal as a token of their esteem [47].

Potain reported in his 1901 paper entitled "De la mensuration du cœur par la percussion et la radiographie: comparaison des deux méthodes" (From the outline of the heart by percussion and radiography: comparison of the two methods) that the outline of the heart by percussion was concordant with that identified using fluoroscopy:

> More than once I had occasion to observe by percussion and radioscopy concordant rapid changes in the volume of the heart. It can be stated, therefore, that both methods give results

> in exactly the same relation to the actual volume of the organ, and this very satisfactorily confirms the value of the percussion. As these results are obtained by absolutely dissimilar means, it is impossible to imagine errors of so diverse origins could coincide exactly and in such a constant manner. (…) Percussion, on the contrary, can be practiced always and everywhere without the aid of any instrumentation and, since it gives identical and equally precise results, it is generally more acceptable [50, p. 419].

He described the method of percussion of the heart (Table 10.1, Fig. 10.1):

> When we want to delineate the boundaries using percussion, the essential point in my opinion and contrary to what we usually do, is to refrain from striking the precordial region and limit percussion to the periphery by following a series of convergent lines which begin at some distance from the usual limit of the precordial dullness and move perpendicular to the line which it circumscribes. If percussion occurs on the part of the lung situated outside the heart and if there is no pulmonary lesion, the sound is full, grave, and substantially equal everywhere. As soon as one reaches the border of the lung, the tone of the percussion sound rises suddenly because the depth of the lung layers vibration suddenly becomes consider-

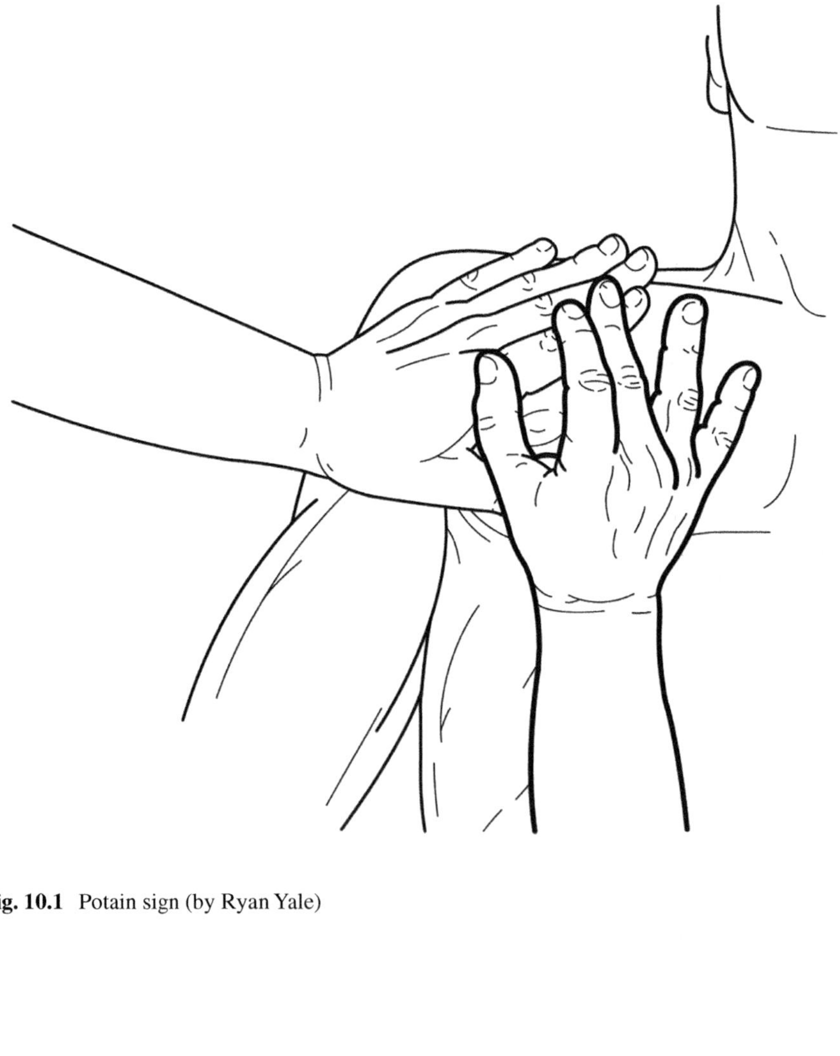

Fig. 10.1 Potain sign (by Ryan Yale)

> ably less. It is this elevation of the tone that warns that one has reached the limit sought. We must stop there and mark this point with a pencil line. To continue farther towards the center of the precordial region is time and trouble lost and unnecessary inconvenience imposed on the patient. That is why I insist on the principle of the method which one could call, the method of peripheral and convergent percussion. It is important to note that it is not a notable diminution of the intensity of the sound to true dullness recognized the moment when we reach the limit of the heart, but a modification of the tone of the noise. This modification is very easy to perceive when one is warned that it is one that must be sought. On the contrary, if we rely on a lesser resonance rather than the higher tone which easily gives the impression of an exaggeration of its intensity, we will not be able to distinguish anything precisely [50, p. 417].

He noted that Professor Jean-Ripler from Lyon believed that percussion of the heart is inaccurate except in patients with pericardial effusion or prominent cardiac hypertrophy. Potain argues that "it is certain that in order to give a precise and comparable results, the delineation of what is known as precordial dullness should be made with a similar method" [50, p. 417]. We are unaware of any studies which evaluated the sensitivity or specificity of this sign.

Teissier Sign

Joseph Teissier (1851–1926) was born in Lyon and completed his aggregation from the Faculty of Medicine in the same city in 1877. The following year he was appointed as *médecin des Hôpitaux* (doctor of Hospitals) in Lyon. He was appointed Professor of Internal Pathology at the Faculty of Medicine in Lyon in 1884. Teissier along with Edmond Weill (1858–1924), and Jean Lépine (1876–1967) started the *Journal de médecine de Lyon* in 1920 [51]. He had numerous accolades including serving as a member of the National Academy of Medicine, France, and the Academy of Medicine, St. Petersburg. Additionally, he served as Officer of the Légion d'honneur, Office of Public Instruction, and Commander of the Order of the Crown and Order of Leopold [52]. He identified a right paravertebral triangular area of dullness corresponding to Grocco's triangle in a patient where there was no corresponding contralateral pleural effusion. The region is located to the:

> [r]ight of the vertebral column, above the line of transverse sound corresponding to the tenth dorsal vertebra which is generally regarded as the lower limit of the thoracic sound. We see with extreme clarity an area of dullness in the form of a right triangle whose base corresponds precisely to this line of lower normal tone, whose small side corresponds to the line of the spinous processes, and whose long side, i.e. the hypotenuse, marks the line of demarcation between the normal pulmonary sound and the zone of the paravertebral diminished sound which we are used to calling at home 'the Grocco Triangle' We have never found that the summit of this triangle exceeds the fourth intercostal spaces [53, p. 97].

He recognized that Grocco triangle was not a pathognomonic finding for a contralateral pleural effusion and may also be found in patients with a large right atrium:

> That dilation of the right atrium is an important factor in the Grocco phenomenon, because it is rational, corresponds to precise anatomical design, and explains the presence of the

> opposite paravertebral triangle in different cases. But I repeat, it seems to me that in this case as in the interpretation of many clinical signs, if they are controlled by multiple actions and various factors, it is necessary to understand what is common in the production of phenomena observed if one does not want to expose oneself to miscalculations. In a general way, we can say that the zone of right paravertebral dullness corresponding to the sign of the paravertebral triangle of Grocco, is observed each time the vibratory capacities of the vertebral column are modified. This occurs whenever the spinal column is in contact with a more or less dense underlying medium (liquid, as in pleurisy, solid, dilated heart or deviated mediastinum). Most often we will have to attribute the reduction in the vibratory capacities of the paravertebral zone to a dilated or deviated right cavity. This zone corresponding to the transverse processes acts a plessimeter through which the finger strikes on these dilated cavities [53, p. 101].

Spodick referred to Teissier sign as "dullness located between the medial border of the right scapula and the vertebral column in pericardial effusion" [54, p. 152]. Although Teissier did not specifically use the term pericardial effusion, he did generally enumerate on other causes for the dullness caused by the heart including, "solid" heart which may correspond to pericardial effusion (Table 10.1). We are unaware of any studies which evaluated the sensitivity or specificity of this sign.

Calvert Sign

There is limited information on William Jephta Calvert (1871–1945). He was born in Englewood, NJ, and served as Assistant Surgeon US Army pathologist to the Board of Health, Professor Clinical Medicine at Baylor University College of Medicine, and member of the Staff of the Texas Baptist Memorial Sanitarium Dallas, Texas [55, 56]. Calvert initially described in 1910 and reported his further experience in 1914, a method for differentiating pericardial effusion from dilation of the heart particularly when cardiac dullness extends to the right sternal border [57, 58] (Table 10.1):

> In pericarditis with effusion the right lobe of the liver is low, varying in its position from the fifth interspace to the sixth rib; in dilatation of the heart the right lobe of the liver is high, varying in position from the fourth to the fifth rib. In each condition a narrow area of relative lung liver dulness is present [58, p. 192].

He accounted for the pathogenesis based on the movement of the heart, ribs, sternum, and liver during the process of embryogenesis:

> In dilatation of the heart are found depressed ribs and sternum, a large right heart, a high position of the liver-fourth to fifth rib, or a continuation of the movements of these organs which normally occurs in the development of the foetus. In pericarditis with effusion there is a small right heart, a slight depression of the ribs, a low position of the liver-sixth to seventh ribs, or a reversion of the foetal position [58, p. 195].

We are unaware of any studies which evaluated the sensitivity or specificity of this sign.

Conner Sign

Lewis Atterbury Conner (1867–1950) was born in New Albany, Indiana, and received his medical degree from College of Physicians and Surgeon of Columbia University in 1890 [59, 60]. He served on staff at New York Hospital and Cornell University Medical College throughout his career beginning in 1894, achieving the rank of Chairman of Medicine for which he served from 1916 to 1932 [61, 62]. He was Chief of the Army Medical Corps Division of Internal Medicine beginning in 1917 and responsible during wartime effort in updating and revising the cardiovascular physical examination disease and diagnosis for determining fitness for duty, translating these findings to civil life [59]. Conner founded The Society for the Prevention and Relief of Heart Disease in 1915, later renamed the New York Heart Association in 1924, and served as its first President [60]. This organization was responsible for the prevention, rehabilitation, psychological aspect, as well as the social and economic consequences of heart disease [59]. He was also the founder and editor-in-chief of the *American Heart Journal* (currently *Circulation-Official Journal of American Heart Association*) from 1925 to 1936 [61, 62]. In addition to his pioneering work in cardiology, he was first to perform a lumbar puncture in the Western Hemisphere and contributed to other therapeutic areas including infectious diseases, thromboembolic disease, disordered respiration associated with central nervous system, and immunologic therapy of pneumonia [59, 60]. The American Heart Association recognized Conner for his accomplishment and contributions to this organization commemorating him by creating the first annual lectureship in his name in 1937 [60]. In a tribute to Dr. Conner, David P. Barr, Office of the Dean of the University Faculty at Cornell University Medical made the following statement:

> Dr. Conner developed a mastery of physical diagnosis which has seldom been equaled. With this invaluable asset he combined qualities of scholarship and perception which enabled him to appreciate and evaluate newer scientific knowledge and to share the enthusiasm and aspirations of his younger colleagues. His learning, his clinical judgment, and above all his integrity, made him the idol of the students and particularly of those chosen young men who were permitted to work with him as interns or residents in the wards of the New York Hospital. To them and to those who have succeeded them, his acumen and skill have become an unforgettable legend [61].

Conner noted variability during percussion and auscultation of the posterior chest wall in patients with pericardial effusion. In addition to the possible presence of "a small area of impaired resonance at the left base close to the spine, with some diminution of the vesicular murmur and a slight change in the voice sound" [63, p. 427], there may also be the more commonly (Table 10.1):

> [a]n extensive area of flatness over both lower chests, with absence of the vesicular murmur and with clear bronchial breathing and bronchophony (or egophony) over the upper and outer border of this area of flatness. Usually the tactile fremitus is not entirely lost even over

> the flat area. Adventitious sounds are commonly lacking, but there may be fine rales along the upper margin of the dull area [63, p. 427].

He found that although this finding is most commonly seen on the posterior left side, it may occasionally be found on the posterior right side [63]. In case where there is a large pericardial effusion the region of flatness to percussion assumes bilaterally the:

> [s]hape of a right-angled triangle, with the apex in the interscapular region, well above the scapular angle, the base corresponding to the base of the thorax, and the oblique side extending downward and outward about to the posterior axillary line: the flatness there shading off gradually into pulmonary resistance. In most cases the triangle of flatness is distinctly smaller on the right side than on the left, but it is rarely lacking entirely when there is even a moderately large area of flatness on the left side [63, p. 428].

This misperception of the differences in sound between the right and left sides may be, "explained by the damping effect upon the normal sound vibrations of the distended pericardial sac lying upon and hugging the bodies of the lower dorsal vertebrae" [63, p. 428]. Conner identified the early left posterior finding in patient with pericardial effusion marked by "appearance of a small area of bronchial breathing just above and within the lower angle of the scapula. This change in breathing has been noted even before any distinct dullness could be detected" [63, p. 428]. He was unable to duplicate the findings of a posterior rectangular dullness outline described by Ewart [63]. We are unaware of any studies which evaluated the sensitivity of specificity of this sign.

Moschcowitz Sign

Eli Moschcowitz (1879–1964) was born in Giralt, Hungary, and received his medical degree from the College of Physicians and Surgeons (Columbia University), New York, in 1900 [64]. He served as Medical Director at Mount Sinai Hospital, Clinical Professor at the College of Physicians and Surgeons, and consulting pathologists at Beth Israel Hospital and Beth El Hospital, Brooklyn, New York [65]. In addition to the sign which bears his namesake, he also described the relationship between anaphylaxis and eosinophilia, thrombotic thrombocytopenic purpura (Moschcowitz disease), and pulmonary hypertension [66]. His work in the field of psychosomatics was instrumental in establishing the relationship between the psychic and disease [66].

Eli Moschcowitz delineated percussion findings for diagnosing a pericardial effusion. From most to least important they include "(1) widening of the area of cardiac flatness, (2) abrupt transition from pulmonary resonance to cardiac flatness, and (3) widening of the cardiac dullness in the second intercostal space" [67,

p. 1663]. The percussion flatness extends to the right of the sternum with an "abrupt transition of pulmonary resonance to cardiac dullness" and as confirmed by radiogram "widening of the cardiac outline in the second intercostal space" [67, p. 1663–1664]. Identification of all three percussion abnormalities enhances the likelihood for diagnosing a pericardial effusion [67]. Thus, Moschcowitz sign refers to the presence of an abrupt transition from pulmonary resonance to cardiac dullness in patients with pericardial effusion (Table 10.1). We are unaware of any studies which evaluated the sensitivity or specificity of this sign.

Dressler Sign

Wilhelm (William) Dressler (1890–1969) was born in Budzanow, Poland, and graduated from the University of Vienna Medical School in 1915. He was Associate Chief of the cardiac clinic in Vienna from 1924 to 1938 [68]. He subsequently served as chief of cardiology at Maimonides Medical Center, Brooklyn, New York [68]. Dressler described in a retrospective study of 29 patients with pericardial effusion for whom cardiac percussion findings were available and diagnosis confirmed in 17 (58%) that using the criteria of marked dullness or flatness on percussion (Table 10.1):

> The finding of an extensive area of flat percussion sound over the sternum has proved, in my colleagues' and my experience, to be the leading diagnostic sign in the presence of pericardial effusion. (...) In most cases, pericardial effusion is indicated primarily by a flat percussion note elicited over the lower half of the sternum. The larger the effusion, the more likely is the flat percussion sound to creep higher up the sternum-indeed, sometimes as high as the level of the second costal cartilage, (...) [o]ther areas of flat percussion sound are observed which yield confirmatory diagnostic evidence. One area is in the third left interspace, extending from the left sternal margin for a distance of from 2 to 4 in. to the left, even beyond the left midclavicular line. Occasionally, it encroaches on the second intercostal space. Another broad area of flatness is observed to the right of the sternum in the fifth intercostal space. Its diagnostic significance increases when it reaches upward into the fourth and third intercostal spaces [69, p. 763].

Dressler sign should not be confused with the better recognized Dressler syndrome, which describes the clinical symptoms of fever and chest pain in patients with pericarditis, pleuritis, or pneumonitis although most commonly occurring after a myocardial infarction (postmyocardial-infarction-syndrome) [70]. He also described with Roesler the ventricular fusion beat occurring during episode of paroxysmal ventricular tachycardia (Dressler beat) and an early electrocardiographic finding in patients with an anterior myocardial infarction [71, 72]. We are unaware of any studies which evaluated the sensitivity or specificity of this sign.

Conclusion

Physicians during this time period mastered the technique of percussion of the precordium and applied it as a means of diagnosing pericardial effusion and adherent pericardium. Importantly, they accounted for and described their findings using a meticulous anatomical approach. The absence of studies evaluating the sensitivity or specificity of these sign provides gaps in our understanding of the usefulness of these signs in clinical practice. They do, however, provide an appreciation of the use of anatomical landmarks and precise description of findings identified on physical examination.

Percussion is often neglected and relegated as being an unimportant and useless part of examination of the precordium. We believe that this bedside technique should be emphasized and taught to students in the context of the historical discovery so as to provide insights and gain an appreciation of the finer details detected on the physical examination. This knowledge reinforces to students that through practice and precision subtleties can be identified on examination. Despite advance imaging of the heart, percussion along with inspection, palpation, and auscultation and the sign identified should supplement and not be supplanted by other imaging techniques used in diagnosis.

References

1. Skinner A. The Origin of Medical Terms. Baltimore: Williams & Wilkins Co; 1949.
2. Sigerist HE. On Percussion of the Chest: being a translation of Auenbrugger's original treatise entitled "Inventum Novum Ex Percussion Thoracis Humani, Ut Signo Abstrusos Interni Pectoris Morbos Detegendi" (Vienna, 1761) by John Forbes. MD (London, 1824). Bull Hist Med. 1936;4:373–403.
3. Piorry PA. De la percussion médiate et des signes obtenus à l'aide de ce nouveau moyen d'exploration, dans les maladies des organes thoraciques et abdominaux. Paris: J.-B. Baillière; 1828.
4. [No author]. Necrolog: Dr. Joseph Čejka. Österreichische Wochenschrift für Wissenschaft, Kunst und öffentliches Leben. 1863;26:31.
5. Josef Čejka. Wikipedia Otevřená encyklopedie. 2018. https://cs.wikipedia.org/wiki/Josef_%C4%8Cejka. Accessed 2 Jan 2019.
6. Čejka J. Ausserordentliche Mitglieder. In: Abhandlungen der Königlichen Böhmischen Gesellschaft der Wissenschaften. Prag: Commission der J. G. Calve'sehen Buchhandlung; 1857. p. 20.
7. Čejka J. Three cases of adhesion of the pericarditis. Dublin Q J M Sc. 1856;21:249–56.
8. Birrer RB, Birrer CD. Medical Diagnostic Signs: A Reference of Eponymic Bedside Signs. Springfield: Charles C. Thomas Publisher; 1982.
9. [No author]. The death of Professor Heinrich von Bamberger of Vienna. N York M J. 1888;48:603.
10. [No author]. Professor Heinrich von Bamberger. Br Med J. 1888;2:1137–8.
11. [No author]. Dr. Heinrich von Bamberger. Reviews Med News. 1888;53:616.
12. [No author]. Obituary: Heinrich von Bamberger. Lancet. 1888;2:1048.
13. Bamberger H. Ueber Perikarditis. Virchow's Arch f path Anat. 1856;9:348–80.

14. Bamberger H. Lehrbuch der Krankheiten des Herzens. Wien: Wilhelm Braumüller K.K. Hofbuchhändler; 1857.
15. Sansom AE. Section III: percussion, Chapter XX: Signs of pericardial effusion. In: The Diagnosis of Diseases of the Heart and Thoracic Aorta and the Pathology which Serves for the Recognition of Morbid States of the Organs of the Circulation. Philadelphia: P. Blakiston, Son & Company; 1892. p. 150–68.
16. Pins E. Ein neues symptom bei Perikarditis. Wien med Wchnschr. 1889;34:248–51.
17. Spodick DH. Acute Pericarditis. New York: Grune & Stratton; 1959.
18. [No author]. Obituary: Arthur Ernest Sansom MD. Lond. FRCP, Lond. Lancet. 1907;1:842–5.
19. Kelly HA, Burrage WL, editors. A Cyclopedia of American Medical Biography, vol. 1. Baltimore: The Norman Remington Company; 1920.
20. Firkin BG, Whitworth JA. Dictionary of Medical Eponyms. Boca Raton: The Parthenon Publishing Group; 2002.
21. Rotch TM. Absence of resonance in fifth right intercostal space diagnostic of pericardial effusion. Boston M & S J. 1878;99:389–93, 421–9.
22. Ewart W. Practical aids in the diagnosis of pericardial effusion in connection with the question as to surgical treatment. Br Med J. 1896;1:717–21.
23. Howard JJ, Crisp FA. Visitation of England and Wales. [London]: privately printed; 1895.
24. [No author]. Medical news: Francis Sibson MD, Lond, FRS. Med Times & Gaz. 1876;2:346,450.
25. [No author]. Obituary: Francis Sibson MD, FRS. Br Med J. 1876;2:446–8.
26. Sibson F, Ord WM. A short account of the life and writings of Dr. Sibson. In: Collected Works of Francis Sibson, vol. 1. London: Macmillan and Co; 1881. p. xix–xliii.
27. Francis Sibson. Lives of Fellows. Royal College of Physicians. http://munksroll.rcplondon.ac.uk/Biography/Details/4047. Accessed 15 Dec 2018.
28. Sibson F, Ord WM, editors. Collected Works of Francis Sibson, vol. 4. London: Macmillian & Co; 1881.
29. Austrian Academy of Sciences. Pins, Emil (Elias) (1847–1913), Mediziner. In: Österreichisches Biographisches Lexikon, vol. 8. Wien: VÖAV; 1979. p. 85.
30. Graham HB. Concerning the capsulated bacteria in the production of acute middle ear affections. Ann Otol Rhinol Laryngol. 1910;19:1018–23.
31. Pins E. Ueber ein neues Symptom der Pericarditis. Wien med Bl. 1889;12:57–8.
32. [No author]. Wilhelm Ebstein. Nature. 1936;138:914.
33. Hurst JW. Portrait of a contributor: Wilhelm Ebstein (1836–1912). Clin Cardiol. 1995;18:115–6.
34. [No author]. Obituary: Wilhelm Ebstein. Br Med J. 1912;2:1426.
35. White FA. Physical Signs in Medicine and Surgery: An Atlas of Rare, Lost and Forgotten Physical Signs. Philadelphia: Museum Press Books; 2009.
36. Ebstein W. Ueber die diagnose beginnender Flüssigkeitsansammlungen im Herzbeutel. Arch f path Anat. 1892;130:418–43.
37. Firkin BJ, Whitworth JA. Ewart sign. In: Dictionary of Medical Eponyms. Boca Raton: The Parthenon Publishing Company; 2002. p. 116–7.
38. [No author]. Obituary: William Ewart MD, FRCP. Br Med J. 1929;2:369–70.
39. William Ewart. Lives of the fellows. Royal College of Physicians. http://munksroll.rcplondon.ac.uk/Biography/Details/1476. Accessed 2 Jan 2019.
40. Ewart W. Practical aids in the diagnosis of pericardial effusion in connection with the question as to surgical treatment. Br Med J. 1896;1:717–21.
41. [No author]. Personnel de la Faculté des sciences et des lettres et école préparatoire de médecine et de pharmacie de Toulouse; de l'école préparatoire de médecine et de pharmacie d'Arras. Bulletin administratif de l'instruction publique. 1867;8:459–60.
42. Germe L. Recherches sur les causes des mouvements du cœur, sur son innervation et son indépendance motrice. Paris: Masson et cie; 1897.
43. [No author]. Nouvelles scientifiques: bibliographie. In: de Parville H, éditeur. La nature, revue des sciences et de leurs applications aux arts et a l'industrie. Paris: Gaston Tissandier, G. Masson; 1897. p. 72.

44. [No author]. Rapports sur le concours du Prise Mathieu Bourceret, en 1897, au nom d'une Commission composée de M. M. Marey, Thasbot et Laborde, rapporteur. Bull Acad Méd. 1897;38:483–9.
45. Vaquez H, Bordet E. The heart and the aorta. In: Macy J, editor. Studies in Clinical Radiology. Homeij JA, translator. New Haven: Yale University Press; 1820. p. 82.
46. [No author]. Exploration of the left auricle. Pacific Rec M & S. 1897;12:244.
47. Knopf SA. Obituaries: Professor Potain. N York M J. 1903;73:162.
48. [No author]. Professor Potain. Lancet. 1901;1:128–9.
49. [No author]. Pierre Karl Edouard Potain, MD. Br Med J. 1901;1:121.
50. Potain P. De la mensuration du cœur par la percussion et la radiographie: comparaison des deux méthodes. Semaine méd. 1901;21:417–9.
51. [No author]. Present state of medical journalism in France. JAMA. 1920;74:963.
52. Joseph Teissier – Académie royale de Médecine de Belgique. Fédération Wallonie-Bruxelles. http://www.armb.be/index.php?id=5018. Accessed 2 Jan 2019.
53. Teissier J. La percussion dorsale du coeur et son application à l'interprétation du phénomène de Grocco. Semaine méd. 1911;31:97–101.
54. Spodick DH. Acute Pericarditis. New York: Grune & Stratton; 1959.
55. Curry JJ. Bubonic Plaque-Report of the plaque in Manila, P.I; from Jan.1, 1900 to June 30, 1900. Boston M & S J. 1901;144:277–9.
56. [No author]. Notes and news. Johns Hopkins Hosp Bull. 1916; 27:27.
57. Calvert WJ. A possible differential sign between cardiac dilation and pericarditis with effusion. In: Transaction of the Section on Practice of Medicine of the American Medical Association at the Sixty-First Annual Session, held at St. Louis Mo; June 7 to 10. Chicago: American Medical Association Press; 1910. p. 46–57.
58. Calvert WJ. A new sign differential between dilation of the heart and pericarditis with effusion. Tex State J Med. 1914–1915;10:192–5.
59. Wooley CF, Schneider D, Lerner AA. Lewis Atterbury Conner appreciation and bibliography: current perspective. Circulation. 1998;98:1449–55.
60. Fisher J. Special report: Lewis A. Conner – Cornell's Osler. Circulation. 2000;102:1062–7.
61. Barr DP. Lewis Atterbury Conner. January 17, 1867-December 4, 1950. Cornell University, Office of the Dean of the University Faculty; memorial statement; Cornell University. https://hdl.handle.net/1813/18346. Accessed 8 Dec 2018.
62. Lewis Atterbury Conner, Yale 1887. The American Heart Association. Lewis A. Conner/Circulation 2000 full article. https://www.ahajournals.org/doi/full/10.1161/01.cir.102.9.1062?HITS=10&hits=10&FIRSTINDEX=0&searchid=1&resourcetype=HWCIT&RESULTFORMAT=&maxtoshow=&fulltext=%22Lewis+A.+Conner%22. Accessed 7 Dec 2018.
63. Conner LA. On the diagnosis of pericardial effusion with special reference to physical signs on the posterior aspect of the thorax. Am Heart J. 1926;1:421–33.
64. Eli Moschcowitz. Archives and Special Collections at the Augustus C. Log Health Science Library of Columbia University. P&S. 1964. 28. https://library-archives.cumc.columbia.edu/obit/eli-moschcowitz. Accessed 24 Dec 2018.
65. Eli Moshcowitz, Internist, is dead, Ex-Director at Mt. Sinai did work in Psychosomatics. New York Times 1964. https://www.nytimes.com/1964/02/24/archives/eli-moshcowitz-internist-is-dead-exdirector-at-mt-sinai-did-work-in.html. Accessed 4 Jan 2019.
66. Aufses AH, Niss B. This House of Noble Deeds: The Mount Sinai Hospital, 1852. New York: New York University Press; 2002.
67. Moschcowitz E. A new sign of pericardial effusion. JAMA. 1933;100:1663–4.
68. Firkin BG, Whitworth JA. Dressler syndrome. In: Dictionary of Medical Eponyms. Boca Raton: The Parthenon Publishing Company; 2002. p. 99–100.

69. Dressler W. Percussion of the sternum, 1: aid to differentiation of pericardial effusion and cardiac dilation. JAMA. 1960;173:761–4.
70. Dressler W. The post-myocardial-infarction syndrome: a report of forty-four cases. AMA Arch Intern Med. 1959;103:28–42.
71. Dressler W, Roesler H. The occurrence in paroxysmal ventricular tachycardia of ventricular complexes transitional in shape to sinoauricular beats; a diagnostic aid. Am Heart J. 1952;44:485–93.
72. Dressler W, Roesler H. High T waves in the earliest stage of myocardial infarction. Am Heart J. 1947;34:627–45.

Chapter 11
Physical Signs and Medical Eponyms of Pericarditis: Auscultation

Introduction

Auscultation is the most widely utilized skill employed during the physical examination in patients with acute and chronic pericarditis as physicians search to detect a pericardial friction rub, the pathognomonic sign of this disease. Auscultation is derived from the Latin word *auscultare* to listen or hear with attention [1]. The word "auscultation" was coined by John Forbes (1787–1861) to describe the method of placing the ear directly against the chest wall [1]. Although René Laënnec (1781–1826) introduced the stethoscope in 1817 as a method of indirect auscultation, he applied this apparatus primarily in the study of lungs and breath sounds coining such terms as "crepitation, pectoriloquy, and aegophony" [1]. Interestingly, it was Jean-Baptiste Bouillaud (1796–1881) in 1824 who is credited for using auscultation as a means for diagnosing diseases of the heart [1]. We begin our discussion on auscultatory sounds of pericarditis by first tracing the origins of the pathognomonic sign of pericarditis, the pericardial friction rub.

Abu Marwan ibn Zuhr (Avenzoar) (c.1093–1162), an Arabian physician, was the first to describe moist and dry types of pericarditis [1]. The sounds of the pericardial friction rub was first reported by Victor Collin (b.1796), Laënnec's assistant, in 1824, and further elaborated by Peter Mere Latham (1789–1875) in 1826 [2–4]. However, it was William Stokes (1804–1878) in 1833 who provided the most comprehensive description of the physical diagnosis of pericarditis [1]. We included an excerpt of the original description of pericarditis and pericardial friction rub written by Collin and Stokes to provide the reader with an appreciation of their contribution to the auscultatory diagnosis of this disease.

Collin described in his short treatise entitled *Des diverses méthodes d'exploration de la poitrine, et de leur application au diagnostic de ses maladies* (Various Methods of Investigating the Diseases of the Chest and Their Application to the Diagnosis of its Diseases) the pericardial friction rub sound:

S. H. Yale et al., *Cardiovascular Eponymic Signs*,
https://doi.org/10.1007/978-3-030-67596-7_11

> The sound resembling the cracking of new leather has only once presented itself to our observation; it was in a man who was carried off by a chronic pericarditis. The sound lasted during the first six days of the disease, and disappeared as soon as the local symptoms announced a considerable effusion into the pericardium. M. Devilliers, internal pupil at the Hospital Saint Antoine, observed it at the same time in the case of a man, who, from other symptoms, seemed to suffer from pericarditis. He was then ignorant that this phenomenon had already been observed in this affection, and did not apply the diagnosis. (...) A second time M. Devilliers had an opportunity of examining the dead body of a man who had presented this noise during the whole time of his stay in the hospital. He discovered a chronic pericarditis which had produced thick false membranes and numerous vegetations over the pericardium and heart [2, p. 72–73]. (...) Perhaps the noise which I have compared to the creaking of leather, is a symptom of this affection; it is one of short duration, limited to a few hours, if the disease is acute, and quickly producing effusion; more durable when the progress is slower. The friction of the two lamina of the pericardium, deprived of the serous fluid by the inflammation, may explain the sound [2, p. 132].

Stokes in the chapters "Contribution to thoracic pathology, article VII" published in 1833, and "Article III of researches on the diagnosis of pericarditis," published in 1834, extensively describe the pericardial friction rub. In article VII subsection, "Diagnosis of pericarditis," he wrote:

> On this subject, however, I have nothing original to offer, but may state that in several cases I have been enabled to verify the observation of Collin, relative to the sound of friction, produced by the rubbing together of the surfaces of the pericardium, when they are covered with unorganized lymph, a sound which he compares to that of the creaking of new leather. But I can state further, that numerous modifications of this sound may be met with. It resembles the creaking of leather in some cases, the rubbing of two very rough surfaces in others. In some it may be confounded by an inexperienced observer with Laennec's "bruit de Rape," and in others, may closely resemble the different modifications of the bruit de soufflet, with which I feel satisfied it has constantly been confounded. In many instances we have observed that the sounds in a single case have undergone a series of modifications, passing from the loudest sound of friction of two very rough surfaces, to a sound similar to the most faint bruit de soufflet; and in two cases we have (on applying the hand) felt the friction of the roughened surfaces of the pericardium in the most distinct manner, causing a violent "fremissement." [5, p. 63].

In article III he summarized the finding in patients with pericarditis:

> I shall now state in the form of propositions, the general results of my researches on this subject: — 1. That in cases of pericarditis with effusion of lymph, the rubbing of the two roughened surfaces causes sounds perceptible to the ear, and vibrations communicable to the hand, by which the disease can be easily and surely recognized, even when all other symptoms are absent. 2. That the more rough is the state of the serous membrane, the more distinct will these signs be. 3. That the sounds accompany the two sounds of the heart in almost all cases. 4. That they are audible generally, only over the region of the heart. 5. That they present themselves with various modifications of character, but often resemble the sounds produced by extensive valvular disease. 6. That they are most distinct when the region of the heart continues with its natural sound on percussion, but that the existence of fluid does not necessarily imply their complete subsidence. 7. That they may re-appear after the absorption of fluid from the bag of the pericardium, or the new supervention of inflammation. 8. That the sounds may continue when the sensation of rubbing is no longer perceptible by the hand. 9. That they are singularly and rapidly modified by direct antiphlogistic treatment to the heart. 10. That by observing the progress and mutations of those signs, we can trace the process of organization, or of obliteration of the pericardial cavity, judge the

> effect of treatment, and accurately ascertain the exact state of the pericardium. 11. That hence, it must be admitted, that, auscultation is of direct utility in pericarditis, and that the diagnosis no longer rests on negative signs [6, p. 60].

Auscultation is an essential technique performed during the physical examination of the heart in patients with suspected pericarditis. It involves attentively listening to different locations over the precordium. In addition to the pericardial friction rub, physicians identified other auscultatory sounds or signs named eponymously to honor their discovery. As eloquently written by David H. Spodick (b.1927): "When pericarditis is suspected, there is no substitute for diligent auscultation" [7, p. 34].

Pericardial friction rubs sounds have also been described as grating or scratching and classically having three components in patients in normal sinus rhythm: presystolic (atrial), systolic, and diastolic. The examiner may detect one, two, or all three components occurring at different times during the course of disease and even within the same day. Of the three components, the diastolic one is the most difficult to detect because it corresponds to the period of filling of the left ventricle whereas the presystolic and systolic occur during active contraction of the atrial and ventricles, respectively.

Auscultation is an important technique for identifying the pericardial friction rub and other adventitious sounds over the precordium in patients with suspected pericarditis. Other auscultatory findings detected as eponymous signs may also assist clinicians to further support the diagnosis and honor their discovery. Recognizing these signs imparts an appreciation for the meticulous attention that physicians employed while listening to the precordium. Our goal is to summarize the history of physicians who observed the sign as originally described and the sensitivity, specificity, and predictive value and its application in more modern day clinical practice. The signs are presented chronologically based on the year that they were first reported.

Signs

Aran Sign

François-Amilcar Aran (1817–1861) was born in Bordeaux, France, and received his doctorate from the University of Paris, followed by an appointment as an associate professor [8]. He was a deputy physician at the Hôtel-Dieu and Saint-Antoine Hospital, Paris, France [8]. In 1843, he published the book entitled *Manuel pratique des maladies du cœur et des gros vaisseaux* (Practical Manual of the Diseases of the Heart and Great Vessels) [9].

In addition to the sign that bears his namesake, his name is also eponymously associated with Duchenne (Aran-Duchenne spinal muscular atrophy). Aran published this work entitled "Recherches sur une maladie non encore décrit du système musculaire: atrophie musculaire progressive" (Research on a not yet described disease of the muscular system: progressive muscular atrophy) in 1850 [10, p. 172].

Table 11.1 Pericardial auscultation eponymous sign

Name	Year	Description of method for eliciting sign	Significance
Aran [11]	1844	Decreased or loss of the second heart sound.	Adhesive pericarditis
Perret and Devic [16]	1889	Dullness at the left base progressing as the pericardial effusion increases without changes to the mitral insufficiency murmur or bronchial breath sounds.	Pericardial effusion
Fisher [21]	1894	Dull, short sound or occasionally a long, diastolic rumbling sound. A shock occurring at the time of the third heart sound is sometimes palpable over the precordium.	Adhesive pericarditis
Josserand [28]	1894	Loud clangorous (click) diastolic sound heard at the left second and third intercostal spaces (pulmonary area) along the left sternal border.	Acute pericarditis
Warthin [29]	1895	Marked accentuation of the second heart sound located at the second left intercostal space (pulmonary area).	Acute pericarditis
Pérez [34]	1896	Increased intensity of the pericardial friction rub located over the midsternum but more predominately to the right occurring during deep inspiration and after raising and lowering the arms over the head.	Adhesive fibro-mediastinal pericarditis
Gorham [38]	1920	Pericardial friction rub occurring within the first 2 days after a coronary thrombosis and myocardial infarction.	Acute pericarditis
Lian [44]	1933	A loud vibrating sound occurring after the second heart sound in protodiastole (pericardial knock), best heard during inspiration with the patient in the left anterior oblique position.	Chronic calcific pericarditis

Aran described in his paper entitled "Recherches sur les adhérences générales du péricarde; nouveau moyen de reconnaitre cette altération" (Research on the general adhesions of the pericardium; new way to recognize this alteration) the absence of the second heart sound at the apex and base of the heart, "[a] new sign, of which no one, to my knowledge, has mentioned before me: I mean the weakening and the more or less complete extinction of the second sound." [11, p. 476]. Thus, Aran sign refers to the loss of the second heart sound in patients with adhesive pericarditis (Table 11.1). We are unaware of any study which evaluated the sensitivity or specificity of this sign.

Perret and Devic Sign

Simon Perret

There is limited historical information on Simon Perret (1847–1901). He served as a physician at the Hôpitaux de Lyon, France, and Associate Professor in the Medical Faculty of Lyon [12, 13]. He was also a member of the National Society of Medicine, Society of Medical Sciences, Paris, and Royal College of Physicians, Edinburgh.

Eugène Devic

Eugène Devic (1858–1930) was born in La Cavalerie, Aveyron, France, received his medical degree in 1886, and was named associate professor at the Medical College of Lyon in 1892 [14]. In 1894, he was a physician at the Hôpitaux de Lyon, followed by serving as the head of the Department of Medicine at hospitals La Croix Rousse and Hôtel-Dieu, Lyon [14, 15]. He published in a variety of therapeutic areas including pediatrics, gastroenterology, infectious disease, neurology, and cardiovascular disease. In addition to the eponymous sign related to pericarditis, his name is perhaps best recognized in conjunction with his student Fernand Gault (1873–1936) in describing the syndrome neuromyélite optique aiguë (currently known by the name Neuromyelitis optica, NMO, or Devic disease), a conditions characterized by the symptoms of acute myelitis and optic neuritis.

Perret and Devic described in their paper "Un nouveau symptôme de la péricardite avec épanchement chez les enfants" (A new symptom of pericarditis with effusion in children):

> [a] symptom that we have just seen three times in the space of six months, and that two consecutive cases has prevented us from avoiding a misdiagnosis. This sign, which falls within the category of objective signs, has, we believe, a real value, it is easy to notice, and it must henceforth revert to the classical symptomatology of pericarditis with effusion. First of all, here are our three observations, collected by Messrs. Pic and Chabaleir, internal members of the department [16, p. 280].

They described pulmonary signs in the three children with acute effusive rheumatic pericarditis and mitral insufficiency murmur:

> Observation 1: [o]n the left lung there is dullness and a mitral murmur which is limited at first to the lower portion of the lung. As the pericardial effusion progresses the dullness evolves to occupy almost the entire lung without accompanying changes to the mitral murmur. Observation 2: [o]n the side of the pericardium dullness appeared at the left lung base without changes to the sound of the mitral murmur or bronchial breath sounds. Observation 3: 1. Mitral insufficiency murmur heard on the front and back of the thorax first appearing towards the spine of the scapula and extending as the effusion progresses. 2 Dullness increased in size and intensity as the effusion increased and eventually occupied the entire height of the left lung and the subclavicular depression, 3 sub-crackling rales on the entire left side [16, p. 283].

Thus, Perret and Devic sign refers to increased dullness in the left hemithorax without effect on the mitral insufficiency murmur or bronchial breath sounds in patients with an enlarging pericardial effusion (Table 11.1). d'Espine described these same pulmonary findings at the left lung base as *pseudo-pleuretiques* (pseudo-pleuritic). That is, an area of dullness and bronchial breath sounds at the lung base medially extending and bordering the ninth rib between the midscapular line and spine. He attributed these findings to the compression of the lung by the enlarged pericardial effusion [17]. Furthermore, these same findings were described and reported by Ewart, Bamberger and Pins in adults under the name Ewart-Bamberger-Pin sign [18]. We are unaware of any study which evaluated the sensitivity or specificity of this sign.

Fisher Sign

Theodore Fisher (1863–1949) received his medical training at Guy's Hospital, London, and junior appointments at Guy's Hospital for Diseases of the Skin, Blackfriars Royal Hospital for Children, and Women and Bristol General Hospital [19]. He served as a pathologist at the Bristol Royal Infirmary and for outpatients at the Hospital for Sick Children and Women [19]. At the time of the publication of the sign that bears his namesake, he was an assistant physician to the East London Hospital for Children, Shadwell [20].

Fisher noted that children with cardiac hypertrophy and an adherent pericardium have an "indrawing of the chest wall in the neighbourhood of the cardiac impulse and Broadbent's sign, i.e. systolic retraction of the hinder and lower part of the left side of the chest." [21, p. 309]. He explained that this finding was based on the "outward thrust of a portion of the comparatively flexible chest wall of a child by a large heart is compensated by the indrawing of other portions, the inward movements near the cardiac apex being possibly dependent upon external atmospheric pressure." [21, p. 309].

Fisher and Graham Steell independently reported in the same month in the *British Medical Journal* and *Practitioner*, respectively, the findings of an adherent pericardium and a "presystolic or diastolic murmur without mitral stenosis." [21, 22]. Fisher reviewed the record of 13 children with an adherent pericardium secondary to rheumatic heart disease, marked hypertrophy and dilation of the heart. In five patients, a "diastolic or presystolic bruit had been present at the apex, yet the necropsy showed that the mitral orficie was dilated and the aortic valves were not thickened." [21, p. 906]. In some of these cases a systolic thrill was also present [21]. Steell also described, in April 1894, two patients with rheumatic heart disease, cardiac enlargement, adherent pericardium, and apex diastolic murmur accompanied by a thrill and reduplication of the second heart sound. Thus he recognized "that even in the absence of aortic incompetence implicit confidence cannot be placed in a diastolic apex-murmur accompanied by thrill as a sign of mitral stenosis. This is a conclusion, which has been forced upon me by the facts related-facts which there is no gain-saying, whatever their explanation." [22, p. 258].

Fisher further elaborated in his 1907 paper entitled "Some features of adherent pericardium" auscultatory findings both a short and sometimes a long rumbling sound at the cardiac apex:

> [d]ull sound when occurring near the first sound, is sometimes described as part of a reduplicated first sound, and when shorter, occurring near the second sound, as part of a reduplicated second sound audible only at the apex. Sometimes this dull sound may be equidistant from the first and second sound, and then under certain conditions of accentuation forms part of a bruit de galop. The diastolic sound may take part in the production of these combinations and of various others. It may be present for a long time or be evanescent. It may be the precursor of, or accompany, progressive valvular disease, be associated with permanent dilatation of the heart in which valvular disease is absent, or may be heard for a brief period during, or after, the presence of some passing condition of ill-health in which we must suppose the heart has shared. Again, the sound may occasionally be audible when there seems to be nothing whatever to account for its presence. I have been speaking of a dull, short sound, but the long, rumbling sound some times audible in cases of adherent

> pericardium is, in all probability, a sound of similar causation — that is to say, it is the short, dull sound much prolonged. (…) A shock occurring at the time of "the third sound of the heart," as the short, dull sound has been called, can, indeed, sometimes be felt by the hand placed over the heart — a sufficient proof, without the evidence of a cardiographic tracing, that there is abnormal cardiac action [23, p. 312].

Thus, Fisher sign refers to the presence of a presystolic sound in patients with adherent pericardium (Table 11.1). Steell name is not eponymously ascribed with this finding even though they both reported it in the same year. We are unaware of any study which evaluated the sensitivity or specificity of this sign.

Josserand Sign

Gabriel Nové-Josserand (1868–1949) was born in Amplepuis, Rhône, France, and received his doctorate in medicine at Lyon in 1893. He was appointed *chef-de-service* in 1897 and associate professor of surgery at the Charity Hospital in Lyon in 1898 [24, 25]. He served as the first professor and chair of pediatric surgery and orthopedy at the University of Lyon from 1921 to 1937 and was the national correspondent to the Academy of Medicine for the division of surgery in 1937 [26]. He was editor of *Revue d'Orthopédie* from 1911 to 1949 and founder of the French Society of Orthopedy, appointed first secretary general in 1918, and served as president in 1922 [27]. Nové-Josserand served as the president of the International Society of Orthopedics and Traumatic Surgery in 1930 and was elected honorary fellow of the Royal College of Surgeons, England, in 1933 [27]. His major area of surgical expertise was in orthopedic surgical repair of bone deformities such as club-foot and spina bifida occulta, congenital repair of malformation of the urinary tract (hypospadias), and devising a pathologic classification of tumors of the bone [27].

Josserand published in 1894 in *Congrès français de médecine* a paper entitled "Les signs de la péricardite aiguë" (The signs of acute pericarditis) where he described an early sign of pericarditis in patients with articular rheumatism (acute rheumatic fever) (Table 11.1):

> When one compares the aortic and pulmonary artery regions during auscultation at the base of the heart during the course of an articular rheumatism, it sometimes happens that in this region, that is, in the second and third intercostal spaces along the left edge of the sternum, the second sound is more intense, striking, and clangorous. It is the opposite of what happens in chronic aortitis where the second sound is more resonant to the right of the sternum. Sometimes the phenomenon is intense enough to translate in a tactile way: the hand placed on the base of the heart perceives an exaggerated diastolic shock at the pulmonary valve area [28, p. 838].

Josserand further stressed the significance of this finding:

> This intensity of the diastolic sound brilliancy must make one carefully search for the existence of the friction which is often found, whereas it would have been missed on superficial auscultation. If it was not initially found, we can predict its occurrence in a period usually varying from one to three days. This sign occurs early, is often transient; disappears within a few days, with the friction complicating and soon replaces the sound. It is therefore a

> phenomenon occurring during the acute, initial, congestive period of pericarditis, and comparable for example to crackling rale in pneumonia [28, p. 839]. (…) There is more: nothing proves in these cases that the pericardium alone is involved; endopericarditis is not uncommon, and endocarditis is known to have no early symptoms. One can generalize the significance of the diastolic sound: it indicates that the heart is globally involved with a severity that is not yet possible to specify and that it is necessary to institute the necessary medication without waiting for later occurrence of a blowing murmur or friction sounds [28, p. 840].

Furthermore, he explained what he believed to be the pathogenesis of this finding:

> In pericarditis, the false membranes preferably develop and friction is heard along the left border of the sternum and above the apex of the heart. It is likely that at this region the underlying myocardium, which continues directly upwards with the infundibulum of the pulmonary artery, is congested, turgid, and that the myocardium is densely covered with pericardial fibrinous exudates, causing the nearby pulmonary valve sounds being amplified to the ear. (…) [s]o there is in the pericarditis a densified heart stump, which amplifies adjacent valvular noises. The importance of this sign lies both in diagnosis and in treatment. In contentious cases where one hesitates between a friction and a blowing sound caused by either anemia or extracardiac condition, the presence of the diastolic resonance will point you towards the first direction [28, p. 839–840].

It is of interest that Warthin published the same finding (the phenomenon described by Josserand one year earlier) in his paper entitled "Accentuation of the pulmonary second sound an important sign in the diagnosis of pericarditis" in 1895 which became recognized and named Warthin sign [29]. Dargein and Plazy also reported this heart sound in two patients, one who subsequently developed pericarditis and the other endocarditis and pericarditis [30]. We are unaware of any study which evaluated the sensitivity or specificity of this sign.

Warthin Sign

Aldred Scott Warthin (1866–1931) received his medical degree in 1891, PhD in 1893, and served as a faculty member at the University of Michigan Medical Center. From 1903 throughout the remainder of his career, he was a professor of pathology and director of the pathological laboratories at the University of Michigan. He served in multiple leadership positions such as being elected as the president of the American Association of Pathologist and Bacteriologist in 1908, Association of American Physicians in 1928, American Association for Cancer Research in 1928, and the American Society for Experimental Pathology in1924 [31]. He was elected Master of the American College of Physician and served as its first vice-president of this organization in 1925 [32]. He was the editor of *Annals of Clinical Medicine* (currently *Annals of Internal Medicine*) [32]. In addition to the sign which bears his namesake, he studied the reticuloendothelial system, discovering and applying a stain, Warthin-Starry, for the identification of Treponema spirochetes in syphilis and hereditary cancer genetics [32].

Warthin described in 1895 in his paper entitled "Accentuation of the pulmonary second sound an important sign in the diagnosis of pericarditis" five cases where there was "marked accentuation of the pulmonary second sound, either with or without the coexistence of peculiar murmurs at the base or apex of the heart" [29, p. 395]. The sound was heard at the second left intercostal space. "It began early, either with the symptoms or preceding them, and continuing through the course of the disease, disappeared finally only after all other signs and symptoms had ceased." [29, p. 397]. Warthin acknowledged, confirmed, and expounded upon Josserand's earlier finding and found that "in our experience it is not transitory, being the very last thing to disappear." [29, p. 397]. He further provided his explanation for the pathogenesis of this clinical finding:

> [i]t must happen that a thickening of the pericardium around the pulmonary artery or a deposit of fibrin in the same region must amplify the sound of the pulmonary valves so long as the condition exists; and this may be present for a long time after the active disease has subsided. It is conceivable then that this accentuation must exist in all cases except the very mildest, in which the pathologic changes take place in only a very slight degree. The intensity of the accentuation of the sound will depend therefore upon the degree and character of change in the muscle and pericardium, and upon the amount and character of the exudate, whereby there is an increased conductivity of the pulmonary sound in the space lying between the valves and the chest-wall [29, p. 398].

Warthin thus recognized that this sign will only be present in cases where the pericardial inflammation is localized to the pulmonary region of the pericardium which he found to be present in the majority of cases. Warthin sign thus refers to accentuation of the second heart sound in patients with pericarditis (Table 11.1). We are unaware of any study which evaluated the sensitivity or specificity of this sign.

Pérez Sign

Jorge (George) Víctor Pérez (1851–1920) was born in Puerto de la Cruz, Tenerife in the Canary Islands [33]. He received his MRCS in 1882 and MB at the University College of Hospital, London, returning to Puerto Orotava, Tenerife for medical practice beginning in 1883 [33]. As summarized by William Ewart, "Dr. Perez was best known to the medical world through his discovery of the characteristic sounds often yielded by fibrous mediastinitis–Perez's sign. He combined with great accuracy special keen nose for therapeutics." [33]. Pérez described an auscultatory finding in the chest in a patient with mediastino-pericarditis:

> [e]ither of the arms was raised over the head and lowered again, that during both movements most extraordinary friction sounds were heard, of a similar nature but much coarser and louder than those which had been heard for years in this case, during deep inspiration and mainly over midsternum, while the patient was having one of her frequently recurring attacks of mediastinal pleurisy and pericarditis [34, p. 407].

Pérez's colleague, Dr. Harris, who examined the patient the latter part of the same year postulated that:

> The most probable explanation of their production appeared to be that the elevation and lowering of the arms moved the main vessel of the arm, and to a less extent also the arch of

> the aorta, and that this movement of the vessels dragged upon adhesion situated round the vessels external to the pericardium, and so produced the crackling sound [34, p. 407].

Thus, this sign refers to the presence of "dry friction-crepitation sound over the external region, and to either side, but chiefly to the right." [34, p. 408] (Table 11.1). We are unaware of any study which evaluated the sensitivity or specificity of this sign.

Gorham Sign

Lemuel Whittington Gorham (1885–1968) was born in Albany, New York, and earned his medical degree from Johns Hopkins University in 1910. In 1913, he was an instructor, and subsequently physician in chief, director of the Department and Professor of Medicine at Albany Medical College, New York, in 1937 [35]. He was the president of the American Clinical and Climatological Association in 1936, appointed member of the New York State Public Health Council in 1940, and director of the Public Health Research Institute in New York City in 1951 [35–37].

Gorham described six patients (autopsy finding in three) with coronary thrombosis and myocardial infarction who subsequently developed fever and a pericardial friction rub, a symptom complex previously described by Sternberg who coined the name for this syndrome "Pericarditis Epistenocardica" which consists of:

> 2. The presence of fever coming on usually in 24 hours, and lasting four or five days. The patients are clear mentally, but restlessness is often extreme. Leucocytosis may be present.
> 3. A pericardial friction rub, frequently of light intensity, developing within the first few days, transitory in nature, often recurrent, and localized over a small area. Such a rub may be readily overlooked, unless one carefully and repeatedly seeks for it. This was present in five of the six cases. Failure to hear it in one case (No. VI) may possibly be explained by the fact that the infarcted area was on the posterior surface of the left ventricle, and that hemopericardium developed [38, p. 123]. (…) Pericardial friction is the most important and characteristic single sign of the syndrome. The difficulty in detecting the friction rub, because of its light quality, its sharply defined localization, and its transitory or recurrent character is to be especially emphasized [38, p. 130].

Thus, Gorham sign refers to the presence of a pericardial friction rub in patients with myocardial infarction (Table 11.1). This sign is best recognized in connotation with Dressler, who also described this phenomenon in 1955 and coined the term "post-myocardial infarction syndrome" [39, 40]. We are unaware of any study which evaluated the sensitivity or specificity of this sign.

Lian Sign

Camille Lian (1882–1969) was born at Treigny, Yonne, France, and received his medical degree in Paris, graduating in 1909 [41]. He was appointed physician of the Hôpitaux in 1919 and associate professor in 1923 [41, 42]. In 1926 with his colleague George Minot (Paris), he developed a phonocardiograph (Lian-Minot) while at the Tenon Hospital, publishing a treatise on phonocardiograpy with Minot and Welti in 1941 [41]. He was an associate of internal pathology at Tenon Hospital in 1928 and was nominated professor of the history of medicine and subsequently professor of clinical medicine in 1942 [41, 42]. Lian was the president of the French Society of Cardiology, member of the Swiss Academy of Medical Science, and recipient of the "Golden Stethoscope Award" by the International Cardiology Foundation [41, 43]. His life study involved the investigation of the heart and arterial vessels with important contributions in heart murmurs and sounds, angina, arrhythmias, heart failure, and myocardial infarction [42].

Lian and his colleagues Maurice Marchal and Jean Pautrat in their manuscript entitled "Un signe clinique de la calcification du péricarde: la vibrance péricardique protodiastolique" (A clinical sign of pericardial calcification: pericardial protodiastolic vibrancy) published in *Bulletins et mémoires de la Société médicale des hôpitaux de Paris,* of a clinical sign in two patients, a heart sound, which they named the protodiastolic pericardial vibrancy believed to be caused by pericardial calcification:

> The sign we describe as a proto-diastolic pericardial vibration is a sound that reaches a surprising true vibrancy, much louder than the normal noises of the heart with which it constitutes a three-beat rhythm. It occurs immediately after the second noise and is a protodiastolic phenomenon. Its high intensity is explained in that it seems to burst immediately under the ear. From the distal tip or the juxta-xiphoid region it is perceived throughout the precordial region and up to the supra-sternal trough during auscultation of the aorta and even in the supraclavicular regions during auscultation of the subclavian artery [44, p. 23].

They recorded the phenomenon of protodiastolic pericardial vibrancy using phonocardiogram and recognized: "Thus, it may be useful to use the three-beat rhythmic record which we did in our two observations to support our clinical diagnosis and to better study protodiastolic pericardial vibrancy." [44, p. 24]. Fluoroscopic examination of the pericardial calcification showed:

> In general, the location at first glance, is found in the two frontal views at the lower edge of the right ventricle. We have seen that in the left anterior oblique position calcification of the right ventricle is continued by a large circle surrounding the whole heart. It therefore seems difficult to talk about localization at the lower edge when in both cases we see a limestone network encompassing the entire heart. We can say that the maximum density of limestone deposit is generally located in the right ventricular region. The density of calcifications is usually low and always projected on the shadow of the heart. This explains why many cases go unnoticed especially radioscopically. (…) But the position of examination of choice is, as we have just established above, unquestionably the left anterior oblique position during complete inspiration [44, p. 22].

They accounted for what they believed to be the pathogenesis of this phenomenon:

> It is therefore likely due to intrapericardial calcifications. We do not know whether these occupy the visceral leaflet, the parietal leaflet of the pericardium separately, or the two leaves contiguous to an intrapericardial symphysis (concretio type). Only a necroscopic examination could determine the nature of the lesion that causes the calcification. We think it is due to chronic pericarditis, sclerosis, and limestone precipitation. (…) We believe that it reflects the vibration of the calcified shell of the heart during its abrupt protodiastolic dilatation. In short, it is a protodiastolic gallop sound vibrating by calcification of the pericar-

> dium. The protodiastolic localization is explained in these two patients by heart failure allowing the ventricular congestion to reach great importance from the beginning of the diastole. (…) Also, it is possible that in all cases of pericardial calcification where this lesion results in an added noise, it is always protodiastolic, even in the absence of any cardiac insufficiency. The added noise would therefore be the translation of the increase of volume which occurs in the hearts at the beginning of the diastole. An increased volume occurs in physiological infancy and adolescence to the sound of the heart in certain insufficiencies, cardiac to a protodiastolic galloping sound, and in the calcification of the pericardium in protodiastolic vibrancy [44, p. 25–26].

Furthermore, they considered the significance of this stethoscopic sign in clinical medical practice:

> The mobility characteristics of calcified plaques allow differential diagnosis with pulmonary or pleural calcification. The pericardial calcified plaques follow the heart during respiratory movements. They are always energized by synchronous beats of the same amplitude during cardiac contractions [44, p. 22]. (…) Therefore, we consider the protodiastolic pericardial vibrancy as a clinical sign intended not to allow a single diagnosis on its own, but to orient the clinician to a probable diagnosis of pericardial calcification and to induce him to perform a detailed radiological examination which will provide a definitive conclusion [44, p. 24].

Thus, Lian sign refers to the presence of vibratory protodiastolic sound or "pericardial knock" occurring in patients with calcific pericarditis (Table 11.1). We are unaware of any study which evaluated the sensitivity or specificity of this sign.

Conclusion

During the cardiac examination, both the diaphragm and bell of the stethoscope should be used to detect both the high- and low-frequency sounds at the mid- to left lower sternal border [45]. If uncertainty remains in the diagnosis, the sound may be further accentuated by placing the patients in the knee and elbow position [45]. Awareness of auscultatory sounds or signs in patients with pericarditis supports the diagnosis of pericarditis, enhances our understanding of the pathophysiology of disease, and provides an appreciation for other findings in addition to pericardial friction sound that may be found in patients with acute or calcific pericarditis. The lack of studies evaluating the sensitivity or specificity of these signs creates gaps in our medical knowledge of how often they are found and how useful they are in clinical practice providing opportunities for further investigation.

References

1. Skinner HA. The Origin of Medical Terms. Baltimore: The Williams & Wilkins Company; 1949.
2. Collin V. Manual for the Use of the Stethoscope: A Short Treatise on the Different Methods of Investigating the Diseases of the Chest. Ryland WN, translator. 3rd ed. Boston: Benjamin Perkins & Co.; 1829.

3. Latham PM. Pathological essays on some diseases of the heart. London M Gaz. 1829;3:209–18.
4. Latham PM. In: Marti R, editor. The Collected Works of Dr. P.M. Latham with Memoir by Sir Thomas Watson, vol. 1. London: The New Sydenham Society; 1876.
5. Stokes W. Contributions to thoracic pathology. Dublin J M & Chem Sc. 1833;3:50–65.
6. Stokes W. Researches on the diagnosis of pericarditis. Dublin J M & Chem Sc. 1834;4:29–60.
7. Spodick DH. Pericardial friction. In: Acute Pericarditis. New York: Grune & Stratton; 1959. p. 34–7.
8. Aran F-A. Wikipedia. https://en.wikipedia.org/wiki/Fran%C3%A7ois-Amilcar_Aran. Accessed 12 Oct 2018.
9. Aran FA. Practical Manual of Diseases of the Heart and Great Vessels. Harris WMA, translator. Philadelphia: Barrington & Geo D. Haswell; 1843.
10. Aran FA. Recherches sur une maladie non encore décrit du systéme musculaire (atrophie musculaire progressive). Arch Gén de Méd. 1850;3:172–214.
11. Aran FA. Recherches sur les adhérences générales du péricarde; nouveau moyen de reconnaitre cette altération. Arch Gén de Méd. 1844;4:466–87.
12. [No author]. Deaths in the profession abroad: S. Perret. Br Med J. 1901:1242.
13. [No author]. Dr. S. Perret. Boston M & S J. 1901;145:724.
14. Miyazawa I, Fujihara K, Itoyama Y. Pioneers in neurology: Eugène Devic (1858–1930). J Neurol. 2002;249:351–2.
15. Moulin T, Clarac F, Petit H, Broussolie E. Neurology outside Paris following Charcot. In: Bogousslavsky J, editor. Following Charcot: A Forgotten History of Neurology and Psychiatry. Basel: Karger; 2011. p. 170–87.
16. Perret S, Devic E. Un nouveau symptôme de la péricardite avec épanchement chez les enfants. Province Méd Lyon. 1889;3:279–93.
17. D'Espine A, Picot C. Péricardite. In: Traité pratique des maladies de l'enfance. Paris: J.-B. Baillière et fils; 1899. p. 745–50.
18. Spodick DH. Pericardial effusion: clinical manifestations. In: Acute Pericarditis. New York: Grune & Stratton; 1959. p. 56–61.
19. Fisher T. Royal College of Physicians. Lives of the fellows. 2009. http://munksroll.rcplondon.ac.uk/Biography/Details/1547. Accessed 6 Jan 2019.
20. [No author]. Dr. Theodore Fisher. Med Press & Circ. 1905;131:550.
21. Fisher T. A diastolic bruit at the apex in the heart disease of children. Br Med J. 1894;1:906–7.
22. Steell G. Diastolic murmur in dilation of the heart without arterial incompetence or auriculoventricular constriction. Practioner. 1894;52:254–8.
23. Fisher T. Some features of adherent pericardium. Clin J. 1907;30:308–12.
24. Medical News. Foreign University Intelligence. 1898:1783. https://play.google.com/books/reader?id=qVBKAQAAMAAJ&printsec=frontcover&pg=GBS.PA1783. Accessed 3 Jan 2019.
25. [No author]. Chronique et nouvelles scientifiques. Lancette française. 1898;71:578.
26. Nové-Josserand G (1868–1949). IdRef. Identfiants et Référentiels pour l'esneignement supérieur et le recherché. https://www.idref.fr/071070060. Accessed 7 Dec 2018.
27. Nové-Josserand G (1868–1949). Royal College of Surgeons. Plarr's Lives of the Fellows. 2013. https://livesonline.rcseng.ac.uk/client/en_GB/lives/search/detailnonmodal/ent:$002f$002fSD_ASSET$002f0$002f338901/one?qu=Josserand&te=ASSET. Accessed 12 Dec 2018.
28. Josserand G. Des signes de la péricardite aigue. In: Congrès français de médecine 1894. Lyon; 1895. p. 838–40.
29. Warthin AS. Accentuation of the pulmonary second sound an important sign in the diagnosis of pericarditis. Med News. 1895;66:395–9.
30. Dargein JG, Plazy L. Péricardite et signe de Josserand. Bull et Mém Soc Méd d Hôp de Par. 1922;46(1):712–3.
31. [No author]. Aldred Scott Warthin, professor of pathology, and director of the pathological laboratories. In: The President's Report for 1930–1931. Ann Arbor: The University of Michigan Press; 1932, p. 367–8.

32. Lynch HT. Alfred Scott Warthin MD, PhD (1866-1931), classic in oncology. Cancer J Clin. 1985;35:345–7.
33. [No author]. Obituary: Dr. George V. Perez. Br Med J. 1920;1:456.
34. Perez GB. A new auscultatory sign of mediastinal affections. Lancet. 1896;2(1864):407–8.
35. L. Whittington Gorham papers, 1901–1967. Archive grid. (cited 2018 December 4). https://beta.worldcat.org/archivegrid/data/319126690. Accessed 11 Nov 2018.
36. Whittington Gorham L. The American Clinical and Climatological Association. p. 250. https://europepmc.org/backend/ptpmcrender.fcgi?accid=PMC2279666&blobtype=pd. Accessed 23 Nov 2018.
37. [No author]. Dr. L. Whittington Gorham. Am J Public Health. 1940;30:1018.
38. Gorham LW. The significance of transient localized pericardial friction in coronary thrombosis (pericarditis, epistenocardica). Albany Med Ann. 1920;41:109–30.
39. Dressler W. A post-myocardial-infarction syndrome: preliminary report of a complication resembling idiopathic recurrent benign pericarditis. JAMA. 1956;160:1379–83.
40. Dressler W. The post-myocardial infarction syndrome. AMA Arch Intern Med. 1959;103:28–42.
41. [No author]. Camille Lian 1882–1969. Br Heart J. 1969;31:789–90.
42. Le Professeur Agrégé Camille Lian de la Faculté de Médecine de Paris. Chanteclair 1928;23e:439. http://www.biusante.parisdescartes.fr/histoire/medica/resultats/index.php?do=page&cote=chanteclx1928x18&p=77. Accessed 7 Dec 2019.
43. Welti H. Le Professeur Camille Lian (1882-1969). Bull Schweiz Akad Med Wiss. 1969;25:202.
44. Lian C, Marchal M, Pautrat J. Un signe clinique de la calcification du péricarde: la vibrance péricardique protodiastolique. Bull et Mém Soc Méd d Hôp de Par. 1933;1:20–8.
45. Perloff JK. Physical Examination of the Heart and Circulation. 2nd ed. Philadelphia: W.B. Saunders Company; 1990.

Chapter 12
Peripheral Arterial Disease

Introduction

A variety of signs have since been described from the time of Charcot as methods to diagnose peripheral arterial disease (PAD) or arterial injury. These signs employed the physical examination skills of observation, auscultation, palpation, or passive and active movements. Signs, also referred to in some cases as tests, were designed and described by physicians possessing keen insight and knowledge of disease pathogenesis. They were so named eponymously to honor physicians' accomplishments. These signs are easy to perform and remain a relevant aspect of the noninvasive bedside assessment of PAD or injury. The accuracy of these signs in clinical practice is either unknown or has not been further studied but, when present, is more commonly identified in patients with more advanced disease. Understanding the historical content behind these signs provides clinicians' background information of these physicians' accomplishments and an appreciation of bedside methods devised in diagnosis. Knowledge of these simple bedside maneuvers enhances physicians' diagnostic acumen, providing clues to the presence of PAD.

This chapter reviews signs as eponymously described by first providing brief historical information of the person and their original description, and second, if known, their accuracy and utility in clinical practice. The signs are presented chronologically based on the year when they were first published.

S. H. Yale et al., *Cardiovascular Eponymic Signs*,
https://doi.org/10.1007/978-3-030-67596-7_12

Historical Background

The word "claudication" originated from the Latin *claudicare,* to limp, or be lame [1]. Although it was first identified in horses, Jean-Martin Charcot (1825–1893) was the first to recognize this condition in humans: "This interesting observation which is the subject of the present communication seems to us to be similar to cases of intermittent claudication caused by arterial obliteration, well known today in horse pathology" [2]. Charcot described the case in Jean Lefébure, a 54-year-old man with a right iliac artery aneurysm and distal obliterated narrowed vascular segment caused by a bullet wound:

> When Lefébure is obliged to walk for more than a quarter of an hour, he develops throughout the entire right lower limb a feeling of weakness accompanied by bewilderment. If he still continues walking, dull pains accompanied by tingling do not take long to appear. They first occur in the penis and from there spread in the right thigh, leg, and foot. This is followed by cramps, general stiffness, and inability to move the leg. He then needs to sit down and rest for several minutes. During this time symptoms dissipated quickly and soon he is able to walk again. After about twenty minutes the symptoms reoccur requiring him to rest. These kinds of bouts of painful paralysis often occur five or six times within an hour. They never happen spontaneously, that is to say when the patient is at rest, lying down, sitting, or standing. Only walking seems to provoke the symptoms. (…) It has not been possible for us to know whether a lower skin temperature or anesthesia is present in the affected limb since attacks of painful paralysis are produced by walking and disappeared after a few minutes with rest leaving no trace of having been present. Their presence over a long time produces within the patient a kind of disability, preventing him from indulging in his usual occupation [2, p. 230].

Charcot believed that the symptoms were the result of ischemia of the affected limb brought on by exercise and proposed that the pain was due to excitation of motor and sensory nerves [2, p. 237].

Signs

Von Wahl Sign

Eduard Georg von Wahl (1833–1890) was born in Pernau, Livonia (present day Latvia), studied medicine at the University of Dorpat (current Tartu University, Tartu, Estonia), and received his doctorate in 1859 [3–5]. He served as a practicing physician at Pet-Paul Hospital from 1860 to 1867 and was head of the surgical department of the Oldenburg Children's Hospital, St. Petersburg, from 1867 to 1876. At the University of Dorpat, he served as chair of state medicine in 1876, professor of surgery in 1878, head of the surgical clinic, and rector from 1881 to 1885 [4–7]. Von Wahl described an auscultatory sound occurring after traumatic arterial injury (Table 12.1):

Table 12.1 Peripheral arterial disease eponymous sign

Name	Year	Description of sign
Von Wahl [8]	1885	Method to determine the type of arterial injury based on auscultation and palpitation: 1. *Partial arterial separation:* Intermittent, isochronous, blowing noises. Pulse below the injured area is weaker than on the normal side. 2. *Long puncture wounds where external bleeding is stopped by coagulation:* A distinct, isochronous noises occurs with the pulse. These wounds typically do not pulsate. 3. *Complete transection of the artery where the ends have retracted into the wound and are temporarily closed or with temporary obliteration of an injured artery laterally by a thrombus:* There is an absence of sound where the continuity of the blood flow is interrupted. No pulse is present distal to the injured area. 4. *Central or peripheral end of a completely separated artery is reopened:* Absent sounds and rapidly growing pulsating hematoma (terminal aneurysms).
Moszkowicz [14]	1907	The extremity is held upright at an angle while a strong tourniquet is strapped around the thigh as high as possible for 5 minutes. When the extremity appears pale, the tourniquet is loosened: 1. In normal arteries and in patients with arteriosclerosis without severe vascular occlusion, hyperemia appears promptly if blood flow is present. 2. In patients with severe vascular occlusion, the hyperemia is less intense and takes longer before it spreads to the entire extremity.
Buerger [23]	1917	Elevate the limb 60–90° above the horizontal until blanching occurs and then lower the limb to the dependent position and observe for rubor.
Adson [34]	1927	Patient elevates the chin or rotates the head to the affected side during inspiration. Symptoms include paresthesia over the distribution of the brachial plexus and absent radial pulse on the affected side.
Samuels [42]	1929	The patient is placed in the reclining position preferably on a low bed or couch. He/she is then instructed to elevate both legs to an angle of 90° and while maintaining this position is asked to rapidly flex and extend both feet. Observe the plantar surface of both feet as the motion is occurring. If there is unilateral arterial disease, the normal pink tint of the skin of the sole gradually fades into pallor color, which remains as long as the feet are held vertical even after the motion has ceased. The healthy foot retains its natural pink color despite prolonged ankle motion.
Fuchsig [45]	1957	Patient sits with legs crossed. There is an oscillatory movement of the foot synchronous with the pulse in patients with occlusive atherosclerotic disease involving the popliteal artery.
DeWeese [51]	1960	Pedal pulse present at rest and absent during exercise when claudication is present.

From the first section of this work it is undoubtedly clear that through the physical examination of the vessel we have an excellent way to recognize, in most cases, the type of injury present immediately after the traumatic event. Through auscultation the remaining symptoms of vascular injury obtain their full diagnostic value. In such circumstances it seems advisable to carry out the examination with the stethoscope each time there is suspicion of arterial injury in order to carefully evaluate for the presence or absence of a sound and its diagnostic significance. Since I do not base my conclusions on theoretical speculations but on experimentally testing and clinically confirmed facts, it seems most appropriate to summarize them in the following brief sentences:

1. In every partial separated artery during auscultation, an intermittent, isochronous, hissing, or scraping noise can be perceived where blood flows to the periphery through the two vessels. This is most evident at the site of the injury, propagating to either side, but most commonly in the direction of the bloodstream. In most cases, the pulse below the injured area is albeit weaker than on the healthy side.
2. At particular sites on the body where external bleeding from a punctured wound is stopped by coagulation, a periarterial hematoma of a greater or lesser extent develops very rapidly at partially injured large arterial trunks. These sites usually have no pulsations, but distinct isochronous noises occurring with the pulse.
3. In complete transection of the artery where the ends have retracted and the wound is temporarily closed, as well as with temporary obliteration of an injured artery laterally by a thrombus, there is in all cases no sound where the continuity of the blood flow is interrupted. The location of the severed artery can be determined with certainty by the absence of the pulse beneath the injured area.
4. When the central or peripheral ends of a completely separated artery are reopened, it is not uncommon to experience a rapidly growing pulsating hematoma (terminal aneurysm) which shows no noise. This rule occurs only in cases where the vein is also injured and yet the arterial blood flows into the venous tracts [8, p. 136–137].

Von Wahl emphasized the significance of his findings:

> The practical meaning seems to me to be obvious. If we are able to diagnose an arterial injury with certainty at the time when the main symptom of the injury, bleeding, is no longer present than Guthrie's theorem: "That no operation ought to be performed on a wounded artery unless it bleeds" is no longer valid. We must take advantage of this period of blood stasis in order to prevent rebleeding, which, according to Fischer's view, leads to a mortality of 60 to 80 percent. It is during this period of stasis that we have to expose the wounded vessel in order to prevent it from rebleeding. It is during this period of inactivity that ligation of the injured vessel can easily be performed and by simultaneously clearing the blood which has flowed into the tissues the course of the wound can be improved. Waiting for a later date reduces the chance of healing dramatically [8, p. 138].

To summarize, in a partially separated artery, a systolic blowing or grating sound is heard, while in complete transection no sounds are identified during auscultation (Table 12.1) [9]. Furthermore, pulsation is palpated in a partial separated artery or in cases when there is reestablished flow in a previously transected artery. Von Wahl emphasized that these findings are important to recognize, as they are methods to determine whether the underlying artery is completely severed, and if so, whether it can safely be repaired so as to avoid secondary rebleeding [8].

Von Wahl's observations of the palpatory and auscultatory findings in arterial injuries were accurate. Blunt or penetrating traumatic injury to an artery may cause hemorrhage, thrombosis, and an intimal flap, as a result of arterial dissection that may prolapse into the arterial lumen and produce auscultatory sounds. Complete arterial transection causes arterial retraction, spasm, hematoma, and absence of sounds. An arterial puncture results in hemorrhage, a large hematoma, and a pseudoaneurysm. As inferred by von Wahl but not named as such, pseudo-aneurysm as well as an arteriovenous fistula, later findings occurring after an injury, may produce a palpable pulsatile mass and/or a bruit [10].

Moszkowicz Sign

Ludwig Moszkowicz (1873–1945) was born in Krakow (Galizien) and studied at the Faculty of Medicine, University of Vienna, Austria, graduating in 1887 [11–13]. He practiced general medicine at Wiener Rudolfinerhaus, Vienna, Austria, from 1898 to 1914 [11, 13]. Moszkowicz habilitated in surgery at the University of Vienna in 1929 and under National Socialism (Nazism), his venia legendi certificate was unjustifiably revoked and he was expelled from the University in 1938 [12].

Moszkowicz described the finding of active hyperemia occurring after temporary occlusion of the circulation (Fig. 12.1):

> In my experiments which primarily involve the lower extremities, I proceeded by first holding the extremity up for a while then lace the thigh with a strong rubber elastic bandage as high as possible for 5 minutes. The extremity becomes completely pale and stands out clearly in color in contrast to the other extremity. If the bandage is loosened after 5 minutes, the hyperemia promptly appears if the circulation is sufficient even in cases of underlying

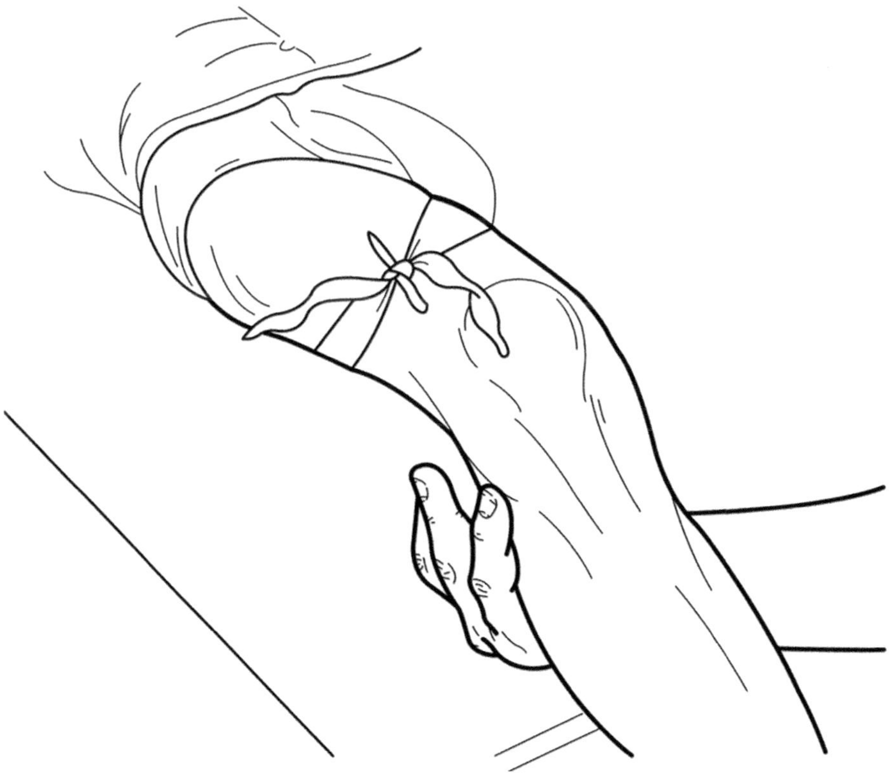

Fig. 12.1 Moszkowicz sign (by Ryan Yale)

> arteriosclerosis. This is quite different in persons in whom paraesthesias, temporary cyanosis, or even more severe symptoms such as intermittent claudication, gangrene, or disturbances of circulation indicate severe occlusion of the arteries. The hyperemia in these cases is weaker and takes longer before it spreads over the extremity. The redness spreads downward progressing slowly and hesitantly, scarcely noticing a change in color before it finally reaches the tips of the toes. Often one sees a single mottled island persisting for a particularly long time due to ischemia. In other cases the skin at times appears marbled, illustrating that it contains a certain number of capillaries supplied by a small artery. Sometimes the hyperemia is seen as normal, spreading out at lightning speed, then falters or progresses slowly. On one side it may already reach down the leg, while on the other side the limb is still quite pale. Precise observation gives a very clear picture of the circulatory conditions of the limb which is particularly blatant when, as in gangrenous pedis, an entire vascular area is usually completely occluded and the hyperemia just stops below the knee or lower leg. One cannot help feel that one can directly see where and in which artery the occlusion is located [14, p. 219–220].

He postulated that the hyperemia is caused by small vessels and capillaries and when present suggests that an adequate blood flow is being supplied to the tissues [14]. He believed that this test was a useful method to diagnose atherosclerosis and other vascular diseases, to distinguish vascular diseases from other painful conditions of the lower extremity, and to determine the site of arterial occlusion on the leg [14]. This sign is presumably best detected in patients with severe PAD and thus lacks sufficient sensitivity to be used as a screening test (Table 12.1). We are unaware of any study, which evaluated the sensitivity or specificity of this sign.

Buerger Sign

Leo Buerger (1879–1943) was born in Vienna and received his medical degree from the College of Physicians and Surgeons (Columbia University) in 1901 [15–18]. He completed a 1-year internship at Lenox Hill Hospital, New York, and another year as an assistant pathologist at Mount Sinai Hospital [19, 20]. Over the next 3 years, he was a surgical intern at Lenox Hill Hospital [20]. From 1905 to 1906, he was a volunteer surgical assistant at the Breslau Surgical Clinic, Poland [15, 16, 18–20]. He returned to the United States and at Mount Sinai served in various roles beginning in 1907 including an assistant surgical pathologist, assistant adjunct surgeon, eventually earning the rank of associate surgeon [15, 19]. He was appointed professor of urologic surgery at New York Polyclinic in 1917, professor of urology at the College of Medical Evangelists (currently Loma Linda University) in 1930 [15, 16, 18, 19], and in New York as a surgeon in private practice in 1934, where he was on staff at Beth David, Bronx, Israel Zion, and Wyckoff Heights Hospitals [15, 19]. Buerger using the single sheath cystoscope designed by Frederic Tilden Brown (1853–1910) in 1899 further improved its performance by creating an outer sheath which now allowed for the passage of other instruments during the procedure. This instrument latter became known as the Brown-Buerger cystoscope [21]. As a description of his character as described by George W. Kaplan:

> It is difficult to learn much of Dr. Buerger's personal life although those who knew him described him as "a genius, brilliant, difficult." It was known that he was disliked by many largely because of his egotism. (…) In 1932 Dr. William J. Mayo wrote of Dr. Buerger, "a man who has done as much as he has for his profession becomes an historical figure in medicine and I think this is true throughout this country and Europe." [20, p. 343].

His name is perhaps best recognized in association with the vascular obliteration of small to medium-sized arteries and veins of the lower extremity in a process referred to as obliterating thromboangiitis [22]. Buerger described an early method for detecting thromboangiitis obliterans and other causes of organic vascular disease prior to the appearance of rubor or erythromelalgia by:

> [i]nduced rubor that manifests itself in the pendent position of the foot after the limb has been previously elevated to the vertical. It is a physiological phenomenon that ischemia or blanching of a limb artificially produced, by an Esmarch or Martin bandage, will be followed by sudden dilation of the capillaries of the peripheral parts when the circulation is allowed to return. Elevating the leg 60 to 90 degrees above the horizontal without the use of any artificial means also causes blanching in the leg whose larger arteries are occluded. When such a blanched limb is then depressed to the pendent position, a similar induced or reactionary rubor becomes manifest. This well-known manifestation may be invoked in the examination of cases for whom impaired circulation due to arterial occlusion is suspected [23, p. 324].

This remains an easily performed bedside test in patients with severe peripheral vascular occlusive disease (Table 12.1). Being confined to patients with severe disease, it lacks sufficient sensitivity to be used as a screening test.

Adson Sign or Adson-Coffey Syndrome

Alfred Washington Adson (1887–1951) was born in Terrill, Iowa, and received his medical degree from the University of Pennsylvania in 1914 [24]. He was a surgical fellow at the Mayo Foundation from 1914 to 1917 (in 1915 named the Mayo Graduate School of Medicine), and joined the staff as a junior general surgeon at the Mayo Clinic, Rochester Minnesota, in 1918 [25–29]. He also received a master of arts degree from the University of Nebraska and master of science from the Mayo Foundation Graduate School, University of Minnesota in 1918. At the Mayo Clinic, he developed the section of neurosurgery in 1919, serving as professor and as first chief from 1921 to 1946 [26–31].

He received doctor of science honorary degrees from the University of Nebraska and St. Olaf College in 1948 [29, 32]. Among his other accomplishments, he was appointed to the Minnesota State Board of Medical Examiners as both president and member of the board in 1929. He was founding member of the American Board of Surgery, American Board of Psychiatry and Neurology, and later the American Board of Neurological Surgery [27, 29, 33]. Adson was the president of the American Society of Neurological Surgeons from 1932 to 1933 [31]. He served on the councils of the Minnesota State Medical Association (President in 1937) and the American

Medical Association (member of the Council on Medical Services and Public Relations) from 1943 to 1951 [27, 29]. He contributed extensively to the field of neurosurgery with particular interest in sympathectomy for the treatment of hypertension and vascular diseases including Raynaud's and thromboangiitis obliterans. Other significant contributions were in the areas of trigeminal neuralgia, cerebrospinal rhinorrhea, and the sign that bears his name [33]. He is also credited for developing surgical instruments (e.g., dissecting forceps, illuminated brain retractor) [26, 27]. As a description of his character:

> Of all the honors that came to him, he appreciated and valued most the final honor conferred to him by the former fellows in neurosurgery just two months before his untimely death. The convening of these younger men brought to him forcibly how much he meant to the entire specialty of neurosurgery and especially to them [27, p. 123]. (…) Ad was home with the young, the old, the famous, and the infamous (…) as well as with men of modest backgrounds and sills. None of the pioneers was quite like Adson, and this was good for all of us [33, p. 54].

Adson and Jay R. Coffey recognized the anatomical relationship between the attachments of the lateral border of the scalenus anticus muscles tendon and either a ligamentous band or completely formed cervical rib to the first rib in causing compressive vasculopathy and secondary neurologic symptoms of the upper extremity on the affected side. Neurologic symptoms caused by compression of the brachial plexus include one or more of the following: tingling, burning, and numbness associated with altered sensation of hyperesthesia and paresthesia located on the medial side of the arm extending to the fingers. Venous involvement resulting from compression of the subclavian vein causes a dusky hue appearance of the arm, hand, fingers, and edema, while compression of the subclavian artery causes a diminished radial pulse and/or atrophy of the upper extremity. Disease severity is proportionate to the degree of occlusion by compression and inversely proportional to the distance between the lateral border of the scalenus anticus tendinous attachment to the first rib and the angle of the cervical rib [34].

Adson and Coffey described a bedside method for reproducing symptoms by further decreasing the width of the space between the lateral border of the scalenus anticus muscle and cervical rib (Table 12.1, Fig. 12.2):

> Diminution in volume of the radial pulse is common; the pulse can be decreased or obliterated by having the patient elevate the chin or rotate the head to the affected side while inspiring air. These symptoms vary in degree, according to the amount of pressure over the subclavian artery [34, p. 845]. (…) [t]his produces paraesthesia over the distribution of the brachial plexus, and frequently, obliteration of the pulse at the wrist on the affected side [34, p. 852].

Other variations in the test include turning the head to the opposite side or performing the Valsalva maneuver when hyperextending the neck [35]. Thus, Adson and Coffey recognized the role of the scalenus anticus muscle and cervical rib in causing symptoms through compression of the subclavian artery, subclavian vein, and brachial plexus (inferior and middle trunks), a condition included as part of a group of disorders that is collectively referred to as thoracic outlet syndrome (Table 12.2) [30, 34, 36]. The test or sign lacks sufficient sensitivity and specificity as it may be found in asymptomatic people [35, 37].

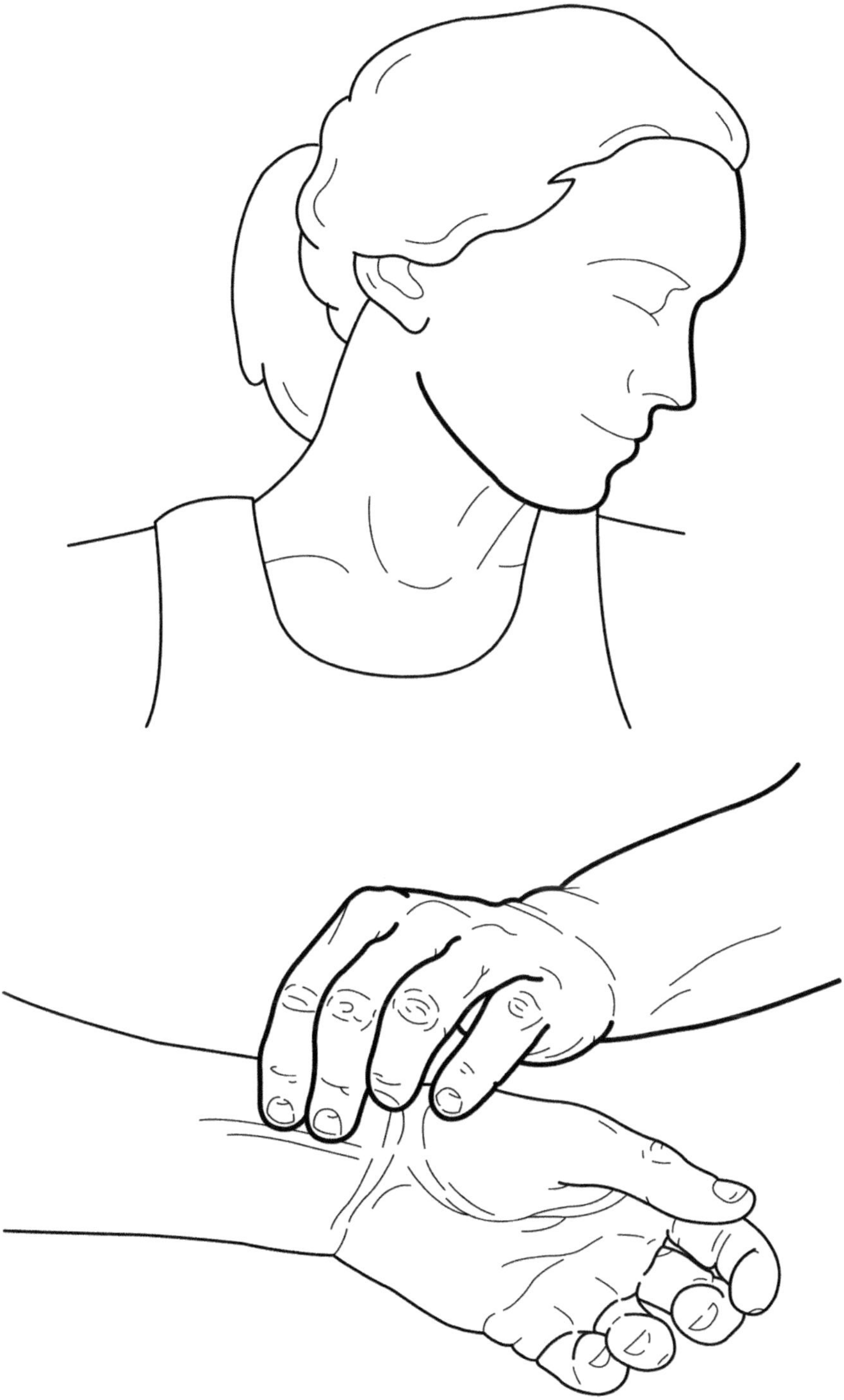

Fig. 12.2 Adson sign (by Ryan Yale)

Table 12.2 Differential diagnosis of thoracic outlet syndrome

Arterial
  Embolism
  Aneurysm

Autoimmune
  Buerger disease
  Cold agglutin disease
  Dermatomyositis
  Mixed connective tissue disorders
  Polyarthritis nodosa
  Polymyositis
  Raynaud disease
  Rheumatoid arthritis
  Scleroderma
  Systemic lupus erythematosus
  Takayasu disease

Compression
  Carpal tunnel syndrome
  Cubital tunnel syndrome
  Adenopathy
  Aneurysm

Lymphatic   Lymphedema
Movement disorder   Cervical dystonia

Musculoskeletal
  Rotator cuff tendinitis
  Cervical spine strain
  Cervical arthritis
  Acromioclavicular joint disorder

Metabolic   Myxedema

Pain syndrome
  Fibromyalgia
  Complex regional pain syndrome

Psychiatric   Psychogenic

Thrombotic
  Acute axillosubclavian thrombosis
  Catheter or pacemaker wire
  Parsonage-Turner syndrome
  Primary and secondary thrombotic disorders

Trauma
  Brachial plexus
  Local repetitive

Tumor
  Pancoast syndrome
  Nerve sheath

Venous
  Postphlebitic syndrome
  Klippel-Trenaunay syndrome
  Central venous stenosis
  AV dialysis fistulas

Samuels Sign

Saul Simon Samuels (1895–1961) was born in Brooklyn, New York, received his medical degree from Columbia University, New York, in 1920, and completed an internship at Mount Sinai Hospital from 1920 to 1923 [38]. In addition to serving as a private practitioner of vascular surgery in New York City, he also was appointed clinical assistant surgeon from 1925 to 1930 followed by a position as chief of the Department of Peripheral Arterial Disease at Mount Sinai Hospital [38]. From 1933 to 1943 he was adjunct vascular surgeon at Bellevue Hospital, NY. His other appointments in New York City included: angiologist at Manhattan General Hospital in 1935, consulting vascular surgeon, Long Beach Memorial Hospital in 1939, attending angiologist at Brooklyn Hebrew Home and Hospital for the Aged in 1940, attending vascular surgeon at the Italian Hospital in 1957, and chief of the Department of Angiology at Stuyvesant Polyclinic and Swedish Hospital in 1958 [38].

At the time of the publication of his book, *Management of Peripheral Arterial Disease* in 1951, he was chief of the Department of Arterial Disease at Stuyvesant Polyclinic Hospital, New York [39]. He was credited for coining the term "angiology" from the Greek "science of the blood vessels" [40]. He also published the books, *The Diagnosis and Treatment of Diseases of the Peripheral Arteries* in 1936 *and Peripheral Vascular Diseases (Angiology)* in 1940, *Management of Peripheral Arterial Diseases* in 1946, and *Diagnosis and Treatment of Peripheral Vascular Disorders* in 1956 [38, 41].

He was founder and editor-in-chief of the journal *Angiology* in 1950 and founding member and first president of the Angiology Research Foundation in New York City in 1954 [38]. He was a recipient of the Lucien Howe Prize and medal for a work on the treatment of peripheral vascular disease. He was a fellow of American Geriatric Society, Academy of Sciences, and Academy of Medicine in New York and a member and honorary member of other societies [38].

Samuels described a method for the early detection of peripheral vascular occlusive disease of the lower extremities (Table 12.1, Fig. 12.3):

> [t]he patient is placed in the reclining position, preferably on a low bed or couch. He is then instructed to elevate both legs to an angle of 90 degrees and while maintaining this position to carry out a fairly rapid motion of flexion and extension of both feet, using the ankle joints as pivots. Three factors are thus employed to produce ischemia; namely, gravity, obstructed arteries, and the squeezing action of the leg and foot muscles involved in the foot motion. Another essential factor in this test is careful observation, in a good light of the plantar surface of both feet as the motion is taking place. If there is unilateral arterial disease, a striking change is soon noted in the appearance of the sole of the affected limb. The normal pink tint of the skin gradually fades into a cadaveric pallor, which remains as long as the feet are held vertical, even after the motion has ceased. The healthy foot retains its natural pink tinge in spite of prolonged ankle motion [42, p. 1572].

He emphasized that attention during the test should be directed toward the plantar surface of the feet. This is an easily performed bedside maneuver used to elicit ischemia in patients with PAD. We are unaware of any study that evaluated the sensitivity or specificity of this sign.

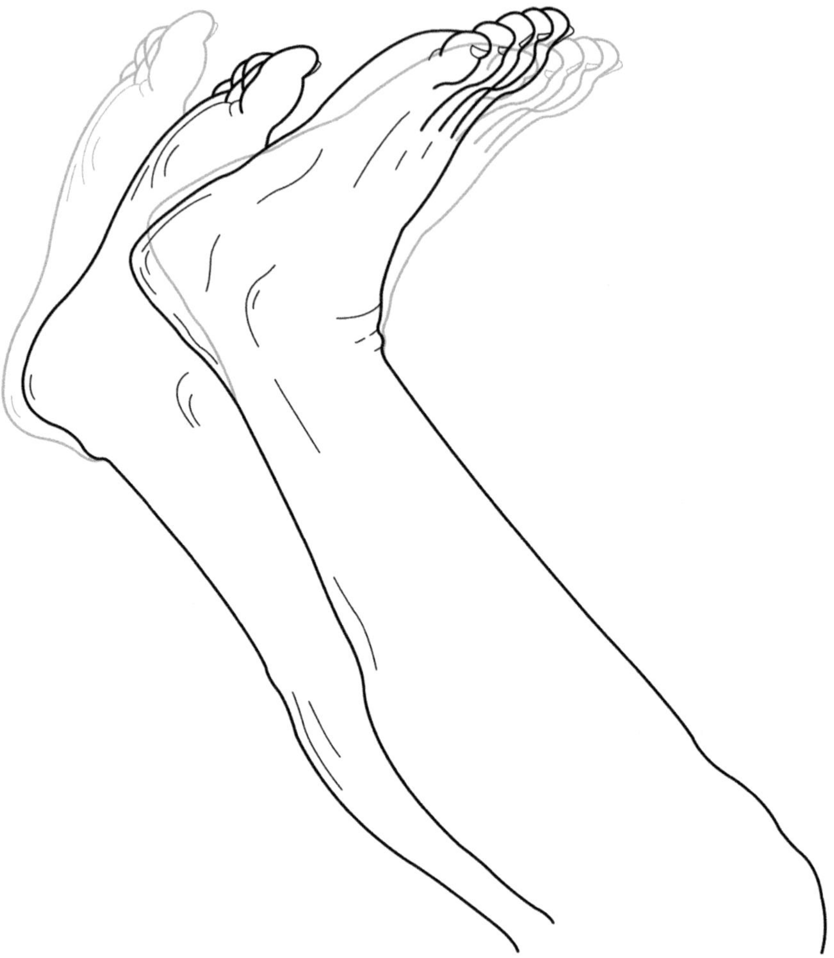

Fig. 12.3 Samuels sign (by Ryan Yale)

Fuchsig Sign

Paul Fuchsig (1908–1977) was born in Schärding, Austria, and received his medical training at the Universities of Kiel, Vienna, and Innsbruck, graduating from the latter in 1931 [43]. He led the first Surgical University Clinic, General Hospital in Vienna from 1932 to 1956, was head of the surgical department at Kaiserin (Empress) Elisabeth Hospital in Vienna from 1957 to 1961, and was appointed professor and chair of the first Surgical Clinic in Vienna in 1961 [43, 44]. Fuchsig identified the following finding (Table 12.1, Fig. 12.4):

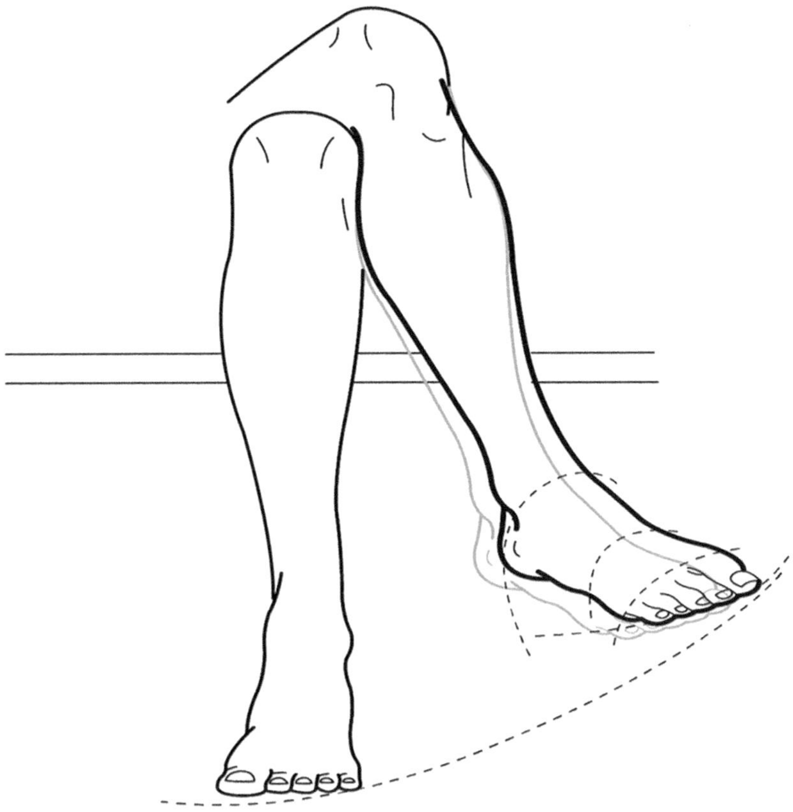

Fig. 12.4 Fuchsig sign (by Ryan Yale)

> If one observes people sitting in the first row of a concert or lecture hall and their legs are crossed, it is generally seen that the foot of the dependent lower extremity moves rhythmically up and down with short but distinct excursions. If one follows the phenomenon it turns out that this oscillation occurs synchronously with the pulse, and is absent only when perfusion to the affected extremity is disturbed. Preliminary clinical experience of such a connection led me for the first time in 1953 to point out that pulse-synchronized foot pendulum was a useful symptom necessitating a focused assessment of the peripheral perfusion [45, p. 936].

To assess whether adequate blood flow is present in the lower extremity, the patient is examined in a sitting or lying position:

> The results are the same in both positions provided that one eliminates a few sources of errors in the case of the patient or the examiner. The patient has to keep the examined leg completely relaxed over the other. In our experience, this relaxation is achieved to a sufficient degree by a distracting conversation with the patient, by counting numbers, or in all circumstances by requiring the patient to tightly grasp the fingers. The examiner, in order to

> avoid seeing an illusion, fixates on an object lying in the direction of sight. This allows him to better perceive any rhythmic movements of the tips of the toes. He simultaneously feels the pulse of the patient's radial artery [45, p. 936].

Fuchsig concluded that pulsesynchronous foot oscillation requires patent blood flow in the popliteal artery, its divisions in the lower leg, or the presence of adequate collateral circulation in the case of an occluded popliteal artery [45]. He recognized that diseases leading to a reduction in muscle tone may cause a false-negative test whereas conditions that cause obstruction of blood flow distal to the popliteal fossa may lead to a false-positive test [45]. Hence, the sign lacks sufficient sensitivity or specificity in diagnosis.

DeWeese Sign

James A. DeWeese, Sr. (1925–2013) was born in Kent, Ohio, and received his medical degree from the University of Rochester School of Medicine and Dentistry. He joined the department of surgery after completing his training in 1956 [46]. At the University of Rochester School of Medicine, he was responsible for establishing the vascular surgery residency program in 1960 and the vascular surgery fellowship in 1984 [46]. He served as a professor of surgery, first chair of cardiothoracic surgery (1975–1991), chief of vascular surgery at the University of Rochester (1987–1991), and adjunct clinical professor of surgery at the Uniformed Services University of Health Sciences in Bethesda, Maryland [46, 47]. In collaboration with James T. Adams (1930–2013), he designed the Adams-DeWeese clip, a plastic clamp affixed to the inferior vena cava that partially interrupted venous blood flow for the prevention of pulmonary emboli [46–49]. His other major area of cardiovascular research involved whole body hypothermia and myocardial preservation [47].

He served as the president of numerous national and international surgical societies including the Society for Vascular Surgery, American Venous Forum, North American Chapter of the International Cardiovascular Society, and Pan Pacific Surgical Society [46, 47]. He was a member of the National Board of the American Heart Association, American Board of Surgery, and Thoracic Board of Surgery. He served on four editorial boards as well as several advisory committees including the advisory council on cardiothoracic and vascular surgery for the American College of Surgeons and committee to the New York State Department of Health [47]. He is the recipient of a number of accolades and distinguished honorary awards from the American Heart Association and Society of Vascular Surgery, the Eastern Vascular Society Lifetime Achievement Award, and the Roswell Park Medal [47, 50]. He was also an honorary member of several national and international societies including the University of Michigan Coller Surgical Society, the Dallas Texas Jesse Thomas Vascular Society, Brazilian Society of Angiology, and the Royal Australian College of Surgeons [50].

A description of his character as described by Jeffrey H. Peters, MD, "He had a remarkable legacy here at the University of Rochester, both in clinical care and education of tomorrow's physicians. He was a wonderful man, doctor and mentor and it is a significant loss for the institution" [47]. (…) Another tribute written about his life: "He was loved and respected by his children and grandchildren for the life lesson they learned from him, and the fun family gatherings each year on Canandaigua Lake. He was so proud of each of them. He will be dearly missed [50]."

DeWeese described the disappearance of the pedal pulse with exercise in 13 patients, with suspected (11 angiographically confirmed) cases of peripheral obstructive atherosclerotic disease, as a method for screening patients with symptoms of intermittent claudication (Table 12.1). He found that "the pedal pulses disappeared when these patients ran in place until claudication developed, whereas the amplitude of the pedal pulses did not decrease in normal extremities" [51, p. 1217]. He recommended that patients with symptoms compatible with intermittent claudication, despite a palpable pulse at rest, undergo assessment by exercise testing in order to exclude the diagnosis of obstructive atherosclerotic disease [50]. DeWeese believed that the decreased pulse found in larger arteries is caused by the shunting of blood to the smaller vasodilated arteries during exercise [51]. The sign remains clinically useful today as a method of screening for peripheral vascular occlusive disease, although this type of evaluation is now routinely performed as part of the noninvasive vascular assessment using ankle-brachial indices with rest and exercise and disease localization based on continuous-wave Doppler waveforms and segmental blood pressures.

Conclusion

Signs of PAD are based on physiological principles that lead to a further reduction in blood flow to arteries already severely occluded. These signs were elicited through exercise, elevation, or compressing the blood supply to a limb through maneuvers or the application and release of a ligature. The accuracy of these signs in clinical practice for the most part has not been well studied although they are more commonly found in patients with severe disease. Knowledge of these signs during the formidable years of training provides broader insights and deeper appreciation for the pathophysiology of disease. The majority of these signs are easily performed bedside tests that further heighten suspicion for the presence of peripheral vascular occlusive disease and remain clinically applicable.

References

1. Skinner HA. The Origin of Medical Terms. Baltimore: The William & Wilkins Company; 1949.
2. Charcot JM. Sur la claudication intermittente observée dans un cas d'oblitération complète de l'une des artères iliaques primitives. Compte-rendu Soc Biol. 1858;10:225–38.

3. [No author]. Deaths of great men in the medical profession during 1890. St. Louis Clinique. 1891;4:138.
4. Election, Eduard von. Biographical dictionary of excellent doctors. Zeno.org Meine Bibliothek. http://www.zeno.org/nid/2000803477X. Accessed 3 May 2019.
5. von Wahl EG. Wikiwand. http://www.wikiwand.com/de/Eduard_Georg_von_Wahl. Accessed 3 Apr 2019.
6. [No author]. Obituary for 1800, Russia. Br Med J. 1890;2:1508.
7. National Archives of Estonia. Eduard Georg von Wahl. Flickr. Rahvusarhiv. 2019. https://www.flickr.com/photos/national_archives_of_estonia/15028731089. Accessed 3 May 2019.
8. Wahl E. Ueber die auscultatorischen Erscheinungen bei Gefässverletzungen und sogenannten traumatischen Aneurysmen. Deutsche Ztschr f Chir. 1885;21:118–38.
9. White FA. Physical Signs in Medicine and Surgery: An Atlas of Rare, Lost and Forgotten Physical Signs. Philadelphia: Museum Press Books; 2009.
10. Shackford SR. Extremity vascular injuries. In: Harken A, Moore E, editors. Abernathy's Surgical Secrets. 7th ed. Philadelphia: Elsevier; 2018. p. 148–53.
11. Moszkowicz L. Wikipedia Wolna encyclopedia. https://pl.wikipedia.org/wiki/Ludwig_Moszkowicz. Accessed 5 May 2019.
12. Moszkowicz L. Gedenkbuch für die Opfer des Nationalsozialismus an der Universität Wien 1938. University of Vienna 2009. https://gedenkbuch.univie.ac.at/index.php?id=435&no_cache=1&person_single_id=34437&person_name=moszkowicz&person_geburtstag_tag=not_selected&person_geburtstag_monat=not_selected&person_geburtstag_jahr=not_selected&person_fakultaet=not_selected&person_kategorie=not_selected&person_volltextsuche=&search_person.x=1&result_page=1. Accessed 19 May 2019.
13. Bauer-Merlinsky J. Ludwig Moszkowicz (1873–1945). In: Die Auswirkungen der Annexion Österreichs durch das Deutsche Reich auf die Medizinische Fakultät im Jahre 1938. Wien: Universität Wien; 1980. p. 160–1.
14. Moszkowicz L. Die Diagnose des Arterienverschlusses bei Gangraena pedis. Mitteilg Grenzgebiete Med Chir. 1907;17:216–28.
15. Luft FC. Leo Buerger (1879–1943) revisited. Am J Med Sci. 2009;137:287.
16. Ellis H, Caine Sir R, Watson C. Leo Buerger (1879–1943). In: Lecture Notes - General Surgery. 13th ed. Oxford: Wiley Blackwell; 2016. p. 422.
17. van Krieken J, editor. Encyclopedia of Pathology. Cham: Springer; 2016.
18. Ellis H. Leo Buerger: Buerger's disease. J Perioper Pract. 2013;23:174–5.
19. Birch CA. Buerger's disease: Leo Buerger (1879–1943). Practitioner. 1973;211:823–4.
20. Kaplan GW. Leo Buerger (1879–1973). Investig Urol. 1974;11:342–3.
21. Brown-Buerger Cystoscope. The British Association of Urological Surgeons Limited. 2019. https://www.baus.org.uk/museum/114/brownbuerger_cystoscope. Accessed 5 May 2019.
22. Buerger L. Thromboangitis obliterans: a study of the vascular lesions leading to presenile spontaneous gangrene. Am J Med Sci. 1908;136:567–80.
23. Buerger L. The pathological and clinical aspects of thromboangitis obliterans. Am J Med Sci. 1917;153:319–28.
24. Sebastian A. A Dictionary of the History of Medicine. London: Informa Healthcare; 2011.
25. [No author]. The general faculty: medical fellows on the Mayo Foundation. Bulletin of the University of Minnesota Annual Register (1916–1917). 1918;20(61):59.
26. Pioneers. Alfred W. Adson 1887-1951. History of surgery and anaesthesia. An ODP' perspective. Ken True. 2001. http://www.historyofsurgery.co.uk/history/html/hp044.html. Accessed 22 Feb 2019.
27. Craig W. Alfred Washington Adson: pioneer neurosurgeon (1887–1951). J Neurosurg. 1952;9:117–23.
28. Adson AW. The Society of Neurological Surgeons. The Society of Neurological Surgeons. 2008–2014. https://www.societyns.org/society/bio.aspx?MemberID=7501. Accessed 3 May 2019.
29. Craig WM. Alfred Washington Adson, 1887–1951. Trans Meet Am Surg Assoc. 1952;70:424–6.

30. Mostofi SB. Alfred Washington Adson, 1887–1951. In: Who's Who in Orthopedics. London: Springer; 2005. p. 1–2.
31. Nelson CW. 75th anniversary of neurosurgery at Mayo. Mayo Clin Proc. 1994;69:612.
32. University of Nebraska Honorary Degrees 1872–2018. 2018. https://www.nebraska.edu/docs/awards/docs/HonoraryDegreesAlpha.pdf. Accessed 3 May 2019.
33. MacCarty CS. Alfred Washington Adson (1887–1951). Surg Neurol. 1977;7:53–4.
34. Adson AW, Coffey JR. Cervical rib: a method of anterior approach for relief of symptoms by division of the scalenus anticus. Ann Surg. 1927;85:839–57.
35. Pryse-Phillips W. Companion to Clinical Neurology. 3rd ed. New York: Oxford University Press; 2009.
36. Illig KA, Thompson RW, Freischlag JA, Donahue DM, Jordan SE, Edgelow PI, editors. Thoracic Outlet Syndrome. London: Springer; 2013.
37. Firkin BG, Whitworth JA. Alfred W. Adson. In: Dictionary of Medical Eponyms. Boca Raton: The Parthenon Publishing Group; 2002. p. 4.
38. White JT. Samuels, Saul Simon. In: The National Cyclopaedia of American Biography, vol. 28. New York: James T. White & Company; 1965. p. 21–2.
39. Samuels SS. Management of Peripheral Arterial Diseases. New York: Oxford University Press; 1951.
40. 59th Annual World Congress International College of Angiology in cooperation with Vascular International Austrian Interventional Cardiology "New Horizons in Cardiovascular Medicine". 2017. https://www.maw.co.at/kongress/dokumente/ICA17_final_program.pdf. Accessed 12 Mar 2019.
41. Samuels SS. The Diagnosis and Treatment of Diseases of the Peripheral Arteries. New York: Oxford University Press; 1936.
42. Samuels SS. The early diagnosis of thrombo-angitis obliterans: a new diagnostic sign. JAMA. 1929;92:1571–2.
43. Paul Fuchsig Wien Geschichte Wiki. DYN Krabina 2014. https://www.geschichtewiki.wien.gv.at/Paul_Fuchsig. Accessed 15 May 2019.
44. Keminger K. Professor Dr. Paul Fuchsig zum 65. Geburtstag. Wien med Wochenschr. 1973;123:125–6.
45. Fuchsig P, Ender R. Das pulssynchrone Fußpendeln, ein Symptom zur Beurteilung der peripheren Durchblutung. Wien med Wochenschr. 1957;107:936–8.
46. Through these portals. A History of the Department of Surgery University of Rochester. 2006. https://www.urmc.rochester.edu/medialibraries/urmcmedia/surgery/documents/surgery-history-sm.pdf. Accessed 20 Mar 2019.
47. URMC's James A. DeWeese, M.D., Helped shape cardiovascular surgery. University of Rochester Medical Center. Monday, November 18, 2013. University of Rochester Medical Center Rochester NY. 2019. https://www.urmc.rochester.edu/news/story/3970/urmcs-james-a.-deweese-m.d.-helped-shape-cardiovascular-surgery.aspx. Accessed 2 May 2019.
48. Adams JT, DeWeese JA. Partial interruption of the inferior vena cava with a new plastic clip. Surg Gynecol Obstet. 1966;123:1087–8.
49. Adams JT, DeWeese JA. Experimental and clinical evaluation of partial vein interruption in prevention of pulmonary emboli. Surgery. 1965;57:82–102.
50. Dr. James A. DeWeese. Published in Rochester Democrat and Chronicle. Nov 15 to Nov 17, 2013. Legacy.com. 2019. https://obits.democratandchronicle.com/obituaries/democratand-chronicle/obituary.aspx?n=james-a-deweese&pid=167999785&fhid=13366. Accessed 2 Mar 2019.
51. DeWeese JA. Pedal pulse disappearing with exercise: a test for intermittent claudication. N Engl J Med. 1960;262:1214–7.

Chapter 13
Pulse

Introduction

Examination of the arterial pulse during the physical examination involves the bedside techniques of observation, palpation and auscultation. Observation involves looking for a visible pulsation and through palpation the waveform (contour) which may be diminished, increased in intensity, or be double peaked, and force (strength) of the pulse is felt. Additionally, by palpation, the frequency and regularity or irregularity of the pulse are felt, and along with auscultation, the presence of a thrill of the arterial pulse is felt or heard. Auscultation is also useful in detecting a murmur.

The pulse is usually detected on arteries which are superficial and more easily accessible – carotid, brachial, radial, femoral, popliteal, dorsalis pedis, and posterior tibial. The brachial artery is best used and palpated applying the examiner's thumb medial to the biceps tendon in the antecubital fossa [1]. The hand that is free from palpation of the artery is used to passively raise or lower the patient's forearm to improve identification of the point of maximal arterial pulsation [1]. The examiner counting the pulse and applying slight, gentle, progressive pressure assesses the arterial waveform. The radial, dorsalis pedis, and posterior tibial arteries are smaller arteries and, thus, the pad of the index finger rather than the thumb is better suited and more sensitive for identifying small movements [1].

Using these examination tools, physicians detected a variety of findings which later become eponymously named to honor their accomplishments. The history of the pulse has been previously discussed in chapter "Pericarditis: Physical Signs and Medial Eponyms of Palpation" on Pericarditis Palpation. Herein, we provide brief historical information of the persons who described pulse signs as originally described, and if known their use and application in clinical practice. The signs are described chronologically based on the year they were reported.

S. H. Yale et al., *Cardiovascular Eponymic Signs*,
https://doi.org/10.1007/978-3-030-67596-7_13

Signs

Hering Sign

Karl Ewald Konstantin (KEK) Hering (1834–1918), father of Heinrich Ewald (HE) Hering (1866–1948), was born in Altgersdorf, Lausitz, Germany, and received his medical degree from the University of Leipzig in 1860, training under the zoologist Julius Victor Carus (1823–1903), and physiologists Ernst Heinrich Weber (1795–1878) and Gustav Theodor Fechner (1801–1887) [2, 3]. After graduation, he was a general practitioner and assistant at the Polyclinic Institute under the aegis of Ernst Leberecht Wagner (1829–1888), professor extraordinary of general pathology anatomy from 1862 to 1865 [3, 4]. In 1862, he habilitated as a private lecturer in Leipzig under the ophthalmologists Theodor Coccius (1824–1897) and Karl Stellwag von Carlon (1823–1904) and in 1865 was appointed chair of physiology and medical physics at the Josephinum (medico-surgical military academy) in Vienna, succeeding the physician and physiologist Carl Ludwig (1816–1895) who accepted an appointment as chair at the University of Leipzig [2, 3, 5]. From 1870 to 1895, he served as chair at the University of Prague, succeeding Jan Evangelista Purkyně (1787–1869) maintaining the bilingual (German-Czech) university culture [3]. In 1895, he once again succeeded Carl Ludwig as chair but now at the University of Leipzig [3].

His other contributions to science include the theory of color vision, visual space perception and binocular vision, memory, the reflex control regulating the volume of the lungs during breathing with Josef Breuer (1842–1924) in 1866 (Hering–Breuer reflex), the control of heart rate through breathing in 1871 (Hering–Lommel sign), and confirmed in 1869 Ludwig Traube's (1818–1876) work published in 1865 on rhythmic variation of blood pressure related to variation in vasomotor tone (Traube–Hering waves) [3, 5–7].

He received doctorates of honorary degrees from the Universities of Göttingen and Prague, von Graefe Medal in 1906, Civil Class of Order (Order of Merit for Sciences and Arts) in 1911, and was a member and honorary member of the Academy of Sciences in 1869 and 1895, respectively [8, 9]. As a description of his character F.B. Hoffman of Marburg wrote:

> It was also not so much a question of representing the laboratory work of the physiologist, who was outstanding in his individual research. It was much more important for me to give at least a brief mention of his thoughts, albeit general, in order to avoid making a somewhat faded impression of one of the deepest and most mature thinkers in our science detached from the rich detailed accomplishments already uniformly summarized. His sharp, critical, yet creative spirit, understood the inner context of things (incidentally, also in his disposition and in his political opinion), is similar to another pastor's son from Lusatia, G.E. Lessing. Just as Lessing rose from critical preoccupation with the day's questions of his time to an ever higher and freer perspective, so Hering (to use his own words) gained his way to the heights of science at the laboratory from which a comprehensive and uninhibited view of his narrow yet unique research was possible. The generosity and breadth of his perspective also partly explains the attraction that his personality exerted on everyone who approached him. Despite all the simple modesty of his nature, everyone had the sense of a

> man whose direction of thought was far from the ordinary. Ewald Hering like his friend E. Mach the first physicochemist, is one of those scouts of science who was looking for their own ways, often challenged and misunderstood by their contemporaries and whose actual purpose is only fully appreciated at a later time [3, p. 541].

Karl Ewald Konstantin Hering observed in his study on dogs that (Table 13.1):

> [h]eart rate increases as long as the lungs remain expanded, but returns to a slower rhythm as soon as the lungs are deflated. This acceleration of the heart rate is generally more obvious the lower the heart rate prior to inflation. It sometimes happens that as the lungs become more inflated the heart rate increases more than threefold [7, p. 335]. (...) Conversely, the heart rate immediately slowed down as soon as inhaled air is expelled from the lungs [7, p. 338].

He proposed a pathogenesis for the findings:

> The increased pulse rate takes place in our experiments when both or at least one vagus nerve is intact. This new and important finding of acceleration of the pulse is not due to direct cardiac irritation, pressure, strain or altered blood circulating in the heart. Furthermore, it is known that the central nervous system participates in this acceleration whose coordination is conceivable in two ways. First, respiration may change the blood flow altering the nerves of the heart located in the medulla oblongata, an assumption we have already proved above to be inadmissible. Thus, there remains only the second possibility, namely that inflation of the lungs causes the cardiac nerves within the central nervous system to be changed by peripheral nerve stimulation and thus acceleration of the heart rate occurs reflexively. What afferent and efferent nerve-fibers are involved here in the conduction of the impulses caused by pulmonary inflation? Acceleration of the heart rate occurs in our experiment because stimulation of the inhibitory nerves to the heart located within the central nervous system is diminished due to irritation of the sensory nerve fibers of the lung. Thus, the tone of the inhibitory fibers is to some extent suppressed. The sensory fibers, which could be excited by the inflation of the lungs are first and foremost those of the lungs, chest-wall, and the diaphragm and finally those of the heart and its immediate surroundings [7, p. 348].

Thus, the Hering sign or reflex is the phenomenon of acceleration of heart rate occurring during inspiration and its slow return during expiration.

Faget Sign

Jean Charles Faget (1818–1884) was born in New Orleans, Louisiana, and received his medical degree and awarded magna cum laude from the School of Medicine in Paris in 1844 with the graduation thesis entitled *Quelques faits anatomiques en faveur de la cystotomie sus-pubienne chez les très jeunes enfants* (Some anatomical facts in favor of suprapubic cystotomy in very young children) [10]. After graduation, he returned to New Orleans to begin medical practice from 1845 to 1865. He served on the New Orleans Sanitary Commission and was a member of the Louisiana Board of Health [11]. He was also a member of the Société Médicale de la Nouvelle-Orléans (elite circle of Paris physicians in New Orleans) promoting his theory on the spread of infectious disease, Société Médicale d'Observation (Society for Medical Observation), Société Anatomique de Paris (Anatomical Society of Paris),

Table 13.1 Pulse sign medical eponyms (1871–1923)

Name	Year	Description of sign
Hering, KEK [7]	1871	Pulse increase with inspiration and decreases with expiration.
Faget [15]	1875	Divergence between the pulse and the temperature–pulse that falls as the temperature rises.
Nicoladoni [26]	1875	Decreased pulse occurring upon digital compression proximal to an arterial-venous fistula.
Israel [30]	1877	Decreased pulse occurring upon digital compression proximal to an arterial-venous fistula.
Schapiro [40]	1881	Decreased blood pressure and increased pulse when standing.
Jorissenne [47]	1882	In early pregnancy, the pulse remains constant with postural changes.
Branham [34]	1890	Decreased pulse occurring upon digital compression proximal to an arterial-venous fistula.
Lommel [51]	1902	Increased pulse during inspiration and decreased pulse during expiration.
Mannkopff [55]	1906	With an assistant feeling the pulse, pressure when applied over a traumatic area or myofascial trigger points causes an increased pulse if the patient feels pain in the affected area. After the pressure ceases and the pain caused by it subsides, the pulse rate returned to normal. The pulse rises again when pressure is reapplied. The subject should remain still and breathe regularly. Pressure applied to the area must be abrupt and short. When the acceleration is very noticeable, the method of simulation should be assessed. No conclusions can be drawn if the pulse does not increase. When the acceleration is mild, it is also inconclusive since the patient by holding his/her breath, moaning, writhing as a result of the pain – real or not – can also mildly change the heart rate.
Aschner [71]	1908	Decreased pulse rate after applying ocular pressure-oculocardiac reflex or phenomenon.
Prével [80]	1917	Pulse that increases when moving from the supine to standing position-orthostatic cardiac acceleration or the abdominal cardiac reflex.
Cantelli [81]	1917	Increased number of heartbeats and pulses occurring during bulbar compression, lasting up to several minutes after removing the stimulus.
Ruggeri [82]	1920	Ocular convergence reflex: 1. The individual is placed in a supine position on the bed, and after a few minutes, the radial pulse is counted. The test begins when the pulse, after repeated counting, remains constant. 2. While an assistant is counting the pulse, the subject is asked to carefully position the tip of the index finger 1 cm away from the nose, corresponding to the midpoint of the glabella line nasal tip. 3. While the subject continues to fixate on the tip of the index finger, and after 10–15 seconds have elapsed, the assistant is asked to count the pulse for 30 seconds.
Laubry [89]	1923	(1) Amplitude of the palpable pulse is uniform in regular atrial flutter and variable in irregular atrial flutter (2). Auscultatory findings of either a third (S_3) or fourth (S_4) heart sound heard in patients with atrial flutter.

and corresponding member of the Société Medicale de Caen (Caen Medical Society) [12]. His character was described in an obituary in the *Journal of the Louisiana State Medical Society* as follows:

> [a] man truly loved and respected by all who knew him, for he was the personification of the ideal gentleman—pure, noble, and true. He was one of the kindest and most generous benefactors of the French, and particularly the Creole population of this city, a class that he so honorably represented. He was one of the most modest of men, though the distinctions, which his learning and great professional attainments conferred upon him, would have infused a very different spirit in the minds of most men. His contributions to medicine have been recognized everywhere as being of a substantial character and lasting value [13, p. 577].

In recognition of his accomplishment in describing the clinical feature of the yellow fever epidemic of 1858, he was decorated Knight of the Légion d'honneur by the French government [10]. Faget reported the finding of decrease pulse occurring on the second day in patients with yellow fever while the temperature remains stationary or rose in his book titled *The Type and Specificity of Yellow Fever Established with the Aid of the Watch and Thermometer with Tables of Pulse and Temperature.* He wrote (Table 13.1):

> Here then is a fever in which, studied with the watch alone, we can perceive neither a period of intense, nor a stationary period; if we should form an opinion regarding it by means of the watch alone, we should it as a fever in which the pulse is always sinking, but after a great and early rise, so rapid and so short, that we are never in time to perceive it [27, p. 16–17]. (…) These reservation being made, it is admissible to perceive in this divergence in the direction of the two line of the pulse and temperature at the commencement, in the majority of the cases of yellow fever, a sign which becomes valuable in the diagnosis of the disease: in two-thirds of the tables, while the line of the pulse descends from the beginning, we see that of the temperature rise for one, two and even three days [14, p. 18–19].

In his 1875 monograph titled *Monographie sur le type et la spécificité de la fièvre jaune établis avec l'aide de la montre et du thermomètre* (Monograph on the type and specificity of yellow fever established with the aid of the watch and thermometer), Faget described what he believed to be the pathognomonic finding of the discordant relationship between the pulse and temperature in patients with yellow fever:

> Today, according to the facts accumulated since and compared, we can affirm that there is only yellow fever, among all the pyrexias, which presents with a febrile condition such that the number of arterial pulsations begins to diminish as soon as it has reached its peak and does not return to normal until after a period of seven days. Such a descending pulse duration appears, I believe, only in yellow fever; the line representing it must therefore be characteristic [15, p. 47].

Thomas Layton (1825–1882), Joseph Jones (1833–1893), and Just Charles Touatre (1838–1901) confirmed the finding of the dissociation between pulse and temperature in yellow fever [10, 16]. Touatre in his book entitled *Yellow Fever: Clinical Notes* wrote about his initial recognition, prior to Faget, of the paradoxical relationship between pulse and temperature with the introduction of the clinical thermometer (French naval centigrade):

> Upon coming to New Orleans to practice medicine in 1865, I had a clinical thermometer in my baggage. I believe that I am one of the first physicians in the United States to have utilized this precious instrument in the diagnosis of fevers. I am sure I was the first in New Orleans to have used it for the study of the march of temperature in yellow fever during the epidemics of 1866, 1867 and the following ones. Hence, I was one of the first to note this divergence between the pulse and the temperature in yellow fever; but it is Dr. Faget who, with his observations and mine, built up the magnificent law which bears his name in all justice, as it is he who first caused it to be known to the medical public by his remarkable treatise, *Monographie sur le type et la spécificité de la fièvre jaune établis avec l'aide de la montre et du thermomètre*, which is a masterpiece of originality and of science and judgment [17, p. 34].

It is of further interest that Daniel Blair in his 1852 book *Some Account of the Last Yellow Fever Epidemic of British Guiana* wrote "In some cases, when the disease determined to the intestines, the pulse became startlingly slow, even on the second day of disease" [18, p. 75]. The incidence and prevalence of this sign in other diseases varies widely which may be due to a variety of factors such as size of the population studied, case definition, when the measurements were obtained during the disease course, and unknown factors influenced by the pathogen and host. For example, prevalence of relative bradycardia in typhoid fever has been found to range from 14% to 63% [19]. In addition to yellow fever, Faget sign is found in a variety of infectious and noninfectious diseases. Thus, if present, Faget sign represents a sensitive but nonspecific clinical finding.

Nicoladoni–Israel–Branham Sign

The Nicoladoni–Israel–Branham sign is the eponymic term ascribed to three surgeons who independently described this sign. Each will be discussed in chronological order from the time when the description of this sign was originally published: Nicoladoni in 1875, Israel in 1877, and Branham in 1890.

Carl Nicoladoni (1847–1902) was born and received his doctor of medicine and surgery degree in Vienna in 1871 [20]. He practiced with Johann von Dumreicher (1815–1889), first surgeon's clinic at the Surgical University Clinic of the General Hospital in Vienna in 1872, appointed clinical assistant in 1873, habiliated in surgery in 1876, and succeeded von Dumreicher in 1880 [20]. He was appointed Chief of the General Surgical Unit and Professor of Surgery in Innsbruck, Austria in 1881, Dean from 1883 to 1884, and first clinician to be named rector of the medical faculty at the University of Innsbruck from 1887 to 1888 [20]. In his final position, Nicoladoni served as Senior Professor of Surgery in Graz, Austria, in 1895 [20, 21].

His areas of interest, research, and contribution in medicine and surgery were extensive encompassing the fields of orthopedics, plastic and reconstructive, urogenital, gastrointestinal, and neurosurgery [20]. In the field of reconstructive surgery, he brought forth the concept of tendon transplantation for treatment of hemiplegia. He successfully completed a pedicle thoracoepigastric flap as surgical treatment for an avulsed thumb in 1897 [22]. He also successfully performed pedicle transfer reconstruction from the fifth finger to thumb and second toe of the foot to replace an amputated thumb in 1898 [20, 21]. He provided detailed description on the anatomy and biomechanics of scoliosis as well as a classification and description of pes calcaneus, pes euqinus paralyticus, pes planus, and hammer toe deformities [20, 23]. He described novel surgical techniques in torsion of the spermatic cord and esophageal diverticulum, resection of an incarcerated gangrenous hernia with enterorrhaphy, and performed the first gastroenterostomy [24]. In a memorial, Erwin Payr (1871–1946) describes Nicoladoni's character as a physician:

> In his profession, he was the most conscientious doctor you can imagine, always friendly with a genuine warm and often touching compassion for the poor. Entrusted to his hand, he knew how to acquire in the shortest possible time the unconditional trust and love of his patients. He was one of those doctors who is never forgotten by his patients [25, p. v].

Nicoladoni reported the case of a 17-year-old male with an extensive network of arterial-venous malformation, vascular ectasias, and cirsoid (plexiform) aneurysms located in his right upper extremity. As described by Nicoladoni:

> The skin in the supraclavicular region showed an extensive translucent venous mesh. The whole area was accentuated rhythmically with each heartbeat. Elevation of this region was caused by prominence on the sternal and clavicular portions of the sternocleidomastoid muscle and internal jugular vein. The left supraclavicular region rose only slightly at each heartbeat. (…) A distinct vibratory sensation was felt on the finger when placed on the most dilated portion of the subclavian artery. This vibration is absent when the artery is completely compressed. It was surprising that as soon as the vibration subsided, the pulse in the subclavian was significantly reduced. There were 96 beats prior to compression and 64 beats following compression [26, p. 255].

At the brachial artery, he found:

> Pulse was 96 beats. As long as it is not compressed, little can be said about its shape and volume. Its actual shape is revealed only when the artery is compressed at various locations from an anterior to posterior direction against the bone. (…) Compression at the bicep tendon, the middle of the upper arm, and axillary fossa, caused the pulse, which remained full and strong to drop to 60 beats. Every vibration and noise above the compressed point disappeared, so that it is now possible to determine the exact location over the aorta where a dull prolonged first and short sharp-pitched second sound is heard [26, p. 256].

At the axillary artery, he reported, "When the wall of the dilated artery is stretched to the point that the sound is loudest, the sudden mechanical slowing of the pulse confirms the diagnosis." [26, p. 267]. Nicoladoni described what he believed to be the pathogenesis of the phenomenon of slowing of the pulse found by compression of the brachial artery and when applying an elastic bandage over the left lower extremity:

> I explained that the marked slowing of the pulse occurring after several heartbeats following compression of the brachial artery is due to the following: As soon as the brachial artery is compressed, a certain portion of the remaining blood still moves through the peripheral arterial system into the right ventricle. The entire system of arteries within the remainder of the body is suddenly supplied by a new source of blood resulting from the compression. These arteries thus attain at that moment a filling exceeding their ordinary state. When the compression is removed, the pulse accelerates to 96 beats [26, p. 265]. (…) Overfilling of

> the remainder of the arterial system by an intervention which involves ligating a large artery trunk should increase, as was to be expected from the outset, lateral pressure and pulse rate. However, in our patient there was a slowing of the pulse, so that only one explanation remains to account for this phenomenon. When compressing the brachial artery the vibratory sound over the subclavian and innominate arteries suddenly ceases so that the aortic sounds now can be clearly heard. Blood flow in the right arm does not drop in the ectatic subclavian artery. After compression, a few rapid heartbeats causes considerable filling in the subclavian artery and with it a large rapid increase in pressure which now fills the widths of formerly lax arterial walls to the maximum. It is believed that a sudden mechanical impulse is transmitted with every stroke of the heart to the vagus trunk slowing cardiac contractions [26, p. 266].

James Adolf Israel (1848–1926) was born in Berlin and completed his medical degree and inaugural thesis on Bright disease at the Friedrich-Wilhelm University, Berlin, in 1870 [27]. During the Franco-Prussian War, he served as a military doctor, and after the war, he continued his studies in Vienna [27]. He returned to Berlin serving as a medical assistant at the Jewish Community Hospital in 1872. He traveled to Edinburgh, Scotland, to learn the antiseptic techniques employed by Joseph Lister (1827–1912), which he incorporated into medical practice upon returning to Berlin [27]. Israel provided the first description of the bacterium genus *Actinomyces* for which the species *Actinomyces israelii* was named for his namesake in 1878 [27]. In 1880, he was appointed head of the surgical department at the university succeeding Bernhard Rudolf Konrad von Langenbeck (1810–1887) and was awarded professorship from the University of Berlin in 1894 [27].

His primary area of professional interest was in the diagnosis and surgical management of urologic and renal disease for which his expertise was sought locally and abroad [28]. Israel was a prolific writer publishing more than 170 manuscripts and books in urology including *Erfahrungen über Nierenchirurgie* (Experiences about Kidney Surgery) in 1894, *Chirurgische Klinik der Nierenkrankheiten* (Surgical Clinic of Kidney Diseases) in 1901, and *Chirurgie der Niere und des Harnleiters* (Surgery of the Kidney and Urethra) in 1925 [27]. He was co-founder of the journal *Folia Urologica* [27, 29].

In 1877, he reported the case of a 9-year-old female with an 8×5 cm ulcer located in the middle of the posterior aspect of the right lower leg with diffuse angioectasias in the region of the anterior tibial artery. He found that upon compressing the femoral, popliteal, or anterior tibial artery (at the point of passage through the interosseous ligament) that:

> Digital occlusion of the femoral artery markedly affected the heartbeat: tension at a point of pressure in the central portion of the artery was considerably increased; the pulse rate dropped from 108 beats per minute to 66, and the heart rhythm became irregular. The same result was obtained with compression of the popliteal or the tibial arteries. In addition to arterial compression, the pulse rate also changed when the leg was placed in a horizontal position. With the patient seated and leg raised vertically, the pulse rate dropped from 108 to 92 beats; with the same body position and legs dependent, the number of heartbeats rose to 116. Blocking the arterial supply of blood after vertical elevation of the leg reduced the pulse number from 92 to 54, i.e., by 38 beats; the same procedure with legs dependent from 116 to 66, so by 50 beats. Thus, slowing of the pulse caused by arterial compression was greatest when the legs were dependent [30, p. 111].

Israel acknowledged the previous finding by Nicoladoni but disagreed with the explanation proposed by him to account for the decreased pulse rate:

> We now turn to discuss the strange phenomenon that has caught our attention during the course of the disease. That is the decreased pulse and irregularity of cardiac contraction upon compression of the arteries leading to the angioectasias. Nicoladoni has made the same observation in two cases of phlebarteriectasia of an upper extremity and tried to explain it. The said author proposed that mechanical irritation leads to stimulation of the vagus nerve. When compressing the brachial artery, the cirsoid subclavian artery is stretched due to the increased blood flow so that it exerts pressure on the vagus nerve. Of course, this explanation is made completely untenable by observation in our case [30, p. 125]. (…) The lowering of the pulse rate was achieved under two conditions: to a lesser extent when the leg was raised vertically (108-92) and to a great extent upon compression by a tourniquet over the femoral artery (108-66-42). The pulse frequency rose again when the leg was dependent (92-116) and after the tourniquet was removed. The increase occurred as the collateral circulation was restored and the angiectatic region filled again. These facts lead to the conclusion that the pulse rate is proportional to the blood filling of the leg. The immediate effect of femoral compression is caused by two factors. First, the arterial flow distal to the compressed extremity is reduced leading to the redistribution of blood to the body by way of the inferior vena cava. Second, because of the increased pressure in the venous system, pressure in the arterial system also increases. The same thing happens but with a lesser severity with vertical elevation of the extremities. Can the increase in arterial pressure be related to the fall in the pulse rate? Nicoladoni denies this question—I believe I have affirmed it [30, p. 125–126].

Harris Miller Branham (1862–1938) was born in Fort Valley, Houston Co., Georgia, and received his medical degree from the College of Physician and Surgeons, Baltimore, Maryland, (current University of Maryland School of Medicine) in 1888, achieving first honors in his class of 95 students [31, 32]. He was appointed Assistant Resident Surgeon at Baltimore City Hospital from 1888 to 1889 and in 1889 was a general medical and surgical practitioner in Glynn County, Brunswick, Georgia [32]. He also served as the city's health officer, US surgeon in charge of the Brunswick Quarantine station, president of the Brunswick Board of Health, member of the Medical Association of Georgia, and member of the Board of Aldermen in Brunswick. He was the first to discover yellow fever in the Brunswick section of Georgia [31, 33].

He reported a case titled "Aneurismal varix of the femoral artery and vein following a gunshot wound" in the *International Journal of Surgery* in 1890 in a 24-year-old man with an accidental gunshot wound located at the "antero-internal aspect of the left thigh about 4 1/2 inches below Poupart's ligament, and ranged downwards, backwards and outwards, lodging under the integument of the postero-external surface of the limb, 6 inches above the knee" [34, p. 250]. He identified 3 days later a palpable slight thrill and auscultatory bruit over the wound which subsequently increased in intensity. Furthermore, he also found on examination of the common femoral artery after the wound had healed (Fig. 13.1):

> The most mysterious phenomenon connected with the case, on which I have not been able to explain myself, or to obtain a satisfactory reason for from others, was slowing of the heart's beat, when compression of the common femoral was employed. (…) This symptom became more marked until pressure of the artery above the wound caused the heart's beat to fall from 80 to 35 or 40 per minute, and so to remain until the pressure was relieved.

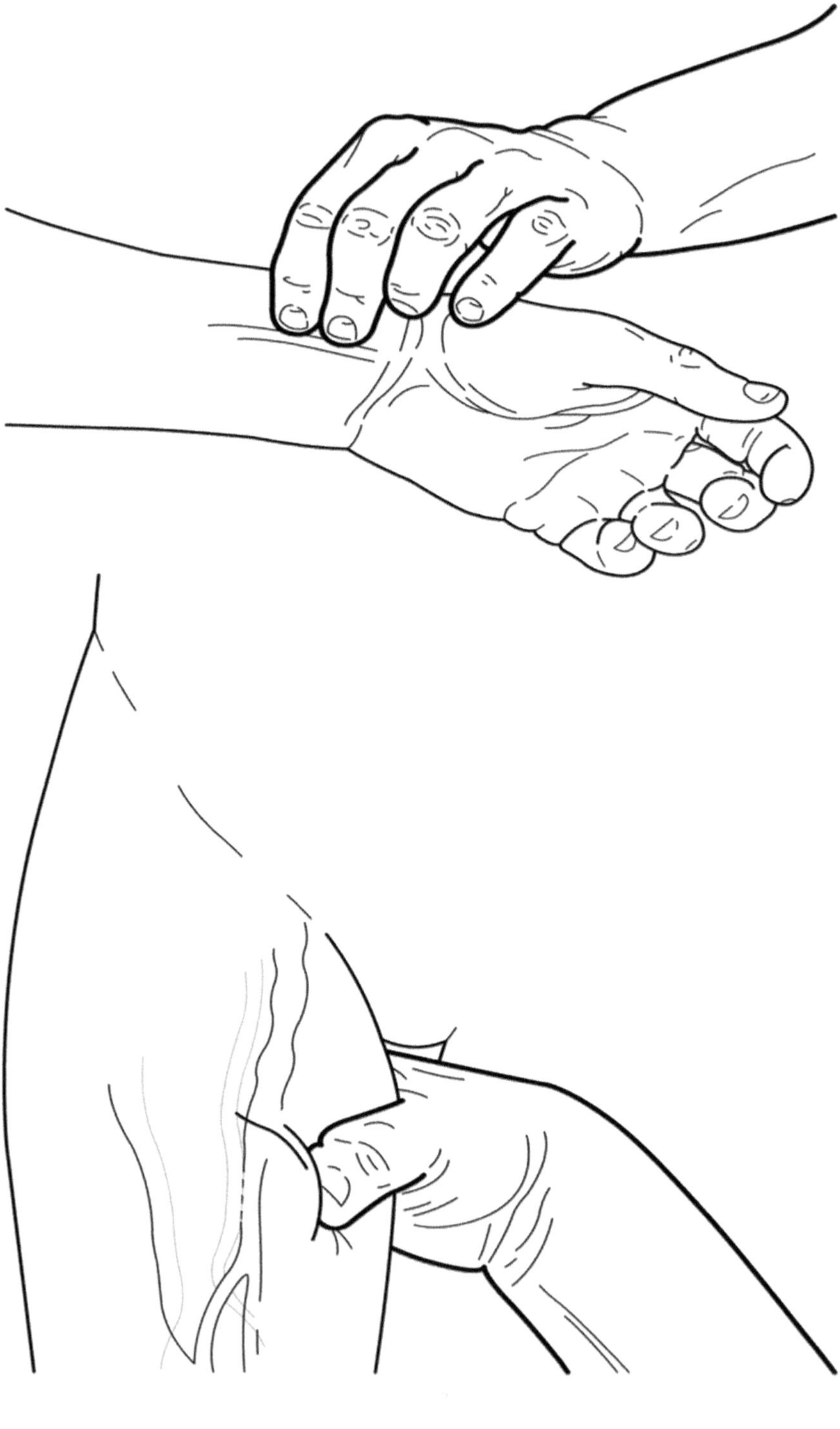

Fig. 13.1 Branham sign (by Ryan Yale)

> Compression of the artery of the sound limb would produce no such effect. Examination of the heart showed it to be free from any valvular trouble [34, p. 250–251].

He identified at the time of surgical repair of the artery 2 months after the injury:

> Upon careful dissection of the vessel it was found that the artery and veins were adherent at the point where the thrill was most perceptible, and that the arterial blood was being pumped into the vein, as shown by the pulsation of that vessel below the wound, and an almost entire absence of the pulsation in the distal portion of the artery [34, p. 251].

His obituary in the *Journal of the Medical Association of Georgia* read:

> Dr. Branham has been credited in press reports as the discoverer of what is known as the "Branham sign" which indicates the "Closure of an arteriovenous fistula by digital pressure results in the slowing of the pulse, increased diastolic pressure and disappearance of the cardiac murmur" [33, p. 35].

To be noted, neither of the last two findings were identified or reported in Branham's manuscript. It was Rudolph Matas (1860–1957), a preeminent vascular surgeon in New Orleans who affirmed that the finding should be known as "Branham sign." Contrarily, Daniel C. Elkin (1893–1958), another vascular surgeon at Emory University, believed at that time that Nicoladoni had previously described this sign [31, 35, 36].

Thus, Nicoladoni (1875), Israel (1877), and Branham (1890), each described the phenomenon of decreased pulse occurring upon digital compression proximal to an arterial-venous fistula (Table 13.1). We recognize that Branham was unaware of the prior publications by Israel and Nicoladoni. This sign has also been reported in cases of thrombotic occlusion of upper extremity AV fistulas designed for hemodialysis access [37]. The current proposed pathogenesis is believed to be due to increase vagal tone caused by increased cardiac contractility and activation of the cardiac baroreceptors in response to (1) increased arterial impedance and (2) decreased effective arterial volume as blood is redirected through higher resistance peripheral vasculature after occlusion of the fistula [37]. The sign has been considered the standard test for the hemodynamic significance of AV fistulas [38]. The sign lacks sufficient sensitivity but is specific marker of high-output heart failure [39].

Schapiro Sign

We were neither able to identify any historical information about adjunct Professor Dr. Heinrich Schapiro's (1852–1901) from the Helena Pawlowna Clinical Institute in St. Petersburg, Russia, nor access his original paper titled, "Klinische Untersuchungen über den Einfluß der Körperstellung und Kompression peripherer Arterien auf die Herztätigkeit" (Clinical studies on the influence of body position and compression of peripheral arteries on cardiac activity) published in Russian in 1881 [40]. However, a summary of this paper was published in *Jahresbericht über die Fortschritte der Anatomie und Physiologie* that same year. In his study, Schapiro examined the relationship between body position and pulse, and blood pressure and pulse in 50 healthy soldiers and determined, "[t]he pulse in the vertical and horizontal body position. He obtained a pulse that was faster standing than supine. The difference in the frequency of the pulse in one or the other body position fluctuated fairly widely (maximum 34, minimum 2, mean 14 beats)." [41, p. 60]. Using the Knoll polygraph, which records the frequency and shape of the pulse curve, he observed the following (Table 13.1):

1. When man moves from the standing to the lying position, the blood pressure in the arterial system is increased.
2. As a result of such an increase in blood pressure, a fairly significant slowing of the pulse is seen in healthy people. On the pulse curve, one can see the features of such a change.
3. Similar deceleration of the pulse and change in the shape of the pulse wave were obtained in the supine position with compression of the femoral arteries. These findings show that in these cases, slowing of the pulse was due to increased arterial blood pressure [41, p. 61–62].

Using the Basch's sphygmomanometer, Schapiro determined the radial artery blood pressure in the standing and supine position and found, "As the table shows, arterial pressure in the horizontal (supine) position is raised considerably (compared to the vertical position). Compression of the femoral arteries produces, as expected a priori, a slight increase in blood pressure as the pulse rate is lowered." [41, p. 62]. In otherwise healthy individuals, there is an initial 3–4 mmHg drop in blood pressure and increased heart rate (10–15 bpm) from the supine to standing position. These changes are sensed and corrected by arterial baroreceptors located in the carotid sinus and aortic arch and involve impulses conducted by way of two pathways: baroreflex and adrenergic [42, 43]. The baroreflex pathway involves afferent nerve impulses from the carotid sinus or aortic baroreceptors synapsing with the nucleus of the tractus solitarius in the medulla oblongata. From here, impulses are conducted to the nucleus ambiguous in the rostral medulla oblongata [43]. The efferent nerve impulses are then sent to the sinoatrial node causing the heart rate to increase [42].

The adrenergic pathways involve sympathetic afferent fibers which run from the nucleus of the tractus solitaries to the rostral and then caudal ventrolateral medulla. The sympathetic efferent fibers continue to the intermediolateral thoracic spinal cord [42]. From here, impulses are conducted to the (1) heart to increase ventricular contraction, (2) arterioles and venules to increasing total systemic vascular resistance through vasoconstriction, and (3) adrenals to activate, in part, the renin–angiotensin system with consequent aldosterone release [44].

Orthostatic hypotension results when these mechanisms fail due to depletion in blood volume, excessive venous pooling, or impairment in autonomic nerves or baroreflex pathways [42]. Thus, the larger fluctuations identified by Schapiro may reflect the imprecision in caliber of the instrumentation or that the soldiers experienced various degrees of orthostasis related to decreased intravascular fluid volume.

Jorissenne Sign

There is limited historical information on Gustave Jorissenne (1846–1924). He was a physician, botanist, archaeologist, and member of the Medical and Surgical Society of Liège, Belgium, and served as Secretary General of the International Congress of Hydrology and Climatology [45, 46].

Jorissenne identified in 1874, "From the first months of pregnancy in an otherwise healthy woman, the heart no longer responds to changes in posture by slowing down or accelerating, it maintains a constant rate" [47, p. 332]. He acknowledged that this finding is an extension of that described by Graves in patients with cardiac hypertrophy, "I had been able to check several times the law of Graves. This illustrious English clinician was the first to indeed notice that in hypertrophy of the heart the pulsation preserves a constant rate in all body positions" [47, p. 329]. Jorissenne described in detail the method for performing this test (Table 13.1):

> At first I thought that prolonged rest prior to the experiment was favorable for the accuracy of tests, but I have since seen this finding multiple times in people who have been walking for either a short or long period of time. I have found it to be advantageous to conduct this test even in the most varied conditions. Therefore, I do not hesitate to say that overexcitation of the heart by a normal or rapid walk does not disturb the physiological law. It is understood that the numbers to be compared must be collected in a limited time, a few minutes at most, unless the conditions remain uniform. However, even though I have said that the best moment for taking this observation is after the patient is awakened from a restful sleep, I realize that it is not always practical. I suppose that it rarely happens that the doctor arrives at just the right time. On the contrary, one would be delighted to have at his disposal a means that could be easily applied in the consulting room if additional provisions are used. We must proceed calmly without intentionally adding undue attention to what we are doing. In fact it is necessary not to provoke emotion since this may cause, within a few seconds after the moment when the unfortunate action occurs, either acceleration or sometimes a noticeable slowing of the heart rate. It is recommended that the radial pulse be counted first in the sitting position. The woman is asked to hang her arm freely to her side to ensure that the findings are uniform. She should lean against the back of the chair sitting comfortably without being excessively stiff or slumping. You should start counting the beats only after a ten or fifteen seconds pause since the movements caused by sitting may result in a momentary acceleration of the heart rate [47, p. 332].
>
> I do not recommend prolonging each observation as this leads to anxiety and may alter the test results. For suggestible women I usually count for half a minute, although that is already too long as a quarter of a minute is usually sufficient. The vertical position is evaluated next. The woman is told not to stand abruptly. When standing the arms should hang to her sides. It is necessary to wait until she is completely calm, that is, for fifteen seconds. Moreover, while palpating the pulse one feels that it slowly becomes regular. The pulse should be counted briefly for a few seconds making sure that its movements are regular.
>
> The patient then lies on either a sofa or a bed depending on the circumstances. The bed is more inconvenient in that the effort to get into it is considerable and excites the heart for a few minutes. For the test to be conclusive, the body including the head must be on a horizontal plane. Then, although this is not absolutely necessary, make sure that the head rests on a more sloping plane. I recall, in fact, the remark of Graves: it is in this position that the decline is most obvious in the absolute physiological state. In these three or four attitudes I would say that the frequency of the pulse at the beginning of pregnancy remains constant. After this

> first test, I believe that it is useful to start again in the opposite direction. I again count the beats in the sitting followed by the vertical position. I can even start from the horizontal to the vertical position always applying the same required precautions. If the person is examined on waking, we first see what happens in the sitting followed by the horizontal position. We end with the vertical position recommending the least possible movements [47, p. 333].

He recognized that the coexistence of other diseases may interfere with or modify the test results:

> In general, the coexistence of other diseases does not allow the diagnosis of pregnancy to be made by this method. However, I showed that it is not always impossible and the question cannot be easily decided as it first seems. Obviously, if considerable hypertrophy of the heart is present prior to pregnancy, uniformity of the pulse already exists. As I had said earlier, it is this disease that the findings and discoveries were made by Graves. Other cardiac conditions are confusing in cases where there is concomitant hypertrophy. (…) Dilation of the heart also makes the heart beats very irregular. In this case the heart beats must be compared rather than counted. Valvular problems do not prevent the heart from being affected by changes in position. (…) However, I will point out that the hypertrophy of the right ventricle does not modify the contractions of the heart. It is necessary that the left ventricle be hypertrophied so that positional changes do not vary its beats. In the latter case, I saw that the pulse remain uniform despite the presence of other serious diseases such as emphysema, bronchitis, asthma, etc. [47, p. 412–413].

Jorissenne concluded based on his observation:

> I conclude (theoretically, because I have not yet had the opportunity to check my predictions) that the invariability of the pulse occurring in a woman suddenly deprived of her period, whereas earlier and more or less recent examinations remained doubtful, is an important finding to support the diagnosis of a pregnancy. I do not know, to tell the truth, whether this invariability occurs in patients with heart disease and one of the described conditions. I doubt it if it is performed in cases of wall thinning, ventricular dilation or tricuspid lesions [47, p. 413].

Thus, Jorissenne sign refers to a pulse that remains fixed with postural changes, a sign of early pregnancy. In fact, during normal pregnancy, the heart rate may increase at rest by 10–20 beats as cardiac output increases. Postural changes from supine to standing causes physiological changes leading to increased cardiac output and heart rate during the first trimester [48].

Lommel Sign

Felix Wilhelm Lommel (1875–1968), son of the physicist Eugen Cornelius Joseph von Lommel (1837–1899), was born in Erlangen region of Franconia and studied medicine in Munich, Würzburg, and Kiel [49]. He served as an assistant to Roderich Stintzing (1854–1933) in 1899 and in 1902 habilitated with his thesis *Clinical Observations on Cardiac Arrhythmia* [49]. He served with Max Erich Richard Matthes (1865–1930) and Dietrich Gerhard (1866–1912) at the Medical Polyclinic, Jena, Germany [49]. He was appointed director of the Medical Polyclinic in 1909 and in 1924 founded the tuberculosis clinic at the University of Jena (Friedrich-Schiller University) [49]. As a description of his character, Kelinsorge, a student of Lommel, wrote:

> As head of the clinic he was always available to provide support to his assistants who often turned to him with confidence involving personal matters. As a teacher, admired due to his short, accurate, humorous and witty remarks woven into the lectures, he made an effort to introduce the patient not as a "case" but as a person [49, p. 1334].

He was elected honorary member of the Berlin Medical Society and Medical Scientific Society at the University of Jena [50]. Lommel in his paper titled "Klinische Beobachtungen über Herzarhythmie" (Clinical observations on cardiac arrhythmia) described the relationship between respiration and pulse rate:

> Although not an arrhythmia, but a slight fluctuation in rhythm. The effect of respiration on the increased pulse rate can be found on clinical examination in many healthy persons. However the magnitude of this effect seems to be particularly different among individuals and probably results from numerous secondary conditions, so that the effect in some can only be detected by the most precise recording of the pulse. In a large number of my investigations in apparently healthy persons there is temporary or permanent complete absence of respiratory fluctuations, so that the pulse was really "rhythmic" in the strict sense of the word. A comprehensive methodological study of conditions whereby respiration alters the pulse in otherwise healthy people was not possible until now [16, p. 468]. (...) The following investigations are intended to show that pulse irregularities caused by respiration are much more common than it is apparently assumed. In most cases these differences are so minor that they are difficult to detect at the bedside, while in other more severe types of arrhythmias, respiration can be used to easily differentiate diseases involving the heart. Under certain circumstances pulse irregularities caused by respiration occur to such an extent that attentive observation is required in order to differentiate them from other arrhythmias. One would expect that the "respiratory" character of the pulse frequency fluctuation should always be easy to ascertain by simple auscultation. Its recognition is often made more difficult by the fact that the clinically most interesting and severe cases of this arrhythmia occur in the setting of normal and often even very shallow respiration in the examples cited [51, p. 470].

Lommel summarized the findings of his observations:

> 1. Many cardiac arrhythmias occur in such a way that in normal conditions there is an acceleration of the heartbeat with inspiration and deceleration during expiration. 2. These arrhythmias are therefore regarded as merely quantitative increases in normal respiratory fluctuations; they likely involve the nervous system. 3. They are not caused by organic heart disease. 4. They account for the arrhythmias occurring in the convalescence of feverish diseases, cardiac neuroses, and in brain diseases where there is irritation of the vagus nerve. 5. The fact that it is purely of nervous origin is important in the differential diagnosis of neurologic and heart disease [51, p. 501].

Lommel sign thus refers to an increased pulse occurring during inspiration and decreased pulse during expiration (Table 13.1).

Mannkopff Sign

Emil Wilhelm Mannkopff (1836–1918) was born in Pasewalk, Prussia, studied medicine at the Friedrich Wilhelm University of Berlin, Julius Maximilian University of Würzburg, Charles University of Prague, and the University of Vienna, and received his doctorate of medicine degree at the University of Berlin in

1858 [52]. In the same year, he was a member of Corps Nassovia Würzburg, a union of current and former students at the Julius Maximilian University of Würzburg whose purpose was to provide a community of academic and nonacademic support to students [52, 53]. From 1859 to1869, he worked as a medical practitioner in Berlin and from 1860 to 1866 served as first assistant and last senior physician at Charité-Universitätsmedizin, Berlin, habilitating in Internal Medicine at the University of Berlin in 1862 [52, 53]. In 1867, he was appointed Chair of Internal Medicine at Philipps University of Marburg, and from 1867 to 1905, Full Professor within the Faculty of Medicine, Pathology and Therapy [52, 53]. He served as Dean of the Medical Faculty in Marburg in 1877, 1881, 1888, and 1907 and rector of the University of Marburg between 1879 and 1886 [52]. In 1884, he became a member of the Leopoldina Academy of Natural Sciences [52, 54]. He was a general physician II class of the Hessen-Kasseler Landwehr and Chairman of the Medical and Dental Examination Commissions in 1892. From 1897 to 1917, he was chairman of the Medical and Dental Examiners and in 1897 was general physician first class [52]. As a description of Mannkopff's character on his retirement, Otto Heβ wrote:

> Mannkopff is a humane doctor at the bedside; his goodness of heart and humanity are probably the personal qualities which are most prominent among all others; how often has he resisted the view that the patient is only "material." For him the physical and mental well-being of the patient is first of all dear to his heart; he often appeared and visited the clinic at night to see severely ill patients [55, p. 927].

Mannkopff reported at a meeting at the Marburg Society of Medicine in 1885 a patient with residual right-sided abdominal pain sustained after trauma with an elevated pulse occurring after palpable pressure:

> With an assistant feeling the pulse, pressure when applied over the traumatic area on the posterior abdominal wall or within the rectum in the direction of the rectovesicalis caused the pulse to rise from 84 to 92 beats and to 120 beats when the patient felt significant pain in the affected area. After the pressure was withdrawn and pain subsided, the pulse rate returned to its earlier value rapidly. The pulse rose again when pressure was reapplied [56].

Rumpf, a colleague of Dr. Mannkopff, assessed "the influence of cardiac activity on painful pressure points in cases of neuralgia and painful pressure" and found "an acceleration of the action of the heart, a brief deceleration, and subsequent acceleration" [57, p. 153]. Rumpf found that in some cases of general neurosis involving neuralgias, there may be a:

> [n]ew or painful pressure point when irritation is accompanied by a change in the activity of the heart and circulation characterized by a, i. simple acceleration of heart activity, ii. initial short-term deceleration with subsequent acceleration, iii. decrease in the pulse size, iv. isolated irregularity of the pulse, v. distinct cyanosis of the face, vi. lowering of the blood pressure, vii. increase in blood pressure. All these findings in cardiac and vascular activity have in common is that with the removal of the painful stimulus, the changes disappear within a short period of time. The first to return to the previous state is the pulse, while blood pressure usually returns to normal more slowly [57, p. 156].

Rumpf thus noted that when performing "Mannkopff maneuver," the following steps should be taken:

> [t]he subject should remain still while looking for Mannkopff sign. Breathing must remain regular and the pressure exerted must be sudden and brief. When the acceleration is very noticeable, you have to consider the method of stimulation. When it is absent, one should not be deceived since the experiment does not allow in this case the ability to draw any conclusion. When the acceleration is mild it has little meaning since the patient, holding his breath, moaning, or writhing as a result of the pain real or not, can to some extent change the rate of cardiac contraction [58, p. 287–288].

Sand believed "that when the signs of Mannkopff and Bechterew are clearly positive, their value is almost absolute regarding the reality of pain or hyperesthesia. It is not obviously caused by hysterical anesthesia" [58, p. 289]. Interestingly, it should be recognized that Cesare Lombroso (1835–1909) was the first to describe in 1867 the relationship between pain and increased pulse rate:

> I observed that the pulse increased steadily and clearly after applying an electrical stimuli to humans. A very painful electric current applied for five seconds five times in six healthy individuals produced in only one person (myself) a decrease of 2 to 4 beats, a difference that is insufficient to calculate. In others an increase of 8, 20, 35 beats was observed [59, p. 116].

Application of a painful stimuli causes acute pain and increased heart rate [60]. There may be sex-related differences since a positive relationship between pain and increased heart rate was found in men but not in women [61–63]. Thus, Mannkopff sign refers to an increased pulse in response to pressure over a painful area (Table 13.1).

Aschner Sign

Bernhard B. Aschner (1883–1960) was born in Vienna and received his medical degree from the University of Vienna in 1907 [64]. He served as an anatomy demonstrator from 1904 to 1907 and apprentice in the I Surgical University Hospital, Vienna, under Emil Zuckerkandl (1849–1910) and Anton von Eiselsberg (1860–1939) [65, 66]. His introduction to Richard Paltauf (1858–1924), Chief of the Department of Experimental Pathology at the University of Vienna, inspired him to take laboratory scientific discoveries directly to the patient's bedside, a term now colloquially referred to as translational medicine. Through this approach, he devised a novel technique using a transbuccal route for hypophysectomy and the oculocardiac reflex, a sign which bears his name [67].

He served in Friedrich Schauta's (1849–1919) Clinic in Vienna in 1908 followed by an appointment as Assistant at the University Clinic in the Department of Gynecological and Obstetrical in Halle an der Saale Germany in 1912 [65, 68, 69]. He was a regiment physician during World War I (1914–1918) and appointed Adjunct Professor for Gynecology and Obstetrics at the University of Vienna [69].

After the War, he was appointed Associate Professor of Gynecology and Obstetrics at Allgemeine Krankenhaus, Vienna [68]. He was persecuted during Nazism and disbarred from the University of Vienna by the National Socialist Party (Nazi Party) because he was Jewish [54]. He emigrated to New York City in 1938 where he was in private practice and held appointments at Stuyvesant and Lebanon Hospitals [68, 69]. In addition to his experimental work on the pituitary gland and contributions as a surgeon, gynecologist, and obstetrician, he was considered a medical historian translating the works of Paracelsus into modern German from 1926 to 1932 [68, 70]. Among his many awards, he was honored during World War I receiving the Knight's Cross of the Maltese Order and Knight's Cross of the Order of Franz Joseph and was the recipient of the Wilhelm Hufeland Award in Germany in 1957, a testimony to his scientific contributions [66, 68].

Aschner described the findings when he applied pressure to the eye in stuporous and anesthetized patients (Fig. 13.2):

> Once while I was pushing on the eye I checked the pulse and found to my great surprise, that it disappeared from under my hand. The slowing of the pulse, the breaking motion (which was also recurring) immediately suggested a vagal stimulation. There were only two possible explanations for this: i. vagal irritation due to intracranial pressure by way of the optic nerve sheaths and cerebrospinal fluid, or, ii. by way of a nerve reflex. (…) Changes in respiration result from pressure on the eye as well as by electrical stimulation of all three trigeminal branches. This manifests in spasmodic inspirations with inspiratory pauses as well as convulsive exhalations and expiratory arrests, the latter occurring particularly during deep narcosis. Furthermore, the vascular center also appears to be involved in that pressure on the eye causes increased blood pressure (excitement of the vasoconstrictor nerves). The influence of the altered respiration on the circulation must also be taken into account [71, p. 1529].

He accounted for the pathophysiology of this finding, "It has now been proven that this phenomenon succeeds by way of a reflex. The afferent sensory nerve of this reflex arm is the trigeminal nerve and the efferent nerve is the vagus and nerves close to it." [71, p. 1529]. Thus, Aschner sign, also referred to as the oculocardiac reflex or phenomenon, is decreased pulse rate caused by bulbar compression (Table 13.1).

Aschner, oculocardiac, or the trigeminovagal reflex is a phenomenon elicited upon direct orbital pressure, traction on the globe contents, or extraocular muscles and has been reported to occur in patients with orbital fractures and ocular trauma, strabismus and cataract surgery, and endoscopic sinus surgery [72–77]. The incidence of this finding varies depending on the patient's age and the case definition used to define a positive response based on the percent reduction in heart rate [78, 79]. It is more commonly found in younger persons, and its presence is modulated by other factors such as hypoxia and hypercarbia [79]. In addition to sinus bradycardia, a number of other arrhythmias have been reported to occur with this reflex including asystole and cardiac arrest [79]. Management includes removing the inciting stimulus.

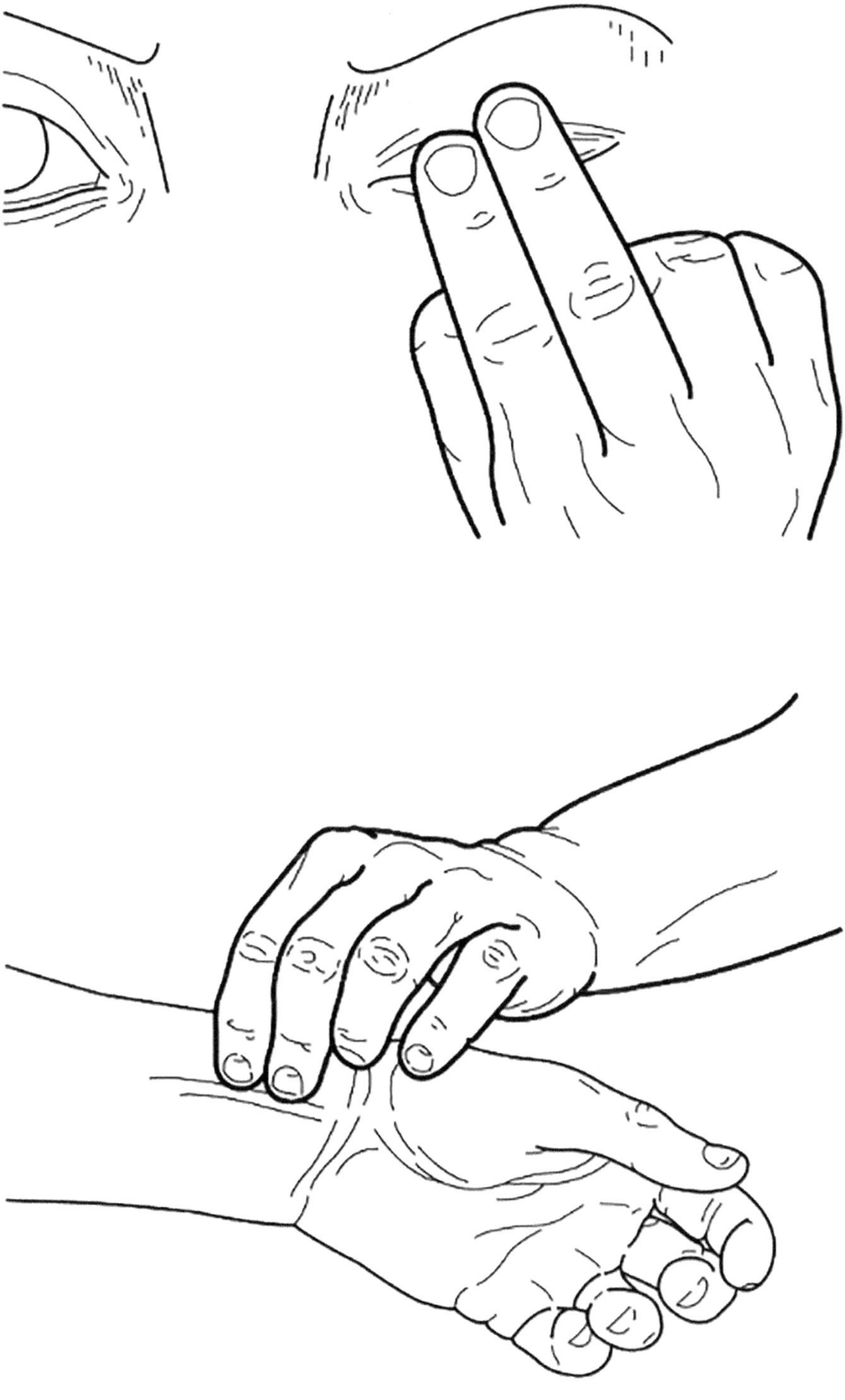

Fig. 13.2 Aschner sign (by Ryan Yale)

Prével Sign

We were unable to identify any historical information on Prével. He found that in certain persons, the pulse increases when moving from the supine to standing position. He believed that this pathological phenomenon of orthostatic cardiac acceleration or the abdominal-cardiac reflex was a condition caused by the movement of the intestines, in particular the stomach:

> In a number of subjects the inverted position causes the pulse to beat slower than in the horizontal position. Observation: In the horizontal position, the fall of the intestines towards the pelvis closely returns to its normal position. In the sitting position, where the stomach and the intestines are only partially affected from gravity, an intermediate number of pulses are obtained compared to the inverted position - the slowest - and in the standing position - the fastest (Observations I and II). Without modifying the upright position or applying a tight belt to the hypogastric region so as to raise the abdominal mass towards the diaphragm, the acceleration caused by standing is seen to diminish or disappear (Observation III) [80, p. 138].

He believed, based on his observations, that the stomach was primary causes for this condition for the following three reasons:

(a) The stomach, as a result of its conformation and its role as an intermittent reservoir of the alimentary tract, is the abdominal organ which most easily follows the effect of gravity.
(b) Orthostatic acceleration occurs after a meal, tends to diminish toward the time of complete evacuation of the stomach, and disappears during fasting in certain subjects.
(c) Acceleration decreases with improvement of the dyspeptic phenomena [80, p.139].

As to the pathophysiology of this reflex, he concluded:

> Orthostatic cardiac acceleration or the abdominal cardiac reflex should be considered as a pathological phenomenon related to a movement of the abdominal organs, in particular, the stomach. This finding depends on two main interacting factors. I believe that this is caused by the overwork of the stomach due to an excessively large food mass and the muscular insufficiency of its abdominal wall. In this context it is interesting to see that a clear relationship exists between the drooping of the abdomen, sub-umbilical protrusion, and the extent of the abdominal-cardiac reflex [80, p. 140-141]. (...) Because the abdominal-cardiac reflex depends on an abnormal state, I believe that the concept of the physiological pulse at least in regards to its many causes must be slightly modified [80, p. 142].

Thus, Prével sign, also referred to as orthostatic cardiac acceleration or the abdominal cardiac reflex, is an abnormal increased pulse that occurs when changing from the supine to standing position (Table 13.1). Similar to Livierato sign, this sign was believed to represent activation of the abdominal sympathetic reflexes.

Cantelli Sign

We were only able to obtain limited historical information on Oreste Cantelli. He was born in 1890 and at the time of his publication was Professor of Special Medical Pathology at the University of Bologna [81]. Normally, compression of the eyeball(s) causes a vagally mediated decrease in the pulse which returns to normal after the stimulus is removed (see Aschner sign). Other authors found an increase in pulse in a variety of conditions such as syphilis, Parkinson's, and pseudo-bulbar palsy [81]. Cantelli reported in his paper "Di una varieta dei riflesso oculo-cardiaco (Riflesso oculo-cardiaco paradossale)," [Of a variety of ocular-reflexes (Paradoxical ocular-reflex)]:

> I happened to observe an increase in the number of heartbeats and pulses during bulbar compression that persisted after termination of the stimulus. In fact, it may take even up to a few minutes to have the heartbeats return to the normal. This phenomenon is opposite of what is normally found; it can also be called "paradoxical" [81, p. 487].

Based on his observation in eight soldiers in a war hospital, he reported:

1. There is a paradoxical ocular-cardiac reflex in which an increase in the number of heartbeats and pulses remains even after bulbar compression has ceased.
2. It is the expression: (a) of a deep lesion of the vagus in its terminations of the nodes of Keith and Flack and (b) an increase in the excitability of the myocardium so that the refractory period decreases.
3. The stimulus that normally starts through the trigeminal nerve following compression of the eyeballs reaches the heart simultaneously by means of the vagus and the sympathetic trigeminal. In these cases, the normal decrease in the number of heartbeats is due to the excess tonicity of the vagus over the sympathetic.
4. The paradoxical response of the heart caused by serious lesions of the cardiac nervous system and the changes that briefly occur cannot be used independently to evaluate and determine prognosis. However, it is always an indication of a latent deficiency in the function of the cardio-vascular apparatus, so it will always be advisable to first remove soldiers suffering from it until a complete and constant healing takes place [81, p. 489].

Thus, Cantelli sign refers to the presence of increased pulse with bulbar pressure (Table 13.1). As previously described, this phenomenon is found in a variety of pathological conditions such as syphilis, Parkinson's disease, and pseudobulbar palsy. This sign is paradoxical since under normal states the pulse decreases with ocular pressure. The sign is believed to be caused by processes that result in vagal nerve insufficiency. We are unaware of any studies which assessed the oculocardiac reflex in these diseases.

Ruggeri Sign

We were unable to identify any historical information on E. Ruggeri. Ruggeri reported his findings on the ocular convergence reflex in normal subjects and patients with a variety of pathological conditions (e.g., tuberculosis, typhus, infectious polyneuropathy). The test is performed as follows (Fig. 13.3):

1. The individual on whom we want to determine the ocular convergence is placed in a supine position on the bed, and after a few minutes, the radial pulse is counted. The test begins when the pulse, after repeated counting, remains constant.
2. While an assistant is counting the pulse, the subject is asked to carefully position the tip of the index finger 1 cm away from the nose, corresponding to the midpoint of the glabella line nasal tip. This observation requires a strong convergence of the eyes followed by a marked miosis, an accommodation effort, and considerable contraction of the orbicularis.
3. While the subject continues to fixate on the tip of the index finger, and after 10–15 seconds have elapsed, the assistant is asked to count the number of pulsations for 30 seconds. It finally remains to establish, based on frequent and repeated counts of the pulse, the time required for it to return to the usual rate [82, p. 1029].

He believed that this test was a useful for determining the neurocardiac function of the heart:

> Referring briefly to the effects of the ocular-convergence reflex on the normal and pathological pulse of some diseased states, I note from this complex research that this maneuver can be a valid diagnostic aid. In fact, it is beyond doubt that in certain diseases such as polyneuritis which I studied, it is useful and indeed necessary to know the neurocardiac state. With common diagnostic measures we are not always able to determine small, latent alterations of oculo-convergence. We are able to detect vague sympathetic discrepancies which is how other obscure cardiac diseases can be identified to determine pathogenic effects. The ocular-convergence reflex occurred in the setting of cardiac-sympathetic excitement in all my cases when a sympathetic or hypofunctional vagal state was obscure. The oculo-convergence reflex identified these functional imbalances leading to tachycardia and more or less profound alteration in the morphology of the sphygmographs. In sympathetic-paresis syndromes, hypervagotonia situations, or in states of true hyposystolia which I observed, the oculo-convergence reflex was inappreciable or absent. Therefore, this test could have a considerable value theoretically revealing vague-sympathetic dysfunction and cardio-dynamic conditions [82, p. 1034].

He provided a hypothesis for the proposed phenomenon:

> I also tried to investigate the cause of the phenomenon. For now I am only allowed to generate hypotheses given the difficulties and gaps in studying ocular sensory–sensory ocular pathways that leads to further questions about the innervation of the iris and the mechanism of the various reflexes. One might think that it was the patient's attention (as shown in the Herz test[1]) that leads to the changes I found in the heart rhythm. At this

[1] Herz or "self-checking test" described by Max Herz (1865–1956) is a method to determine the cardiac function and distinguish it from neurosis. In this method, the pule is first counted, the elbow and wrist are supported by the examiner's left hand, while the examiner's right hand passively flexes and extends the right forearm while counting the pulse. During the movement, the patient is requested to direct his/her "attention" to the slow movement of the forearm. In normal person, the pulse does not change, while in those with neurosis or heart failure, the pulse increases or decreases, respectively [85].

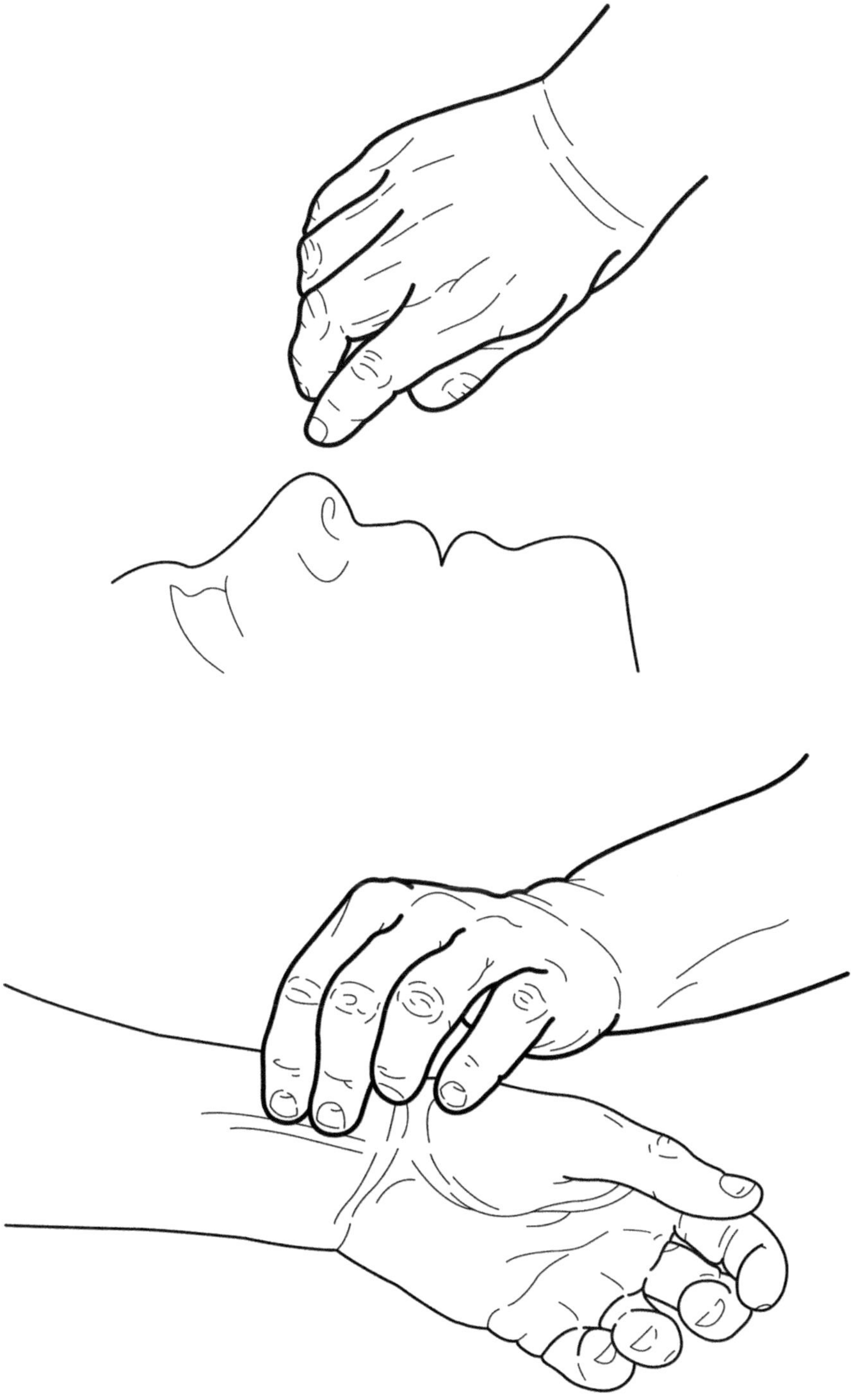

Fig. 13.3 Ruggeri sign (by Ryan Yale)

> hypothesis, however, I immediately objected since in the same subjects where the phenomenon was obvious, the intense visual attention of an object without the intervention of protracted convergence never ended the phenomenon. Another mechanism, therefore, must be sought. The fixation point (end of the index finger, located in the middle third of the glabella line-nasal tip at a distance of one cm) requires convergence, accommodation, a contraction of the exaggerated and protracted orbicularis oculi simultaneously, and complex rhythmic excitations of all terminal branches of the visual apparatus. Such reflex excitations after reaching the mesencephalic nuclei could either stimulate the bulbar cardiac excitatory center or travel instead, by the numerous communicating sympathetic branches, through the cervical ganglion superior to the heart, or follow the sympathetic fibers contained in the vagus to the center of cardiac automatism on the Keith and Flack [sinoatrial] node. This node responds to the stimuli by either accelerating or slowing depending on the intensity of the stimulus and sympathetic state of the subject. The limited research which I have done only allows me to draw hypothetical conclusions as described above. Further research will better able to delineate the issue [82, p. 1034].

The terms accommodation reflex, accommodation-convergence reflex, and near reflex are used to describe the findings in response to coordinated near vision and involve convergence of both eyes, contraction of the ciliary muscles causing a change in the lens shape, and pupillary constriction [84]. Ruggeri sign refers to the presence of tachycardia occurring while attempting to fix a near object during extreme convergence (Table 13.1). We are unaware of any studies which evaluated the sensitivity or specificity of this finding.

Laubry Sign

Charles Laubry (1872–1960) was born in Saint-Florentin in the Yonne, France, and served as *externe des Hôpitaux* in 1894 and *interne des Hôpitaux* in 1899 under Émile Charles Achard (1860–1944) at the Tenon Hospital [85]. He worked with Henri Vaquez (1860–1936) at Saint-Antoine Hospital in 1904 [86, 87]. In 1911, he was nominated *médecin des Hôpitaux* and served at the old Broussais Hospital, Paris, in 1925 [87]. Laubry was elected municipal councilor of Flogny-la-Chapelle, France, and appointed to the Hospital of Bicétre, Paris [86]. During World War I, he served as a surgeon and ophthalmologist and was assigned to the medical and surgical group of the fifth region [86]. In 1921, he led the department of the Hôpital de la Rochefoucauld, followed by appointments to Cochin in 1922, Boulogne-sur-Seine in 1924, and finally at Broussais Hospital, Paris, France, in 1925 [85, 86, 88]. It is at this latter hospital where he conducted his most novel work on congenital heart disease and cardiovascular radiology [88].

Laubry served as editor for *Archives des Maladies du Coeur and des Vaisseaux* (Archives of Diseases of the Heart and Vessels) in 1936 and in the same year founded the Société française de Cardiologie (French Society of Cardiology), serving as its first president [85, 87]. He was named honorary professor in 1941, member of the National Academy of Sciences in the section of Medicine and Surgery of the Institute of France in 1933, member of the Academy of Sciences in 1945, served as the first President of the International Society of Cardiology and organized the 1st World Congress of Cardiology, Paris, and was elected Fellow to the Royal College of Physicians, London in 1953 [85, 86, 88]. As a description of his character:

> It is difficult to convey to those who never knew him personally, a sufficient idea of the man himself, of the extraordinary power that his personality exercised over all those around him and of the great affection and admiration with which he was universally regarded. (…) As a physician, Laubry was a supreme advocate of the Hippocratic art, and his humanity, sympathy, and understanding of mankind inspired confidence and affection in every kind of patient from Clemenceau to the most humble and illiterate inmate of the Broussais. No matter how trivial or how serious the illness, Laubry's presence at the bedside had a magical effect in calming anxiety and dispelling fear. To him, medicine was a part of life and demanded knowledge of the complete patient, his body, his mind, and his heart [87, p. 215]. (…) In the course of his long career, Laubry received many honors and distinctions, and his innumerable scientific contributions have left their mark on the cardiology of his day, but his pupils and friends will remember him not so much for what he did as for what he was, a great physician, an inspiring teacher, and a most lovable man [87, p. 218].

Laubry, Routier, and Van Bogaert describe two clinical signs found in three patients with atrial flutter to confirm the diagnosis (Table 13.1):

1. Anisorhythmia regular or irregular flutter. There are two types: periodic or alternating type and aperiodic or irregular type.

   (a) Periodic anisorhythmia: The alternating type seems to occur frequently in regular and fast flutter. (…) The ventricles fill normally during diastole since the number of atrial systoles in these regular flutters is fixed and occur at the same intervals between the ventricular contractions. (…) [a]t certain moments, there are smaller pulsations of an alternating couple leading to a transient bradycardia.

   (b) Aperiodic anisorhythmia: In aperiodic type, the amplitude is unequal in all pulsations. This disordered anisorhythmia is well known in the complete arrhythmia (atrial fibrillation) and in the very irregular atrial tachycardias. (…) It is obvious that diastolic pauses of different lengths result in different ventricular filling times and consequently systoles of variable volume and pulses of unequal amplitude. (…) The mechanism of this anisorhythmia is probably similar to that of the usual alternating pulse. It is in fact, an alternation of the regular sequence of large and small pulsations. However, the amplitude of each of them varies continuously thus giving the misleading appearance of a disordered anisorhythmia. In other words, all the large and small pulsations instead of always being equal to one another, as is the rule in the alternating pulse, vary continuously in amplitude [89, p. 329].

   In summary, the disordered anisorhythmia is of interest since it is an intrinsic sign of an arrhythmia. This sign is clearly detected even within the slightest irregularities that escape auscultation. In some regular flutters (checked regularity on the electrocardiogram), an alternating oscillating or variable pulse takes on the appearance of a disordered anisorhythmia [89, p. 332].

2. During diastole, there is a third sound with two normal sounds and a continuous variable rhythm. This third sound does not occur at the same time during diastole. (...) [i]s found at a point on the chest where there is a shock heard by auscultation or ventricular heave felt by palpation. What characterizes this three-beat rhythm is the extreme variability of the ratios of the sound added with the two normal sounds occurring in the same position, conditions, and examination. This sound disappears and reappears immediately after the normal rhythm is replaced with either a doubling of the first sound, or a presystolic or protodiastolic gallop depending on whether the dull sound occurs after the first sound or second sound [89, p. 333].

They noted that the sound was not found in all cases of irregular flutter. They postulated that:

> Therefore, in addition to the variable interference of the two dissociated rhythms of the atrium, a special condition of the ventricular is required to produce this three-beat rhythm. That is to say a certain energy of the atrial systole and a particular state of the myocardium wall making it capable of rendering or transmitting a sound [89, p. 333].

They postulated the cause for the sound:

> If our auscultation corresponds well to the graphic image that we have just analyzed, we must ask ourselves how the diastolic filling as well as atrial systole produces the additional noise. To produce a noise you first need a force then something that is likely to vibrate under its impulse. The force here is the flow of blood from the atrium into the ventricle. This flow has a certain lively force especially marked at the two ends of the diastole: at the opening of the auriculo-ventricular valves at the beginning of the diastole, and then at the time of the atrial systole at the end of the diastole. The first generated wave is diastolic filling, while the second wave, normally presystolic, is the atrial filling. (…) The variable three-beat rhythm, without being a characteristic sign of flutter, is nonetheless a valuable sign for the diagnosis of this arrhythmia [89, p. 338].

Thus, Laubry and colleagues described several signs. One is in reference to the amplitude of the palpable pulse which is the uniform in regular rhythm atrial flutter and variable in irregular rhythm atrial flutter. Second, they described the auscultatory findings of either a third (S_3) or fourth (S_4) heart sound heard in patients with atrial flutter.

Conclusion

Assessment of the frequency and character of the pulse assisted physicians to detect a variety of physical findings later eponymously named to honor their accomplishments. Compression, postural changes, and elevation or depression of the extremities lead to activation or inhibition of autonomic nervous system mechanism causing acceleration or depression of the pulse. It is through these keen maneuvers that physicians accounted for potential pathophysiologic mechanisms responsible for alterations of the pulse.

References

1. Perloff JK. The arterial pulse. In: Physical Examination of the Heart and Circulation. 2nd ed. Philadelphia: W.B. Saunders Company; 1990. p. 57–102.
2. Zuntz N. Ewald Hering. Deutsche med Wchenschr. 1918;44:215–6.
3. Hofmann FB. Ewald Hering. München med Wchenschr. 1918;65:539–42.
4. Baumann C. The physiologist Ewald Hering (1834-1918): curriculum vitae. Strabismus. 2013;21:195–9.
5. Tschmerak AV. Nachruf auf E. Hering. Med Klin. 1918;14:329–31.
6. Hering E. Die Selbsteuerung der Atmung durch den Nervous Vagus. Sitzungab d k Akad d Wissensch Math naturw, Cl. Wien; 1868. p. 672–7.
7. Hering E. Über den Einfluss der Atmung auf den Kreislauf Zwiete Mitteilung. Über eine reflketorische Beziehung zwischen Lung und Herz, Sitzungab d k Akad d Wissensch Math naturw, Cl; Wien; 1871. p. 333–53.
8. Trincker D. Hering, Ewald. In: Neue Deutsche Biographie, vol. 8. Berlin: Duncker & Humblot; 1969. p. 617–9.
9. Hering KEK. Orden pour le Mérite für Wissenschaften und Künste. http://www.orden-pourlemerite.de/mitglieder/karl-ewald-konstantin-hering. Accessed 2 Jan 2020.
10. Kelly HA, Burrage WL. A Cyclopedia of American Medical Biography. Baltimore: The Norman, Remington Company; 1920.
11. Faget JC. Wikipedia the free encyclopedia. 2019. https://en.wikipedia.org/wiki/Jean_Charles_Faget. Accessed 4 May 2020.
12. Atkinson WB. A Biographical Dictionary of Contemporary American Physicians and Surgeons. 2nd ed. Philadelphia: D.G. Brinton; 1880.
13. Necrology. Journal Louisiana State Medical Society. New Orleans Med and Surg Jour 1884-1885;12:577.
14. Faget JC. The Type and Specificity of Yellow Fever Established with the Aid of the Watch and Thermometer with Tables of Pulse and Temperature. Paris: J.-B. Baillière; 1875.
15. Faget JC. Monographie sur le type et la spécificité de la fièvre jaune établis avec l'aide de la montre et du thermomètre. Paris: J.-B. Baillière et fils; 1875.
16. Duffy J. The Rudolph Matas History of Medicine in Louisiana, vol. 11. Baton Rouge: Louisiana State University Press; 1962.
17. Touatre J. Yellow Fever: Clinical Notes. Translated from the French by Charles Chassaignac, MD. New Orleans: New Orleans Medical and Ltd; 1889.
18. Blair D. Some Account of the Last Yellow Fever Epidemic of British Guiana. 3rd ed. John Davy, editor. London: Longman, Brown, Green and Longmans; 1852.
19. Ye F, Hatahet M, Youniss MA, Toklu HZ, Mazza JJ, Yale S. The clinical significance of relative bradycardia. WMJ. 2018;117:73–8.
20. Gurunluoglu R, Shafighi M, Huemer GM, Gurunluoglu A, Piza-Katzer H. Carl Nicoladoni (1847–1902): professor of surgery. Surgical Retrospections. Ann Surg. 2004;239(2):281–92.
21. Foucher G. Osteocutaneous reconstruction and pedicled toe transplantation in Central Europe. In: Reconstructive Surgery in Hand Mutilation. London: Martin Dunitz Ltd; 1997. p. 10.
22. Fang F, Chung KC. An evolutionary perspective on the history of flap reconstruction in the upper extremity: flap reconstruction of the traumatized upper extremity. Hand Clin. 2014;30:109–23.
23. JWW. Upson: insomnia and nerve strain. Am J Med Sci. 1909;137:437.
24. Mostofi SB. Carl Nicoladoni, 1847-1902. Who's Who in Orthopedics. London: Springer; 2005.
25. Payr E. Carl Nicoladoni: ein Nekrolog. Deutsche Ztshr f Chir. 1908;68:1–12.
26. Nicoladoni C. Phlebarteriectasie der rechten oberen Extremität. Arch f klin Chi. 1875;18:252–73.
27. Israel JA. Veröffentlicht von Onmeda-Redaktion. 01 April 2014 Onmeda.de für meine Gesundheit 1926.

28. [No author]. The reform advocate. America's Jewish Journal. 1916;50:789.
29. Israel JA, German surgeon. https://www.sciencesource.com/archive/James-Adolf-Israel-German-Surgeon-SS2515414.html. Accessed 20 Feb 2020.
30. Israel JA. Beobachtung einiger bemerkenswerther Phänomene nach Unterbindung der A. femoralis. Arch klin Chir. 1877;21:109–31.
31. Sharma A, Swan KG. Branham's bradycardia reaction. Ann Vasc Surg. 2010;24:295–8.
32. Branham, Harris Miller, MD. In: Georgia, comprising sketches of counties, towns, events, institutions, and person arranged in cyclopedic form. Allen D. Candler and Clement A. Evans editors. 1906. p. 219–20.
33. [No author]. Obituary: Harris Miller Branham. J Med Assoc Ga. 1939;28:35.
34. Branham HH. Aneurismal varix of the femoral artery and vein following a gunshot wound. Int J Surg. 1890;3:250–1.
35. Boland FK. The First Anesthetic: The Story of Crawford Long. Athens: University of Georgia Press; 1950.
36. Hurst W, Harris H. Branham. In: Profiles in Cardiology. Hurst JW, Conti CR, Fye WB editors. Mahwah, NJ: Foundation for Advances in Medicine and Science, Inc; 2003, p. 183–4.
37. Huang HD, Waks JW, Josephson ME, Zimetbaum P. Persistent sinus node suppression caused by thrombotic occlusion of an arteriovenous fistula: a report of two cases. Heart Rhythm Case Rep. 2015;1:190–2.
38. Summer DS. Hemodynamics and pathophysiology of arteriovenous fistulas. In: Vascular Surgery, vol. 2. 4th ed. Philadelphia: W.B. Saunders; 1995. p. 1166–91.
39. Lanken PN, Manaker S, Kohl B, Hanson CW. Intensive Care Unit Manual. Paul N Lankin editor. Philadelphia: Elsevier; 2013.
40. Schapiro G. Klinische Untersuchungen über den Einfluss der Körperstellung und Compression peripherer Arterien auf die Herzthätigkeit. Arzt Red Manassein Bd U. 1881;10-11:13-30. [article in Russian].
41. Schapiro. Physiologie der Bewegung, der Wärmebildung und der Sinne. Herz, Gefhasse. Jahresbericht über die Fortschritte der Anatomie und Physiologie 1881;2:60–3.
42. Low PA, Tomalia VA. Orthostatic hypotension: mechanism, causes, management. J Clin Neurol. 2015;11:220–6.
43. Ricci F, De Caterina R, Fedorowski A. Orthostatic hypotension: epidemiology, prognosis, and treatment. J Am Coll Cardiol. 2015;66:848–60.
44. Robertson D. The pathophysiology and diagnosis or orthostatic hypotension. Clin Auton Res. 2008;18(Suppl 1):2–7.
45. Jorissenne G. Wikipedia. La encyclopedia libre. 2018. https://es.wikipedia.org/wiki/Gustave_Jorissenne. Accessed 12 Aug 2019.
46. [No author]. International congress of hydrology and climatology. Med Rec. 1908;23:308.
47. Jorissenne. Nouveau signe de la grossesse. Arch de Tocol. 1882;21:327–42, 397–417, 733–45.
48. Del Bene R, Barletta G, Mello G, Lazzeri C, Meccacci F, Paretti E, et al. Cardiovascular function in pregnancy: effect of posture. BJOG. 2001;108:344–52.
49. Kleinsorge H. Prof. Dr. med. Felix Lommel 80 Jahre. Dtsch Gesundheitsw. 1955;10:1333–4.
50. Kleinsorge H. Felix Lommel zum 90. Geburtstag. Med Klin. 1965;60:1467–8.
51. Lommel F. Klinische Beobachtungen über Herzarhythmie. Deutsches Archiv für klin Med. 1902;72:465–503.
52. Mannkopff EW. Marburger Professorenkatalog online. Archiv der Philipps-Universität Marburg. November 2017.
53. Mannkopff E. Wikipedia die freie enzyklopädie. https://de.wikipedia.org/wiki/Emil_Mannkopff. 2020. Accessed 4 Mar 2020.
54. Leopoldina. Amtliches organ der Kaiserlichen Leopoldino-Carolinischen deutschen akademie der naturforscher.1893;29:14.
55. Heβ O. Emil Wilhelm Mannkopff: zu seinem 70. Geburtstage. Deutsche med Wchsnschr. 1906;32:926–7.
56. Schmidt-Rimpler. Aerztlicher Vereim zu Marburg, Sitzung vom 14. Januar 1885. Berliner klin Wchnschr. 1886;23:147.

57. Rumpf. Die Beeinflussung der Herztätigkeit und des Blutdrucks von schmerzhaften. Münch med Wochenschr. 1907;54:153–6.
58. Sand R. Stimulation de la douleur. In: La stimulation et l'interprétation des accidents du travail. Paris: Maloine; 1907. p. 286–93.
59. Lombroso C. Algometria elettrica nell'uomo sano ed alienato. In: Annali Universali di Medicina. Milano; 1867. p. 102–21.
60. Terkelsen AJ, Mølgaard H, Hansen J, Andersen OK, Jensen TS. Acute pain increases heart rate: differential mechanisms during rest and mental stress. Auton Neurosci. 2005;121:101–9.
61. Tousignant-Laflamme Y, Rainville P, Marchand S. Establishing a link between heart rate and pain in healthy subjects: a gender effect. J Pain. 2005;6:341–7.
62. Valencia C, Morales F, Gurovich A. Gender differences in cardiovascular reactivity to experimental pain assessment in pain-free adults. J Pain. 2019;20:558–9.
63. Walker LS, Stone AL, Smith CA, Bruehl S, Garber J, Puzanovova M, Diedrich A. Interacting influences of gender and chronic pain status on parasympathetically medicated heart rate variability in adolescents and young adults. Pain. 2017;158:1509–26.
64. Dr. Bernhard Aschner. Geni. 2019. https://www.geni.com/people/Dr-Bernhard-Aschner/6000000018569068317. Accessed 26 Sep 2019.
65. Bettendorf G. Aschner, Bernhard. In: Zur Geschichte der Endokrinologie und Reporducktionsmedizin. Bettendorf G. editor, Berlin: Springer; 1995. p. 15–6.
66. HE. Bernhard Aschner. Martin-Luther-Universität Halle-Wittenberg. 2020. https://www.catalogus-professorum-halensis.de/aschnerbernhard.html. Accessed 15 Sep 2019.
67. Medvei VC. The birth of endocrinology. In: A History of Endocrinology, Part II. Lancaster, England: MTP Press Limited; 1984. p. 289–352.
68. Absolon KB. Dr. Bernhard Aschner: surgeon, scientist, and scholar (1883-1960). Surgery. 1960;48:979–83.
69. Porsch H. Bernhard Aschner. Memorial Book for the victims of the National Socialism at the University of Vienna in 1938. https://gedenkbuch.univie.ac.at/index.php?id=index.php?id=435&no_cache=1&L=2&person_single_id=32749. Accessed 2 Sep 2019.
70. Castiglioni A. The Renaissance. In: A History of Medicine. Translated from the Italian and New York: Alfred A. Knopf; 1941. p. 408–503.
71. Aschner B. Ueber einen bisher noch nicht beschriebenen Reflex vom Auge auf Kreislauf und Atmung. Wien klin Wchnschr. 1908;21:1529–30.
72. Başağaoğlu B, Steinberg A, Tung IT, Olorunnipa S, Maricevich RS. Oculocardiac reflex as a late presentation of orbital floor fracture. J Craniofac Surg. 2018;29(7):e720–2.
73. Reddy SS, Landry JP, Douglass K, Venugopalan PP. A case of ocular cardiac reflex in a child with blunt ocular trauma. BMJ Case Rep. 2014;bcr2014206246. Published 2014 Nov 24.
74. Ha SG, Huh J, Lee BR, Kim SH. Surgical factors affecting oculocardiac reflex during strabismus surgery. BMC Ophthalmol. 2018;18(1):103.
75. Baek HI, Park BC, Kim WH, Son WS. Oculocardiac reflex during the endoscopic sinus surgery. Am J Otolaryngol. 2010;31(2):136–8.
76. Seshubabu G. The oculocardiac reflex in cataract surgery in the elderly. Br J Ophthalmol. 1998;82(5):589.
77. Van Brocklin MD, Hirons RR, Yolton RL. The oculocardiac reflex: a review. J Am Optom Assoc. 1982;53(5):407–13.
78. Dewar KM. The oculocardiac reflex. Proc R Soc Med. 1976;69(5):373–4.
79. Dunville LM, Kramer J. Oculocardiac reflex. In: StatPearls. Treasure Island, FL: StatPearls Publishing; 2020.
80. Prével M. Le réflexe abdomino-cardiaque: essai sur l'un des facteurs de l'accélération cardique orthostatique. Paris méd. 1917;23:138–43.
81. Cantelli O. Di una varietà del riflesso oculo-cardiaco (Riflesso oculo-cardiaco paradossale). Riforma Med. 1917;33:487–90.
82. Ruggeri E. Modificazioni del polso per l'Ocuylo-convergenza protratta in alcuine con dizioni morbose (Di un nuovo riflesso oculo-cardiaco). Riforma Med. 1920;36:1029–34.
83. Herz M. Eine Funktionsprüfung des kranken Herzens. Deutsche med Wchnschr. 1905;31:215–8.

84. Motlagh M, Geetha R. Physiology, accommodation. In: StatPearls. Treasure Island: StatPearls Publishing; 2020.
85. Mouquin M. Laubry Charles. Comité des travaux historiques et scientifiques. Institut rattaché à l'École nationale des chartes. Fiche créée le 16 janvier 2013, https://cths.fr/an/savant.php?id=112622. Accessed 2 Aug 2019.
86. Debré MR. Notice sur la vie et les travaux de Charles Laubry (1872–1960), membre de la section de médecine et chirurgie: déposée en la séance du 23 mars 1964. Paris: Institut de France; 1964. p. 91–110.
87. Bedford DE. Charles Laubry, 1872-1960. Br Heart J. 1961;23:215–8.
88. Trail RR. Charles Laubry. Lives of the fellows. Royal College of Physicians. vol. V, p. 239. http://munksroll.rcplondon.ac.uk/Biography/Details/2654. Accessed 1 Aug 2019.
89. Laubry C, Routier D, Van Bogaert A. Deux signes cliniques nouveaux de la tachycardie auriculaire. Archives des Maladies du Coeur. 1932;25:321–38.

Chapter 14
Pulsation

Introduction

Pulsation in clinical medicine refers to the alternating outward displacement and inward retraction of an organ or structure. Pulsations found during the physical examination are an observed or palpable phenomenon. Those occurring in relationship to an aneurysm are covered in chapters "Aneurysms", "Physical Signs and Medical Eponyms of Pericarditis: Inspection", and "Pulse". Presented in this chapter are the remaining eponymous pulsations that include those found at the internal jugular vein, temporal artery, or left atrium.

Signs

Bamberger Sign

Historical information on Heinrich von Bamberger (1822–1888) has been previously described based on another sign which he identified in patients with pericarditis (see chapter "Physical Signs and Medical Eponyms of Pericarditis: Percussion"). Bamberger believed that there are two types of internal jugular venous pulsations:

> So far it was believed that the jugular vein could only be seen in the case of tricuspid valve insufficiency. Accordingly, I regarded it as a pathological sign of the latter. This view, as newer observations have shown me, is erroneous or rather is valid only in certain cases. You have to be able to differentiate two types of pulsation of the jugularis, the one I call Vein Pulse and other the pulsation of the Bulb. In the latter case, the cervical valves are sufficient, but in the former they are insufficient [1, p. 233]. (…) Regarding the auscultatory phenomena they behave differently in the two types of venous pulses. In pulsation of the bulb, I found a clear, albeit dull, systolic tone in all cases, which sometimes, especially with strong cardiac activity, can be felt clearly with the finger. Its greatest intensity is at the exact location of the valve and is, beyond a doubt, the jugular vein valve sound. With decreasing

S. H. Yale et al., *Cardiovascular Eponymic Signs*,
https://doi.org/10.1007/978-3-030-67596-7_14

> strength and intensity of the heart movement, both the clarity of the pulsation at the bulb and that of the valve sound decrease accordingly and may even temporarily disappear [1, p. 234]. The typical venous pulse with an insufficient valve is sometimes accompanied by no auscultatory phenomenon. More commonly, especially with strong cardiac activity, a systolic noise is heard and vibrations felt on the finger. Both the noise and vibrations always seemed to me to be clearest and strongest at the place where the valves are located. Therefore, I have no doubt that insufficient valves are the source of the noise at the jugular vein [1, p. 235].

Bamberger was the first to graphically record the venous pulse. He showed that "inspiration corresponded to lowering and expiration to an elevation of the pulse curves." [1, p. 240]. Thus, Bamberger recognized that internal jugular venous pulsations may occur in insufficiency and non-insufficiency of the tricuspid valve, differentiated their features, and presumed pathogenesis [2] (Table 14.1).

Danis Sign

We were unable to locate any historical information on Dr. Léon Danis. One should not confuse his name with Léon Denis, a spiritual philosopher who also focused on the meaning of death. He presented his findings first in a seven-page booklet entitled *D'un signe certain et immédiat de la mort réelle* (Of a certain and immediate sign of real death) in 1869 [3], then an abstract of his findings appeared in the *London Medical Record*, describing a sign of death that involves:

> [d]enudation and section of the artery–by a surgeon. This axiom is laid down by Dr. Danis, and will not be disputed by physiologists. 'The artery empty, the heart is dead; the heart dead, the whole body has ceased to live'. (…) The temporal artery, by reason of its nearness to the surface may be selected for the operation, as also for the slight degree in which it retracts. When the artery has been exposed, its colour should be observed; after death it becomes of a yellowish or orange colour; during life it has the colour of surrounding textures. Its pulsations, if any exist, may then be observed; but it may be noted that the sudden exposure to the air sometimes stops the pulsations; from this, however, it will soon recover, if life be not extinct. In the dead body, the artery will gape when divided, and little or no blood will flow, other than a few coagula. If the blood should flow by jets, a compress will restrain it. If it be objected that the patient may be too feeble for the heart to propel the blood, then it follows that it is too feeble to supply the brain with blood, and death must follow [4].

Thus, Danis sign is an archaic and outdated term for determining the presence of death. It is of interest for historical purposes only (Table 14.1).

Table 14.1 Signs of medical eponyms of pulsation in cardiovascular disease

Name	Year	Description of sign
Bamberger [1]	1863	Visual venous pulsations in the internal jugular vein.
Danis [3]	1869	Surgically expose and observe the temporal artery for pulsation.
Inverted Broadbent [16]	1933	Visible and palpable pulsation in the left posterior lateral intercostal spaces.

Inverted Broadbent Sign or Broadbent Inverted Sign

Several references suggest that the terms "Broadbent sign" and "Broadbent inverted sign" are synonymous and are eponymously attributed to findings described in association with adherent pericardium [5, 6]. Others attribute Broadbent inverted sign to "pulsation synchronizing with ventricular systole on the posterior lateral wall of the chest in gross dilation of the left atrium" [7, 8], posterior-lateral systolic pulsation of the left hemithorax secondary to an aneurysm of the left ventricle [9], or pulsations involving the left posterior lateral wall in patients with left ventricular hypertrophy [10]. Our evaluation showed that Sir William Henry (WH) Broadbent, father of Walter B (WB), and John Francis Harpin (JFH) Broadbent described left lateral chest wall retraction at the 11th and 12th ribs caused by adherent pericardium [11–13] (see chapter "Pericarditis: Physical Signs and Medial Eponyms of Inspection") and Sir WH and JFH Broadbent described a left lateral pulsation occurring at the second or third parasternal intercostal space in patients with aneurysm involving the anterior arch of the aorta (see chapter "Aneurysms") [14, 15]. Based on the date of publications, Sir WH Broadbent should be eponymously honored for these initial discoveries.

Ramón Lorenzo observed and palpated in a patient, "One of the symptoms presented by our patient is what we call 'inverted Broadbent sign', that is, a perfectly visible and palpable pulsation in the left posterior lateral intercostal spaces." [16, p. 469]. Lorenzo believed that "The enlargement of the left atrium would alter the conditions of the elastic wall-lung balance causing a certain degree of atelectasis of the latter." [16, p. 469]. He postulated:

> In the case of severe mitral regurgitation these increases and decreases in volume are synchronous with systole and ventricular diastole. Atrial pulsation are transmitted through the air to the elastic and atelectatic tissue of the left lung, which in turn transmits them to the posterior and lateral wall of the left hemithorax making them perceptible to inspection and palpation [16, p. 470].

Thus, there are two Broadbent signs and an inverted Broadbent sign. The former refers to either (i) the tugging or retraction of left false ribs posteriorly occurring during systole in patients with adherent pericardium or (ii) left lateral pulsation occurring at the second or third parasternal intercostal space in patients with an aortic aneurysm involving the anterior arch [11–15]. In contrast, the inverted Broadbent sign refers to the visible and palpable pulsation in the left posterior-lateral intercostal space occurring in patients with left atrial enlargement and severe mitral regurgitation (Table 14.1). Presumably the name was chosen as it was opposite to the retraction, but in the same location on the chest wall, initially described by Sir WH and JFH Broadbent.

Conclusion

Visual and palpable pulsation in the left-posterior intercostal space on the chest wall, temporal artery, and internal jugular vein provided additional clues to physicians regarding the underlying disease process or in the case of the temporal artery a confirmatory sign of death. Bamberger's observations and contributions related to the internal jugular vein were important in that it lead to the recognition that other disease processes such as tricuspid stenosis as well as junctional, premature ventricular contraction, and complete heart block, in addition to tricuspid insufficiency, may cause venous pulsation.

References

1. Bamberger H. Beobachtungen über den Venenpuls. Wurzb med Ztschr. 1863;4:232–48.
2. Kelly A. Venous phenomena. North N Y Med J. 1896;63:72–7.
3. Danis L. D'un signe certain et immédiat de la mort réelle. Paris: Adrien Delahaye; 1869.
4. Kesteven WN. Danis on a certain and immediate sign of death. London Med Rec. 1874;2:226.
5. Broadbent, Sir William H. The free dictionary by Farlex (cited. 3 Aug 2019). Available from: https://medical-dictionary.thefreedictionary.com/Broadbent+syndrome. Accessed 12 Jul 2020.
6. Bartolucci S, Forbis P. Broadbent. In: Stedman's Medical Eponyms. 2nd ed. Baltimore: Lippincott Williams & Wilkins; 2005. p. 101.
7. White FA. Physical Signs in Medicine and Surgery: An Atlas of Rare, Lost and Forgotten Physical Signs. Ocala: Museum Press Books; 2009.
8. Robertson WE, Robertson HF. Diagnostic Signs, Reflexes and Syndromes. Philadelphia: F.A. Davis; 1940.
9. Birrer RB, Birrer CD. Medical Diagnostic Signs: A Reference Collection of Eponymic Bedside Signs. Springfield, IL: C. Thomas; 1982.
10. Farkin BG, Whitworth JA. Dictionary of Medical Eponyms. Canforth, NJ: The Parthenon Publishing Group; 1987.
11. Broadbent WH. Adherent pericarditis. Trans Med Soc. 1898;21:109–22.
12. Broadbent JFH. Adherent Pericardium. London: Baillière, Tindall and Cox; 1895.
13. Broadbent WH, Broadbent JFH. Adherent pericardium. In: Heart Disease with Special Reference to Prognosis and Treatment. London: Baillière, Tindall and Cox; 1897. p. 220–5.
14. Broadbent WH. The pulse in aneurism. In: The Pulse. London: Cassell; 1890. p. 227–35.
15. Broadbent WH, Broadbent JFH. Heart Disease and Aneurysm of the Aorta with Special Reference to Prognosis and Treatment. 4th ed. New York: William Wood & Company; 1906.
16. Lorenzo R. El signo de Broadbent invertido en un caso de dilatación aneurismática de la aurícula izquierda. Rev Méd Lat Amer B Air. 1933–34;19:469–78.

Chapter 15
Sound

Introduction

Auscultation is the term derived from the Latin *auscultare* meaning to listen or hear with attention [1]. The term "auscultation" was first coined by Anuce Foës (1528–1595) to describe the immediate or "direct method" of placing the ear directly against the chest wall when translating Hippocrates' (c.460 BC–c.370 BC) *Opera Omnia* [1]. It was René Laënnec (1781–1826) who is credited for developing the stethoscope in 1816, reporting his results to the French Academy of Sciences in 1818, and published the findings in his book *De L'Auscultation Médiate* in 1819, thus paving the way for indirect auscultation [1, 2]. Covered in this chapter are adventitious sounds including gallop and splitting of the second heart sound, fetal heart sounds, and those either transmitted to the abdomen or heard within the precordium in patients with ruptured viscus or appendicitis, respectively.

Signs

Mayor Sign

Georges François Isaac Mayor (1779–1854) was born in Château de Bière, Canton Vaud, Switzerland, and received his certification for medical practice at the College of Medicine, Lausanne, Switzerland in 1802 [3]. His son, also named Georges François Isaac Mayor (1818–1899), was a physician who practiced in Geneva, Switzerland [4]. From 1802 to 1808, he practiced medicine in Vevey, Switzerland [5]. He was granted a medical degree from the University of Montpellier in 1808, expedited because of his prior training, certification, and recommendations [3, 5]. It was at Montpellier where he met Georges Cuvier (1769–1832) who sparked his interest in natural history [3]. In 1808, he returned to Geneva, Switzerland,

S. H. Yale et al., *Cardiovascular Eponymic Signs*,
https://doi.org/10.1007/978-3-030-67596-7_15

Table 15.1 Sounds of medical eponyms

Name	Year	Description of sign
Mayor [6]	1818	Auscultation of the fetal heartbeat by immediate auscultation when the ear is placed against the gravid uterus.
Bouillaud [15]	1835	Metallic tinkling or ringing sound in patients with cardiac hypertrophy.
Sansom [16]	1881	Splitting of the second heart sound in moderate-to-severe mitral stenosis.
Mannaberg [29]	1894	Accentuation of the pulmonic component of the second heart sound in acute appendicitis.
Claybrook [33]	1914	Cardiac and pulmonary sounds heard on auscultation of the abdomen in cases of a ruptured viscus.

continuing his medical practice [5]. He was the recipient of the Geneva Civil Rights Award for his services performed during the typhoid epidemic of 1814, founding member of the Swiss Society of Natural Sciences in 1815, and cofounder of Musée academique Genève in 1818 and Society of History and Archaeology in 1838 [3–5]. He along with Berger served as cosecretary of the Société du Samedi, a local physician organization [3]. He was also a member of the Faculté de Medicine de Genève and cofounder of the *Journal de Genève* in 1826 [3, 5]. His interest extended into the fields of forensic medicine, archaeologist (found the Veyrier station from Magdalenia in 1833), and Geneva's city government (member of municipal, administrative, and Grand Council) [5]. Mayor was the first to identify the fetal heartbeat in 1818:

> Mr. Mayor, a clever surgeon of Geneva, who seemed to us very interested in his relations with the art of childbirth, and with forensic medicine. He discovered that one can recognize with certainty whether a child who has come to near term is living or not, applying the ear to the belly of the mother; if the child is alive, one hears the beatings of his heart very well, and is easily distinguished from those of the pulse of the mother [6, p. 249–250].

Thus, Mayor sign refers to immediate auscultation of the fetal heartbeat by applying the ear directly against the abdomen during pregnancy (Table 15.1).

Bouillaud Sign

Jean-Baptiste Bouillaud (1796–1881) was born at Bragette near Angoulème, France, and studied medicine at École Polytechnique, Paris, beginning in 1814, intern at the Paris Hospital in 1818, and qualified with a medical degree in 1823 [7–10]. In 1823, he served as an intern under the auspices of René Joseph Hyacinthe Bertin (1757–1828) at the Hôpital Cochin, Paris. Bouillaud obtained his agrégé degree and was elected to the Académie de Médecine in 1826 and appointed the Chair of Clinical Medicine, La Charité, Paris and Hôpital de la Pitié in 1831 [7, 8, 10]. He was elected member of the Chambre des Députés (Chamber of Deputies) for Angoulême, France, in 1840, Officer of the Légion d'honneur, France in 1847 (Commander in 1868), and Dean of the Medical Faculty of Medicine, Paris, in 1848

[7, 8]. Bouillaud was president for the Académie des Sciences (Academy of Sciences) in 1862 and First International Congress of Medicine in 1867, and served as a member of the French Academy of Sciences in 1868 [7, 8, 10].

Bouillaud made significant contributions to the fields of cardiology and neurology. He coined the term "endocarditis" and described the anatomical changes found in this inflammatory disease, recognized the relationship between acute generalized articular rheumatism (rheumatic fever) and endocarditis and pericarditis (endopericarditis), retraction of the precordium in cases of adhesive–constrictive pericarditis (Bouillaud sign), cancer and venous thrombosis, splitting of the second heart sound and its relationship to closure of the aortic and pulmonic valves in mitral stenosis (Bouillaud sign), open snap of mitral valve in mitral stenosis, venous hum in chlorosis (anemia), and gallop rhythm [7]. Additionally he studied congenital heart disease and further contributed to the understanding of localization of cerebral deficits [11–14]. As a description of his character as written in his obituary in the *Medical Times and Gazette:*

> [g]ifted with eloquence and a highly combative disposition, while possessed of no mean appreciation of the value of his own labours, there was scarcely a discussion of importance in which he did not take part in the *Bulletin* in those prolonged discussions which Frenchmen seem never to weary in listening to [9, p. 616]. (…) It was felt that there had passed away one of their medical glories of the epoch, and one who amidst a life of controversy, had yet endeared himself to all who knew him, and had cast great lustreon the famous school to which he belonged [9, p. 617].

Bouillaud described the method for reproducing the sound of the metallic tingling of the heart:

> Nothing is easier than to imitate the metallic tingle of the heart. If you apply the palm of your hand to your ear and you lightly strike the back of that hand with the finger of the other hand, you will hear a ringing quite similar to the one we report. The same phenomenon will occur if one finger of the hand is applied to the ear while the other one strikes the part of the head on which it is supported, an experiment already indicated in the work of M. Laennec. The same phenomenon occurs remarkably similar to one walking on a floor in an apartment where a complete silence reigns and the two hands are applied against the ears by their palmar surface. It is to indicate the resemblance of the tingling, determined by the percussion of the heart against the pectoral walls, with that which took place in the preceding experiments that M. Filhos has designated it under the name of auriculo-metallic tinkling. The metallic tingling due to the shock of the heart does not differ from that obtained when the chest is struck in a region which corresponds to a vast cavern filled with air and communicating with bronchi through an opening in the shape of a neck. We can, by a more direct experience, imitate the sound of metal tinkling of the heart. Here it is: apply the ear to a given region of the chest, then strike with a finger another part of this cavity and you will hear a metallic tinkling perfectly similar to that produced by the shock of the heart against the chest. In either case the conditions are absolutely the same except with percussion, instead of it being practiced by the heart from inside out in the experience above, is practiced from outside in through the finger [15, p. 194–195].

Bouillaud elaborated on the significance of this finding:

> The metallic tingling produced by the heart is transmitted through the pectoral walls and intra-thoracic organs following the law which governs the propagation of the other noises which we previously studied. I heard it very distinctly in the region of the infraspinous fossa

> of the left scapula in two individuals with very extensive pneumonia of the left lung. As known, this is a disease that increases the lungs density and easily transmits sounds [15, p. 195].

Thus, Bouillaud sign refers to the metallic tinkling of the heart or the S4 sound heard in cases of cardiac hypertrophy (Table 15.1). Another sign named after Bouillaud describes the depression or retraction of the precordium occurring in patients with adherent pericardium (see Chapter 8, Physical Signs and Medical Eponyms of Pericarditis: Inspection).

Sansom Sign

Historical information on Arthur Ernest Sansom (1838–1907) has been previously described based on another sign he identified in patients with an aortic aneurysm (see Chapter 1, Aneruysm). Sansom is credited for identifying and explaining the pathogenesis for reduplication or splitting of the second heart sound:

> It is undoubted that by far the most common condition in which double sound is heard is mitral stenosis [16, p. 200]. (…) It is obvious, therefore, that mitral stenosis is a condition which especially disposes to reduplication of the second sound, and it is *à priori* probable that in this form of valve lesion there should be some special reason for its manifestation [16, p. 203]. I consider, then, that there is a theory of auricular causation of reduplication of the second sound which is well worth considering and that we have before us as plausible explanations of the phenomenon. A) That it is due to non-simultaneous closure of the semilunar valves in the aorta and the pulmonary artery, respectively. B) That it is the effect of a sudden tension of the mitral valves after the normal second sound [16, p. 202].

Sansom postulated the pathogenesis for this finding in the case of mitral stenosis:

> It appears to me most probable that reduplication of the second sound which occurs in mitral stenosis is apparent, not real, and that it is caused (as is apparent reduplication of the first sound) by sudden tension of the mitral valves [16, p. 204]. (…) In reduplication of the first sound (so-called) this tension is effected by the auricle just before the ventricular systole, and the mechanism for its production postulates a hypertrophied auricle with an inconsiderable degree of stenosis of the mitral aperture. In reduplication (so-called) of the second sound the tension of the mitral curtains is effected early in diastole. The moment the ventricle becomes relaxed after its systole, the blood, retained in a state of tension (the pressure in the pulmonary circuit being heightened) in the left auricle enters with force into the ventricular cavity, and, finding its way on the parietal side of the curtains of the mitral valve, causes these to bulge towards the centre of the ventricle, and in so doing occasions the click of valve-tension, which click, coming so soon after the second sound, closely resembles a reduplication of the latter. The extrusion of the blood being continued, and the force causing such extrusion being reinforced by the auricle, the presystolic murmur is produced [16, p. 205].

What must be kept in mind was that Sansom described this phenomenon prior to the advent of phonocardiography and echocardiography. Although splitting of the second heart sound may be found in mitral stenosis, the reduplicated second sound more commonly resembles the pulmonic closure and the opening snap of the mitral valve [17] (Table 15.1).

Mannaberg Sign

Julius Mannaberg (1860–1941) was born in Budapest, Hungary, and received medical degree from the University of Vienna in 1884 [18, 19]. He worked for Moritz Kaposi (1837–1905), a dermatologist at the Vienna General Hospital in 1887 and from 1887 to 1895 for Herman Nothnagel (1841–1905), an internist at the First Medical Clinic [19, 20]. Here he studied bacteriology which led to the discovery of streptococci as a cause of acute Bright's disease (acute nephritis). He achieved the rank of first assistant at the First Medical Clinic in 1894 [21, 22]. From 1890 to 1892, he was the recipient of the Oppolzer Travel Scholarship to study malaria during the summer months in Istria, Dalmatia, Croatia, Slavonia and Austro-Hungarian monocracy [20, 23]. He published several books related to his findings including *Die Malaria-Parasiten: Auf Grund Fremder und Eigener Beobachtungen Dargestellt* in 1893 [24], *The Malarial Parasites: A Description* based upon observations made by the author and by other observers in 1894 [25], *Die Malaria-Krankheiten* in 1899 [26], and *Nothnagel's Encyclopedia of Practical Medicine: Malaria, Influenza and Dengue* with Leichtenstern and Stengel in 1905 [27].

Mannaberg habilitated at the University of Vienna in 1895 and served as a general internist beginning in 1898, achieving the rank of extraordinary Professor of Medicine in 1902 and Director of the Vienna General Polyclinic from 1917 to 1930 [18, 19]. He was elected to the Royal Society of Tropical Medicine in 1909 [28]. During World War II, he was persecuted as a Jew by the Nazis [18].

In his review of 88 patients with perityphlitis (appendicitis) seen at the Hofrath Nonnagel clinic from 1882 to 1892, Mannaberg identified the finding of "accentuation of the pulmonary sound" in 10 (11%). Since that time, an additional 13 cases of uncomplicated acute perityphlitis were seen, and:

> Among these, the pulmonary sound was accentuated 4 times very loudly, 7 times considerably louder than the second aortic sound; in the two remaining cases the pulmonary as well as the aortic sounds were present. If I exclude the last two from the series of positive cases, a ratio of 11:13 remains [29, p. 210].

Mannaberg accounted for the difference found in the cases reporting:

> It will hardly seem strange that the symptom in question has been perceived so much more often than has been the case in our older case histories. Despite all the accuracy and objectivity in describing the symptoms, the observer's attention is always directed to the point where the disease is located. Therefore it is understandable that we usually immediately assess the status of the heart in perityphlitis in a fairly superficial manner. Incidentally, in the majority of cases I asked my esteemed boss to confirm the findings in order to keep myself personally as free as possible from subjective influence. Therefore, I hold myself entitled to the statement that accentuation of the pulmonary second sound frequently occurs in perityphlitis. As far as I am aware, this finding has hitherto not been previously reported in the literature [29, p. 210].

Mannaberg was unable to explain the pathogenesis of his findings:

> I must confess that I lack any clue as to the explanation for the increase of blood pressure in the small series of patients with perityphlitis. (...) I must therefore forgo an explanation

> of the symptom for the time being. (…) Further observations may teach us, as with the symptom mentioned here in a large number of perityphlitis and other pathological conditions in the abdomen, whether this claim has diagnostic value [29, p. 211].

Thus, Mannaberg sign refers to increased intensity of the pulmonic component of the secondary heart sound in patients with acute appendicitis (Table 15.1).

Claybrook Sign

Edwin Brown Claybrook (1871–1930) was born in Westmorland County, Virginia, and received his medical degree from the University College of Medicine (currently Virginia Commonwealth University School of Medicine), Richmond, Virginia [30]. He served as surgeon for the Western Maryland railroad [31]. He was founder of the Allegany Hospital, member of the Cumberland Board of Health, fellow of the American College of Surgeons, president of the Allegany County Medical Society, and member of the Southern Medical Society [30–32].

Claybrook initially reported in 1904 at the 106th annual meeting of the Medical and Chirurgical Faculty of Maryland, the method to identify whether there is rupture of bowel in cases where there is no visible evidence of injury:

> It consisted in the transmission of the heart and respiratory sounds, so that they could be heard all over the abdomen almost as well as over the chest. The ear was all that was needed to elicit the symptom, and if it was of any special value it was doubly valuable on that account, for often the very life of these patients depends upon the attitude of the doctor who first sees them [33, p. 105–106]. (…) [t]he sign is clear and distinct when it is present and can be elicited without any instrument whatever by anyone who has one good ear. I therefore think it should always be looked for, and when it is present the abdomen should be opened as soon as the patient can be moved to a hospital, or if that is impossible, or too time consuming, as soon as it can be done at home [33, p. 106].

Claybrook described when the sign is present, its duration, and pathogenesis:

> It is present soon after the reception of the injury, and has been noted as early as a half hour after the reception of injury. It continues in unoperated cases as long as twenty-four hours after injury, to my personal knowledge, and may last for days. I believe that it is due to the irritation of the parietal peritoneum by the sudden outpouring of foreign material, as bowel content, blood and urine, into the abdominal cavity [33, p. 106].

Thus, Claybrook believed that rupture of one of the abdominal viscera causes the presence of fluid exudate or blood in the abdominal cavity and the transmission of cardiac and respiratory sounds over the abdomen and chest (Table 15.1). We believe it was the presence of free air within the abdomen accompanying rupture of a viscus that accounted for the increased intensity of cardiac and respiratory sounds.

Conclusion

Laennec acknowledged Hippocrates' use of immediate auscultation as a mechanism to listen to succussion splash in hydropneumothorax. He was bewildered, somewhat dismayed, and humbled that Hippocrates did not further bring this science to the forefront when he wrote:

> If Hippocrates had prosecuted this line of enquiry further, there is no doubt that he would have discovered many valuable truths, had might perhaps have arrived at mediate auscultation itself. But he seems to have proceeded no further than to announce the incorrect observation above quoted, and which his successors appear to have totally disregarded. This seems at first wonderful; and yet nothing is of more common occurrence: It is not given to any man to comprehend all the relations and all the consequences of the most simple fact; and we know that nature's secretes are more frequently betrayed by fortuitous circumstances than obtained by the force of our scientific efforts [34, p. 24–25].

With the development of the stethoscope, a new age was born for the bedside examination of the heart. Auscultation remains the cornerstone and primary skill required in cardiovascular assessment. Through training and practice, determination of the pitch, frequency, loudness, duration of the heart sounds, extra heart sounds (e.g., gallop, clicks and rub), and characteristic of heart murmurs (e.g., patterns, quality, location, radiation, respiratory variation) is used to differentiate and identify the origin of these sounds. The signs described in this chapter as well as from prior chapters on murmurs and the pulse assist physicians in identifying the underlying cause of disease. We recognize the need for further study in order to better understand their role in clinical medicine.

References

1. Skinner HA. The Origin of Medical Terms. Baltimore: The Williams & Wilkin Company; 1949.
2. Laennec RTH. De l'auscultation médiate; ou traité du diagnostic des maladies des poumons et du cœur, fondé principalement sur ce nouveau moyen d'exploration. Paris: Chez J.A. Brosson et J.S. Claudé; 1819.
3. Mayor FI. Copepod cryptography. In: Damkaer DM, editor. The Copepodologist's Cabinet: A Biographical and Bibliographical History, vol. 1. Pennsylvania: American Philosophical Society; 2002. p. 213–5.
4. [No author]. Nécrologie: Dr. I. Mayor Variétés. Rev méd de la Suisse Rom. 1899;19:364–5.
5. Mayor, François-Isaac. Historisches Lexikon der Schweiz. http://www.hls-dhs-dss.ch/textes/d/D14538.php. Accessed 2 May 2020.
6. Collective. Notices des séances de l'Academie royale des sciences de Paris. In: Bibliothèque universelle des Sciences, Belles-Lettres, et Arts, vol. 9. Genève: Imprimerie de la Bibliothèque Universelle; 1818. p. 241–51.
7. [No author]. Obituary. Med News. 1881;39:766.

8. Silverman BD. Profiles in cardiology: Jean Baptiste Bouillaud. Clin Cardiol. 1996;19:836–7.
9. [No author]. Obituary: Professor Bouillaud. Med Times Gaz. 1881;2:616–7.
10. Rolleston JD. Jean Baptiste Bouillaud (1796–1881): a pioneer in cardiology and neurology. Proc Roy Soc Med. 1931;24:37–46.
11. Jacyne LS. Construing science. In: Lost Words – Narratives of Language and the Brain, 1825–1916. Princeton: Princeton University Press; 2000. p. 22–5.
12. Garrison FH. The nineteenth century: the beginning of organized advancement of science. In: An Introduction to the History of Medicine. Philadelphia: W.B. Saunders; 1914. p. 328–593.
13. Lilllicrap D. Introduction to a series of reviews on cancer-associated thrombotic disease. Blood. 2013;122:1687–8.
14. Eling P, Brunia K. Who was the red dean? J Hist Neurosci. 2017;26:111–8.
15. Bouillaud J. Traité clinique des maladies du coeur: précédé de recherches nouvelles sur l'anatomie et la physiologie de cet organ, vol. 1. Paris: J.-B. Baillière; 1835.
16. Sansom AE. On the causes and significance of reduplication of the sounds of the heart. Proc M Soc London. 1881;5:191–210.
17. McKusick V, Webb GN, Humphries JO, Reid JA. On cardiovascular sound: further observations by means of spectral phonocardiography. Circulation. 1955;11:849–70.
18. Jabloner HC. Blimlinger E, Hatschek C, Sutter FG, Zetter P. Dem Bundesminister für Kunst und Kultur, Verfassung und öffentlichen Dienst wird empfohlen, das im Dossier der Kommission für Provenienzforschung "Sammlung Dr. Julius Mannaberg" (3/2014). http://www.provenienzforschung.gv.at/beiratsbeschluesse/Mannaberg_Julius_2014-07-03.pdf. Accessed 5 Apr 2020.
19. Julius Mannaberg. Wien Geschichte Wiki. July 31 2019. https://www.geschichtewiki.wien.gv.at/Julius_Mannaberg. Accessed 25 Mar 2020.
20. Wyklicky H. Mannaberg, Julius. Deutsche Biographie. 16 (1990), pp. 57. https://www.deutsche-biographie.de/pnd127464840.html#ndbcontent, https://www.deutsche-biographie.de/sfz57787.html. Accessed 15 May 2020.
21. Mannaberg, Julius (1860–1941), internist OBL. Australian Biographical Lexicon. Austrian Center for Digital Humanities and Cultural Heritage. http://www.biographien.ac.at/oebl/oebl_M/Mannaberg_Julius_1860_1941.xml. Accessed 10 Feb 2020.
22. Tyson J, Smith AJ. Diseases of the kidneys, bladder and suprarenal capsules. In: Sajous CE, editor. Annual of the Universal Medical Sciences and Analytical Index. Philadelphia: F.A. Davis Company; 1889. p. 3–4.
23. Mannaberg J. Biographisches Lexikon hervorragender Ärzte des neunzehnten Jahrhunderts. Berlin: Urban & Schwarzenberg; 1901.
24. Mannaberg J. Die Malaria-Parasiten: Auf Grund Fremder und Eigener Beobachtungen Dargestellt. Wien: Alfred Hölder; 1893.
25. Mannaberg J. The Malarial Parasites. London: New Sydenham Society; 1894.
26. Mannaberg J. Die Malaria-Krankheiten. Wien: Alfred Hölder; 1899.
27. Mannaberg J, Leichtenstern O, Stengel A. Nothnagel's Encyclopedia of Practical Medicine: Malaria, Influenza and Dengue. London: W.B. Saunders; 1905.
28. [No author]. Year Book – Royal Society of Tropical Medicine and Hygiene. London: Royal Society of Tropical Medicine and Hygiene; 1991.
29. Mannaberg J. Ueber Accenturung des II. Pulmonal-tones bei Perityphlitis. Zentralbl innere Med. 1894;15:209–11.
30. [No author]. Death of Dr. Edwin Brown Claybrook, B & O surgeon at Cumberland for thirty-on years. B & O Magazine. 1930;18:31.
31. [No author]. Int J Med Sci. 1931;44:345.
32. Allegany County Medical Society. Medical society meetings. Bull Med Chir Fac Maryland. 1919;11:134.
33. Claybrook EB. A new diagnostic sign in injuries of the abdominal viscera. Surg Gyn Obstet. 1914;18:105–6.
34. Laennec RTH. Chapter III of immediate auscultation. In: Treatise of the Disease of the Chest and on Mediate Auscultation. Forbes J, translator. 3rd ed. London: Thomas & George Underwood; 1829. p. 24–7.

Chapter 16
Venous Thrombosis: Venothromboembolic Disease of the Lower Extremities

Introduction

Prior to the advent of advanced imaging techniques, physicians devised a variety of physical examination maneuvers, described as signs of medical eponyms, as methods to detect lower extremity deep vein thrombosis (DVT) and pulmonary embolism (PE) or venothromboembolism (VTE). Eponyms are present in the medical literature because they often reflect a simpler and concise way of describing a phenomenon. They are honorific terms ascribed to individuals for their accomplishments, which may include identifying such things as a disease, structure, sign, test, procedure, syndrome, maneuver, medical device, or surgical technique. Eponyms are derived from the name of a person, but not necessarily the first, who reported, described, or significantly contributed to the clinical understanding of the occurrence. The use of eponyms remains controversial and important questions have been raised regarding their appropriateness. Although there have been instances where eponyms were abandoned, the remainder are by and large embedded within the established and contemporary medical literature making their disappearance unlikely.

Physicians used a variety of techniques, described as signs of medical eponyms, as a bedside method for diagnosing DVT as detected through observation, palpation, compression, movement, pressure, sphygmomanometer, or maneuvers performed during the physical examination. The historical context of medical innovation is also tightly interwoven with advances in imaging, which has further led to the evolution of a number of eponyms in PE. Eponymous signs of venous thrombosis of the lower extremities were devised based on enumerating distinct

---

Reprinted, in part, from Thromb Res vol 182, Ye F, Tekiner H, Yale ES, Mazza JJ, Stalvey C, Yale SH, Venothombembolic signs and medical eponyms Part I, pages 194–204;2019, with permission from Elsevier.
Reprinted, in part, from Thromb Res vol 182, Ye F, Tekiner H, Yale ES, Mazza JJ, Stalvey C, Yale SH, Venothombembolic signs and medical eponyms Part II, pages 205–213;2019, with permission from Elsevier.

S. H. Yale et al., *Cardiovascular Eponymic Signs*,
https://doi.org/10.1007/978-3-030-67596-7_16

clinical features found on physical examination including swelling, increased temperature, pulse, venous pain, and tenderness. Symptoms when present are caused by functional obstruction and/or inflammatory changes within the vessel wall.

Physical signs are considered unreliable methods alone for detecting DVT. For those signs that have been studied, there are a number of methodological limitations hindering the ability to draw meaningful conclusions about their accuracy and validity in clinical practice. Nevertheless, some findings when present and used in conjunction with other key signs, symptoms, and aspects of the patient's history may be useful in furthering supporting the clinical suspicion and likelihood of VTE. These signs also provide the means to better recognize the relationship between clinical findings and VTE. The acquisition of historical knowledge about these signs is important as it further enhances our understanding and appreciation of the diagnostic acumen that physicians were required to employ to diagnose VTE prior to the advent of advanced imaging methods.

This chapter provides the readers with a historical perspective and framework of the three factors, as described by Rudolf Virchow, required for thrombosis formation followed by brief biographical information, signs as originally described, and if available, their sensitivity and specificity. Reviewed are both common and less frequently encountered VTE eponyms identified during the physical examination and on radiologic imaging. We divided this chapter into two parts with the first focusing on venothromboembolic disease of the lower extremity and second on cerebral venous thrombosis. We present these signs chronologically based on the year they were first reported. Our goal is to recognize those pioneers whose aim was to advance the field of medicine by identifying methods to diagnose VTE, provide insights regarding the anatomical relationship and pathophysiological processes proposed for each sign, and determine the application of the sign in clinical practice.

Historical Background

Prior to Rudolph Virchow's (1821–1902) description of the three phenomena that account for thrombosis in the pulmonary artery, physicians already began to recognize the importance of movement of blood, inflammation, and substances within blood that lead to the development of a thrombus [1–10]. It was Aristotle (384 BC–322 BC) who initially postulated the existence of factors in blood that promote coagulation and thrombus formation, "There is another kind of ines or fibre that is found in the blood, but not in the blood of all animals alike. If this fibre be left in the blood, the blood will coagulate; if it be removed or extracted, the blood is found to be incapable of coagulation." [11, p. 515]. Virchow is credited for eloquently synthesizing these concepts, based on his own experimental work in dogs' pulmonary arteries, into three principles that have stood the test of time and recalled by physicians as "Virchow's triad." These factors encompass the phenomenon of stasis of blood flow, inflammation, and hypercoagulability of blood. Virchow's name is of historic importance and most highly recognized among physicians as being associated with

VTE. To provide the reader with a perspective regarding his work, we briefly describe his experimental findings and contributions to this field of medicine.

Galen of Pergamon (c.130 CE–c.200 CE) originally introduced the word "thrombosis" which was Greek for "curdling" [12]. However, Virchow is credited for first coining the term "thrombosis" to describe a blood clot when editing *Gesammelte Abhandlungen zur Wissenschaftlichen Medicin* (Collected Treatises on Scientific Medicine) collated in 1910 into a single work entitled *Thrombosis und Embolie* (Thrombosis and Emboli):

> When I was editing the *Handbook of Special Pathology and Therapy* (vol. 1, p. 156), I worked on the section of obstruction and grafting in the vascular system, and decided to introduce a new name. I chose the name thrombosis, as a way to have satisfied the medical terminology [13, p. 482].

Virchow was also the first to use the term "embolia" when describing the processes whereby a loose body or thrombus is propagated in the bloodstream:

> For the question naturally arises how far particular disturbances that can be designated by the name pyaemia may, in the consequence of softening the thrombi, be evoked in the body. To this we may answer that secondary disturbances certainly frequently occur, but not so much by the immediate introduction into the blood of the liquefied softened masses as by the detachment of larger or smaller fragments from the end of the softening thrombus which are carried along by the blood current and driven into remote vessels. This gives rise to the very frequent process upon which I have bestowed the name *Embolia* [14, p. 204].

He reported based on autopsy studies that pulmonary emboli arise from venous thrombi:

> It remains to be explained how primary spontaneous coagulation of blood occurs in the pulmonary artery, since this mode of genesis has been established as a fact by eminent investigators. Such coagulation would be quite similar to what we see occurring spontaneously in the body veins and right heart, and thus, as there, the same conditions would have to be established for their formation. Of course, I limit myself here to the actual primary occurrence of clots, regardless of previous diseases of the lung parenchyma or the vessel walls. I explain from the outset that I am not against the possibility of blood clotting in the pulmonary arteries at all, but only against the possibility of such coagulation developing under the same conditions, or, as one says, for the same reasons as in the veins of the body. If such a possibility existed, an argument which I have made earlier and in which I still believe would be entirely true, namely, that in all cases where old, primary clots were found in the pulmonary artery, upon closer examination, the origin in the veins can be shown. Therefore, pulmonary clots never occur without venous clot and the existence of the former is sure proof of the occurrence of the latter [15, p. 252].

In a series of experiments, he introduced several different foreign substances into the pulmonary artery and accounted for three possible consequences of obstruction within this artery [13, p. 456]:

1. Phenomena of irritation of the vessel and its neighborhood
2. Phenomena of blood clotting
3. Phenomena of the interruption of the bloodstream

Virchow also described the mechanism leading to inflammation of the vessel wall and propagation of a clot:

> My experiments on the artificial obstruction of the pulmonary arteries as well as those about the obstruction of the body's arteries have, in part, shown another way for developing disease. Emboli acting as mechanical or chemical irritating bodies in the vessel walls lead

> to secondary inflammation, which varies according to the nature of the stimulus and can extend far beyond its original location. (…) Previously, we repeatedly identified primary inflammation of the vessel wall and consequent thrombus formation. Here we must dwell on it even more specifically, because it is precisely this form which most closely resembles the doctrinaire notions of phlebitis, arteritis, and endocarditis, and which has been studied by most investigators, without, however, finding a corresponding solution. Here arises the question of how inflammation of the vessel wall produces coagulation of blood. For we cannot allow the view that the mass that fills the vascular lumen is an exudate of the vessel wall. But as for this form of thrombosis we must reject both the view of Cruille, that the coagulation of the blood is the first effect of inflammation, and Rokitansky's statement that the exudate emerging from the wall of the vessel causes blood to coagulate. No one has seen such an exudate. Thus, it will be shown with certainty that inflammation brings its first findings not in the coagulation of the blood, but rather in the alteration of the vessel walls [13, p. 615].

Therefore, a careful analysis of Virchow's work shows that his results were in reference to the pulmonary artery and embolus and not the deep veins of the legs. His discussion and conclusions were in reference to the consequences of thrombosis and propagation of a thrombus (embolus) rather than the development of a clot. He also erroneously believed that a thrombus leads to inflammation, rather than a thrombus occurs as a result of inflammation. Nevertheless, it could be inferred that by determining the consequence of a thrombus, he indirectly discovered and synthesized the properties and conditions that cause VTE.

Signs

Trousseau Sign

Armand Trousseau (1801–1867) was born in Tours, Indre-et-Loire, France, and received his doctorate from the Hôpital Générale, Paris, in 1825 [16]. He was an associate professor in the Faculty of Medicine, Paris, in 1827, and recipient of the Légion d'honneur in 1837. He along with H. Belloc in 1837 were the recipients of the prize essay from the Royal Academy of Paris for their monograph entitled *Traité pratique de la phthisie laryngée, de la laryngite chronique et des maladies de la voix* (A Practical Treatise on Laryngeal Phthisis, Chronic Laryngitis, and Disease of the Voice) [17, 18]. In 1839, he served as a physician at the Hôpital St. Antoine followed by an appointment as Chair of Therapy and Pharmacology [16]. He was appointed professor of the medical faculty and physician at the Hôtel Dieu, Paris, in 1850 [19]. Following his mentor Pierre-Fidèle Bretonneau (1778–1862), he adopted the use of tracheostomy for patients with croup, diphtheria, laryngo-pharyngeal swelling, and suffocation, writing a monograph describing this procedure and intubation in 1851 [20]. He was elected member of the French Academy of Medicine in 1856 and served as chair of Therapeutics and Medical Matters at Charité Hospital in 1864 [16, 21]. Among his other accomplishments, he introduced thoracentesis in 1834, described gastric vertigo, and signs that bear his name related to tetany and thrombophlebitis in patients with cancer [22]. He wrote a series of monographs on clinical medicine delivered at Hôtel-Dieu in Paris in 1861 applying a novel approach to disease based on a case-based study method [21]. In a description of his attributes and character, he was described as:

> [e]xtremely interesting as a professor of materia medica, and impressive as a clinical lecturer. His impressive, chaste, and elegant diction, charmed and fixed the attention of his auditors, equally with the clearness of his thoughts. (…) He pointed out to his most intimate medical friends and favorite pupils the different symptoms and physical signs of his disease, commenting upon the progressive development of the gastric tumor from day to day preceding his death, with the same precision and impressiveness that characterized his clinical lectures in the wards of the hospital [23].

Trousseau acknowledged the occurrence of thrombi in patients with tuberculosis and recognized their occurrence in patients with cancer (Table 16.1):

> A long well known fact that the blood of cachectic persons has a strong tendency to coagulate explains the frequency of coagula in the vessels of tuberculous patients who have reached the cachectic stage of their disease. I wish also to recall to your recollection some of the facts which prove that the same spontaneous coagulation is common in cancerous patients and gives rise to phlegmasia alba dolens. In Saint-Bernard's ward, I had frequent opportunities of observing this phenomenon in women affected with cancer of the uterus. Patients of this description in the last stage of their disease present with symptoms of cachexia, and then, all at once, the inferior extremities become swollen soon after which the saphenous and crural veins can be felt to be hardened. In such cases, it is found on examination after death that their hard condition is owing to cruoric or intravascular fibrin clots [24, p. 286-287]. (…) I have long been struck with the frequency with which cancerous patients are affected with painful edema in the superior or inferior extremities, *whether one or the other was the seat of cancer*. The frequent concurrence of phlegmasia alba dolens with an appreciable cancerous tumor led me to inquiry whether a relationship of cause and effect did not exist between the two, and whether the phlegmasia was not the consequence of the cancerous cachexia. I have since had an opportunity of observing other cases of painful oedema where there existed a cachexia referable neither to the tubercular diathesis, puerperal state, nor chlorosis. At autopsy I found visceral cancer but during life there was no appreciable cancerous tumor. I have thus been led to the conclusion that when there is a cachectic state not attributable to tuberculous diathesis or to the puerperal state, there is probably a cancerous tumor in some organ [24, p. 287].

Thus, Trousseau sign refers to the presence of superficial and deep venous thrombosis in patients with malignancy.

Trousseau sign of malignancy also known as Trousseau syndrome has been named to describe the presence of spontaneous, recurrent, or migratory, venous, and arterial thrombosis at multiple sites (including the superficial veins), microangiopathic hemolysis, nonbacterial thrombotic endocarditis, and cardiac emboli in patients with a known or occult malignancy [25, 26]. We are not aware of any study that evaluated the sensitivity or specificity of the sign. The other well-known sign or phenomenon ascribed to Trousseau is the presence of carpal spasmodic contraction of the hands and digits that occurs after the arterial pulse is occluded for 5 minutes by a sphygmomanometer in patients with tetany and rickets [27]. In this phenomenon the fingers are flexed at the metacarpophalangeal joint and extended at the proximal and distal interphalangeal joints with the thumb flexed and adducted into the palm.

Table 16.1 Venothromboembolism eponymous signs of the lower extremities

Name	Year	Description of sign	Sensitivity	Specificity
Trousseau [24]	1873	Thrombosis at superficial and deep veins in patients with malignancy.	Unknown	Unknown
Mahler [28]	1895	Increased pulse rate without a corresponding rise in temperature.	Unknown	Unknown
Rieländer [38]	1906	Pain elicited with palpable pressure under the inguinal ligament and same side of the abdomen.	Unknown	Unknown
Michaelis [32]	1911	Subfebrile rise in temperature is indicative of a thrombosis.	Unknown	Unknown
Ducuing [48]	1929	Pain elicited with gentle palpable pressure under the inguinal ligament, iliac fossa, popliteal fossa or calf.	Unknown	Unknown
Denecke [57]	1929	Sharp pain located in the posterior region of the plantar arch in the sole of the foot occurring upon standing after prolonged bedrest.	Unknown	Unknown
Olow [59]	1930	Calf is grasped between the knee, lower and middle third of the leg (where the triceps surae forms the Achilles tendon). Sign is positive if pain is felt when forward moderate pressure is applied anteriorly toward the tibia.	Unknown	Unknown
Payr [81]	1930	Pain on pressure over the medial plantar aspect of the foot at the calcaneus inferior to the ankle. Early sign of lower extremity thrombosis being in some cases the only symptom occurring immediately or within 24 hours prior to the development of edema, leg swelling, calf infiltration, and increased resistance of the calf muscle upon passive dorsiflexion of the foot.	Unknown	Unknown
Meyer [83]	1932	Pain upon the compression of posterior tibial vein against the tibia.	Unknown	Unknown
Krieg [85]	1935	Pain upon pressure over the vein in the adductor canal, groin, lower leg, calf, or sole of the foot.	Unknown	Unknown
Westermark [97]	1938	Absent vascularity on chest radiograph in pulmonary embolism.	14%	92%
Pilcher [100]	1939	In patients with an unexplained rise in temperature, uncover both legs for 10 minutes. If thrombus is present, the leg is warmer on the affected compared to the unaffected leg.	Unknown	Unknown
Hampton [107]	1940	Irregular humped shape shadow on chest radiograph in pulmonary infarction.	22%	82%
Homans [113]	1941	Irritability behind the knee, posterior muscle, soleus, and gastrocnemius muscle on forced dorsiflexion of the foot. Incomplete dorsiflexion or involuntary flexion of the knee as the forefoot is flexed.	10–54%	39–89%

(continued)

Table 16.1 (continued)

Bisgaard [136]	1941	Infiltration of the calcaneo-malleolar region causing a deep pressure pain.	Unknown	Unknown
Bauer [140]	1941	Restlessness of the leg and transitory aching of the calf.	Unknown	Unknown
Bancroft [149]	1945	Both knees are semi-flexed with the feet resting on the bed. Palpation of the affected leg reveals edema. Pain is elicited when the gastrocnemius muscle is compressed against the posterior surface of the tibia.	Unknown	Unknown
Moses [152]	1946	Three-part test. Part 1: Using the fingers, firm pressure is applied compressing the calf in an anterior direction to identify the area of venous tenderness. Part 2: Calf is firmly compressed from side to side between the fingers and palm of the hand. Part 3: Brief neurologic examination (alteration in cutaneous sensation, position and vibratory sensation and deep tendon reflexes). Pain elicited by direct compression of an area in the deep posterior calf with the fingers in an anterior direction toward the tibia (part 1 but not part 2) is considered a positive test for DVT. The presence of pain when the calf is compressed between the fingers and palms in the lateral direction suggests involvement of the superficial tissue or muscle rather than the veins.	38%	88%
Neuhof [157]	1947	Patients' heels on bed, knees flexed, and calf muscle relaxed. Palpation reveals thickening and infiltration deep to the gastrocnemius muscle.	Unknown	Unknown
Bailey [161]	1947	Fingertip pressure is applied over each saphenous opening. Using a stroking motion, the finger in the other hand moves inferiorly following the course of the femoral vein. A positive sign is the presence of unilateral segment of localized tenderness.	Unknown	Unknown
Rosenthal [163]	1948	Passively extend the foot up to 45 degrees. If no pain occurs, then plantar flex the toes while holding the foot in extension. Alternatively, the entire test can be performed with both motions occurring simultaneously. A positive test is the presence of pain located lateral to the anterior tibia crest particularly at a point 3 inches above the distal tibia.	Unknown	Unknown
Pratt [166]	1949	Dilated superficial veins located over the tibia.	Unknown	Unknown

(continued)

Table 16.1 (continued)

Name	Year	Description of sign	Sensitivity	Specificity
Lawrence [170]	1950	Coughing, sneezing, or laughing increases pain in an inflamed area in the lower extremity. In cases of either early DVT or in proximal thrombosis, compression of the greater saphenous vein close to the saphenofemoral junction causes pain to disappear when coughing. In case of DVT below the knee, this same maneuver causes the pain to disappear in 50% of cases.	Unknown	Unknown
D'Alessandro [173]	1951	Marked diminution or absence of the femoral pulse.	Unknown	Unknown
Louvel [175]	1952	Pain in an inflamed superficial venous segment in the lower extremity induced by coughing.	Unknown	Unknown
Bellini [179]	1953	Disappearance of the femoral pulse as detected through sphygmanometer and oscillometer and its reappearance using trinitric (nitroglycerin)	Unknown	Unknown
Castañeda [180]	1953	Difference in consistency between the diseased (hard) calf compared to a normal calf caused by muscular edema. Also is described the sign of the toe in which compression of the edge of the first joint of the first toe causes sudden sharp pain in patients with phlebothrombosis.	Unknown	Unknown
Lowenberg [181]	1954	The patient's pain threshold is first determined by inflating a pneumatic cuff on the arm rapidly to 250 mmHg. If pain is experienced, then a reduced pain threshold is detected. A pneumatic cuff is placed over the calf or thigh and slowly inflated (10–15 seconds) to 180 mmHg pressure. If pain is elicited before this, the end point has been reached and the cuff is deflated. Pain, grimacing, or withdrawal of the limb beneath the inflated cuff at 80, 100, or 120 mmHg (60–150 mmHg) is a positive cuff test. In patients with a reduced pain threshold, pain response below 180 mmHg may indicate a false-positive result.	20%	85%
Rose [188]	Unknown	A small region of the skin is pinched due to the presence of thickening of the dermis and subcutaneous tissue caused by early edema.	Unknown	Unknown
Ortiz-Ramírez [162]	1955	Patient recumbent and extremity slightly flexed. A sphygmomanometer cuff is applied above the knee and inflated to 40 mmHg. Pain most commonly occurring in the popliteal region is a positive test and disappears with the deflation of the cuff.	Unknown	Unknown

(continued)

Table 16.1 (continued)

Popkin [193]	1960	Patient recumbent with pain occurring when pressure applied using the index finger or thumb over the anteromedial surface of the leg compressing the tissues between the fingers and underlying bone.	Unknown	Unknown
McLachlin [122]	1962	Unilateral swelling of the left ankle.	73%	Unknown
Lisker [134]	1964	Bone tenderness upon percussion using the flexed fingers on the broad subcutaneous surface of the tibia, medial to the tibia crest.	Unknown	Unknown
Peabody [200]	1964	Patient supine and examiner places the thumb against the second metatarsals on the plantar surface of the feet. Using pressure, raise the feet approximately 20 inches off the bed. The examiner observes for evidence of plantar flexion by noting the relative position of the first metatarsals medially.	17%	98%
Change [205]	1965	Chest radiograph shows widening of the descending pulmonary artery.	Unknown	Unknown
Pataro [207]	1965	Patient in the prone or supine position with the leg flexed on the thigh at a 45° angle. Unidigital pressure is applied at equidistant points from the midline of the calf. A positive test is the presence of fixed-point tenderness detected on the calf.	Unknown	Unknown
May [210]	1969	Patient supine, blood pressure cuffs are placed on both calves and inflated to 150 mmHg. Healthy people report that the pressure is uncomfortable. However, on the thrombosed leg, the patient reports pressure pain, grimaces, and spontaneously withdraws the leg at 80–120 mmHg.	Unknown	Unknown
Davies [211]	1972	Patients' knee flexed to 90° and the foot resting on a flat surface. Palpation of the calves is conducted using the palmar aspect of the hands gently lifting the muscle up and down in order to detect a difference in weight and hardness of the calf muscles caused by intramuscular inflammatory edema.	Unknown	Unknown
Corrigan-Strachan [212]	1973	Inability to fully extend the knee when flexed in the range of 20–25 degree.	Unknown	Unknown
Sigg [214]	1979	Knee extended and downward pressure is applied to the patella using the palmar aspect of one hand while the other hand lifts the heel. A positive test is the presence of pain in the popliteal fossa. This pain can also be provoked by vigorous pressure on the patella with the leg extended on a firm support.	57%	62%
Palla [217]	1983	Chest radiograph shows widening of the descending pulmonary artery.	Unknown	Unknown
McConnell [222]	1996	Regional pattern of abnormal RV wall motion with akinesia of the mid-RV free wall.	70–93%	33–94%

Mahler Sign

There is limited historical information on Richter A. Mahler (1863–1941). His manuscript entitled *Thrombose, Lungenembolie und plötzlicher Tod* (Thrombosis, pulmonary embolism and sudden death) during the postpartum period was part of a two-volume collection of papers written by physicians at the Dresden Gynecology Clinic, Budapest, in 1895 and edited by Professor G. Leopold, Medical Council of Obstetrics and Gynecology [28]. Charles G. Cumston publication "Pulmonary embolus following in operative interference" in 1908 contained a translation of Mahler's original work (Table 16.1):

> In a typical thrombosis the pulse rises and continues to rise while the temperature remains perfectly normal. If there is edema, a thrombotic strand may be palpable, or, if pulmonary symptoms arise the pulse beat reaches its highest point and occasionally the temperature goes up at the same time. While the temperature will be found to fall during the next few hours, the pulse will remain rapid for several days. Sometimes the recognition of thrombosis is made more difficult by a gradual increase in the pulse rate simultaneous with a slight rise in temperature at the very commencement of the process. In such cases however, the diagnosis is pretty certain when there is a marked divergence between the pulse and temperature curves. On the other hand, there are cases where the gradual increase in the pulse rate is not marked, the temperature is normal, and then, again, there may be a small and very rapid pulse. In these cases one should also take into consideration the possibility of a thrombosis [29, p. 287].

Mahler believed that extensive thrombosis within the pulmonary circulation leads to an increased cardiac output and more frequent and weaker contractions of the heart, and that the pulse increases proportionally to the extent of resistance caused by the size of the thrombus and decreases with the formation of collateral circulation [30]. He found that the pulse increases disproportionate to the temperature; after an initial increase, the temperature falls while the pulse steadily increases [31].

Michaelis in his publication on "Prodromalerscheinungen der puerperalen und postoperativen Thrombose und Embolie" (Prodromal signs of puerperal and postoperative thrombosis and embolism) described the relationship between temperature and thrombosis and wrote about the significance of Mahler's sign:

> Zurhelle in Bonn in 1908 dealt with a publication from the Fritsch clinic, especially on thrombosis and embolism after gynecological surgery. This extremely thorough and solid work, which I will have to consult more often, also contains a critique of the sign: "Our observations," it says, do not reveal the significance of Mahler's symptom for the prognosis of a possible thrombosis, and it is, as stressed by others, by no means a characteristic symptom seen. (…) Hell comes in a work from the Herffschen clinic to a similar judgment. Herff himself declared at the 11th Gynecologists Congress, "There is no Mahler sign." [32, p. 73].

Singer found in 35 postpartum cases that a gradual increase in pulse precedes the development of a thrombus and embolism in about 90% of patients, and in a typical case the pulse increases while the temperature remains normal [33]. Richter found that 63% of patients with thrombosis and embolism were positive for Mahler's sign, 34% were indeterminate, and in 2% the sign was completely absent [34]. In an observational study of the pulse and temperature over the first six postpartum days in 125 women with and 2190 women without symptoms of thrombophlebitis, Dilhos and Mach found no difference between the groups in the frequency of occurrence of the "step-like accelerated pulse" or Mahler sign [35]. They also found no difference in the rise of temperature (Michaelis sign) between each group. Regarding the significance of Mahler and Michaelis sign, K.I. Sanes wrote:

> Each of them considers his symptoms pathognomonic of oncoming thrombosis. If such symptoms could be found they would be of great value but unfortunately only a small number of authors confirm Mahler's and Michaelis's claims, most of them discussing these symptoms either deny their existence entirely or consider them rare. These prodromal symptoms therefore cannot be relied upon, although it is worthwhile bearing them in mind and to take advantage of them when they do appear [36, p. 118].

Rieländer in his paper entitled "Ueber Venenthrombosen im Wochenbett" (About venothrombosis in the puerperium) reported that:

> If we examine our cases for the presence of Mahler's sign, we find that in about two thirds of cases, depending on the extent of the thrombosis, it can be detected more or less clearly; in the other cases it is either absent, or it can not be discerned that the overall impression of the pulse curve is already controlled by some febrile disease. It is especially pronounced in case where thrombus symptoms on one leg disappears, only to reappear on the opposite leg. Yes, in these cases, without any other symptoms being present apart from a slight pain in the limb, it could already be seen from the renewed increase in the pulse curve that now the illness also passed to the other side [37, p. 366; 38, p. 163].

This is believed to be an early sign of thrombosis, present before other symptoms occur, and is found in situations where an overt febrile process is not identified [38]. This sign lacks sufficient sensitivity or specificity to be useful when used alone during the clinical examination. However, in the appropriate clinical setting its presence should heighten consideration for the diagnosis.

Rieländer Sign

Wilhelm August Rieländer (1875–1926) was born in Erfurt, Germany, and graduated from the School of Medicine in 1899. After serving as a voluntary assistant for 2 months in 1900, he was subsequently appointed resident in the gynecology clinic at the University Women's Hospital in Marburg, Germany [39]. Between 1903 and 1911, he served as a head of the training of midwifery students and in 1904 received his habilitation in Midwifery and Gynecology [39]. He became chief physician at a field hospital during World War I, and retired as a second midwife teacher in 1920 [39].

Rieländer reported that "pain in the groin, especially under Poupart's ligament" along with "pain to pressure on the corresponding side of the abdomen" is a symptom found in thrombosis of the leg during the puerperium period [38]. This sign lacks sufficient specificity and does not enhance the diagnostic accuracy of the physical examination [40] (Tables 16.1 and 16.2).

Table 16.2 Specific location of the sign of venous thrombosis in the lower extremity

Site in lower extremity
Inguinal ligament
Ducuing
Rieländer
Thigh
Bailey
Bellini
Krieg
D'Alessandro
Lawrence
Louvel
Lowenberg
Popliteal
Ducuing
Homans
Ortiz-Ramirez
Sigg
Leg
Bauer
Bellini
Ducuing
Meyer
Krieg
Lawrence
Lisker
Louvel
Pilcher
Popkin
Pratt
Rosenthal
Calf
Bancroft
Davies
Ducuing
Homans
Moses
Neuhof
Casteñeda-Uribe
Krieg
Lowenberg
Olow
Pataro
May
Foot
Bisgaard
Denecke
Krieg
McLachlin
Payr
Peabody

Michaelis Sign

We were only able to identify limited historical information on Hans Michaelis who served as a gynecologist in Königsberg, Prussia (current Kaliningrad, Russia) [41]. He described in his paper titled "Prodromalerscheinungen der puerperalen und postoperativen Thrombose und Embolie" (Prodromal signs of puerperal and postoperative thrombosis and embolism) the relationship between temperature and thrombosis:

> If I were asked how do you explain these small temperature increases? The expression of what kind of process should they be attributed?, I would say it is a sign that a thrombus is there, which is not organized in the normal way, but is perhaps in the process of dissipating from which even the smallest particles are already crumbling and circulating in the blood. However, without any bacterial involvement the softening can be explained by the increase in temperature. (…) I do not claim that any unexplained occurrence of subfebrile temperatures indicates an embolic risk, but I must say again according to my observations puerperal postoperative thrombosis and embolisms do not occur out of the blue; there is a premonitory symptom in the form of subfebrile temperatures. If this occurs, one must think of the possibility of thrombosis or embolism and act accordingly [32, p. 75].

Michaelis believed that the temperature is altered prior to thrombosis and embolism. According to Michaelis not "every subfebrile temperature is an index of the onset of thrombosis, but anything over 37.5 °C suggests the necessity for caution and close supervision of the patients, guarding them against any violent movement, any excitement, or fright, and keeping the bowels loose with oil injections, a mild laxative, and suitable diet." [42, p. 549].

Faris [43] in a retrospective and prospective cohort of 144 patients who underwent radioactive fibrinogen scan for the detection of calf vein thrombosis found that 20 of 40 patients with thrombi met their case definition of fever as defined by a temperature between 37.4 °C and 38.0 °C, duration of not less than 2 days, absence of fever 24 hours before the suspected DVT and its occurrence after postoperative days 1 and 2. The high false-negative rate was believed to be primarily attributed to thrombi not detected or those of a shorter duration [43]. In a study of 137 patients over the age of 35 years undergoing major abdominal surgery, Doppler ultrasound was performed every other day beginning on the first postoperative day through day 19 or until the patient was fully ambulating. DVT was identified in 8 patients, with fever and DVT present in only 2 patients [44]. In a study previously discussed under Mahler sign, Dihos and Mach also found no difference in the rise of temperature (Michaelis sign) between each group [35]. This prodromal sign appears to lack sufficient sensitivity or specificity when used alone during the clinical examination (Table 16.1). However, in the appropriate clinical setting when other signs and symptoms are present, its presence should heighten consideration for the diagnosis.

Ducuing Sign

Joseph Ducuing (1885–1963) was born in Toulouse, France, and received his Laureate from the Faculty of Medicine, University of Toulouse in 1912 [45]. He served as a physician in the surgical ambulance in Châlons-en-Champagne and Saint-Gaudens from 1914 to 1916 [45]. At the Hôpitaux de Toulouse, he was appointed chief operating physician in 1919, associate professor of general surgery in 1920, and professor and chief surgeon at the Faculty of Medicine in 1922 [45]. He was selected as the director of the Anticancer Centre (Centre Claudius Regaud) in 1929 and founded the regional association for the fight against cancer in 1932 [45]. He was appointed Chair of the Surgical Clinic of Cancer from 1938 to 1940 [46]. He served at the Purpan Hospital in 1946, and was appointed President of the French Association for Cancer Studies in 1952 [47]. The Warsaw Hospital was renamed "The Joseph Ducuing Hospital" in 1979 in his honor [45]. He recorded in his book *Phlébites, Thromboses et Embolies Post-Opératoires* (Phlebitis, Thromboses and Postoperative Embolism) the finding that:

> [p]hlebitis of the leg causes spontaneous pain in three main regions, inguinal, popliteal, and the calf. This pain is most often mild, but it is sometimes severe, deep, dull, gravitational, and continuous, with some intermittent twinges lasting a few days and gradually improving. We have again seen spontaneously painless postoperative phlebitis with pain expressed by gentle pressure on the groin, the popliteal fossa, or the calf. We insist in particular on a small pain sitting behind the inguinal ligament or in the iliac fossa that we systematically look for in all our patients. This pain is of great diagnostic value to us especially when it is located on the left side or when it is associated with either a very slight ballooning of the abdomen, a shiny and edematous condition of the skin, or a slightly exaggerated circulation of the veins [48, p. 99].

There is no consensus in the literature what constitutes Ducuing sign. It has been described in relation to ballottement, shaking, or a back and forth movement of the calf [49–52]. Other authors described Ducuing sign in reference to pain on compression or palpation of either the calf or groin [53–55]. The utility of this sign in clinical practice is unknown (Tables 16.1 and 16.2).

Denecke Sign

Kurt Denecke (1903–1991) studied medicine at the Universities of Göttingen, Würzburg, and Munich, Germany, passing his state medical examination in 1927 [56]. He completed a medical assistant year at Otten (Old Town Hospital) in Magdeburg and from 1928 to 1930 at Aschoof in Freiburg [56]. He received his doctorate based on the paper titled "Condylenfrakturen der Tibia" (Condylar fractures of the tibia) in 1928. He started his surgical training in Schmieden, Frankfurt, in 1930 followed by additional training in 1931 at Goetze and Erlangen [56]. He served as a first senior physician at the Surgical University Clinic, Erlangen, Germany, in 1948, a position which he formerly held prior to WWII in 1937 [56]. He was appointed associate professor at the University Hospital in 1952 [56].

Denecke was the acting director of the clinic in 1954, and chief physician of surgery at the Surgical Clinic, City Hospital Fürth, in 1956 [56].

While serving as a professor of surgery and chief physician at Klinikum Fürth, Denecke described the finding of lower extremity venous thrombosis in his paper entitled "Der Plantarschmerz als Frühsymptom einer beginnenden Thrombose der unteren Extremität" (Plantar pain as an early symptom of incipient lower extremity thrombosis):

> It has been observed that in certain cases, patients who were bedridden for a long time and accidentally get up will experience a sharp pain in the soles of the foot. This pain was usually localized to the posterior area of the plantar arch. Strikingly about 24 h later the clinical symptoms of lower leg thrombosis occur in the affected leg [57, p. 1912].

As to the pathogenesis of the pain, Denecke hypothesized that flexion of the foot causes entrapment of the nerve or pressure on the vascular and nerve bundles leading to ischemia or congestion and dilation of the vessels in the nerve bundles [57]. Hence, he believed that the pain is caused by mechanical mechanisms initiated by foot flexion. He found that plantar thrombosis was found in 2 of 22 cases where there was no clinical evidence of thrombosis of the leg. Conversely, plantar thrombosis was identified in 7 patients, all of whom had clinically diagnosed femoral vein thrombosis. He recommended that in patients with suspected lower extremity thrombosis that patients should routinely be assessed for pressure pain on the medial half on the dorsum of the foot immediately distal to the toes [57]. The utility of this sign in clinical practice is unknown (Tables 16.1 and 16.2).

Olow Sign

John Olow (1883–1948) was born in Malmö, Sweden, and received his medical license in 1910 and doctorate of medicine in 1913 from Lund University [58]. He held a clinical teaching position in obstetrics and gynecology in 1914 and served as first-class marine physician in 1917 [58]. He was appointed professor of obstetrics and gynecology at the Upsala, Sweden Gynecological Clinic, and senior physician in the Obstetrics and Gynecology Department at the Academic Hospital in 1923 [58]. Olow served as a professor of obstetrics and gynecology at the Karolinska Institute, Stockholm, and chief physician and director at the General Maternity Hospital in 1931 [59]. He described an early maneuver for detecting thrombosis of the leg (Fig. 16.1):

> The calf is grasped below the knee between the lower and middle third of the leg, where the triceps surae muscle forms the Achilles tendon. Forward moderate pressure is applied against the tibia. Thrombus is present if the patient feels pain. (…) In general, this sign is present from a few hours to a few days before the appearance of the classic symptoms of thrombosis. However, in some cases, the sign is ephemeral, and so, if you examine it only once or twice you can miss it. If you repeat the exam once or twice a day, it almost always appears on one or the other occasion [59, p. 159–160].

Thus, pain on the pressure of the calf at the junction of the gastrocnemius muscle and Achilles tendon is referred to as Olow sign. The utility of this sign in clinical practice is unknown (Tables 16.1 and 16.2).

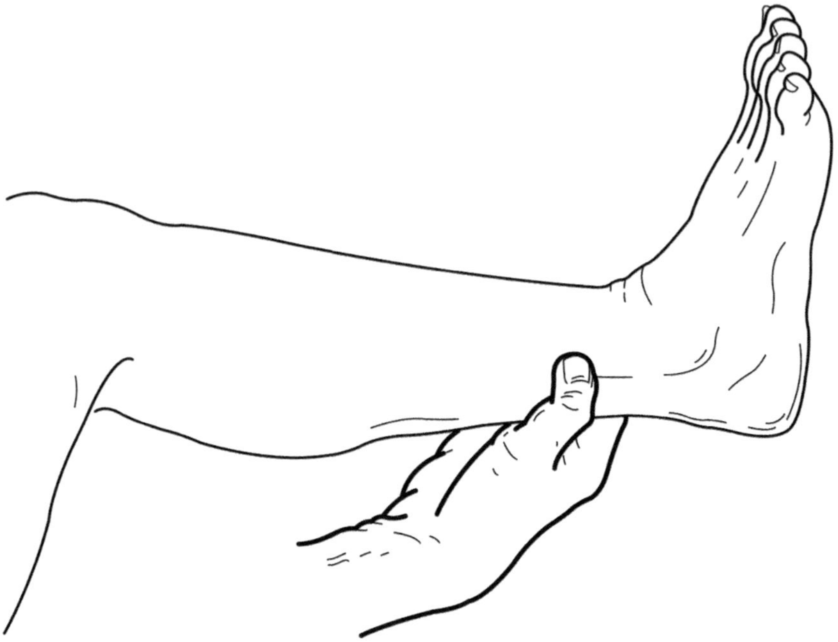

Fig. 16.1 Olow sign (by Ryan Yale)

Payr Sign

Erwin Payr (1871–1946) was born in Innsbruck, Austria, in 1871 and completed his medical training at the University of Innsbruck in 1894 [60, 61]. That same year, he served as an assistant in internal medicine and surgery at the Institute of Pathological Anatomy in Vienna [62, 63]. He served as primary physician in the Surgical Gynecological Department at the Graz Municipal Hospital until in 1906 and was subsequently appointed chair, Department of Surgery, at the University of Greifswald Paul Leopard Friedrich in 1907 [60, 61]. He was appointed ordinarius professor of surgery in Königsberg (Prussia) in 1910 as well as in Leipzig from 1911 to 1936 where he also served as the director of the University Clinic [60, 62]. Payr made a number of extraordinary contributions in multiple therapeutic areas in medicine and surgery. His surgical expertise spanned the fields of orthopedics, neurosurgery, organ transplantation, abdominal, urogenital, otolaryngology, and thyroid surgery [63–78].

Gerhard Tschmarke, an assistant at the Surgical University Clinic of Leipzig under the auspices of Payr as director, reported in their paper titled "Erfahrungen über den Fußsohlendruckschmerz als Frühsymptom der Thrombose" (Experience of foot sore pressure pain as an early symptom of thrombosis) that in 152 postoperative cases, thrombosis was found in 21 (13%) patients. Pain in the sole of the foot was the first among other signs found in 5 of 16 cases and in the remaining was detected simultaneously with the appearance of mild subjective or objective signs of

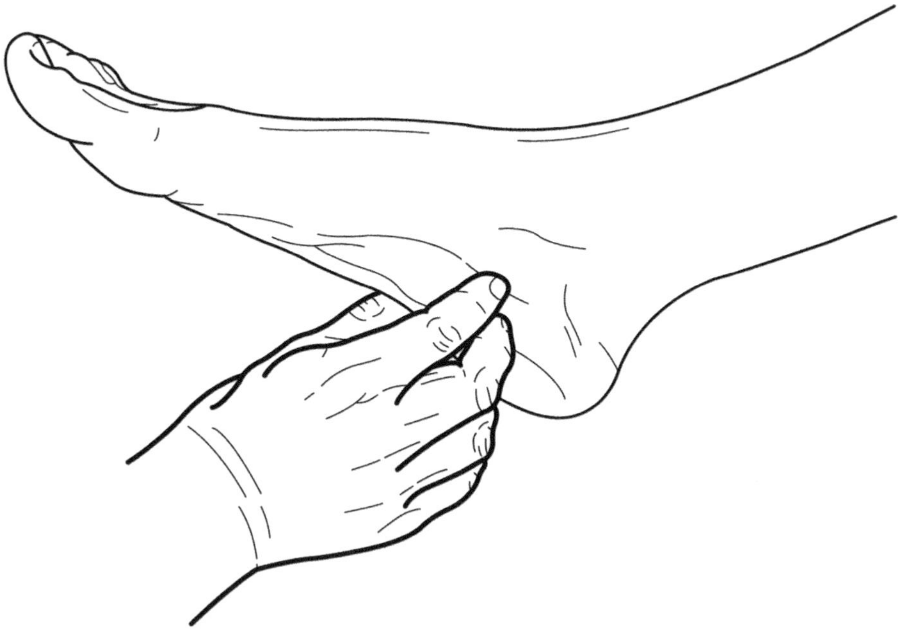

Fig. 16.2 Payr sign (by Ryan Yale)

thrombosis. The sign was absent in 5 cases of thrombosis [79, 80]. He believed that thrombosis in the lower extremity begins at the rete plantar venosum located in the plantar aspect of the feet which contains particularly large numerous vessels [80]. In the description of the physical finding Payr stated (Fig. 16.2):

> Since I have been careful I find more and more often in people with otherwise uncertain picture of a thrombosis and in those with small pulmonary embolism without a clear area of origin of the clot, a noticeable pressure sensitivity on the inside of the sole of the foot from the heel bone just below the inner ankle. A little later the area over the posterior tibial vein, between the tibia and achilles tendon, is sensitive with mild edema and patients sometimes complain of pressure sensitivity over the heel. Passive dorsiflexion of the foot causes pain either alone or with simultaneous pressure on the deep calf veins. On closer examination however, the point of pain is most pronounced at the location described. (…) This foot pressure soreness is a "warning" sign of a developing thrombosis and may indicate a threatening embolism. (…) I find these early symptoms of deep vein thrombosis very important. (…) [81, p. 971].

Tschmarke concluded:

> In the absence of any objective sign of thrombosis one will rarely be inclined to add weight to the patient's information about a sensation of tingling or numbness in the foot, tension in the calf, or heaviness in the lower leg. However, if this information occurs simultaneously with positive evidence of foot pressure soreness then one is more likely to be prepared for the occurrence of thrombosis and not be surprised if within 24 hours or later, the first flawless objective signs of are detectable. Foot pain in the sole of the foot is therefore indeed an early sign of the thrombosis developing in the lower leg [80, p. 926].

Tschmarke acknowledged the importance of recognizing plantar pressure pain as an early manifestation of thrombosis:

> In fact, in the majority of cases, the subjective and objective manifestations of thrombosis were and remain so minor that without the alarming symptom of pressure pain, numerous thromboses would not have been recognized. In the majority of cases, it was only the sudden onset of this symptom that prompted a more detailed examination for objective signs of developing thrombosis, or the rather vague subjective signs of an in-depth examination. Then, either immediately or within the next 24 hours after the onset of pressure pain, it was possible to detect objective signs of the existing thrombosis, such as edema, measurable swelling, calf infiltration, increased resistance of the calf musculature against passive dorsiflexion of the foot. The striking difference in the data on the frequency of postoperative thrombosis is therefore likely to be a proof of the subtlety of the symptom [80, p. 925].

This sign has been reported to lack sufficient specificity and does not increase the diagnostic accuracy of the physical examination [40] (Tables 16.1 and 16.2). It should be recognized that another sign which bears his name is associated with diseases involving the knee. Payr sign of the knee is an increased pain in the medial knee when downward pressure is applied to the knee while the patient is sitting. This sign may be found in patients with disease involving the medial meniscus and its posterior horn [27].

Meyer Sign

There is little historical information identified about Otto Meyer (1896-?) who practiced medicine in New York City. As a well-known specialist of phlebitis and its complication, he published the book entitled *Phlebitis: The Hidden Cause of Most Leg and Foot Ailments* in 1940 [82]. In 1932, Meyer described in his paper titled "Symptomenkomplex und Therapie des Ulcus phlebiticum" (Complex symptoms and therapy for phlebitic ulcers) (Fig. 16.3), "The most precise tender point on the posterior tibial vein is located at the lower third of the leg when pressure is applied pushing the vein against the medial surface of the tibia." [83]. Thus, Meyer sign refers to compression of the posterior tibial vein at the lower third of the leg against the medial side of the tibia. The utility of this sign in clinical practice is unknown (Tables 16.1 and 16.2).

Krieg Sign

Erich Krieg (1902–1970) was born in Germany. He was elected the first president of the German Association for Phlebology (later German Society for Phlebology) and served as chairman of the society whose goals were to train and develop theory and standards for physicians practicing phlebology [84]. In 1959, he was elected the first president of the International Union of Phlebology in 1959 [84]. Since 1975, the Erich Krieg Prize has been awarded to scientists whose work in phlebology

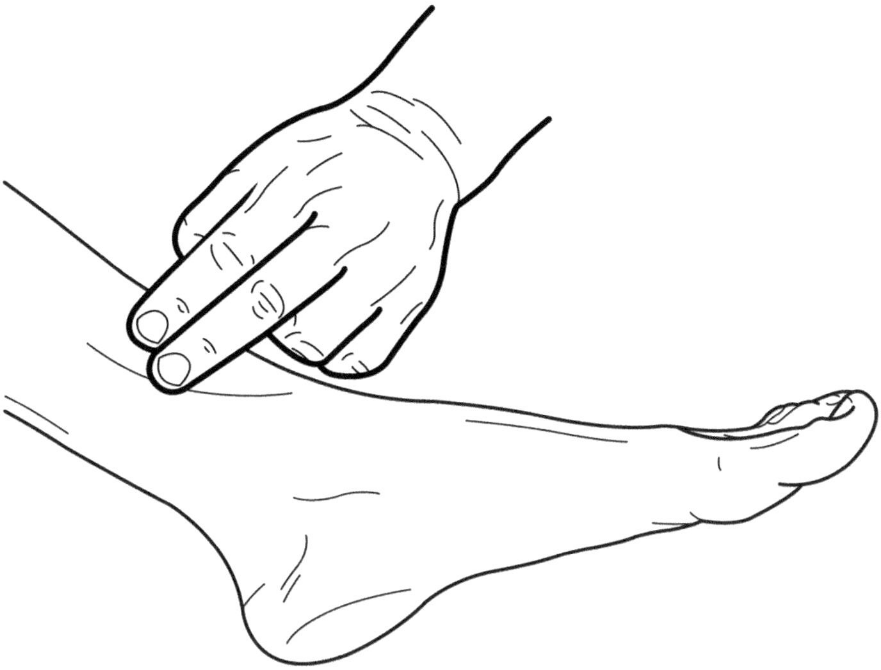

Fig. 16.3 Meyer sign (by Ryan Yale)

serves to advance science and practice [84]. Krieg in his description of venous thrombosis reported that:

> The most valuable early sign is pressure pain in the vein. It can clearly be detected up to 24 hours prior to the appearance of clear signs of thrombosis. It occurs on the thigh mostly in the area of the adductor slit or in the groin, on the lower leg, calf or sole of the foot [85, p. 777].

Thus, pain on pressure over the distal end of the adductor canal (subsartorial or Hunter canal) is a positive sign for the presence of thrombosis of the thigh [86]. We are unaware of any study that assessed the sensitivity and specificity of this sign. The utility of this sign in clinical practice is unknown (Tables 16.1 and 16.2).

Neumann Sign

We have purposely omitted the name Robert Neumann (1902–1962) from Tables 16.1 and 16.2 containing eponymous names due to the atrocities he committed against humanity in the concentration camps as a member of the Schutzstaffel (SS), a paramilitary organization under the Nazi party [87–89]. We have rightfully stated that medical eponyms are intended to be honorific term(s) used to acknowledge the person(s) whom the discovery is attributed. Their use should be reserved and restricted to honor only those individuals who uphold the principles of the Hippocratic oath—*primum non nocere* or "first, do no harm." The honor should not be bestowed upon an individual, regardless of his/her other altruistic lifetime accomplishment(s), to someone who intentionally harmed others by committing research under unethical circumstances or who was involved in atrocities against humanity. Thus, the eponymic sign ascribed to Neumann is ethically inconvenient to be used in medical discourse.

Robert Neumann was born in Nüssdorf, Silesia, and received his medical degree in medicine and musicology at the Universities of Wroclaw and Hamburg, Germany, in 1929 and doctorate from the University of Hamburg in 1930 [88]. In 1932, he was appointed assistant, in 1934 senior physician, and in 1935 director at the Pathology Institute of the Robert Koch Hospital in Berlin [89]. He received his habilitation and qualified as an adjunct professor in 1936 [88]. He joined the SS in 1933, was SS-Untersturmführer (second lieutenant) between 1936–1937, and promoted to SS-Obersturmführer (first lieutenant) in 1938 [88–90]. He was also a member of Lebensborn e.V. (Nazi hygiene and health ideological practices) as well as the National-socialist German Worker's Party (NDSAP) in 1937 which propagated anti-Semitic and nationalism beliefs [90]. In 1940, he established the Pathological Institute at Tongji University in Shanghai, China, a mission established for "cultural-political reasons," and served as its director in 1941 [89]. From 1945 to 1948 he was retained as an allied prisoner [94, 96] and in 1948 worked as a scientific employee for STADA pharmaceutical company, Tübingen, Germany, later serving as the head of the hospital in Reutlingen, Germany [90].

He identified in 163 autopsies of the lower extremities that thrombosis was identified in 100 patients. The lower leg was involved in 87% of these patients with the second most common site being the plantar vein in the foot (71%). He found that the malleolar veins, which connect the plantar from the lower leg veins, were infrequently thrombosed. Thus, Neumann postulated that thrombi originate more commonly in the calf and less frequently in the plantar region. Based on their point of origin, he described a benign and malignant type of venous thrombosis. The benign type originates in the calf and is characterized by an increasing frequency with advancing age, slow progression and multiple, non-fatal pulmonary emboli. The malignant type originates in the plantar veins, occurs early in life, rapidly progresses and ascends to the femoral veins, and is more likely to cause fulminant lethal pulmonary emboli [91].

He proposed that thrombi occur based on the concept of coherent segmentation. The segmentations occur at points where the vein is crossed-over by ligaments, tendons, and bone. Two crossovers named "proximal" and "distal" plantar vein points, caused by segmentation of the veins in the plantar region, are responsible for lateral plantar vein thrombosis. He believed that their identification is important for the early detection of the malignant type of venous thrombosis. The "distal foot pressure pain" was postulated to occur even earlier than the "proximal plantar pressure pain." He further emphasized that people with flat arch (pes planus) are more likely to develop segmented thrombus in the lateral plantar vein compared to those with a normal or high arch (pes cavus) [91].

He described the method for detecting these points: "The proximal plantar vein point is easy to find; it lies close to the malleolus internus next to the calcaneus." [91, p. 722]. To identify the distal point:

> The patient is ideally placed in a prone position. The sole of the foot must - which is important - be at a right angle to the longitudinal axis of the lower leg. The greatest width of the sole of the foot above the heel and over the tarsal bones are divided in half, and the two half points of the plantar skin are connected by a line. Then the medial highest points of the internal malleolus and the medial heads of the metatarsals are marked by crossed lines. A ruler is placed at these two points, the distance of these two points is measured, and at the point of bisection of this line, the vertical is established (by applying a straight rod or pencil to the half point and the medial side of the foot). The distal plantar vein point lies where this perpendicular intersects the halo line of the sole of the foot [91, p. 722].

He believed that the "foot pressure pain" of Payr as described by Tschmarke is a very sensitive sign of early thrombus in the foot and calf and is located exactly after the "proximal plantar venous point." He noted that the "distal foot pressure pain" may appear even earlier than the "proximal plantar pressure pain." He called for further investigation to confirm his findings [91]. The utility of this sign in clinical practice is unknown.

Westermark Sign

Nils Johan Hugo Westermark (1892–1980) was born in Stockholm, Sweden, and received his medical degree in 1919 from Karolinska Institute School [92, 93]. He was a sailor representing Sweden on the boat Sans Atout when he competed in the 1912 Summer Olympics winning the silver medal in the 8-meter class [94]. He served in the Department of Radiology in Sabbatsbergs Hospital (1920–1921), Karolinska Radium Hospital (1922–1923), St. Eriks Hospital (1922–1929), and St. Görans Hospital (1930–1957) [93]. He received his PhD in radiology in 1930 and was appointed associate professor at Karolinska Institute that same year, followed by the title of professor in 1955 [93]. He served as a secretary general of Nordisk Förening för Medicinsk Radiologi (Northern Association for Medical Radiology) in 1933 and between 1946 through 1947 delivered a series of lectures at the University of Minnesota at the Center for Continuation Study on thoracic radiology compiled into a textbook entitled *Roentgen Studies of the Lung and Heart* [95, 96].

Westermark published in "On the roentgen diagnosis of lung embolism" the radiographic appearance of embolism of the pulmonary artery in patients without pulmonary infarction in 1938:

> [i]schaemia of the distributed area of the pulmonary artery on the peripheral side of the embolus or emboli has appeared on the radiogram as a local and well defined clarified zone with diminished or absent vascularization. In an area corresponding to the site of the embolus and on the central side of this the vascular design has been well maintained but seems to stop abruptly. (…) It is clear, therefore, that lung embolism without infarction leads to anemia and diminished vascularization and not hyperaemia and increased vascularization as assumed by previous authors such as Assmann and Frimann-Dahl [97, p. 366-367].

Westermark sign possesses a high specificity (92%) but has a low sensitivity (14%) for the diagnosis of pulmonary embolism. It has a positive predictive value of 38% and a negative predictive value of 76% [98]. Thus, the presence of this radiographic finding suggests the presence of pulmonary embolism; however, its absence does not exclude the diagnosis (Table 16.1).

Pilcher Sign

Robin Sturtevant Pilcher (1902–1994) was born in Middlesex, England, and received his medical degree at the University College of London in 1927 where he subsequently spent his entire medical career. In 1938, he was appointed professor of surgery and from 1938 to 1967 director of the Professional Surgical Unit [99]. He served as the chairman of the Court of Examiners of the Royal College of Surgeons in 1965 and in 1967 was appointed fellow of the Royal College of Physician (FRCP) [99].

Pilcher reported that thrombosis of the leg is diagnosed based on the findings of delayed cooling on exposure, pain, tenderness, and slight fullness and cyanosis of the superficial veins. The delayed cooling test is performed by:

> A patient has an unexpected rise of temperature and the legs are exposed for ten minutes, even if they look normal. A marked difference of temperature is suggestive of thrombosis, the thrombosed leg being warmer, and I do not remember any case showing this sign alone which did not subsequently develop others [100, p. 629].

He emphasized, "This test is vitiated by operation or inflammatory lesions of the limb in question" [100]. Hall and Clark reported, using a thermocouple, a temperature difference of 1 °C or more in 14 of 28 patients with a positive scan for DVT detected by ^{125}I-fibrinogen scanning and clinical examination [101]. In experiments in 5 dogs that underwent temporary occlusion of the right femoral vein, there was a drop in skin temperature, lasting for up to 24 hours suggesting the presence of a thrombus, followed over the next 8 days by a small rise in temperature [102]. Provan in a qualitative study of 468 patients assessing for increased skin temperature of the leg found a hot leg in 40 patients without clinical symptoms suggestive of DVT and 36 patient with physical signs (local calf tenderness, edema or femoral vein tenderness) and presumed DVT [103]. He found that a hot leg and subsequent signs of venous thrombosis occurred within a period of 1 to 7 days (average 3 days) [104]. He concluded:

> The statistical evidence given does not prove that the relation between a warm leg and deep venous thrombosis is causal, but in the absence of any other suggested factor it seems very likely to be so. (…) The use of this sign may draw attention to venous thrombosis, and, in this series, raises the diagnosis rate from 7.3% to 10.5% [104, p. 336].

This sign lacks sufficient sensitivity or specificity when used alone during the clinical examination. However, in the appropriate clinical setting its presence should heighten consideration for the diagnosis (Table 16.1).

Hampton Sign

Aubrey Otis Hampton (1900–1955) was born in Copeville, Texas, and received his medical degree from Baylor University Medical School, Texas, in 1925, and radiology training at the Massachusetts General Hospital, Boston, Massachusetts in 1926 [105]. He was appointed chief of the Department of Radiology at Massachusetts General Hospital in 1941 and subsequently chief of radiologic service at Walter Reed Hospital from 1942 to 1945 [105, 106]. After World War II, he led the Department of Radiology at Garfield Hospital, Washington, D.C., and served as a radiology consultant at Walter Reed Hospital [106, 107]. He was than appointed chief consultant and medical director of radiology of the Veteran's Administration [105], and created a radiologic pathology fellowship at the Armed Force Institute of Pathology [105]. Hampton and Benjamin Castelman described the radiographic shape of a pulmonary infarction:

> The medial or cardiac margin of an infarct is convex toward the heart, presents a serrated margin, and, if the central roentgen ray is tangent to it, a convex, slightly irregular "hump"-shaped shadow is produced. When the lateral costophrenic margins of the lung are involved, the posteroanterior view of the chest shows the "hump"-shaped shadow. When the anterior and posterior costophrenic margins are involved, the "hump" shadow is seen only in the lateral view [107, p. 312]. (…) The cardiac margin of the infarct is rounded or "hump"-shaped instead of pointed [107, p. 313].

Hampton's hump has a moderately high specificity (82%), but has a low sensitivity (22%), with a positive predictive value of 29% and a negative predictive value of 76% for the diagnosis of pulmonary embolism [108]. The presence of Hampton's sign suggests the presence of pulmonary infarct but its absence does not exclude the diagnosis (Table 16.1).

Homans Sign

John Homans (1877–1954) was the fifth generation of physicians in his family to have received his undergraduate education at Harvard University in 1899, graduating from Harvard Medical School as class valedictorian in 1903 [109, 110]. He completed a surgical internship at the Massachusetts General Hospital followed by serving as an assistant to Maurice Richardson, Mosely Professor of Surgery at Harvard from 1903 to 1908 [111]. He received further training under the aegis of Dr. Cushing at Johns Hopkins University School of Medicine, Baltimore, on experimental hypophysectomy in the Hunterian Laboratory from 1908 to 1909. Cushing, then surgeon in chief at the Peter Brigham Hospital in 1910, appointed Dr. Homans in 1912 as one of his principal associates [110]. From 1918 to 1919 he served as a major in the Army Medical Corps as chief of an operating team in the evacuation hospitals [111]. In 1946, he retired as a clinical professor of surgery, emeritus.

Throughout his career, he published multiple scientific manuscripts including in 1931 the first edition of *A Textbook of Surgery* and the monograph, *Circulatory*

Diseases of the Extremities, in 1939. He was a founding member of the Society of Vascular Surgery [109]. For his accomplishments throughout his career, he was honored by his name being bestowed—John Homans Chair of Surgery at Harvard Medical School and the John Homans Lectureship in the Society of Vascular Surgery (SVS) in 1950 [112].

Among his many accomplishments, he was the first to advocate for the ligation of the femoral vein in the groin below the saphenofemoral junction to prevent pulmonary emboli [109] and contributed extensively to the pathogenesis and treatment of lymphatic and venous ulcers in the legs [110]. As described by Daniel C. Elkin:

> His great contribution to the field of vascular surgery lies not only in the originality of his observations but in his willingness to share his knowledge with all who would listen. He has never been dogmatic about the method of treatment, realizing the changes that time brings about. Most men who record an original observation and propose a method of treatment usually refuse to modify their beliefs. For many years an advocate of femoral-vein ligation in treating bland thrombosis, he was willingly accepted and practiced anticoagulant therapy [111, p. 999].

Homans described the dorsiflexion sign in 1941 in his paper "Exploration and division of the femoral and iliac veins in the treatment of the thrombophlebitis of the leg" as a "discomfort behind the knee on forced dorsiflexion of the foot." [113, p. 179]. In describing the course of disease, he wrote:

> The swelling and cyanosis, if any, always disappear in a few days, but the dorsiflexion sign usually lasts for a week or more. (…) If, on the other hand, when the patient first gets up, the discomfort, edema and especially the dorsiflexion sign reappear, the superficial femoral vein is at once exposed and divided [113, p. 179–180].

He further stated, "This type of thrombosis, though difficult of identification, can often be diagnosed, whether or not embolism has occurred, by a combination of clinical symptoms with discomfort behind the knee on forced dorsiflexion of the foot." [113, p. 184].

Allen et al. in their study of 202 patients treated by femoral vein interruption at Massachusetts General Hospital coined the term "Homans sign" for his namesake who first described it. In a footnote, they said, "Dr. John Homans calls it the dorsiflexion sign. It is carried out by dorsiflexion of the foot with the knee straight. If the patient complains of pain or soreness in the calf muscle when this is done the sign is interpreted as positive for venous thrombosis" [114, p. 732]. In 1944 in his paper "Diseases of the veins" commenting on Allen et al. findings, Homans said (Table 16.1, Fig. 16.4):

> I prefer to call it the dorsiflexion sign,—this was found to be present in 42 per cent. I regard this dorsiflexion sign as having a greater degree of importance than would be judged from this analysis. Actually, dorsiflexion of the feet is intended to bring out, on the side of the venous thrombosis, some degree of irritability of the posterior muscle, the soleus and gastrocnemius. Discomfort need have no part in this reaction. Dorsiflexion may be less complete in response to an equal degree of upward pressure on the affected side as compared with the normal, or the patient may involuntarily flex the knee as the forefoot is forced upward, to release the tension on the posterior muscle. If one looks on the dorsiflexion sign as evidence of even the faintest irritability of the posterior muscle, the early stage of the thrombosis occurring with and about them,-the sign will probably be found present more frequently than either tenderness or swelling [115, p. 53].

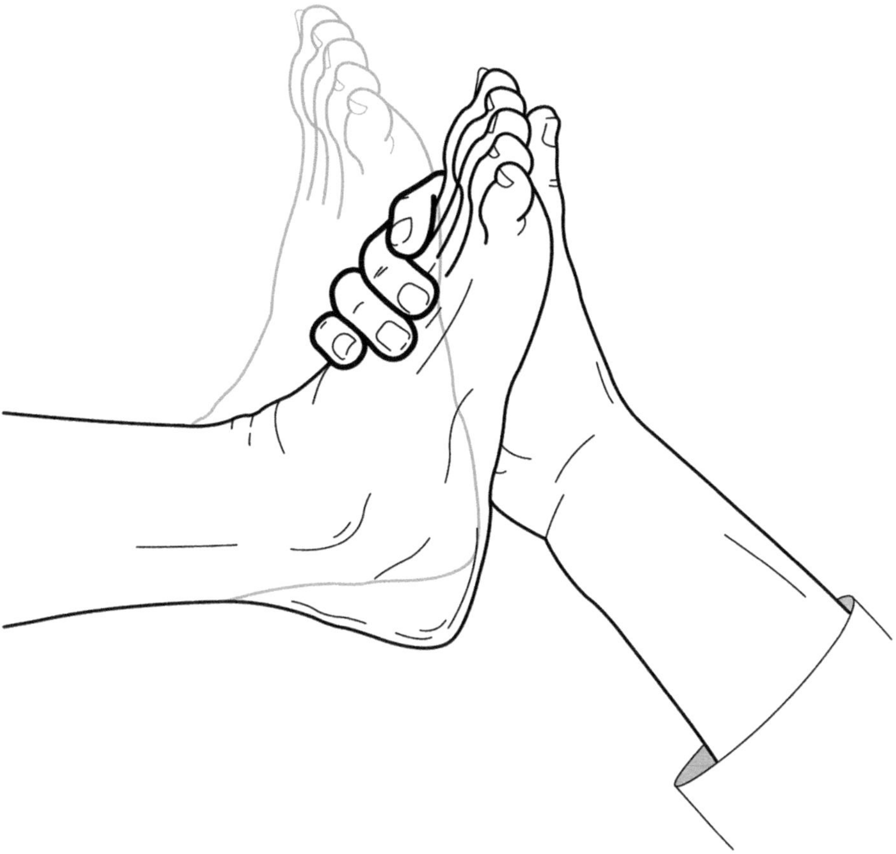

Fig. 16.4 Homans sign (by Ryan Yale)

Thus, Homans' original description for a positive test included "irritability" of the calf muscle, incomplete dorsiflexion of the foot, and/or involuntary flexion of the knee upon forced dorsiflexion of the foot. It is of historical interest that Tschmarke in this 1931 paper reported an objective sign of existing thrombosis of "[i]ncrease resistance of the calf musculature against passive dorsiflexion of the foot." [80, p. 925].

Several textbooks and manuscripts when describing Homans sign stated that the knee should be flexed, in a slightly flexed position, or at a 30° angle [116–119]. Other authors used the term "abrupt" or "sudden" when performing ankle or foot dorsiflexion with pain occurring in the calf or popliteal region [120–127]. As delineated by Homans, discomfort (slight pain) is not required for a positive test and occurs behind the knee, and irritability involves the soleus and gastrocnemius muscles [122–127]. Multiple studies investigated the accuracy and utility of Homans sign in the clinical diagnosis of DVT and identified that the sensitivity ranges from 10 to 54% and specificity is 39 to 89% [122, 128–132]. One study showed that Homans sign was more commonly found in patients with suspected DVT and a negative venogram than in those with a positive venogram [136]. Additional studies by O'Donnell, Haeger, and Molloy showed no differences for the presence of Homans sign in patients with or without venographically confirmed DVT [127, 132, 133].

Homans, despite his objection to assigning his name and limitations of this sign, undoubtedly remains the most widely recognized eponym attributed to venous thrombosis of the calf. The wide range of sensitivity and specificity found in Homans sign is attributed to a number of factors including conditions in the leg that cause a false-positive rate such as tenderness of the calf, muscle, fascia, nerves and subcutaneous tissues caused by a herniated intervertebral lumbar disk, Baker's cyst, calf muscle spasm, and shortened heel cord as well as not performing the sign as originally described, thus limiting the interpretation and conclusions of this sign [125, 134].

Bisgaard Sign

There is limited historical information about Holger Ove Bisgaard (1880–1943). He was born and lived in Glamsbjerg, Denmark [135]. Inscribed in his tombstone are the words "Many were cured. He gave back the joy of living," in reference to his method for treating a venous leg ulcer [135].

Bisgaard in his book entitled *Ulcus und Eczema cruris, Phlebitidis sequelae usw* (Ulcus and Eczema Cruris, Phlebitidis Sequelae, etc.) described the treatment of a venous leg ulcer using a combination of leg elevation, elastic support combined with deep firm massage around the ulcer. He identified early findings found in patients with lower extremity phlebitis and in those who develop a venous ulcers of the lower extremity caused by venous insufficiency and stasis (Fig. 16.5):

> [i]n the lower extremities of patients who are bedridden or when dealing with elderly persons, abnormalities of some kind can often be demonstrated. There may be infiltrations in the muscles that cause rheumatoid-type pain, stiffness of the joints and infiltration in their environment, but the most common anomaly is undoubtedly the infiltration of the calcaneomalleolar region, which I have for the sake of simplicity would like to call it 'backdrop'. From here it often spreads out into the neighboring regions especially towards the back of the ankle. (…) The infiltration in this setting, which appears to be present in virtually every ulcer or eczema in this region, cannot always be seen or felt but always manifests as a deep pressure pain. (…) This provokes the pathognomonic symptom of this condition; a facial expression that lies approximately in the middle between smiles and weeping [136, p. 16].

Bisgaard described the etiopathogenesis for the infiltration of the ankle:

> The acute onset of infiltration is seen in debilitating conditions of various kinds such as occurring after birth and surgery, and often as a precursor to phlebitis or phlegmia and presumably as its direct cause. This acute infiltration should never be underestimated; on the contrary, it should be accorded the greatest importance as the first source for embolisms. At this stage, it is still easily possible to eliminate it by massage and intensive movement of the ankle joint [137, p. 21]. (…) This is based exclusively on clinical observations that I have made in many years on a large number of patients. It may be justified if I point to the new pathological-anatomical examinations (Rössle, Voegt, Neumann, Frukholm, et al.) that find thrombosis in exactly the same regions (thigh, ankle, and calf) which I found infiltrations [136, p. 22].

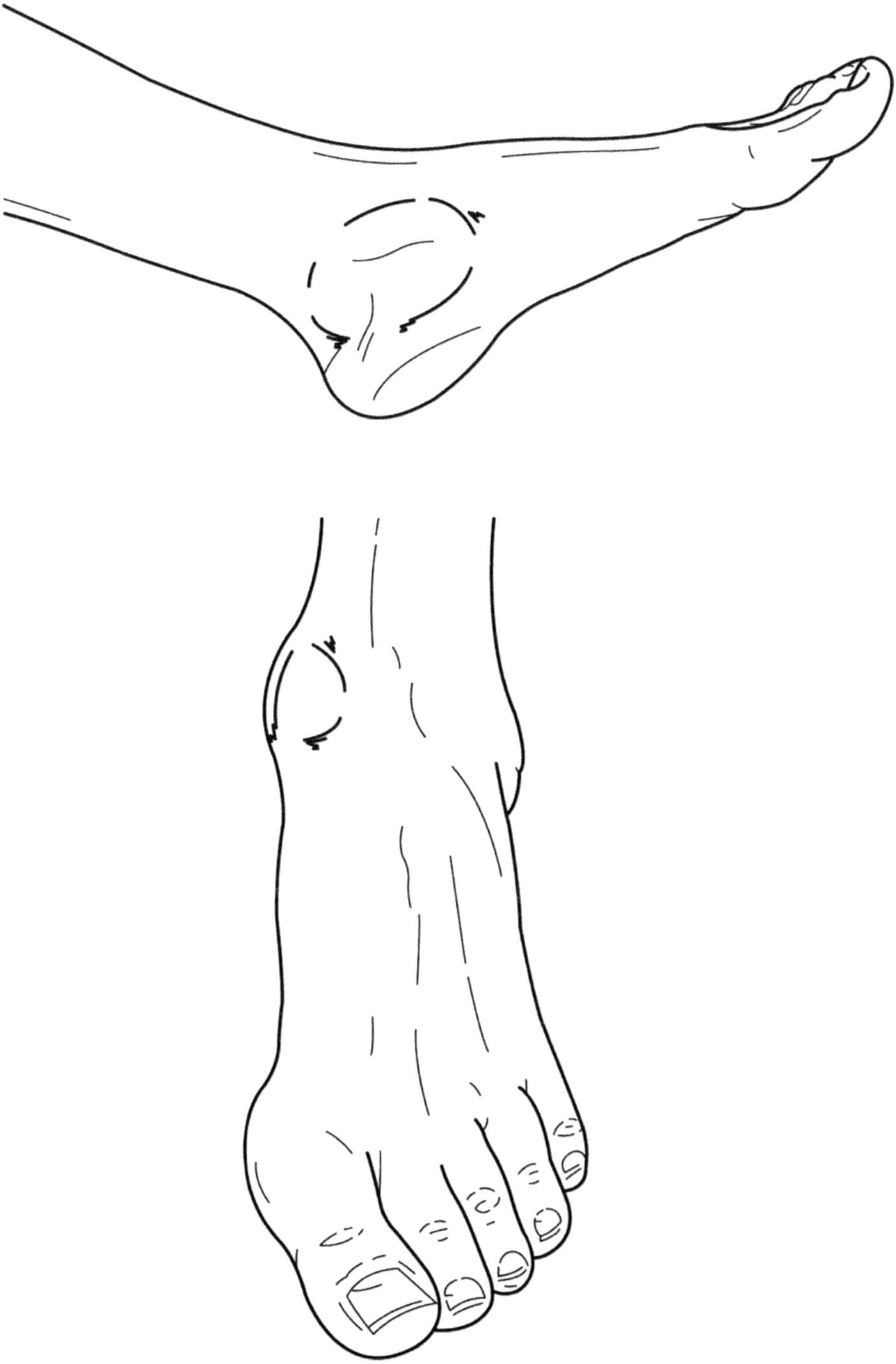

Fig. 16.5 Bisgaard sign (by Ryan Yale)

Bisgaard recommended that vigorous massage and mobilization was the best method to prevent thrombosis and embolism. Bisgaard sign is said to be neither sensitive nor specific for the diagnosis of DVT [137] (Tables 16.1 and 16.2).

Bauer Sign

Gunnar Bauer (1895–1970) graduated from medical school from the University of Lund and Karolinska Institute, Stockholm, Sweden [138]. He completed his training in cardiothoracic surgery at Sabbatsberg and Malmö Hospitals in Sweden [138]. He spent several years in Sveg, Northern Sweden, followed by service as a chief-surgeon at Mariestad General Hospital in Mariestad, Sweden, where he spent the remainder of his career [138]. He made significant contributions that led to a better understanding of DVT by applying the technique of standing descending venographic studies in patients with acute thrombosis and venous incompetence of the legs. He also pioneered the use of heparin to treat VTE and promoted early ambulation to prevent post-thrombotic syndrome [138]. Bauer's venographic work paved the way to an enhanced knowledge of the evolving thrombotic and post-thrombotic syndrome. He demonstrated that thrombosis of the lower extremity starts in the calf veins and that the post-thrombotic syndrome occurred due to the patency of the popliteal and femoral venous valves [138]. He also distinguished post-thrombotic deep venous reflux from idiopathic valve incompetence. He and Knut Haeger in 1963 formed the Soceitas Phlebologica Scandinavica at Mariestad, Sweden, and described the symptom of restlessness and tenderness of the calf muscle as an early sign of DVT [139]. According to Bauer:

> Heed must be given to the slightest unexplained rise in the pulse rate or the temperature, to any unmotivated general restlessness, to the least signs of pulmonary infarction and to the faintest signs of a pathologic condition of the legs, such as a transitory aching in the calf, lasting perhaps only a few hours, a slight change in the color of the skin, a small increase in the firmness of the calf muscle or a tender spot, found only with difficulty, on the back of the lower part of the leg [140, p. 466-467].

Thus, Bauer sign refers to restlessness of the leg and transitory aching of the calf in patients with DVT. The utility of this sign in clinical practice is unknown (Tables 16.1 and 16.2).

Bancroft Sign

Frederic Wolcott Bancroft (1880–1963) graduated from Johns Hopkins University Medical School in 1906 [141–143]. He served as an assistant surgeon in 1914 and instructor of clinical surgery at Columbia University College of Physicians and Surgeons, New York City, in 1946 [144]. He was appointed chairman of the Committee on Fractures of the American College of Surgeons in

1922 and from 1922 to 1946 as associate professor of clinical surgery at Columbia-Presbyterian Medical Center [145]. Bancroft served as the director of surgery at Lincoln Hospital, New York City, from 1924 to 1926 and from 1926 to 1936 surgical director, Fifth Avenue Hospital, associate professor of clinical surgery at Columbia University, attending surgeon at the United States Veterans Hospital No: 81, and consulting surgeon at Lincoln Hospital [141, 146]. He was professor of clinical surgery at the Columbia University College of Physicians and Surgeons from 1926 to 1946 and professor of clinical surgery at the New York Medical College from 1947 until his death [141]. In 1936, he was elected to the Board of Governors of the American College of Surgeons for a three-year term [147] and was a surgical director of the New York City Hospital from 1936 to 1946 [141]. His expertise spanned the fields of vascular and orthopedic surgery. He was the founding member of the American Board of Surgery [148]. He was described by Preston Wade, "He was loved by his many friends and associates, and few teachers have had more loyal and dedicated young surgeons who looked to him as their greatest stimulation in the practice of surgery. His life was truly one dedicated to all of the best ideals in surgery." [141, p. 17]. In his paper on "Proximal ligation and thrombectomy for phelebothrombosis of the femoral and iliac veins," Bancroft reported that (Fig. 16.6),

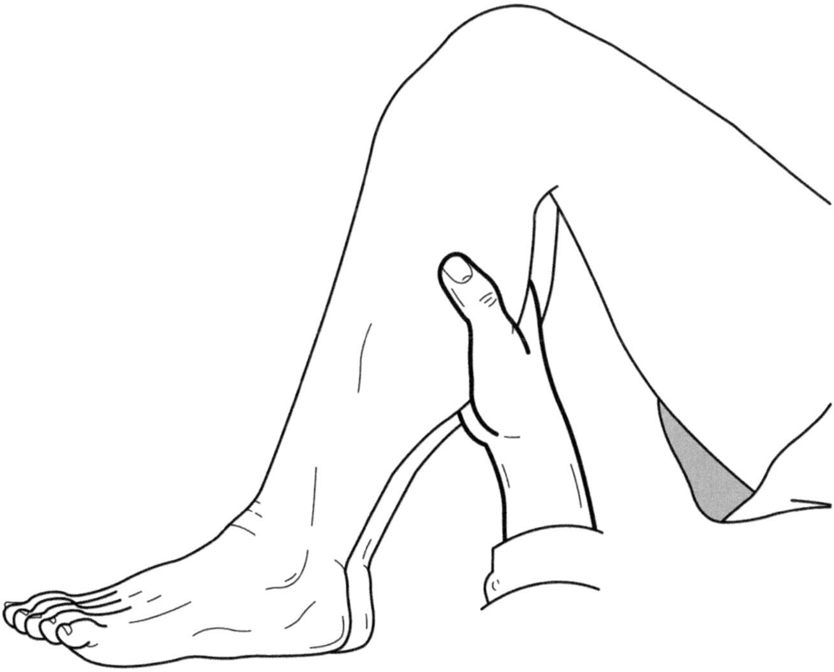

Fig. 16.6 Bancroft sign (by Ryan Yale)

> Homans has described the sign, which is now given his name; if the foot is flexed dorsally it compresses the gastrocnemius muscle, and pain is experienced in the calf. I have also found that if one semiflexes both knees, with the feet resting on the bed, the calf of the affected side gives one the feeling of a deep edema, and, as the gastrocnemius muscle is compressed against the posterior surface of the tibia, pain is elicited [149, p. 176].

Thus, compression of the gastrocnemius muscle against the tibia is a positive Bancroft sign. This sign has been reported to be neither sensitive nor specific for the presence of thrombosis [150] (Tables 16.1 and 16.2).

Moses Sign

William Russell Moses (1916–2005) was born in Spartanburg, SC, and received his medical degree from George Washington University, D.C., in 1938 [151]. Moses completed an internship and residency at Union Memorial Hospital in Baltimore, Maryland. In 1941, he served as the chief of surgery at Gallinger Municipal Hospital (later became known as D.C. General which closed in 1953) [151]. He also served as an adjunct clinical professor in the Department of Surgery at George Washington University School of Medicine [151]. He had a medical practice in Washington in 1941 and served as a founding member of the Falls Church Medical Center in 1965 [151].

Moses described a three-part method for testing the skin, subcutaneous tissue, fascia, and calf muscle independent of the deep vein. During the first part of the test, firm pressure of the fingers is used to identify the area of venous tenderness located on the calf by direct compression in the posterior-anterior direction. During the second part of the test, the calf is firmly compressed from side to side between the fingers and palm of the hand (Fig. 16.7):

> In the presence of bland venous thrombi, the skin, subcutaneous tissue, fascia and muscles show little, if any, tenderness on firm compression, whereas direct pressure on the veins, as executed in the first maneuver causes definite pain. On the other hand, the superficial tissues are extremely tender at the second test if the tenderness resides in their layers. These two stages do not, however, rule out tenderness of the deep calf nerves, such as is present in a peripheral neuritis. The third part of the test is therefore a brief neurologic examination, with a search for alteration of cutaneous sensation and an evaluation of position sense of the toes, the vibratory sense and the deep reflexes [152, p. 290].

Thus, pain elicited by direct compression of the deep posterior calf with the fingertips in the posterior-anterior direction is considered a positive test for DVT. The presence of pain when the calf is compressed between the fingers and palms in the lateral direction suggests involvement of the superficial tissue or muscle rather than the veins [152, 153].

Moses found that this test correctly identified thrombus in all of 12 patients with operative proven thrombosis [152]. In 31 patients with a positive test and suspected phlebothrombosis, thrombus was identified by direct visualization within the vein in 14 patients. In the remaining 17 patients, there was radiographic evidence of pulmonary emboli with infarction in 12 patients [152]. In 65 patients with suspected phlebothrombosis, the sign was negative in all with no evidence for thrombosis

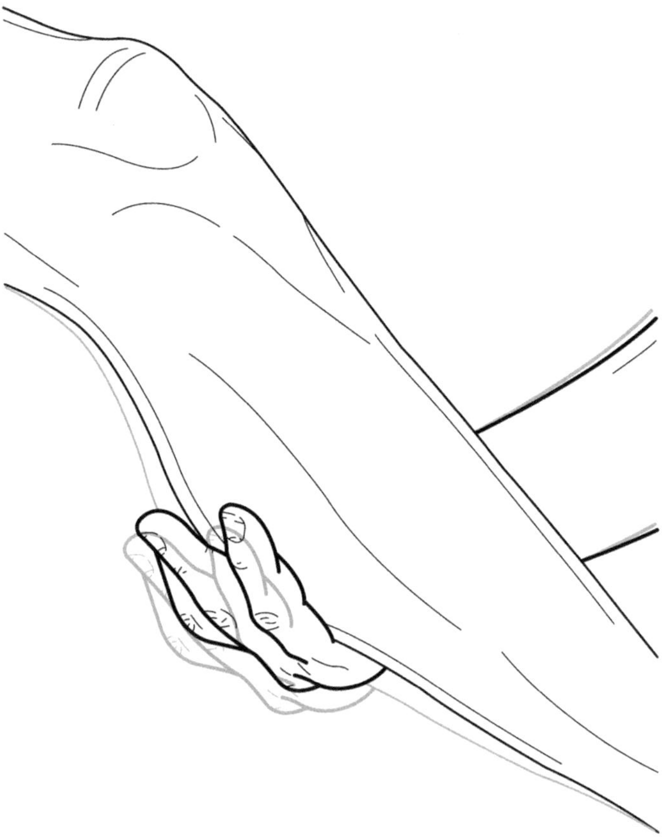

Fig. 16.7 Moses sign (by Ryan Yale)

found on subsequent follow-up [152]. In a study of 105 clinically suspected cases of deep and superficial thrombophlebitis among 92 patients, Felder reported that Moses sign was identified in 56 (53%) patients [117]. The sign was found to have a sensitivity and specificity of 38% and 88%, respectively [154]. The high specificity of the sign suggests that a positive test increases the likelihood of DVT. Its absence does not exclude the diagnosis (Tables 16.1 and 16.2).

Neuhof Sign

Harold Neuhof (1884–1964) received his medical degree in 1905 from the College of Physicians and Surgeons of Columbia University, NY. He completed his internship and residency at Mount Sinai, New York City, and was appointed to the Physicians and Surgeons Division of Surgical Service at Bellevue Hospital, NY, in 1910 [155]. From 1913 to 1923, he was a member of the neurosurgical service at Montefiore Hospital, NY, and subsequently served as an attending surgeon and

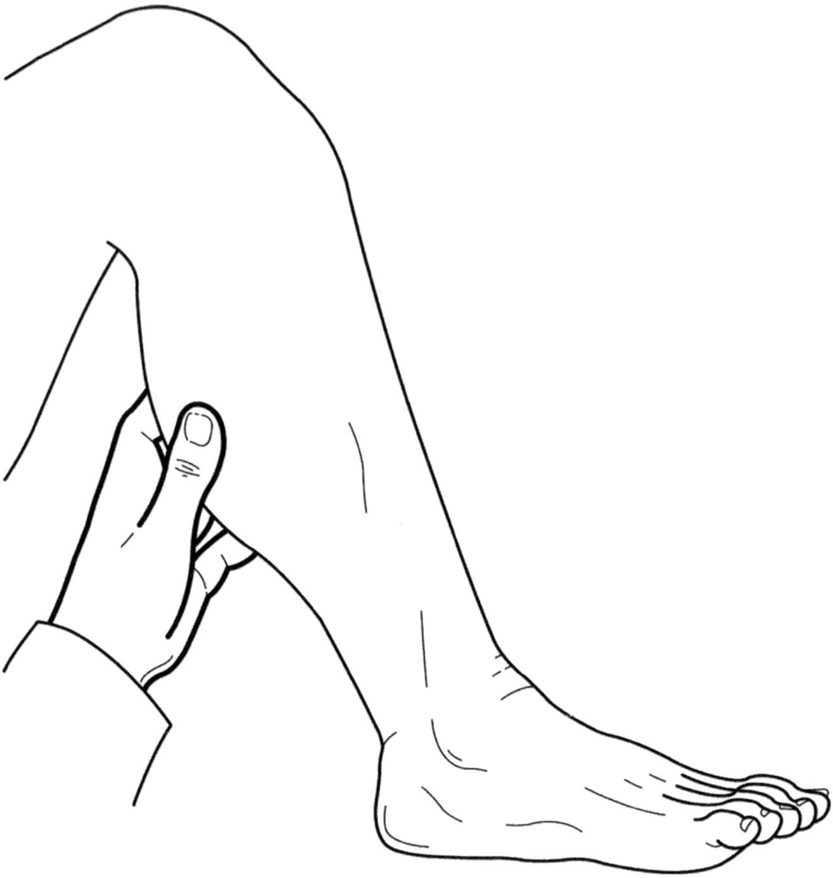

Fig. 16.8 Neuhoff sign (by Ryan Yale)

chief of the Surgical Division from 1923 to 1932. From 1932 to 1946, he was appointed chief in the Department of Surgery at Mount Sinai Hospital, NY, and consultant surgeon and director emeritus of the Department of Surgery at The Mount Sinai Hospital beginning in 1946 [156]. He was subsequently appointed director of the Division of Surgery at Beth-El Hospital in Brooklyn, NY, retiring from this position in 1959 [155, 156].

He made significant contributions to the field of medicine and surgery including his literary contributions to lung cancer, mediastinitis, thrombophlebitis as well as the transplantation of the kidney of a lamb into a human. With colleagues in his department, they developed a comprehensive pathophysiological and surgical approach to lung abscesses. His other contributions include serving as a founding member of the American Board of Surgery and American Board of Thoracic Surgery [155]. He was a fellow of the New York Academy of Medicine, American College of Surgeons, and member of American Association for Thoracic Surgery and American Surgical Association. He was a member of the societies of Surgery, Thoracic Surgery, and Cardiovascular Surgery in NY [155]. He described in 1947 (Fig. 16.8):

> A sign which I regard to be valuable (and which apparently is not mentioned in the literature) is infiltration to be felt on palpation of the deep calf musculature. With the patient's heels resting on the bed, the knees flexed and the calf muscles relaxed, palpation reveals thickening and infiltration deep to the gastrocnemius. The area of infiltration, of greater or lesser extent, is vertically disposed. It usually is tender, although tenderness varies with different patients. The area of infiltration, which corresponds to the general region of the deep veins of the calf, may coexist with subjective signs of venous thrombosis or may be present alone [157, p. 114; 158, p. 6].

He reported, "It is of interest to note that characteristic infiltration of the calf was present in all cases in which Homans' sign was positive, but was also present in a number of cases in which no other objective evidence of venous thrombosis existed." [157, p. 114]. (…) "Two objective signs of value and frequently present are infiltration of the calf and increase in circumference of the calf" [157, p. 115; 158, p. 6]. We are unaware of any study that evaluated the sensitivity or specificity of this sign. Neuhof found that this finding was present in all patients whom Homans sign was present as well as in other patients which there was no other objective evidence for venous thrombosis [157]. The utility of this sign in clinical practice has not been confirmed (Tables 16.1 and 16.2).

Bailey Sign

Henry Hamilton Bailey (1894–1961) received his medical training at the London Hospital Medical School qualifying in 1916. After World War I, he served as a house surgeon and surgical registrar in London and was recognized for fellowship in the Royal College of Surgeons in 1920 [159]. He worked as an assistant surgeon at the Liverpool Royal Infirmary in 1925, Dudley Road Hospital in Birmingham and Bristol Homeopathic Hospital in 1930, Bath Homeopathic Hospital in 1931, and latter posts at the Royal Northern Hospital in Holloway, North London in 1932 and several other hospitals in London [159]. He was a prolific writer, writing or editing 15 books including *Emergency Surgery* (1920), *Demonstration of the Physical Signs in Clinical Surgery* (1927), and *A Short Practice of Surgery* with RJ McNeil Love (1932). His books were unique because of the clarity of presentation and incorporation of the use of illustration and photography to explain disease or techniques [159]. His other accolades include hunterian professor of the Royal College of Surgeons, Fellow of the American College of Surgeons, member of the Société d'Urologie (French Society of Urology), and a vice-president of the International College of Surgeons [160].

Hamilton Bailey wrote in his textbook *Physical Signs in Clinical Surgery* in patients with suspected thrombophlebitis:

> 1. Apply finger-tip pressure over each saphenous opening, and with a stroking motion, run the finger down the course of each femoral vein. Observe if there is unilateral tenderness. 2. Let the patient draw up her knees and lie quietly, relaxing the muscles. Palpate the entire leg from the feet upward, seeking a localized area of muscular resistance combined with deep tenderness (Frykholm). 3. Palpate deeply in the popliteal spaces, after which ask the patient to lower the legs on the bed [161].

Ortiz-Ramirez and Serna-Ramirez described a new sign of provoked pain and compared this sign with other signs of presumed deep phlebitis including Bailey sign in 32 persons. Fourteen of 32 patients had a positive Bailey sign [162]. They did not, however, describe how Bailey sign was performed. We believe that Bailey sign refers to femoral venous tenderness upon palpable pressure throughout the course of the femoral vein after compressing the saphenous venous junction in patients with venous thrombosis. The utility of this sign in clinical practice has not been confirmed (Tables 16.1 and 16.2).

Rosenthal Sign

We were unable to identify any historical information on Randolph Rosenthal. At the time of the publication of his physical finding, he served in the Peripheral Vascular Disease Department at the Bronx Hospital, NY [163]. He described the foot extension sign as a bedside diagnostic method for detecting DVT of the leg which (Fig. 16.9):

> [c]onsists simply of passively extending the foot 45 degrees or less, depending on the maximum painless mobility of the ankle joint and, if this elicits no pain in the patient, plantar flexing the toes while the foot is held in extension by the examiner's hand. At present the author's practice is to combine these two movements into one, (…) by grasping the toes, flexing them in a plantar direction, and automatically extending the foot up to 45 degrees or less at the same time [163, p. 1148].

The test is considered positive if:

> [t]he maneuver elicits pain anywhere just lateral to the anterior crest of the tibia, but especially at a point three inches above the distal end of the tibia, where the position of the anterior tibial vein is most superficial in its course. It is at this point that foot extension produces maximum compression of the anterior tibial vein [163, p. 1148].

Thus, Rosenthal sign is pain located lateral to the anterior tibial crest particularly at a point 3 inches above the distal tibia elicited on either extension of the foot to an angle of 45 degree or when flexing the toes while the foot is held in extension. The utility of this sign in clinical practice has not been confirmed (Tables 16.1 and 16.2).

Pratt Sign

Gerald Hilary Pratt (1906–1979) was born in Montello, Wisconsin, and received his medical degree from the University of Iowa in 1928. He was a clinical associate professor of surgery at the New York University School of Medicine and attending surgeon at St. Vincent's Hospital and Medical Center, St. Clare's Hospital and Health Center and Doctor's Hospital, NY [164].

In 1948, Pratt reported on the presence of three dilated veins over the tibia as an early sign of thrombosis of the deep veins of the leg [165]. In his 1949 paper on "An

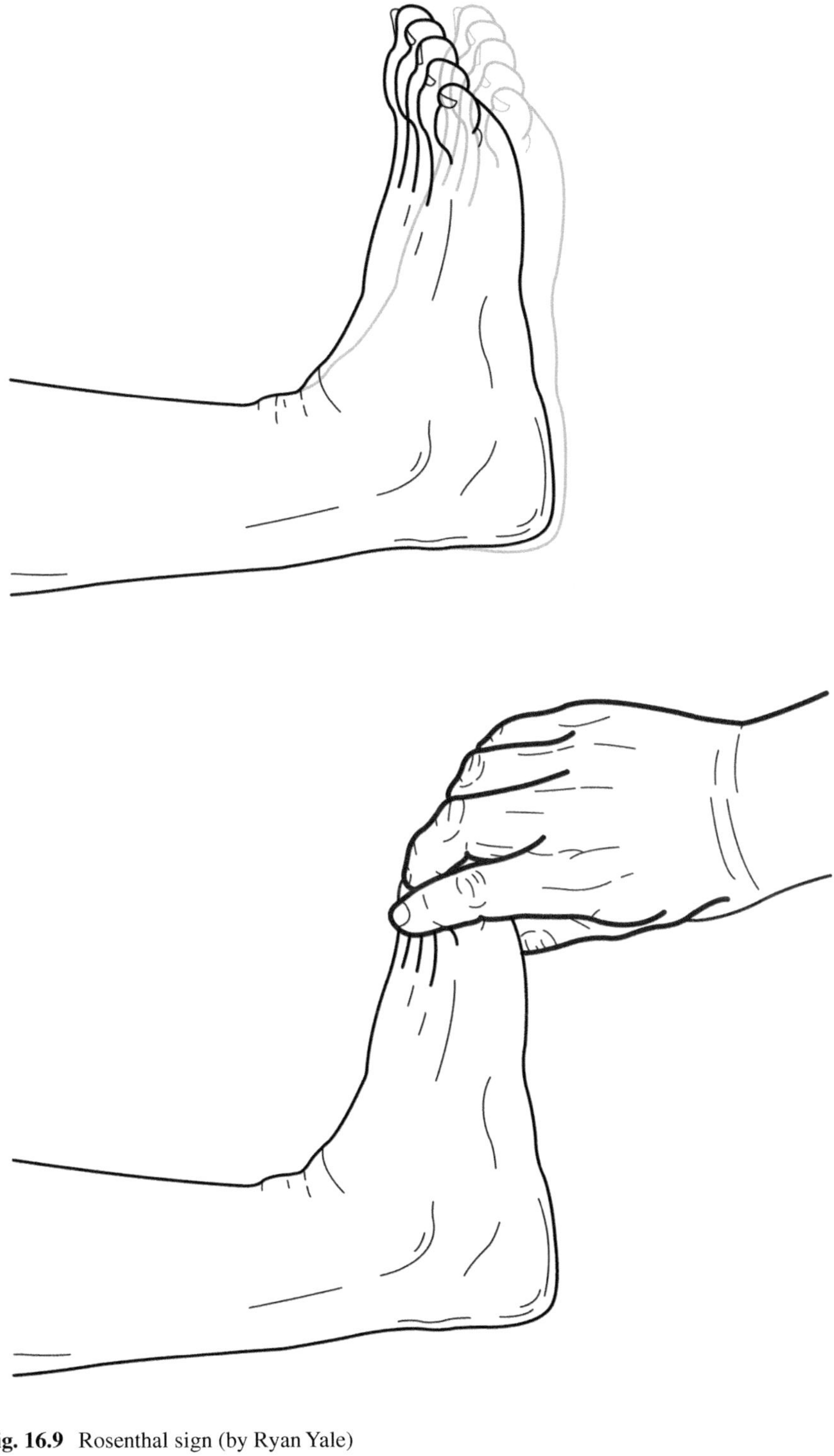

Fig. 16.9 Rosenthal sign (by Ryan Yale)

early sign of femoral thrombosis," he stated, "Since then, this phenomenon has been observed so consistently that the term 'sentinel' veins has been coined for this finding." [166, p. 477]. He attributed the pathogenesis to "These three small veins over the tibia empty into the saphenous and the anterior tibia vein system are superficial and unsupported but musculature and therefore dilate very early." [166, p. 476–477]. He found that the sign was present in 84 of 109 patients with thrombosis of the leg and that it is present earlier than Homans' sign [166]. This signs is believed to be neither sensitive nor specific, thus limiting its diagnostic value in clinical practice [167, 168] (Tables 16.1 and 16.2).

Lawrence Sign

Elias D. Lawrence (1905–1994) received his medical degree from the University and Bellevue Hospital Medical College in 1929 and completed his internship at Barnett Memorial Hospital in Paterson, New Jersey, from 1929 to 1930 [169]. At the time of the publication of his sign, he was an associate surgeon at Barnett Memorial Hospital. He described the cough-pain sign as a method for diagnosing acute superficial thrombophlebitis of the legs:

> I have noticed that in many cases the pain in the inflamed area was increased by coughing, sneezing, or laughing. In these cases, compression of the greater saphenous vein close to the saphenofemoral junction resulted in the disappearance of the pain on coughing. This was found to be present in practically all patients who were seen early or when they are involved as at the knee or proximal; and in about 50 per cent of the cases with involvement below the knee. I have called this the "cough-pain sign" [170, p. 164].

He reported that the sign may be absent in cases in which there is resolution of the inflammatory process or if the superficial thrombophlebitis is below the knee. He believed that if the cough-pain sign remains positive after compressing the greater saphenous vein, it may be caused by communicating veins. Thus, Lawrence sign or the "cough-pain" sign refers to the presence of pain located at the site of an inflammatory superficial thrombosis of the lower extremity elicited by factors that increase venous pressure (e.g., coughing, sneezing, laughing). The utility of this sign in clinical practice has not been confirmed (Tables 16.1 and 16.2).

D'Alessandro Sign

Arthur Joseph D'Alessandro (1911–1983) graduated from Columbia University College of Physician and Surgeons, New York City, in 1935 [171]. At the time of reporting his sign, he served as an assistant surgeon in the peripheral vascular service at Presbyterian Hospital and Newark City Hospital, and was affiliated with St. James Hospital in Newark, NJ [172, 173]. He served as a member of the American Medical Association, Academy of Medicine of New Jersey, and fellow of the American College of Surgeons (FACS) [171]. Upon his retirement, he was recognized as an emeritus member of the Essex County component of the New Jersey Medical Society. He described a number of important signs and symptoms of thromboembolism and stated:

> To these I should like to add a fairly constant, simple, and early sign that I have found to be of great value in my clinical practice. In the past five years, I have become increasingly aware, particularly on palpating the femoral pulse preparatory to vein ligation, of the significance of marked diminution or even absence of the femoral pulse in the affected extremity. This phenomenon has invariably been present, even in the absence of other appreciable signs or symptoms (…) [173, p. 1759-1760].

He postulated that arterial vasospasm was the physiologic mechanism responsible for the deceased femoral pulse and that this finding occurs early, prior to edema or swelling of the lower extremity [173]. The utility of this sign in clinical practice has not been confirmed (Tables 16.1 and 16.2).

Louvel Sign

Jacques Louvel (1898–1983) was born in La Ferté-Macé, Normandy, France. He finished his internship at Hôpitaux de Paris, and later served as a chief physician of the cardiology clinic at the University [174]. Inspired by his masters Vaquès and Laubry, Louvel published several articles related to cardiovascular pathology as well as preventive and curative therapy of phlebitis [174]. Louvel and Laubry described at the March 16th 1952 French Session of Cardiology entitled "Sur un symptôme peu connu de thrombophlébite" (On a less-known symptom of thrombophlebitis) (Tables 16.1 and 16.2):

> [a] simple test, which we have used for nearly fifteen years and which we feel it is important to make others aware. This is pain caused by coughing in the presence of thrombophlebitis. When a subject complains of an intense pain in the leg, with or without dilatation of the superficial veins, with more or less marked edema, with or without pain on dorsiflexion of the foot is told to cough, and if cough causes pain in a suspected area of the vein, the diagnosis is phlebitis. The sign thus makes it possible to prove the venous and inflammatory origin of pain. This sign, when one is lucky to have it at the beginning of or during an evolving phlebitis episode, is the factor that guides the clinician on the possible extension of the inflammatory process. Thus, we were able to follow, step by step, even in the depth of the thigh, the ascending progression of a venous thrombus [175, p. 630].

Louvel noted that the sign can be useful in the diagnosis of superficial venous thrombosis but is also useful in determining response to treatment as "its total disappearance allowed us to confirm, in difficult cases, the extinction of the inflammatory process." [175, p. 630]. They described the usefulness of the sign in treatment:

> When the coughing sign causes pain in a segment of the saphenous vein it is usually possible to suppress the symptom by exerting a digital pressure on the anastomotic saphenofemoral junction. This is an indication for venous ligature. If however, despite compression of the saphenous junction, the pain of the underlying venous thrombosis is still present by coughing, it is because there is another valvular failure originating below the saphenofemoral junction communicating with the vein. Thus, the physician must identify the second site of failure and apply venous ligature [175, p. 631].

Thus, Louvel found that the sign can be used for diagnosing, treating, and determining response to treatment and its absence to confirm resolution of the inflammatory process [175]. They reported that this sign is present in only 40% of cases. Lawrence previously reported in the *Journal of Medical Society of New Jersey* in 1950 a positive "cough-pain sign" is an indication for venous ligature [170]. This sign is unreliable in the diagnosis because it lacks sufficient sensitivity and is nonspecific [176, 177].

Bellini Sign

We were unable to identify any historical information on Dr. Ettore Bellini. At the time of the publication of his physical finding, he served at the Ospedali Civili Riuniti di Venezia Prima Divisione Medica diretta dal Primario Prof. Angelo Spanio (United Civilian Hospital of Venice First Medical Division directed by Prof. Angelo Spanio) [178]. He reported in a communication to the Venetian Medical-Surgical Society session on January 29th 1953 the finding of "a not infrequent observation in phlebitis disease, namely the detection and disappearance of the femoral and popliteal pulses" [179, p. 72]. He assessed the thighs and legs of 50 patients daily using a sphygmomanometer and oscillometer to measure the pressure and pulse, respectively. In patients with DVT, he found an increase in minimum pressure values (sometime caused by increasing the minimum or lowering the maximum pressures), decrease in differential pressure, and a decrease in the oscillometric curve and index compared to the unaffected thigh and leg or previous values in the same limb if both legs developed thrombosis. He also performed what he referred to as the "trinitric" (nitroglycerine) test as a method for distinguishing vasospastic from previous or co-existing arterial disease. A positive test was reported as a reappearance or increase in the affected limbs pulse rate and oscillometric index, reappearance or lowering of the maximum and minimum pressure, or increase of the differential pressure. Furthermore, to distinguish a coexisting or autonomous functional arteriopathy he found that the reaction to trinitrine resolved in 30 minutes compared to those with DVT that persisted for at least 6 hours [179]. He concluded that phlebopathy induced a reflex mechanism and transient arterial vasospasm. The utility of this sign in clinical practice has not been confirmed (Tables 16.1 and 16.2).

Castañeda Sign

We were unable to identify any historical information about Manuel Castañeda-Uribe. At the time of the description of his physical finding he served as the head of the vascular surgery service at the General Hospital of Mexico and Sanatorium no.

1 of the IMSS [180]. Castañeda-Uribe presented his findings at the Mexican Association of Gynecology and Obstetrics in 1953 [180]:

> In phlebothrombosis edema does not occur early, but begins the third or fourth day and is localized to the supramalleolar region. However, there is another type of edema that is located in the calf muscles, infiltrating them, named "sign of the calf" (Castañeda Uribe), which is of a hard consistency that occurs when there is thrombosis of the veins of the leg due to ascending progression from the foot [180, p. 495].

Thus, Castañeda sign refers to the palpatory hard calf caused by muscular edema in patients with venous thrombosis. He also described the sign of the toe, in which compression of the edge of the first joint of the first toe causes sudden sharp pain in patients with phlebothrombosis (Tables 16.1 and 16.2, Fig. 16.10). The utility of these sign in clinical practice has not been confirmed.

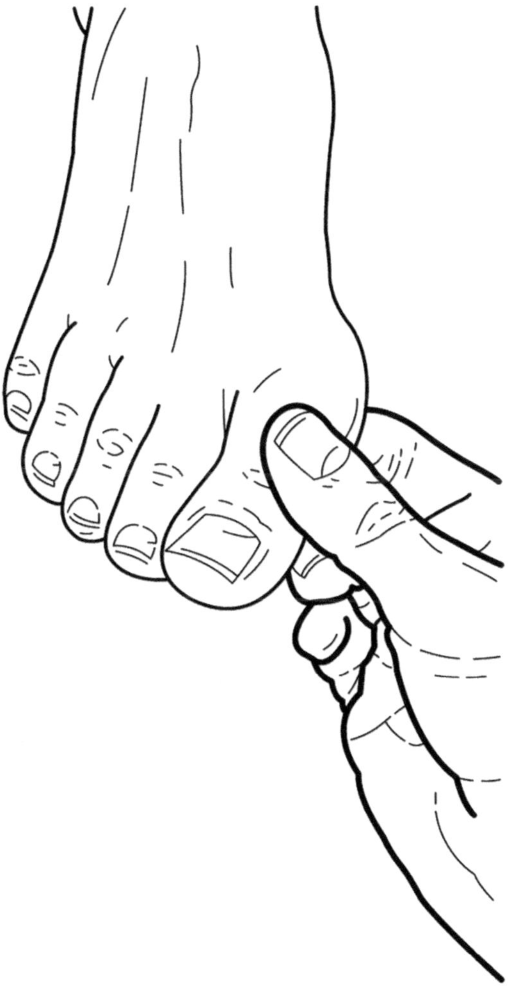

Fig. 16.10 Castañeda sign (by Ryan Yale)

Lowenberg Sign

We were unable to identify any historical information on Dr. Robert I. Lowenberg (1917–2000). He practiced as a vascular surgeon in the Department of Surgery, General Service at Grace-New Haven Community Hospital, Connecticut [181]. Lowenberg developed a sphygmomanometer cuff pain test for diagnosing and predicting the onset of phlebothrombosis. His findings were first reported in *Science* in 1954:

> A pneumatic cuff is distended over the calf or thigh slowly to 180 mmHg pressure. If pain is elicited before this, the end point has been reached and the cuff is deflated. A positive cuff test is indicated by pain beneath the inflated cuff at 80, 100, or 120 mmHg. A negative test that becomes positive a few days post-operatively or several days after a patient has been put to bed with a myocardial infarction is presumed evidence of intravascular clot and should be treated as such [181, p. 883].

He expanded upon this further with more detailed information included in his publication in the *Journal of the American Medical Association* that same year (Tables 16.1 and 16.2):

> In patients suspected of having phlebothrombosis, the pneumatic cuff is placed about the calf or thigh and slowly distended; distention of the cuff should be accomplished in 10 to 15 seconds. Normally patients do not register discomfort below 180 mmHg over the calf or thigh. In the presence of phlebitis, the patient will complain bitterly of pain at a level of significantly below the normal [182, p. 1567].

The technique involved as described by Lowenberg:

> In performing the test, the patient's threshold for pain must first be determined. In order to accomplish this, the oscillometer cuff is placed on the arm and rapidly distended to two hundred fifty millimeters of mercury. The average patient experiences no pain at this pressure. The test is then performed by similar compression successively of the lower limbs above and below the knee. A blood pressure cuff or an oscillometer cuff serve equally well for this study. A level of one hundred eighty to two hundred millimeters of mercury pressure has been found proper for the lower extremity. If pain is experienced as indicated by the patient's withdrawing the limb, wincing, or crying out, the cuff is immediately deflated. This is considered a positive test. For the purpose of checking the patients' reliability, the test may be safely repeated within a minute or two. The same response should be elicited within twenty millimeters of mercury pressure. (…) In patients with a reduced pain threshold, a pain response at levels below 180 mmHg must be given special interpretation relative to the pain-response level on the upper extremity [183, p. 142].

A positive sphygmomanometer cuff test occurs if pain occurs between 60 to 150 mmHg. For confirmation he recommended repeating the test with the new value being within 10 mmHg of the previous one [182]. Lowenberg acknowledged that false-positive results are found in patients with muscle cramps, trauma, superficial phlebitis, and intermittent claudication and that no false-negative results were identified. He also recommended that the cuff test not be performed in patients with superficial thrombophlebitis since it may elicit pain and exacerbate the disease [183].

Haeger identified a sensitivity of 20% and specificity of 85% for this sign among 72 patients with suspected DVT [127]. A false-positive test may occur in patients with varicose veins, pregnancy, trauma, and muscle injuries [153]. Barner et al.

studied the utility of the Lowenberg test at the calf in three groups of patients: 1) 230 hospitalized admission, 2) 107 postoperative patients, 3) 50 venographically confirmed DVT. In this study the cuff was distended at a rate of approximately 20 mmHg per sec. A positive Lowenberg test was detected in 25 hospitalized patients, none of whom had or developed DVT. In the postoperative group, the Lowenberg test did not assist in establishing the diagnosis of DVT; a false-positive test was found in 22 patients. In the third group of patients with venographically confirmed DVT, Lowenberg test showed a false-negative and false-positive rate of 22% and 26%, respectively. Hence, in select patients with equivocal leg tenderness, a positive Lowenberg test on one leg, with a normal response on the contralateral side, may assist in confirming the presence of DVT [184]. Makin studied Lowenberg test in 55 patients and found that this test was not useful in diagnosing DVT [185]. Overall, Lowenberg sign has been reported to be neither sensitive nor specific for the diagnosis of DVT [186].

Rose Sign

We were only able to identify limited historical information about S.S. Rose. He was a member of the Department of Surgery at the University of Manchester and Withington Hospital, Manchester [187]. He served as the vice-chairman on the Organizing Committee of the First United Kingdom Meeting of the Union International de Phlébologie (International Union of Phlebology) in 1985, and was chief editor of the *Journal of the International Society for Cardiovascular Surgery* from 1983 to 1987 [187, 188].

We were unable to identify the original reference to this sign. Bailey described, Rose sign, in his textbook *Physical Signs in Clinical Surgery* as the method for identifying early edema in patients with suspected DVT. This involves: “pinch up a small portion of skin. In very early edema there is a resistance that is not present on the normal side, owing to thickening of the dermis and subcutaneous tissue.” [189, p. 819] (Fig. 16.11). The utility of this sign in clinical practice has not been confirmed (Table 16.1).

Ortiz-Ramírez Sign

Teófilo Ortiz-Ramírez was born in 1901 in Morelia, Michoacán, Mexico, and received his medical degree in 1924 from the Autonomous National University of Mexico (UNAM) where he remained as a member of the Faculty of Medicine. Here he earned the titles Professor of Introductory to Clinical Medicine from 1929 to 1932, Pathology Physiology in 1930, and Clinical Medicine beginning in 1933 [190]. He also led the Section of Experimental Biochemistry, Consulting Department,

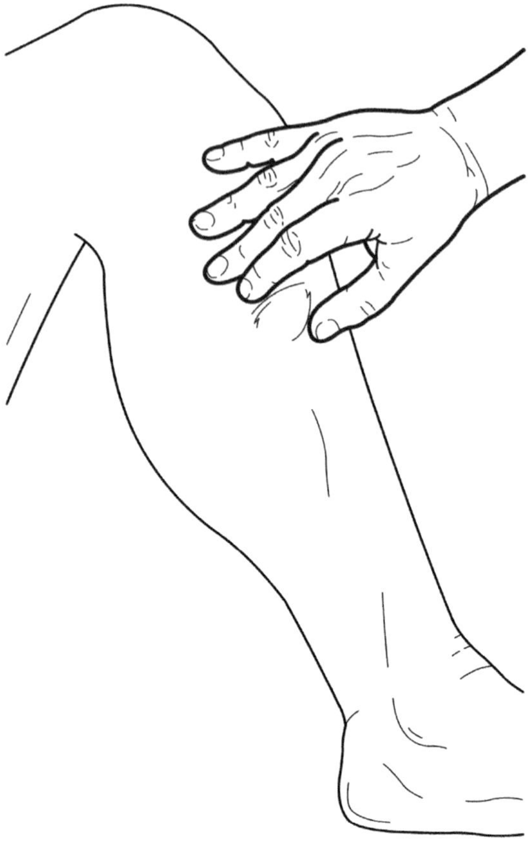

Fig. 16.11 Rose sign (by Ryan Yale)

Chemistry and Pharmacy at various times at the National Department of Health, Mexico, between 1927 and 1935. In 1955, he was a professor at UNAM [190]. Among his other accomplishments, he was founding president of Mexican Society of Cardiology between 1945 and 1946, member of the National Academy of Medicine and the National Institute for Cardiology, and general director of the Interamerican Society of Cardiology [190].

Teófilo Ortiz-Ramírez and Serna-Ramírez described a method for detecting phlebitis in the lower extremities (Tables 16.1 and 16.2, Fig. 16.12):

> With the patient in the recumbent position and the extremity to be explored slightly flexed, a sphygmomanometer mercury cuff was applied above the knee, with a pressure of around 4 cm Hg. The venous hypertension provoked pain in some place, most often in the popliteal region of the calf in cases of deep phlebitis. The pain increased during the 5 minutes of the test, sometimes it was similar to pain occurring spontaneous, and disappeared almost instantaneously after releasing the pressure [162, p. 367].

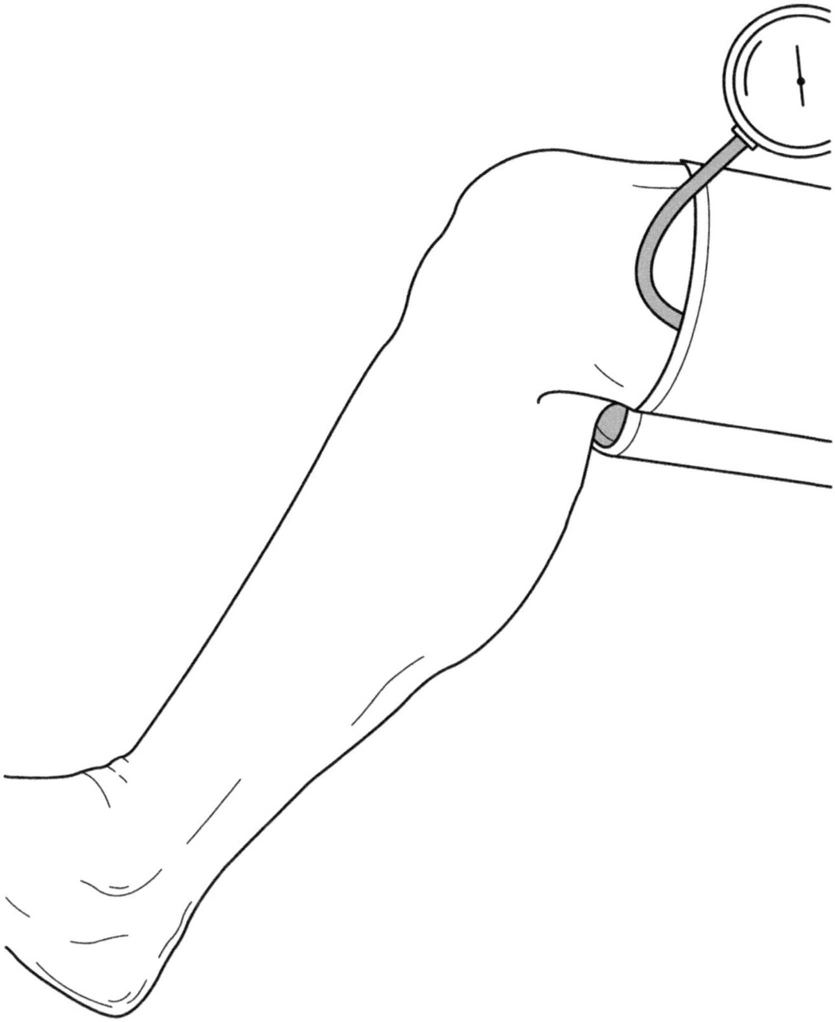

Fig. 16.12 Ortiz-Ramirez sign (by Ryan Yale)

They reported that a positive sign requires that the pain appears or increases with pressure and decreases with release of the sphygmomanometer. The "cuff sign" was found in 32 (100%) with phlebitis as compared to 81% identified by Homans sign [162]. Ortiz-Ramírez postulated that compression of the thigh causes within 1–2 minutes distention of the venous system and pain [162]. Ortiz-Ramírez and Serna-Ramírez believed that the pain in patients with thrombophlebitis is caused by venous distention and that the sign was not pathognomonic for DVT since it was assessed in a non-homogenous population and venous thrombosis was not definitively confirmed [162].

Popkin Sign

There is limited historical information available about Roy J. Popkin. He received his medical degree from the University of Minnesota in 1930 [191], and served as an attending in medicine and later as the chief of the Peripheral Vascular Clinic at the Cedars of Lebanon Hospital, Los Angeles, California [192]. He described the "finger pressure test" in patients with venous stasis of the lower extremities (Fig. 16.13):

> [b]est performed with the patient recumbent and the shoes and stockings removed. Sufficient pressure is applied with the index finger or thumb over the anteromedial surface of the leg compressing the tissues between the fingers and underlying bone. The pain is usually more intense distally and disappears proximally. The intensity of the pain produced frequently surprises the patient. It is often unexpected. The complaint of pain and evidence of pitting are found more often in the afternoon or when the patient has been up and about for several hours [193, p. 301-302].

Popkin reported that this sign was present in a variety of conditions associated with venous insufficiency or obstruction causing venous stasis. He hypothesized that the source of pain may be due to afferent fibers along the veins. This sign is believed to be a sensitive but nonspecific finding in DVT. The utility of this sign in clinical practice has not been confirmed (Tables 16.1 and 16.2).

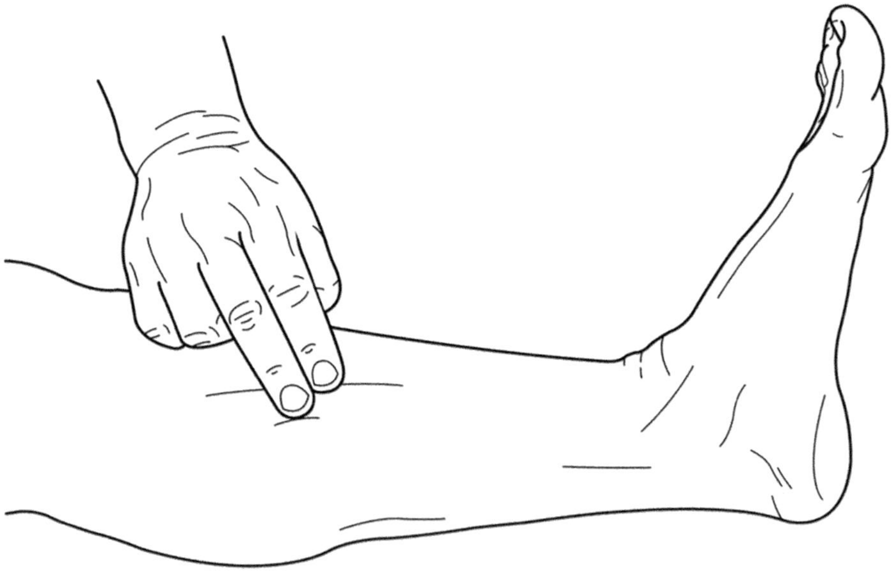

Fig. 16.13 Popkin sign (by Ryan Yale)

McLachlin Sign

John Adams McLachlin (1915–2004) received his medical degree from the University of Western Ontario in 1940. He served during WWII as a surgeon (Lieutenant Commander) in the Royal Canadian Navy, followed by positions as chief of surgery at St. Thomas-Elgin General Hospital and instructor at the University of Western Ontario [194]. At the time of the publication of the sign which bears his name he worked at Westminster Hospital, Department of Veterans Affairs, and the Departments of Medical Research and Surgery at the University of Western Ontario [122]. He was awarded the Queen's Jubilee Medal for his dedicated service to the community and was a recipient of the Research Gold Medal by the Royal College of Physicians and Surgeons. McLachlin was a senior member of the Canadian Medical Association, fellow of the Royal College of Surgeons of Canada (FRCSC), and fellow of the American College of Surgeons (FACS) [195].

McLachlin et al. reported in their paper entitled "An evaluation of clinical signs in the diagnosis of venous thrombosis" that (Tables 16.1 and 16.2):

> Unilateral swelling of the ankle is, by far, the best single test in the clinical diagnosis of venous thrombosis. If asymmetrical swelling of the ankle is noticed, the diagnosis of venous thrombosis must be suspect. (…) It must be emphasized, however, that swelling of the ankle seems to be of diagnostic validity for the left leg only [122, p. 741].

MacLachin et al., in their small necropsy series showed that an increase in circumference of the left ankle, identified in 83% of patients, was the only finding among local tenderness, changes in skin temperature, Homans dorsiflexion sign, and venous dilation useful in detecting DVT [122]. Langersedt assessed the clinical diagnosis of DVT using plebography as the reference standard among 307 of 396 patients with suspected disease who underwent physical examination, ^{99m}Tc-plasmin test, and phlebography. They found that pitting edema was the most common sign identified in 80% of patients with DVT with a sensitivity of 73% in contrast to increased circumference of the thigh and calf (62% and 59% respectively), tissue consistency (57%), increased skin temperature (49%), hematoma (41%), exudate of the knee joint (23%), and Homans sign (42%) [196]. Thus, leg swelling is a sensitive but non-specific finding in DVT [197].

Lisker Sign

We were able to identify only limited historical information about Samuel Lisker. At the time of the publication describing his sign, he served as an assistant professor of medicine and director of the Division of Peripheral Vascular Diseases and Clinic at Graduate Hospital, University of Pennsylvania, Philadelphia [134]. Edward W. Knox, MD, MRCPI, a fellow of Dr. Lisker, described the clinical findings of

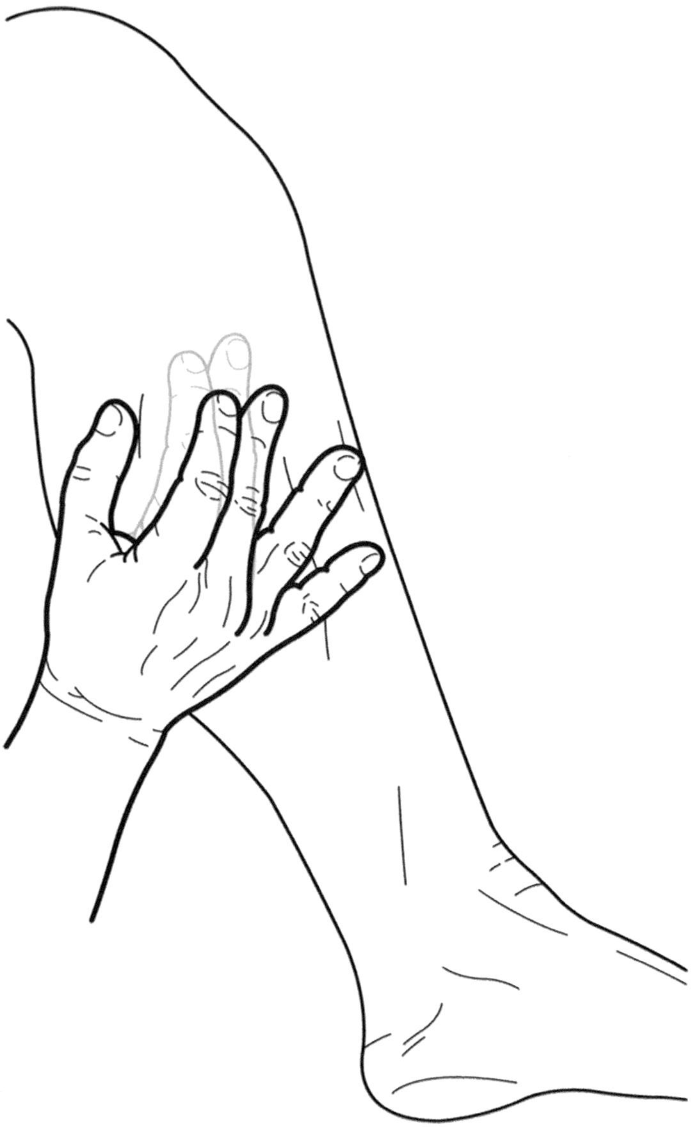

Fig. 16.14 Lisker sign (by Ryan Yale)

thrombophlebitis in a series of 20 unselected patients at the University of Pennsylvania [134]. In this series he used the tibial tap sign or Lisker sign that involved percussing using the flexed fingers on "the broad subcutaneous surface of the tibia medial to the crest" [134, p. 30] (Fig. 16.14). A positive sign is the presence of bone tenderness. In cases where the sign was uncertain percussion tenderness over the patella is compared to tibia. The tibia test is considered insignificant if tenderness is equivalent over both sites. In Knox's series, tenderness over the upper third of the tibia resolved faster than the lower two-thirds. Furthermore, he noted that tenderness presents more acutely and is more common in the lower two-thirds of the tibia. He hypothesized that bone tenderness was caused by increased interosseous pressure due to venous thrombosis and obstruction of venous blood flow [134].

Knox identified a positive Lisker sign in 26 of 34 (76%) lower extremities with DVT. Tenderness was found distributed throughout the tibia in fourteen patients, more severe in the lower two-thirds in ten, and upper area in two patients [134]. This sign is said to be present in 65% of patients with thrombophlebitis [198]. The utility of this sign in clinical practice has not been confirmed (Tables 16.1 and 16.2).

Peabody Sign

Dr. Charles Newton Peabody (1925–2011), born in Detroit as a son of a physician father, received his medical degree from Harvard University in 1946 [199]. At the time of his publication he was a member in the Department of Surgery, Framingham Union Hospital, Framingham, Massachusetts [200]. Peabody later became an assistant professor at Boston University School of Medicine. He was a navy veteran of the Korean War and remained a member of the Naval Reserve until his retirement as a commander in 1976 [201]. He also published a book entitled *Zab: Brevet Major Zabdiel Boylston Adams (1829–1902): Physician of Boston and Framingham* (1985) [202]. Peabody described the plantar flexion spasm technique as a later sign to diagnose thrombophlebitis (Fig. 16.15):

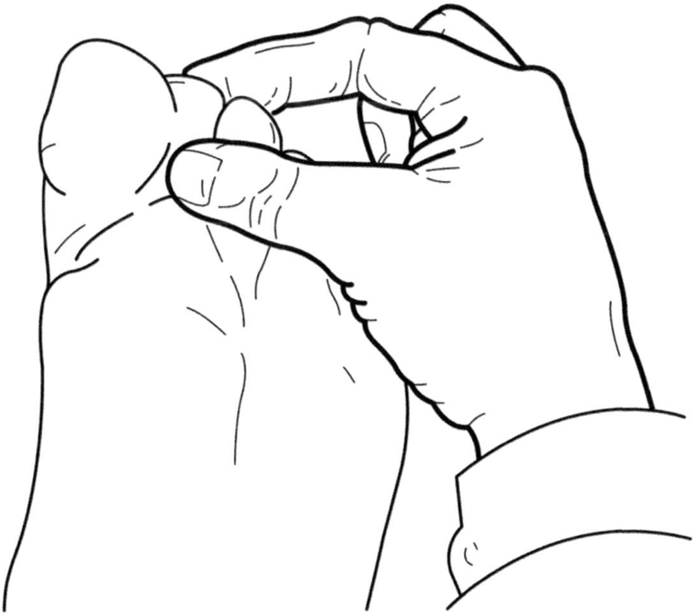

Fig. 16.15 Peabody sign (by Ryan Yale)

> The examiner stands at the end of the bed with the covers pulled back and the legs exposed. The feet are placed opposite each other. The examiner then places both his thumbs against the ends of the second metatarsals on the plantar surface of the feet. He then applies enough pressure against the bottom of the foot so that he can raise the feet off the bed about 20 inches. He observes the difference in plantar flexion by looking down at the feet. This is done by noting the relative position of the medial side of the end of the first metatarsals. When the internal malleoli are touching or nearly opposite each other, the bunions in the normal person will remain opposite each other. But if there is calf muscle spasm, the bunion in the diseased foot will be more plantar flexed [200, p. 434].

He postulated that thrombophlebitis causes a low-grade spasm of the gastrocnemius and soleus muscles resulting in plantar flexion of the foot. The degree of plantar flexion seen was proportionate to the amount of resistance caused by spasm of the gastrocnemius muscle. In 25 patients with thrombophlebitis, Peabody found the plantar flexion sign in 20 (80%), calf tenderness in 24 (96%), Lowenberg's sign in 21 (84%), and Homans and plantar flexion signs in 20 (80%). The sign is believed to be as reliable as Homans and Lowenberg signs [200]. Others report that the sign is neither sensitive nor specific for DVT [203]. However, another study showed its sensitivity and specificity to be 17% and 98%, respectively [154]. Richards et al. reported that Peabody sign was present in 19 of 150 patients with a false-positive rate of 11% (2 of 19 patients) [204]. The high specificity of this sign, if confirmed, suggests that its presence should heighten suspicion for DVT. Its absence, however, does not exclude the diagnosis (Tables 16.1 and 16.2).

Change Sign

There is limited historical information available about C.H. Joseph Change and Clayton Davis. Change was a member in the Department of Radiology at West Virginia University School of Medicine, Morgantown, West, Virginia. Davis, coauthor of this manuscript, was a fellow of the American College of Surgery (FACS) and associate chief of surgery, Man Memorial Hospital Man, West Virginia [205]. They reported:

> The most consistent roentgen sign of pulmonary embolism in our patients were dilation of the descending pulmonary artery, parenchymal densities and pleural fluid. The earliest consistent sign was widening of a previously normal descending pulmonary artery. This sign usually appeared within 24 hours of the onset of chest pain and shows its maximal measurement within two or three days. Dilation of the descending pulmonary artery persists for a period of one to two weeks and usually returned to normal in three to four weeks [205, p. 146].

In their series of 23 consecutive patients with pulmonary infarction all patients were found to have dilation of the right (19) or left (4) descending pulmonary arteries. The size of the right descending pulmonary artery ranged from (17–22 mm [normal upper limit on inspiration 16 for adult males and 15 mm for adult females]) and of the left descending pulmonary artery ranged from 17 to 26 mm [normal range <17 mm] [205]. The utility of this sign in clinical practice has not been confirmed (Table 16.1).

Pataro Sign

Vicente Francisco Pataro (1907–1983), professor of surgery at the Faculty of Medicine in Buenos Aires, was one of the most important figures of Argentine surgery of the twentieth century. He was born in Buenos Aires on March 2, 1907 and received his medical degree from the Faculty of Medicine of the University of Buenos Aires [206]. In 1935, he initially served in Room V of the Pirovano Hospital, and later became head of Surgical Clinic at the Dr. Ricardo Finochietto Polyclinic, Avellaneda, Buenos Aires [206]. Pataro also served as a surgical consultant of the Naval Hospital of Buenos Aires from 1962 until his death. He was an honorary member of numerous national and foreign scientific societies, founder and president (1954–1957) of the Argentine Society of Angiology, and editorial board member of *The Journal of Cardiovascular Surgery* [206].

Sfarcich described in his paper titled "La presión unidigital de pantorrilla como signo thrombosis venosa aguda de los miembros inferiors" (Calf unidigital pressure as a sign of acute venous thrombosis of the lower limbs) a sign that was initially described in 1954 in the *Interpoliclínicos Days of the National Institute of Social Medicine*:

> The sign taught by Dr. Vicente F. Pataro, which he calls McBurney's calf, is in our opinion the most useful sign in the investigation of acute venous thrombosis. It is the first one that appears and the last to disappear after treatment. When the calf is painful and when systematically investigated a fixed point of pain is always found. It is similar to that which occurs in acute appendicitis–although the entire right iliac fossa is painful, there is a point of exquisite pain named McBurney's point. That's why Dr. Pataro called this one McBurney's sign of the calf. The obvious value of this sign is that a calf can hurt for several reasons, but the well-located and fixed painful point is an unambiguous sign of acute venous thrombosis [207, p. 1945].

The test is performed as follows: "The patient is placed in the prone or supine position with the leg flexed on the thigh at a 45° angle. (…) To assess for the presence of pain, unidigital pressure is applied at equidistant points from the midline of the diseased calf" [207]. Sfarcich compared this sign to Homans, Olow, Lowenberg, and Ramirez signs in 121 patients with DVT and found it to be present in 100% and was always the first sign to appear [207]. The utility of this sign in clinical practice is unknown (Tables 16.1 and 16.2).

May Sign

Robert May (1914–1984) was born in Klagenfurt, Kärnten, and studied medicine in Innsbruck, Austria, from 1933 to 1938 [208]. He was taught phlebology by René Lehriche and C.L. Olivier in Paris and completed his surgical training in Vienna and London [208]. In 1956 he was head of the Vascular Department at Krankenhaus der Kreuzschwestern (Hospital of Cross Sisters), University of Innsbruck, Austria [208], and in 1982 was named Professor of Phlebology [208]. In 1979 he was editor of the textbook *Chirurgie der Bein- und Beckenvenen* (Surgery of the Veins of the Legs and Pelvis) [209].

May reported in his paper titled "Frühdiagnostik peripherer venöser und arterieller Durchblutungsstörungen" (Early diagnosis of peripheral venous and arterial circulatory disorders) a method for detecting venous thrombosis:

> With the patient lying, blood pressure cuffs are placed on both calves. Both cuffs are inflated to 150 mmHg. Healthy people report that the pressure is uncomfortable. However, on a diseased leg, the patient reports a pressure pain, grimaces and spontaneously withdraws his leg at 80-120 mmHg [210, p. 444].

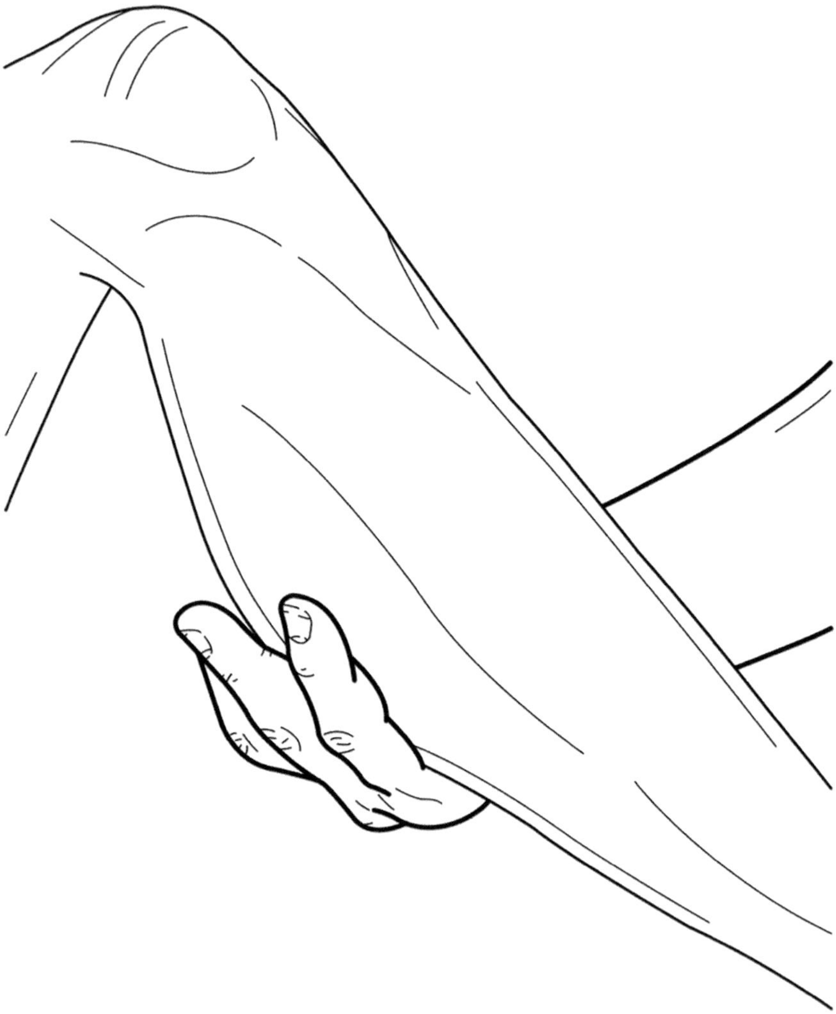

Fig. 16.16 Davies sign (by Ryan Yale)

Thus, May sign refers to the presence of pain or discomfort at a sphygmomanometer cuff pressure of 80 to 120 mmHg rather than at 150 mmHg. The utility of this sign in clinical practice is unknown (Tables 16.1 and 16.2).

Davies Sign

There is limited historical information available about Ieuan John Treharne Davies. At the time of his publication he was a member in the Department of Medicine, University Hospital of Wales [211]. He described a method for detecting DVT in the calf (Fig. 16.16):

> Palpation of the calves should be performed with the flat of the hand by gently lifting the muscle up and down with the knee flexed to 90° and the foot resting on the bed. Palpation is aimed at detecting a difference in weight of the calf muscles and a difference in hardness of the muscles due to intramuscular inflammatory oedema [211].

Thus, Davies sign refers to the difference in weight and hardness of the calf muscles when the knee is flexed to 90 degrees. The utility of this sign in clinical practice is unknown (Tables 16.1 and 16.2).

Corrigan-Strachan Sign

There is limited historical information about Drs. Corrigan or Strachan. At the time of the publication Thomas Corrigan and Colin J.L. Strachan were members of the Department of Surgery at King's College Hospital Medical School, London, and

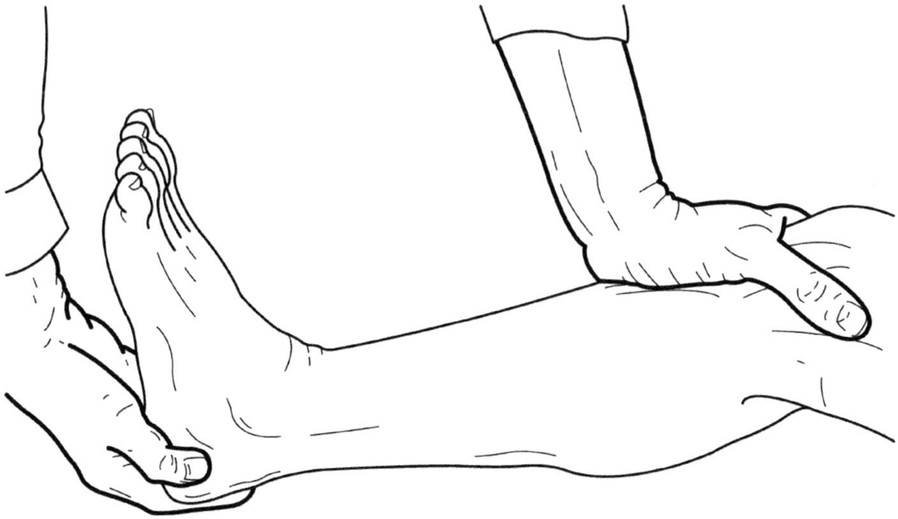

Fig. 16.17 Sigg sign (by Ryan Yale)

Mater Misericordæ Hospital, Dublin, Republic of Ireland [212]. They described two patients with extensive DVT with or without superficial thrombosis in which the knee was flexed in the range of 20–25 degree, "short of full extension and the patient was unable to extend it beyond this point" [212]. They reported that DVT "should be kept in mind in the presence of a flexed knee of recent onset whether no joint lesion is found" [212]. They attributed this finding to muscle spasms and/or sciatic neuritis. The utility of this sign in clinical practice is unknown (Table 16.1).

Sigg Sign

Dr. Karl Sigg (1912–1986) was born in Basel, Switzerland, and completed his medical training in this same city. In 1939, he established a practice for the management of venous diseases [213]. He was head of the Polyclinic for Venous Diseases at the University Gynecological Clinic Basel, Honorary President of the Swiss Society for Phlebology, and honorary member of the German Society for Phlebology [213]. In 1958, he published his book titled *Varicen - Ulcus Cruris und Thrombose: Neue Wege zur Nichtoperativen Behandlung* (Varicose leg ulcers and thrombosis: new ways to nonoperative treatment).

Wupperman described a sign of pain in the knee-joint during hyperextension for diagnosing DVT that he dedicated in gratitude to his revered teacher Karl Sigg. The maneuver is performed as follows (Fig. 16.17):

> Pressure applied to the patella using the palm of one hand and simultaneously lifting the heel using the other hand, causes a strong pain in the popliteal fossa. This pain can also be provoked by vigorous pressure on the patella with the leg stretched out on a firm support [214, p. 725].

In patients with phlebographically proven thromboses a mean positive accuracy of 0.83 and a mean specificity of 0.56 were found for Sigg sign [214]. Sigg sign, compared to Lowenberg, Bisgaard, Payr, Homans, Deneke, Pratt signs, and pressure pain in the calf, showed the highest observed overall mean positive postoperative accuracy (0.57), while the overall specificity did not differ (0.62) [214]. Thus, Sigg sign refers to the pain in the popliteal fossa when palpatory pressure is applied to the patella with one hand and the opposite hand elevates the heel of the foot. Sigg sign lacks sufficient specificity and in general does not further enhance the diagnostic accuracy of the physical examination for DVT [41] (Tables 16.1 and 16.2).

Palla Sign

Antonio Palla received his degree in medicine and surgery from the University of Pisa in 1974 [215]. He served at the CNR Institute of Clinical Physiology and Second Medical Clinic in 1963, was an assistant at the at the Institute of Clinical Medicine from 1977 to 1980, appointed chair of the Department of Respiratory

Diseases at the University of Pisa in 1980, and named ordinary professor of respiratory disease at the University of Pisa in 2001 [216, 217]. He was a member of the European Respiratory Society, American College of Chest Physicians, Italian Society of Respiratory Medicine (SIMeR), and International Alliance of Patients' Organizations (IAPO) [215]. Palla was editor of the *Journal of Nuclear Medicine-Allied Sciences*, member of the Board of Directors of "Thrombosis and Arteriosclerosis," and on the editorial committee of the *Quarterly Journal of Nuclear Medicine* [215]. His areas of specialty include respiratory diseases, in particular, tuberculosis, and nuclear medicine at the University of Pisa.

Palla et al. conducted a quantitative radiographic analysis of the right descending pulmonary artery in 73 (118) patients with confirmed pulmonary embolism (61 scintigraphy and 12 pulmonary angiography) and in 85 (147) patients with unconfirmed suspicion of pulmonary embolism (perfusion lung scan). They found that:

> [t]he enlargement of descending pulmonary artery may be useful to raise the suspicion of pulmonary embolisms. As documented here, the descending pulmonary artery was wider in patients with confirmed pulmonary embolism than in those without confirmation. The typical "sausage" appearance of the descending pulmonary artery, easily recognizable without any measurement, was present in about one-fourth of the patients with confirmed pulmonary embolism and its was never observed in patients in whom the original clinical suspicion of pulmonary embolism was rejected subsequently [217, p. 517].

It is of historic interest that transient enlargement of the pulmonary artery had been previously described by Fleishner in 1958 [218]. It was Palla and colleagues who performed the first accurate and quantitative analysis of the descending pulmonary artery in pulmonary embolism. The sensitivity or specificity of the sign is unknown [98, 217, 219] (Table 16.1).

McConnell Sign

Michael V. McConnell received his medical degree from Stanford University, California, in 1990 and completed his internship and residency in Internal Medicine at Bingham and Women's Hospital, Harvard Medical School, Massachusetts, followed by a fellowship in Cardiology and Cardiovascular Imaging at Brigham and Women's' and Beth Israel Hospitals, Boston in 1996 [220]. From 2000 to 2015 he served as the director of the Cardiovascular MRI Program and from 2010 to 2013 was the director of Preventive Cardiology Clinic in the Stanford Division of Cardiovascular Medicine [220]. From 2008 to 2015, he served as the director of the NIH Training Program in Cardiovascular Imaging at Stanford (CVIS) and from 2014 to 2015 served as the director of the Cardiovascular Health Innovation [220]. He is a clinical professor of medicine in cardiovascular medicine where he has appointments in preventive medicine and cardiovascular imaging. His current focus involves using technology as a means to prevent, detect, and manage disease as Head, Cardiovascular Health Innovations at Verily Life Sciences [221]. In a study cohort of 41 patients and validation cohort of 85 patients McConnell and colleagues found in the right ventricle (RV):

> Among patients with acute pulmonary embolism and RV dysfunction, there is a distinct, regional pattern of abnormal RV wall motion. Both quantitative and qualitative analyses of 2-dimensional echocardiograms in patients with acute pulmonary embolism revealed normal wall motion of the RV apex but akinesia of the mid-RV free wall [222, p. 472].

They reported a sensitivity, specificity, positive, and negative predictive values of 77%, 94%, 71%, and 96%, respectively. Another study identified that the sensitivity, specificity, positive, and negative predictive values of the McConnell sign for the diagnosis of pulmonary embolism were 70, 33, 67, and 36%, respectively [223]. Using ECHO-CG the PPV of McConnell's sign was 57% (CI, 45–67%) [224]. Finally, in 137 patients free from known cardio-respiratory disease, a sensitivity of 93% with a specificity of 81% was found [225]. Evidence suggests that the sign may be detected in patients with a high clinical suspicion for pulmonary embolism (Table 16.1).

Conclusion

The physical examination is limited in some cases in its ability to identify DVT because of a reduced or absent inflammatory infiltrate, collateral circulation and partial occlusion of the vessel. Surprisingly, with the exception of a few signs, there is a paucity of studies that assessed their accuracy and reliability in diagnosing venous thrombosis. Furthermore, for those signs which have been studied, a variety of methodological limitations affect the interpretation of studies including a small sample size, misinterpretation of a positive test, not describing the method of performing the sign, improperly performing the test as originally described and intended, testing in a population without a validated control group, retrospective study, small sample size, and type of imaging study used as the gold standard to confirm the diagnosis Therefore, further studies are required to assess the validity of these signs in clinical practice. Nevertheless, despite gaps in knowledge regarding their validity and reliability they remain historically important since many were conceived during the time prior to the advent of noninvasive laboratory and imaging techniques that have tremendously facilitated the accurate diagnosis of VTE.

The use of eponymous terms probably cannot be avoided in the scientific literature and in daily patient care, but when cited should be appropriately used as originally described to avoid misrepresentation and to ensure their appropriate application. The use of eponyms confers historical, literary, and cultural information that reaches beyond and therefore conveys the dignity of a broader educational background and understanding. Accurate knowledge of eponyms of VTE and a familiarity with the clinicians and their stories provides interesting background information and in some instances, an easier milieu for remembering their sign. Although most eponyms are infrequently used by clinicians, the information conveyed by these signs may lead to further proficiency in clinical skills and performance and may assist in considering VTE when used in conjunction with the history and other clinical signs and symptoms. Further interest to rigorously studying these signs, although supplanted when routine use and availability of duplex ultrasonography to screen patients for DVT became commonplace in medical practice, provides opportunity to understand their role in clinical medicine.

References

1. Paré A. The Works of That Famous Chirurgion Ambrose Parey. London: Th. Cotes and R. Young; 1649.
2. Wiseman R. Severall Chirurgicall Treatises. London: E. Flesber and J. Macock; 1676.
3. Forrester JM. Malphighi's De Polyp Cordis: an annotated translation. Med Hist. 1995;39:477–92.
4. Hunter J. Observations on the inflammation of the internal coats of veins. Tr Soc Improve M Chir Knowl. 1793;1:18–29.
5. Haller AV, Cullen W, Wrisberg HA. First Line of Physiology. Cullen W, translator. Edinburgh: Elliot & Robinson; 1786.
6. Baillie M. Of uncommon appearances of disease in blood vessels. Tr Soc Improve M Chir Knowl. 1793;1:119–37.
7. Hodgson J. On the diseases of veins, inflammation of the veins. In: A Treatise on the Diseases of Arteries and Veins Containing the Pathology and Treatment of Aneurisms and Wounded Arteries. London: Moyes Greenviile Street, Hatton Gardon; 1815. p. 511–7.
8. Hewson W. Properties of the blood – of the separation of the serum; the colour of the crassamentum; and of the causes of the coagulation of the blood. In: Gulliver G, editor. The Works of William Hewson. London: Sydenham Society; 1746. p. 1–30.
9. Andral G. Essai d'hématologie pathologique. Dublin J M Chem Sc. 1843;23:288–99.
10. Rokitansky C. Abnormal conditions of the veins. In: Swaine WE, Sieveking E, Moore CH, Day GE, editors. A Manual of Pathological Anatomy, vol. 4. London: Sydenham Society; 1852. p. 235–76.
11. Aristotle. Volume IV Historia Animalium by D'Arcy Wentworth Thompson. In: The Works of Aristotle. Ed. Translated into English by JA Smith and WD Ross. Oxford: Claredon Press;1910.
12. Anning ST. The historical aspects of venous thrombosis. Med Hist. 1957;1:28–37.
13. Virchow R. Phlogose und Thrombose in Gefässsystem. Gesammelte Abhandlungen zur Wissenschaftlichen Medicin. Frankfurt A.M.: Verlag von Meidinger Sohn & Comp; 1856.
14. Virchow R. Purulent cysts in the heart, cellular pathology as based upon physiological and pathological histology. In: Twenty Lectures Delivered in the Pathological Institute of Berlin during the Months of February, March and April 1858. Chance F, translator. London: John Churchill; 1860. p. 196–219.
15. Virchow R. Gesammelte Abhandlungen zur Wissenschaftlichen Medicin. Frankfurt A.M.: Verlag von Meidinger Sohn & Comp.; 1862.
16. Fresquet JL. Armand Trousseau (1801–1867). Historia de la medicina.org. In: Epónmos y biografias médicas. 2008. http://www.historiadelamedicina.org/trousseau.html. Accessed 2 Mar 2019.
17. Trousseau A, Belloc H. Traité pratique de la phthisie laryngée, de la laryngite chronique et des maladies de la voix. Paris: Baillière; 1837.
18. Trousseau A, Belloc H. A Practical Treatise of Laryngeal Phthisis, Chronic Laryngitis, and Disease of the Voice. Warder JA, translator. Philadelphia: A. Waldie; 1839.
19. Medvei VC. The History of Clinical Endocrinology. New York: The Parthenon Publishing Group; 1993.
20. Trousseau A. Nouvelles recherches sur la trachéotomie pratiquée dans la période extrême du croup. Paris: Felix Malteste et c.; 1851.

21. Moore MD, Fahey TJ. Armand Trousseau, 1801-1867. In: Pasleka JL, Lee JA, editors. Surgical Endocrinopathies: Clinical Management and the Founding Figures. Cham: Springer; 2015. p. 177–9.
22. Firkin BG, Whiteworth JA. Dictionary of Medical Eponyms. Boca Raton: The Parthenon Publishing Company; 2002.
23. [No author]. Death of Trousseau and Follin. Med Times & News Med Rec. 1868;2:264.
24. Trousseau A. Phlegmasia alba dolens. In: Cormack JR, Bazire PV, editors. Lectures on Clinical Medicine. Philadelphia: Lindsay & Blakiston; 1873. p. 281–332.
25. Samuels MA, King ME, Balis U. Case 31-2002: a 61-year-old man with headache and multiple infarcts. N Engl J Med. 2002;347(15):1187–94.
26. Callander N, Rapaport SI. Trousseau's syndrome. West J Med. 1993;158:364–71.
27. Birrer RB, Birrer CB. Medical Diagnostic Signs: A Reference Collection of Eponymic Bedside Signs. Springfield, IL: Charles C. Thomas Publisher; 1982.
28. Mahler RA. Thrombose, lungenembolie und plötzlicher Tod. In: Leopold G, editor. Geburtshülfe und Gynäkologie. Arbeiten aus der Dresdener Frauenklinik in Dresden. Hirzel. (VIII, 391 S. Lex. 8) e/ 24. Leipzig; 1895, p. 72–120. [Original reference not accessible].
29. Cumston CG. Pulmonary embolus following operative interference. Boston M S J. 1908;158:284–7.
30. Zurhelle E. Thrombose und embolie nach gynäkologischen Operationen. Archiv f Gynäkologie. 1908;84:443–512.
31. Hoffmann A. Thrombose, lungembolic und plötzkucher Tod; von Mahler aus Budapest (p. 72-120). Schmidt's Jahrb. 1895;247:104–5.
32. Michaelis H. Prodromalerscheinungen der puerperalen und postoperativen Thrombose und Embolie. München med Wochenschr. 1911;58:73–6.
33. Singer. Thrombose und Embolie im Wochenbett, mit besonderer Berücksichtigung der gonorrhoischen Infection. Arch f Gynäk. 1898;56:218–63.
34. Richter A. Thrombose und Embolie im Wochenbett, sowie die auf derselben Grundlage beruhenden Lungenerkrankungen der Wöchnerinnen. Arch f Gynäk. 1904;74:102–44.
35. Dlhos E, Mach AM. Diagnostická cena Mahlerovho príznaku. Cesk Gynekol. 1963;28:225–7.
36. Sanes KI. Septic pelvic thrombophlebitis. Tr Am Ass Obst & Gynec. 1912;25:107–37.
37. Fehring WB. Venous thrombosis in the puerperium by Dr. Rieländer. Marburg Surg Gynecol Obstet. 1907;5:365–6.
38. Rielander A. Über venethrombosen im wochenbett. Monatschr f Geburtsh u Gynäk. 1906;24:154–69.
39. Gundlach F. Catalogus Professorum Academiae Marburgensis (1527–1910). Marburg: Elwert; 1972.
40. Lanzer P, Topol EJ. Pan Vascular Medicine: Integrated Clinical Management. Berlin: Springer-Verlag; 2001.
41. Pschyrembel W. Pschyrembel klinisches Wörterbuch, mit klinischen Syndromen und Nomina Anatomica. Berlin: Walter de Gruyter; 1986.
42. [No author]. Current medical literature: premonitory signs of thrombosis. JAMA. 1911;56:549.
43. Faris J. Temperature chart analysis in the diagnosis of deep vein thrombosis. Am Heart J. 1974;87:259–60.
44. Rickford CR, Negus D. The early detection of postoperative deep vein thrombosis: an assessment of Doppler ultrasound, physical examination and temperature chart. Br J Surg. 1975;62:182–5.
45. Ducing J. Wikipédia L'éncylopédie libre. 2016. https://fr.wikipedia.org/wiki/Joseph_Ducuing. Accessed 2 May 2018.
46. Arlet J. Éloge de monsieur le doyen Lazortes. 2015. http://academie-sciences-lettres-toulouse.fr/wp-content/uploads/2017/10/2015-1-Eloge-Lazorthes.pdf. Accessed 2 May 2018.
47. Boure R. Inventaire des hommages rendus aux chercheurs Toulousains par leurs pairs (années 1880–2010): attributions de noms, publications dédiées et galeries de portraits. 2017. https://

pastel.hypotheses.org/files/2017/04/Inventaire-Pastel-numérique-R.Boure-.pdf. Accessed 15 May 2018.
48. Ducuing J. Phlébites thromboses et embolies post-opératoires. Paris: Masson et Cie; 1929.
49. Schneider FA, Siska IR, Avram JA. Clinical Physiology of the Venous System. New York: Kluwer Academic Publishers; 2003.
50. Janzen R. Pain Analysis: A Guide to Diagnosis. Baltimore: Williams & Wilkins; 1970.
51. Nüllen H, Noppeney T, Diehm C. Venöse Thromboembolien. Berlin: Springer-Verlag; 2014.
52. Ringelstein EB. Prävalenz der tiefen Beinvenenthrombose bei Patienten mit wahrscheinlicher paradoxer Embolie im Vergleich zu Patienten mit anderer Insultätiologie. Inagural-dissertation zur erlangung des doctor medicinae der medizinischen fakultät der Westfälischen Wilhelms-Universität Münster vorgelegt von Schomacher, Guido aus Beckum 2007. https://kipdf.com/inaugural-dissertation_5ad8729f7f8b9a688b8b45bc.html. Accessed 12 May 2018.
53. Kochen MM. Management der tiefen Beinvenenthrombose Veränderungen in Diagnostik und Therapie im Zeitraum von 1990 bis 2003. Inaugural-Dissertation zur erlangung des doktorgrades der medizinischen Fakultät der Georg-August-Universität zu Göttingen vorgelegt von Felix K. Schlehahn Aus Leipzig Göttingen. 2007. https://ediss.uni-goettingen.de/bitstream/handle/11858/00-1735-0000-0006-AF41-C/schlehahn.pdf?sequence=1. Accessed 12 May 2018.
54. Solares JIF, Garcia JLP, Hernandez CM, Vargas MF. Diagnóstico de la trombosis venosa profunda y de la tromboembolia pulmonar. Documento de Consenso CEFyL Semergen. Recomedaciones sobre profilxis, diagnóstico y tratamiento de la enfermedad tromboembólica venosa en atención primaria. http://www.capitulodeflebologia.org/download/Mailings/Consenso-ETEV-en-Atencion-Primaria.pdf. Accessed 18 May 2018.
55. Segno di Laurel. http://happyslide.net/doc/323165/segno-di-laurel. Accessed 20 May 2018.
56. Friess H, Demir IE, Ceyhan GO. Vereinigung der Bayerischen Chirurgen (1911-2011): Zur 100. Jubiläums-tagung der vereinigung. München; 2011. http://www.vereinigung-bayerischer-chirurgen.de/content/files/100-jahre-vbc-buch.pdf. Accessed 10 May 2018.
57. Denecke K. Der Plantarschmerz als Frühsymptom einer beginnenden thrombose der unteren Extremität. München med Wchnschr. 1929;76:1912–3.
58. Olow J. https://sv.wikipedia.org/wiki/John_Olow 2018. Accessed 15 Mar 2019.
59. Olow J. Sur un détail concernant le diagnostic de la thrombose crurale. Acta Obstet Gyn Scan. 1930;10:159–62.
60. Haeseker B. Dr. J.F.S. Esser and His Influence on the Development of Plastic and Reconstructive Surgery. Rotterdam: Erasmus Universiteit; 1983.
61. Garrison FH. An Introduction to the History of Medicine. 3rd ed. Philadelphia: W.B. Saunders Company; 1921.
62. Jurasz AT. I jego szkoła chirurgiczna. Uniwersytet Medyczny im. Karola Marcinkowskiego w Poznaniu. Fakty UMP. Dwumiesięcznik informacyjny. 2016;4:6–8.
63. Linetskiy SV, Hubálková H, Staňková H, Šmucler R, Mazánek J. Ozone and its usage in general medicine and dentistry. Prague Med Rep. 2008;109:5–13.
64. Health Technology Assessment Unit a Medical Development Division Ministry of Health. Ozone Therapy. Health Technology Assessment Unit Medical Development Division Ministry of Health MOH/PAK/110.06 (TR). 2005 http://www.moh.gov.my/update2017/1009.pdf. Accessed 30 Apr 2018.
65. Pardeep S, Kirtika S, Neha S, Nidhi D. Review of ozone and its role in prosthodontics. Sch J Dent Sci. 2017;4:226–32.
66. Pagadala S, Tadikonda DC. Ozone therapy a frontier in periodontics: a review. Int J Adv Res. 2015;3:652–7.
67. Drumi W, Drumi C. Emerich Ullmann (1861-1937): not only a pioneer of kidney transplantation. J Nephrol. 2004;17:461–6.
68. Wicht JH. Renal transplant survey: how standardized is a standard kidney transplant. Thesis: Master of Medicine (MMed) in Surgery. University of Cape Town; 2016. https://open.uct.ac.za/bitstream/handle/11427/24507/thesis_hsf_2017_wicht_jonathan_h.pdf?sequence=1. Accessed 4 Mar 2019.

69. Hamilton D. A History of Organ Transplantation: Ancient Legends to Modern Practice. Pittsburgh: University of Pittsburgh Press; 2012.
70. Schindler OS. Surgery for anterior cruciate ligament deficiency: a historical perspective. Knee Surg Sports Traumatol Arthosc. 2011;20:5–47.
71. Sanchis-Alfonso V, Monllau JC. The ACL-Deficient Knee: A Problem Solving Approach. London: Springer Verlag; 2013.
72. Payr E. Der heutige stand der Gelenkchirurgie Verhandlungen der Deutschen Gesellschaft für Chirurgie. Arch f klin Chir. 1927;148:404–521.
73. Milojević AJ, Radojčić BS, Meljnikov ID. Hydrocephalus-history of surgical treatment over the centuries. Istorija Medicine. 2012;7:119–25.
74. Sivayoham IS. Camero-venous shunt for secondary glaucoma following orbital venous obstruction. Br J Opthalmol. 1968;52:843–5.
75. Payr E. Wikipedia: the free encyclopedia. 2017. https://en.wikipedia.org/wiki/Erwin_Payr. Accessed 10 Apr 2018.
76. Crolley VE, Gibbins N. One hundred years of external approach medialisation thyroplasty. J Laryngol Otol. 2017;131:202–8.
77. Spiegel HU. Aus dem Universitätsklinikum Münster Klinik und Poliklinik für Allgemeine Chirurgie [From the University Hospital Münster Clinic and polyclinic for general surgery]. Direktor: Univ. Prof. Dr. Norbert Senninger Abteilung Chirurgische Forschung Leiter: Prof. Dr. Dipl. Ing. H.U. Spiegel Die Entwicklung der "Chirurgischen Forschung" in Deutschland. Inaugural-Dissertation zur Erlangung des doctor medicinae dentium der Medizinischen Fakultät der Westfälischen Wilhelms- Universität Münster vorgelegt von Neumann, Michaela, Brigitte aus Berlin; 2016. https://d-nb.info/991641264/34. Accessed 8 May 2018.
78. Payr E. Austria-Forum. 2020. https://austria-forum.org/af/AustriaWiki/Erwin_Payr. Accessed 8 May 2020.
79. Tschmarke G. Erfahrungen über den Fußsohlendruckschmerz als Frühsymptom der thrombose. München med Wohnschr. 1931;11:2135.
80. Tschmarke G. Erfahrungen über den Fußsohlendruckschmerz als Frühsymptom der Thrombose. Chirurg. 1931;3:924–7.
81. Payr E. Gedanken und Beobachtungen über die Thrombo-Emboliefrage. Centrabl f Chir. 1930;57:961–78.
82. Meyer O. Phlebitis: The Hidden Cause of Most Leg and Foot Ailments. New York: Savoy Book Publishers; 1940.
83. Meyer O. Symptomenkomplex und Therapie des Ulcus phlebiticum. München med Wohnschr. 1932;79:551.
84. Petter O, Holzegel K. Zur Geschichte der deutschen Phlebologie. Torgau: Kopielski Druck und Medien; 2005.
85. Krieg E. Zum klinischen Bild der infektiösen Fernthrombose. München med Wohnschr. 1935;82:776–8.
86. Hunter WC, Sneeden VD, Robertson TD, Snyder GAC. Thrombosis of deep veins of the leg: its clinical significance as exemplified in 251 autopsies. Arch Int Med. 1941;68:1–17.
87. Strous RD, Edelman MC. Eponyms and the Nazi era: time to remember and time for change. Isr Med Assoc J. 2007;9:207–14.
88. Neumann Robert Dr. Startseite / 1933-1945 Täter und Mitläufer / 1933–1945 BiografienN. http://www.tenhumbergreinhard.de/1933-1945-taeter-und-mitlaeufer/1933-1945-biografien-n/neumann-robert-dr.html. Accessed 10 Apr 2018.
89. Hildebrandt S. The Anatomy of Murder: Ethical Transgressions and Anatomical Science during the Third Reich. New York: Berghahn Publications; 2016.
90. Robert Neumann (Pathologie). Wikipedia - Die freie Enzyklopädie. 2020. https://de.wikipedia.org/wiki/Robert_Neumann_(Pathologe). Accessed 7 May 2020.
91. Neumann R. Ursprungszentren und Entwicklungsformen der Bein-Thrombose. Arch f path Anat. 1938;301:708–35.
92. Maizlin ZV, Westermark N. Sans Atout and olympic medal. In: Wonders of Radiology. Scotts Valley, California: Create Space Publishing; 2010. p. 138–41.

93. Maizlin ZV, Cooperberg PL, Clement JJ, Vos PM, Coblentz CL. People behind exclusive eponyms of radiologic signs, Part II. Can Assoc Radiol J. 2010;61:44–53.
94. Nils Westermark sailor and radiologist. https://upclosed.com/people/nils-westermark/. Accessed 2 Feb 2019.
95. Westermark N. Archive.today. SR/Olympic Sports. Sports Reference LLC. 2000-2015 http://archive.li/iBYNv. Accessed 3 Feb 2019.
96. Westermark NJH. Roentgen Studies of the Lungs and Heart. Minnesota: University of Minnesota Press; 1948.
97. Westermark N. On the roentgen diagnosis of lung embolism. Acta Radiol. 1938;19:357–72.
98. Sreenivasan S, Bennett S, Parfitt VJ. Westermark's and Palla's signs in acute pulmonary embolism. Circulation. 2007;115:e211.
99. Robin Sturtevant Pilcher. Lives of the fellows. Royal College of Physicians. http://munksroll.rcplondon.ac.uk/Biography/Details/3567. Accessed 15 May 2018.
100. Pilcher R. Postoperative thrombosis and embolism. Lancet. 1939;234(6055):629–30.
101. Hall CM, Clark CG. Clinical signs in deep-vein thrombosis. Br J Surg. 1971;58:101–4.
102. Keaveny TV, White C, Belzer FO. Skin temperature, blood flow, and venous occlusion. J Cardiovasc Surg. 1970;11:219–23.
103. Provan JL. The early diagnosis of deep venous thrombosis. Proc R Soc Med. 1964;57:1149–50.
104. Provan JL. Raised skin temperature in the early diagnosis of deep-vein thrombosis of the legs. Br Med J. 1965;2(5457):334–7.
105. Maizlin ZV, Cooperberg PL, Clement JJ, Vos PM, Coblentz CL. People behind exclusive eponyms of radiologic signs, Part I. Can Assoc Radiol J. 2009;60:201–2.
106. Schatzki R, Lingley JR. Aubrey O. Hampton, 1900-1955. Am J Roentgenol, Radium Therapy Nucl Med. 1956;76:396.
107. Hampton AD, Castleman B. Correlation of post mortem chest teleroentgenograms with autopsy findings with special reference to pulmonary embolism and infarction. Am J Roentgenol. 1940;43:305–26.
108. Worsley DF, Alavi A, Aronchick JM, Chen JY, Greenspan RH, Ravin CE. Chest radiographic findings in patients with acute pulmonary embolism: observations from the PIOPED study. Radiology. 1993;189:133–6.
109. Yao JST. The Society of Vascular Surgery John Homans lectureship. J Vasc Surg. 1996;23:1077–80.
110. Barshes NR, Belkin M. The Homans family in American surgery. Ann Surg. 2015;261:416–20.
111. Elkin DC. John Homans lecture. N Engl J Med. 1951;245:997–1000.
112. Veith FJ. A look at the future of vascular surgery. J Vasc Surg. 2016;64:885–90.
113. Homans J. Exploration and division of the femoral and iliac veins in the treatment of the thrombophlebitis of the leg. N Engl J Med. 1941;224:179–86.
114. Allen AW, Liton R, Donaldson GA. Thrombosis and embolism: review of 202 patients treated by femoral vein interruption. Ann Surg. 1943;118:728–39.
115. Homans J. Diseases of the veins. N Engl J Med. 1944;231:51–60.
116. DeGowin EL, DeGowin RL. Bedside Diagnostic Examination. New York: MacMillan Publishing Company; 1981.
117. Felder A. Evaluation of the various clinical signs of thrombophlebitis and experience in therapy with anticoagulants. Surg Gynecol Obstet. 1949;88:337–50.
118. Anand S, Wells P, Hunt D, Brill-Edwards P, Cook D, Ginsberg JS. Does this patient have deep vein thrombosis? JAMA. 1998;279:1094–9.
119. Seidel HM, Ball JW, Dains JE, Benedict GW. Mosby Guide to the Physical Examination. St. Louis: Mosby; 1999.
120. Dunphy JE, Botsford TW. Examination of the blood vessels and lymphatics. In: Physical Examination of the Surgical Patient and Introduction to Clinical Surgery. Philadelphia: W.B. Saunders Company; 1975. p. 228–57.
121. Kahn SR. The clinical diagnosis of deep venous thrombosis: integrating incidence, risk factors, and symptoms and signs. Arch Intern Med. 1998;58:2315–23.
122. McLachlin J, Richards T, Paterson JC. An evaluation of clinical signs in the diagnosis of venous thrombosis. Arch Surg. 1962;85:738–44.

123. Urbano FL. Homans' sign in the diagnosis of deep vein thrombosis. Hosp Physician. 2001;37:22–4.
124. Sandler DA. Homans' sign and medical education. Lancet. 1985;326(8664):1130–1.
125. Shafter N, Duboff S. Physical signs in the early diagnosis of thrombophlebitis. Angiology. 1971;22:18–30.
126. Naib BA, Salih NA. Accuracy of color duplex imaging (CDI) in diagnosis deep vein thrombosis (DVT) versus clinical prediction index. IJSR. 2013;2:66–70.
127. Haeger K. Problems of acute deep venous thrombosis: the interpretation of signs and symptoms. Angiology. 1969;20:219–23.
128. Hirsh J, Hull RD, Raskob GE. Clinical features and diagnosis of venous thrombosis. J Am Coll Cardiol. 1986;8:114B–27B.
129. Wheeler HB. Diagnosis of deep vein thrombosis: review of clinical evaluation and impedance plethysmography. Am J Surg. 1985;150:7–13.
130. Cranley JJ, Canos AJ, Sull WJ. The diagnosis of deep venous thrombosis: fallibility of clinical symptoms and signs. Arch Surg. 1976;111:34–6.
131. Johnson WC. Evaluation of newer techniques for the diagnosis of venous thrombosis. J Surg Res. 1974;16:473–81.
132. O'Donnell TF Jr, Abbott WM, Athanasoulis CA, Millan VG, Callow AD. Diagnosis of deep venous thrombosis in the outpatient by venography. Surg Gyneco Obstet. 1980;150:69–74.
133. Molloy W, English JJ, O'Dwyer R, O'Connell J. Clinical findings in the diagnosis of proximal deep vein thrombosis. Ir Med J. 1982;75:119–20.
134. Knox EW. Deep thrombophlebitis of the lower limbs. Ulster Med J. 1964;33:28–35.
135. Miles B. Candles in Denmark. London: John Murray Publishers; 1958.
136. Bisgaard H. Ulcus und Eczema cruris, Phlebitidis sequelae usw: Studien über die statischen Erkrankungen der unteren Extremitäten und ihre Behandlung. Kopenhagen: Munksgaard; 1941.
137. Zink C. Dictionary of Obstetrics and Gynecology. Dyer KR, translator. Berlin: Walter de Gruyter & Co.; 1987.
138. Wiersema AM. The history of heparin, part II: the early development and road to clinical use. In: Periprocedural Prophylactic Antithrombotics in Arterial Procedures: The Road to Consensus. Ede, Netherlands: GVO/Ponsen and Looijen; 1964. p. 43–81.
139. Eklöf B. Presidential address: the dynamic approach to venous disease-following in the footsteps of Gunnar Bauer and Robert Kistner. J Vasc Surg. 2005;42:369–76.
140. Bauer G. Venous thrombosis, early diagnosis with the aid of phlebography and abortive treatment with heparin. Arch Surg. 1941;43:462–72.
141. Wade PA. Frederic Wolcott Bancroft. In: Curry GJ, Cohn I, Wade FV, editors. Profile in Trauma. Springfield, IL: Charles C. Thomas; 1969. p. 15–7.
142. [No author]. New York Med J. 1906;83:1306.
143. [No author]. Catalogue of Officer and Graduates Columbia University from the Foundation of King's College in 1754. 16th ed. New York: Columbia University; 1916.
144. [No author]. Columbia University Bulletin of Information: Annual Reports of the President and Treasurer to the Trustees with Accompanying Documents for the Year ending June 30, 1917. New York: Columbia University; 1917.
145. Peltier LF. Fractures: A History and Iconography of Their Treatment. San Francisco: Norman Publishing; 1990.
146. [No author]. Reprints from the Surgical Service New York City, Fifth Avenue Hospital. New York City; 1928.
147. [No author]. Bancroft FW. New York Physician 1936;6:13.
148. [No author]. Columbia-Presbyterian Medical Center. The Center Annual Report. 1962;4:155.
149. Bancroft FW. Proximal ligation and thrombectomy for phlebothrombosis of the femoral and iliac veins. Ann Surg. 1945;121:175–84.
150. Rajagopalan S, Mukherjee D, Mohler ER. Manual of Vascular Diseases. Philadelphia: Lippincott Williams & Wilkins; 2004.

151. Moses WR. Washington area surgeon. Wash Post 2005. http://www.washingtonpost.com/wp-dyn/content/article/2005/12/15/AR2005121501914.html. Accessed 12 May 2018.
152. Moses WR. The early diagnosis of phlebothrombosis. N Engl J Med. 1946;234:288–91.
153. Shafer N, Duboff S. Physical signs in the early diagnosis of thrombophlebitis. Angiology. 1971;22:18–30.
154. Holohan TV. Plethysmography: Safety, Effectiveness and Clinical Utility in Diagnosing Vascular Disease. Pennsylvania: Diane Publishing; 1996.
155. Touroff AS, Aufses AH. In memoriam Harold Neuhof 1884-1964. J Mt Sinai Hosp. 1964;31:13–4.
156. [No author]. Obituary: Neuhof-Dr. Harold. New York Times. Jan 9 1964. https://www.nytimes.com/1964/01/09/obituary-1-no-title.html. Accessed 2 May 2018.
157. Neuhof H. Venous thrombosis and pulmonary embolization, Part 1: diagnosis of venous thrombosis in the lower extremities. J Mt Sinai Hosp. 1947;14:110–21.
158. Neuhof H. Venous Thrombosis and Pulmonary Embolism. New York: Waverly Press; 1948.
159. Ellis H. Henry Hamilton Bailey. J Audiov Media Med. 1996;19:185.
160. Bailey HH (1894–1961). Royal College of Surgeons. Plarr's Lives of the Fellows. 2015. https://livesonline.rcseng.ac.uk/biogs/E004873b.htm. Accessed 10 May 2020.
161. Bailey H. Early diagnosis of thrombophlebitis decubiti. Clin Med (Northfield). 1947;54:302.
162. Ortiz-Ramírez T, Serna-Ramírez R. New early diagnostic sign of phlebitis of the lower extremities. Am Heart J. 1955;50:366–72.
163. Rosenthal R. A diagnostic sign for anterior tibial vein thrombosis. N Y State J Med. 1948;48:1148–52.
164. Dr. Gerald Pratt, surgeon, dies at 73. The New York Times. 7 Feb 1979. https://www.nytimes.com/1979/02/07/archives/dr-gerald-pratt-surgeon-dies-at-73-cardiovascular-specialist-was-an.html. Accessed 15 Jun 2018.
165. Pratt GH. Surgical management of venous clotting. Surg Clin North Am. 1948;28:341–52.
166. Pratt GH. An early sign of femoral thrombosis. JAMA. 1949;140:476–7.
167. Van Beek EJR, Büller HR, Oudkerk M. Deep Vein Thrombosis and Pulmonary Embolism. Oxford: Wiley-Blackwell; 2009.
168. Deep vein thrombosis. Űltima atualizacão. BMJ Best Practice; 2016. http://bp.api.bmj.com/best-practice/monograph/70/diagnosis/step-by-step.html?locale=pt_BR. Accessed 10 May 2018.
169. [No author]. Dr. Elias D. Lawrence. Quarterly of the Alumni Association of the New York Medical College. 1940;2:7.
170. Lawrence ED. The cough-pain sign in acute superficial thrombophlebitis. J Med Soc N J. 1950;47:164–6.
171. [No author]. Obituaries: Dr. Arthur J. D'Alessandro. J Med Soc N J. 1983;80:64.
172. [No author]. Announcements for the one hundred and first session 1941–1942. New York University Bulletin. 1941;41:31.
173. Alessandro AJD. An early clinical sign of venous thrombosis. JAMA. 1951;14:1759–60.
174. [No author]. Bull Acad de méd. 1984;168:700.
175. Louvel J, Laubry JJ. Sur un symptôme peu connu de thrombophlébite. Arch Mal Coeur Vaiss. 1952;45:630–2.
176. Solaiman FA, Kim ESH. Venous thromboembolism and hypercoagulable state. In: Griffin BP, editor. Manual of Cardiovascular Medicine. 4th ed. Philadelphia: Lippincott Williams & Wilkins; 2013. p. 446–58.
177. Kim ESH, Bartholomew JR. Venous thromboembolism. In: Askari AT, Lincoff AA, editors. Antithrombotic Drug Therapy in Cardiovascular Disease. New York: Humana Press; 2010. p. 331–50.
178. Bellini E. Communicazione alla Societa Medico-Chirurgica Veneziana. Seduta del 29 Gennaio; 1953.
179. Bellini E. Un segno precoce nella diagnostica delle trombosi venose degli arti inferior. G Sci Mediche. 1953;8:71–8.

180. Castañeda-Uribe M. Diagnóstico diferencial entre tromboflebitis y flebotrombosis. Ginecol Obstet Mex. 1953;8:381–5. [Reproduced: Ginecol Obstet Mex. 2008;76:493–6].
181. Lowenberg RI. A new clinical test for intravascular clot. Science. 1954;119:883.
182. Lowenberg RI. Early diagnosis of phlebothrombosis with aid of a new clinical test. JAMA. 1954;155:1566–70.
183. Lowenberg RI. Use of the cuff pain test in the early diagnosis of phlebothrombosis. J Am Podiatry Assoc. 1958;48:141–3.
184. Barner HB, DeWeese JA. An evaluation of the sphygmomanometer cuff pain test in venous thrombosis. Surgery. 1960;48:915–24.
185. Makin GS. Assessment of a simple test to detect postoperative deep venous thrombosis. Br J Surg. 1968;55:822–4.
186. Subramonia S, Lees TA. Clinical assessment of venous disease. In: Labropoulos N, Stansby G, editors. Venous and Lymphatic Diseases. Boca Raton: CRC Press; 2006.
187. Negus D, Jantet G, editors. Phlebology '85: Proceedings of the First United Kingdom Meeting of the Union Internationale de Phlébologie (London, 16-20 September 1985). London: John Libbey Publishing; 1986.
188. Rose SS. Cardiovascular surgery. J Cardiovasc Surg. 1993;1:6.
189. Bailey H. Physical Signs in Clinical Surgery. 13th ed. Bristol: John Wright & Sons; 1960.
190. Teófilo Ortiz Ramírez. John Simon Guggenheim Memorial Foundation. 1935–1936. https://www.gf.org/fellows/all-fellows/teofilo-ortiz-Ramírez/. Accessed 18 Jan 2019.
191. [No author]. Annual members: Roy J Popkin MD. Medical Bulletin University of Minnesota. 1971;43:13.
192. Halpern A. The third annual meeting of the American College of Angiology. Angiology. 1957;8:477–83.
193. Popkin RJ. Venous stasis of the lower extremities: a simple clinical test. Am Pract Dig Treat. 1960;11:301–2.
194. McLachlin JA. National Library of Scotland. Naval forces of the Dominions (Canada) 1735 Royal Canadian Naval Volunteer Reserve (List "A"). 1943;2: 283.
195. [No author]. Alumni news: Dr. John A McLachlin. UWOMJ 1966;36:131.
196. Lagerstedt C. Diagnostic and Therapeutic Aspects of Deep Vein Thrombosis. Lund: Lund University; 1992.
197. Ng KC. Deep vein thrombosis: a study in clinical diagnosis. Singap Med J. 1994;35:286–9.
198. Kennedy D, Setnik G, Li J. Physical examination findings in deep venous thrombosis. Emerg Med Clin North Am. 2001;19:869–76.
199. Peabody CN. Harvard Magazine. 1998;101:129.
200. Peabody CN. An objective sign of thrombophlebitis. Angiology. 1964;15:434–5.
201. Harvard University Obituary and Death Notice Collection – 69. 18 Jan 2011. http://www.genealogybuff.com/ma/harvard/webbbs_config.pl/noframes/read/69. Accessed 18 Jun 2018.
202. Peabody CN. Zab: Brevet Major Zabdiel Boylston Adams, 1829-1902: Physician of Boston and Framingham. Boston: Francis A. Countway; 1984.
203. van Beek EJR, Büller HR, Oudkerk M. Deep Vein Thrombosis and Pulmonary Embolism. Oxford: John Wiley and Sons; 2009.
204. Richards K, Armstrong JD Jr, Tikoff G, Hershgold EJ, Booth JL, Rampton JB. Noninvasive diagnosis of deep venous thrombosis. Arch Intern Med. 1976;13:1091–6.
205. Change CH, Davis C. A roentgen sign of pulmonary infarction. Clin Radiol. 1965;16:141–7.
206. Sfarcich DB, Vicente F. Pataro (1907–1983). Rev Argent Cirug Card. 2009;7:160–1.
207. Sfarcich DB. La presión unidigital de pantorrilla como signo de trombosis venosa aguda de los miembros inferiors. Pren Méd Argent. 1965;52:1945–6.
208. Petter O, Holzegel K. Zur Geschichte der deutschen Phlebologie. Torgau: Kopielski; 2005.
209. May R. Chirurgie der Bein- und Beckenvenen. Hirsch HJ, translator. Philadelphia: Saunders; 1979.
210. May R. Frühdiagnostik peripherer venöser und arterieller Durchblutungsstörungen. Z Allg Med. 1969;45:442–50.

211. Davies IJT. Clinical signs of deep-vein thrombosis. Lancet. 1972;299(7745):321.
212. Corrigan TP, Strachan CJ. New physical sign of acute deep vein thrombosis. BMJ. 1973;4(5887):296.
213. Sigg K. The treatment of varicosities and accompanying complications (the ambulatory treatment of phlebitis with compression bandage). Angiology. 1952;3:355–79.
214. Wuppermann T, Rienhoff O, von Schweder HW, Jobst U, Jester HJ. Ein neues klinisches Thrombosezeichen bei tiefer Beinvenenthrombose: das Sigg'sche Zeichen. Münch med Wschr. 1979;121:725–6.
215. Palla A. Giovani e giovanissmi in pneumologia. European Respiratory News. http://www2.unipr.it/~respdis/palla.htm. Accessed 9 May 2018.
216. Incarcio importante per Palla. Lo pneumologo nominato professore ordinario a Pisa. Il Tirreno Edizione Versila. 2011. http://iltirreno.gelocal.it/versilia/cronaca/2011/05/26/news/incarico-importante-per-palla-1.2503290?refresh_ceIn. Accessed 2 May 2018.
217. Palla A, Donnamaria V, Petruzzelli S, Rossi G, Riccetti G, Giuntini C. Enlargement of the right descending pulmonary artery in pulmonary embolism. AJR. 1983;141:513–7.
218. Fleischner FG. Pulmonary embolism. Can Med Assoc J. 1958;78:653–60.
219. Lee DS, Vo HA, Franco A, Keshavamurthy J, Rotem E. Palla and Westermark signs. J Thorac Imaging. 2017;32:W7.
220. Michael V, McConnell, MD, MSEE. Stanford profiles. http://med.stanford.edu/profiles/Michael_McConnell/. Accessed 20 May 2018.
221. Verily Life Sciences LLC, 2018. https://verily.com. Accessed 20 May 2018.
222. McConnell MV, Solomon SD, Rayan M, Come PC, Goldhaber SZ, Lee RT. Regional right ventricular dysfunction detected by echocardiography in acute pulmonary embolism. Am J Cardiol. 1996;78:469–73.
223. Casazza F, Bongarzoni A, Capozi A, Agostoni O. Regional right ventricular dysfunction in acute pulmonary embolism and right ventricular infarction. Eur J Echocardiogr. 2005;6:11–4.
224. Vaid U, Singer E, Marhefka GD, Kraft WK, Baram M. Poor positive predictive value of McConnell's sign on transthoracic echocardiography for the diagnosis of acute pulmonary embolism. Hosp Pract. 1995;41(2013):23–7.
225. Nazeyrollas P, Metz D, Jolly D, Maillier B, Jennesseaux C, Maes D, Chabert JP, Chapoutot L, Elaerts J. Use of transthoracic Doppler echocardiography combined with clinical and electrocardiographic data to predict acute pulmonary embolism. Eur Heart J. 1996;17:779–86.

Chapter 17
Venous Thrombosis: Cerebral Venous Thrombosis

Signs

Gerhardt Sign

Historical information about Carl Jakob Christian Adolph Gerhardt (1833–1902) has been previously discussed under the section pericarditis, where he described another sign which bears his namesake. Gerhardt found in 96 autopsies in children, thrombosis of the cerebral sinus in 7, all occurring in children less than 6 months of age. In his paper "Ueber Hirnsinusthrombosis bei Kindern" (about cerebral sinus thrombosis in children), he described in detail his observations in three of these children (Table 17.1, Fig. 17.1):

> We are unable to find any characteristic findings for these more general neurologic phenomena that characterizes the disease in question. They do not always have clear discernible symptoms. In almost all our cases we find an unequal filling of the external jugular veins which in many if not most cases makes it possible to diagnose cerebral sinus thrombosis.

Table 17.1 Eponymous signs of cerebral venous thrombosis

Name	Year	Description of sign	Sensitivity	Specificity
Gerhardt [1]	1857	In a child with a previously bilaterally filled jugular veins, the external jugular vein on one side appears severely dilated while the opposite external jugular vein due to a cerebral vein thrombosis is collapsed.	Unknown	Unknown
Griesinger [2]	1862	In transverse sinus thrombosis, there is a painful swelling located behind the mastoid process.	Unknown	Unknown
Crowe [10]	1912	In unilateral cerebral sinus thrombosis, engorgement of the retinal vessels in both fundi occurs when the jugular veins on the contralateral healthy side is compressed.	Unknown	Unknown

S. H. Yale et al., *Cardiovascular Eponymic Signs*,
https://doi.org/10.1007/978-3-030-67596-7_17

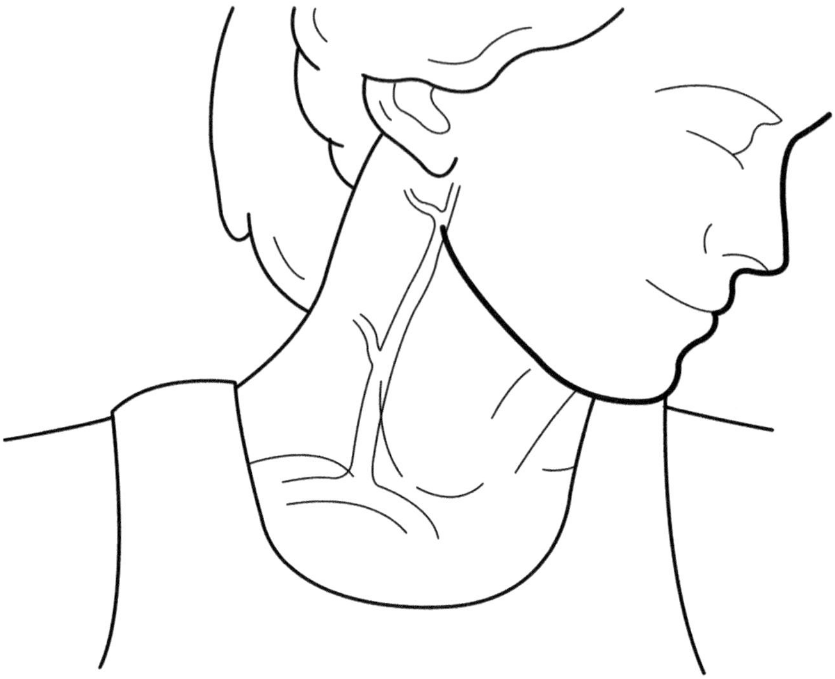

Fig. 17.1 Gerhardt sign (by Ryan Yale)

> This finding can in any case be all the more certain when a direct sign can explain the symptoms. (…) The diagnosis of cerebral sinus thrombosis can be made, with some degree of distinctness and consistency, in cases with severe cerebral symptoms caused by an acute gastrointestinal catarrhal if one observes in children, with previously uniform filled jugular veins, that one external jugular vein is collapsed while the other appears to be severely dilated. In fact, the side which is predominantly affected will be the one in which the vein is collapsed. (…) in the absence of this symptom, thrombosis cannot be ruled out with certainty – it is a symptom that should be applied positively and never negatively [1, p. 488].

Gerhardt also found that the external jugular vein on the thrombosed side is less prominent during inspiration [1]. Thus, Gerhardt sign refers to a collapsed internal jugular vein in cases of cerebral venous sinus thrombosis.

Griesinger Sign

Historical information about Wilhelm Griesinger (1817–1868) has been previously chronicled under the section pericarditis, where he described another sign which bears his namesake. Griesinger described a complication occurring in patients with otitis interna (Table 17.1, Fig. 17.2):

> Since my work in 1860, I had five new cases of thrombosis of the sinus transversus. In three of these, attention was paid to the sign of an unequal filling of the jugular veins as

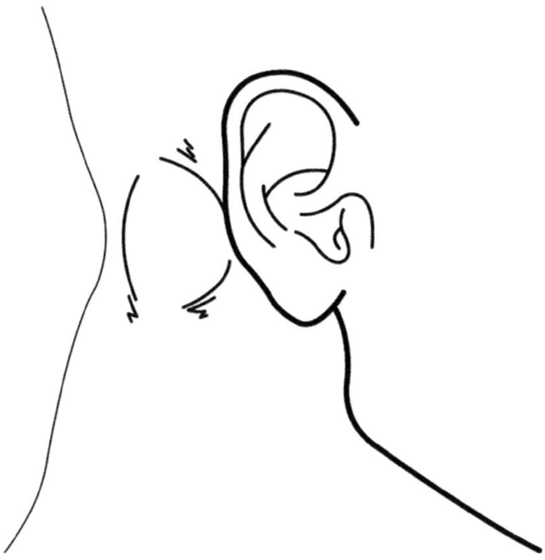

Fig. 17.2 Griesinger sign (by Ryan Yale)

> stated by Gerhardt but never found. In one cases I observed a condition which may serve as a new as yet unknown indirect sign of the thrombosis of the sinus transversus. If present, which in any case is rare, it involves a circumscribed painful edema, a small phlegmasia dolens behind in the ear when the thrombosis spreads through the emissary and leaks into the sigmoid fossa [2, p. 447].

He described the pathogenesis and pathologic findings of mastoid swelling in a patient with encephalitis occurring in March 1862:

> Ulrich Ott (a case of repeated encephalitis with vastly distended blood coagulation located within the internal cerebral veins which undoubtedly played the main role), at the time of an exacerbation of encephalitis, rapidly developed a severe headache after a general convulsive seizure. To the left (side of encephalitis) a soft, non-pulsating, extremely painful, and sensitive swelling, was found around the periphery of the left mastoid process. (...) The transverse sinus, from its point of inflection to the foramen lacerum, was firmly filled with a tenacious, gray-walled fibrin clot adhering to the wall. Within the sigmoid fossa, a circa 1 mm. thick veins (emissaries), were completely filled with a firm, adherent clot extending outward into the mastoid process. In order to account for the swelling of the emissary veins by the thrombosis, one would have to explain how these veins conducts blood out of the sinus even though no primary area on the outside is affected by its obstruction. The emissary veins connect the sinus with the posterior ear veins. Where the blood flows in the emissary vein it comes from the side of the stronger pressure. Thus, thrombosis of the emissary can very easily continue into one of the posterior ear veins, directly from where this edema arise [2, p. 447].

Schwartze believed that Griesinger and Gerhardt signs are not pathognomonic for the diagnosis of cerebral venous thrombosis:

> The symptoms cited by Gerhardt and Griesinger as sinus thrombosis are not reliable. The former attaches great importance to a weaker filling of the jugular vein, which receives its blood from the clogged sinus transversus. However, the uneven filling of the jugular veins does not seem to allow a firm conclusion on the location of the existing thrombosis in the

> cerebral sinus. As early as 1859 in the Journal for Teething Diseases of Behrend and Hildebrand (1859–331), I cited a case in which the opposite relation to the filing state of the veins took place [3, p. 219]. (...) Even more uncertain is the utilization of the symptom raised by Griesinger of a painful edema on the mastoid process. This occurs contrary to what Griesinger believes only rarely occurs, namely the propagation of thrombosis through the emissary leading from the sigmoid sinus through the mastoid foramen to the surface of the skull. It is well known that such edema occurs at the mastoid and transversus into the cavities of the petrous bone. It occurs in cases of inflammations of the soft tissue of the middle and outer ear even without there being any other reason to assume inflammation and thrombosis of the transverse sinus [3, p. 220].

Thus, Griesinger sign refers to painful edematous swelling located behind the mastoid process in patients with thrombosis of the transverse sinus caused by otitis media.

Crowe Sign

Samuel J. Crowe (1883–1955) was born in Washington County, Virginia, and received his medical degree in 1908 from John Hopkins Medical School [4, 5]. After graduation, he was appointed Assistant in Surgery where he worked in the Hunterian Laboratory under the aegis of Harvey Cushing (1869–1939) [4]. After a year as an assistant resident in neurosurgery, he returned to the Hunterian Laboratory to continue his work with Cushing on the study of the pituitary gland [4]. In 1912, he was appointed Associate in Surgery at John Hopkins [6]. At the request and encouragement of William Stewart Halsted (1852–1922), Crowe remained at Hopkins rather than continuing his planned neurosurgical career with Cushing at Harvard and transitioned, as per Halsted's requests, to the field of laryngology. Here he was appointed director of the newly founded Division of Otology and Laryngology [7]. He served in this capacity throughout his career from 1912 to 1952. He is credited for building the first modern clinic of otolaryngology in the United States [4, 5]. Here he recruited a group of scientists whose research focus was on deafness [4]. From 1935 to 1936, he served as president of the American Otological Society [8]. He was honored posthumously as the recipient of the honorary D.Sc. degree from the Johns Hopkins University [9].

Crowe described a method for determining whether there is an anomaly of the intracranial venous circulation, unilateral acute thrombotic or another condition causing obstruction of venous outflow from the sigmoid sinus or jugular bulb (intracranial sinus vein), or internal jugular vein by direct visualization of the retinal veins. In 50 healthy persons examined, he observed the following (Table 17.1):

1. No appreciable evidence of stasis is seen in the retinal or supraorbital veins when one internal jugular is compressed with the finger.
2. Pressure on both internal jugular veins at the same time produces a marked dilation of the veins of the fundi and of the anastomotic vessels connecting the intracranial with the extracranial venous circulation.

3. When the pressure is suddenly released on one side, while it is maintained on the other, the engorged veins of the anastomotic system and the fundi will be immediately empty [10, p. 322].

Based on these principles, in cases of sinus or internal jugular vein thrombosis, he found:

> Since a sinus thrombosis offers a more or less complete obstruction to the outflow of blood into the internal jugular vein on the same side, it naturally follows that in such cases there will be unmistakable evidence of stasis as a result of compressing, with the finger, the internal jugular veins on the opposite side [10, p. 323].

They described the method for performing the examination:

> It is very important while making this examination that the patient should breathe freely and normally; that the collar should be loosened so as to expose the neck and upper part of the chest; and that the fundi should be examined by the direct method; or with an electric ophthalmoscope, while an assistant compresses the internal jugular veins with the tips of the fingers. The compression, however should not be maintained longer than absolutely necessary for it may be possible in this way to rupture a disease vein or dislodge a portion of a thrombus [10, p. 322].

In unilateral sinus thrombosis, engorgement of the bilateral retinal vessels occurs when the jugular veins on the contralateral healthy side is compressed. Under normal conditions it is necessary to compress both jugular veins in order to induce engorgement of the bilateral sinuses.

Thus, Crowe sinus refers to the presence of retinal vein engorgement elicited upon compressing the contralateral internal jugular vein in cases of lateral sinus thrombosis.

References

1. Gerhardt C. Ueber Hirnsinusthrombosis bei Kindern. Deutsch Klinik. 1857;9(45–46): 438–9, 445–9.
2. Griesinger W. Beobachtungen über Hirnkrankheiten: zur Lehre von den Hirnkrankheiten aus Otitis interna. Archiv der Heilk. 1862;3:437–58.
3. Schwartze H. Fälle von Entzündung und Thrombose des Sinus transversus und des Sinus petrosus inferior bei Otitis media purulenta. Archiv f Ohren-, Nasen-u Kehlkopf. 1873;6:219–27.
4. Dr. Samuel J Crowe. Otolaryngology-head and neck surgery. Johns Hopkins Medicine. https://www.hopkinsmedicine.org/otolaryngology/our_team/directors/crowe.html. Accessed 10 Apr 2019.
5. The Samuel James Crowe Collection. The Alan Mason Chesney Medical Archives of the Johns Hopkins Medical Institutions. https://medicalarchives.jhmi.edu:8443/papers/crowe.html. Accessed 10 Apr 2019.
6. [No author]. Faculty changes: Dr. Samuel J. Crow. JAMA. 1912;58:1952.
7. Francis HW, Papel I, Lina I, Koch W, Tunkel D, Fuchs P, et al. Otolaryngology-head and neck surgery at Johns Hopkins: the first 100 years (1914–2014). Laryngoscope. 2015;125:S1–S35.
8. Program of the One hundred twenty-sixth annual meeting. American Otological Society, Inc. April 17–18, 1993. Century Plaza Hotel and Tower, Los Angeles, CA. https://www.americanotologicalsociety.org/assets/prog/1993.pdf. Accessed 20 Mar 2019.

9. Honorary Degrees Awarded at The Johns Hopkins University. Headlines@Hopkins Commencement 2003. http://pages.jh.edu/news/commence03/honorary/chrono.html. Accessed 20 Mar 2019.
10. Crowe SJ. An aid for the diagnosis of conditions associated with an obstruction to the outflow of blood from the brain; with special reference to sinus thrombosis of otitic origin. Johns Hopkins Hosp Bull. 1912;23:321–3.

Chapter 18
Vital Signs

Introduction

Pulse, respiration, temperature, and blood pressure or "vital signs" are routinely performed as part of the cardiovascular assessment and considered the earliest objective fundamental aspect of the physical examination. The term "vital signs" specifies the presence of those bodily functions considered an essential component of life. These signs are historically important to recognize and provide important insights into methods and techniques for diagnosing various disease states. These objective findings along with other key components assist clinicians in narrowing the differential diagnosis or determining the cause of the underlying disease. Included in this discussion are signs found in patients with hyperthyroidism as detected by blood pressure and temperature as well as bleeding disorders that may be surreptitiously discovered when blood pressure is measured using a sphygmomanometer cuff. Additionally, some of these signs may be clinically useful providing important insights into potential mechanisms of disease. Thus, it is important that clinicians learn how to properly perform, identify, and apply these signs. Included in this chapter on vital signs is a brief historical background of the person who described the sign, the sign as originally described, and if available, the sensitivity, specificity, and predictive values of the signs.

Historical Background

Pulse and respiration, two components included as part what we commonly refer to as "vital sign," were long in use before they were technically recognized as important in diagnostic decision making in the nineteenth century. A report by Edward Seguin (1812–1880) published in 1866 in the *Chicago Medical Journal*

S. H. Yale et al., *Cardiovascular Eponymic Signs*,
https://doi.org/10.1007/978-3-030-67596-7_18

was believed to be the earliest method of recording and graphing temperature, respiration, and pulse as a method to visually study these components during the course of pneumonia:

> The cases are accompanied by a diagram, fac simile of the tables of "Vital Signs," used at the bedside to make the daily record of temperature, pulse-beats and respiration. This one only differs from ours in that on it are represented the curves for three cases, whereas usually but one case is put upon a table [1, p. 193].

It was Harvey Cushing (1869–1939) who in 1903 called for including blood pressure in the medical record:

> At the present time, largely owing to the convenience of our timepieces, pulse-rate is commonly recorded alongside of the temperature and perhaps of the respiration on our clinical charts, to the utter neglect of a numerical record of that vascular quality which in many condition is incomparably of greater clinical consequence, namely, arterial tension [2, p. 252].

The term "vital" is derived from the Latin *vitalis* or belong to life. The word *vitalis* is an abbreviated form of *vita* derived from *vivere* meaning to live [3]. A sign is found on physical examination as detected through observation, palpation, percussion, or auscultation. Thus, the term "vital sign" is an objective and measurable finding based on those functions essential or required for life. With the use of more modern technology, pulse oximetry, a measure of blood oxygen saturation, could also be considered a "vital sign" as oxygenation similar to respiration is measurable and essential [4].

Signs

Rumpel-Leede Sign

Carl August Theodor Rumpel (1862–1923) was born in Gutersloh, Germany, and received his medical degree from the University of Marburg in 1887 [5]. He served as a staff member at the Hamburg-Eppendorf Hospital in 1892 [5]. In 1913, he was appointed first director of Barmbecker Hospital and chief physician at the Second Medical Service of Allgemeines Hospital [5, 6]. With Alfred Kast (1856–1903) and Eugen Fraenkel (1852–1925), he co-authored the patho-anatomical atlas *Pathologisch-anatomische Tafeln nach frischen Präparaten mit erläuterndem anatomisch-klinischem Text* (Pathological–anatomical panels of fresh specimens with explanatory anatomical-clinical text) [7]. He presented his paper titled "Photographien von Scharlachkranken mit multiplen Hautblutungen" (Photographs of scarlet fever with multiple skin hemorrhages) at a meeting of the Ärztlichen Verein in Hamburg, Germany, in 1909 [6, 8]:

> These hemorrhages also occur spontaneously on the forearm and elbow regions where the exanthem is most dense and are arbitrarily produced by mechanical stimuli, especially by applying Biers compression bandage on the upper arm. This is useful in the differential

> diagnosis of scarlet fever. (…) they have not been observed, at a certain maximum pressure, in other infectious diseases such as measles, rubella, and diphtheria [8, p. 2297].

Carl Stockbridge Leede (1882–1964) was born in Washington State, received his medical degree from University of Munich in 1908, and completed his postgraduate training in Hamburg and Munich, Germany [9]. He served in Vienna as an assistant professor to Dr. Rumpell at Eppendorfer Hospital in Hamburg, Germany, between 1908 to 1999 [9]. He was certified in medicine by the American Board in 1937, and was a member of the American Association for the Advancement of Science. He later served as a physician at the Children's Hospital in Seattle, Washington [9]. As stated by Dr. Leede, Dr. Rumple:

> At the behest of Mr. Oberartz, Dr. med Rumpel pointed out the diagnostic significance of the phenomenon at a meeting of the medical association on June 13, 1909. He systematically identified cases of scarlet fever by means of a rubber band fixed around the upper arm so that the veins emerged clearly while the pulse was diminished on palpation. Several hundred cases of scarlet fever were examined with the findings of pronounced hemorrhage on the skin [10, p. 294].

Leede, an assistant in the department of the general hospital at the Eppendorf Hospital under the aegis of senior physician Dr. Rumpel, discussed in his 1911 paper entitled "Hautblutungen durch Stauung hervorgerufen als diagnostisches Hilfsmittel beim Scharlach" (Skin bleeding elicited by congestion as a diagnostic aid in scarlet fever) the difficulty in confirming a diagnosis of scarlet fever in the absence of the exanthema. Leede and colleagues identified in patients with scarlet fever undergoing venipuncture that "distal to the congestion caused by the bandage, there were small and sometimes quite large petechiae and in some cases suffusion-like bleeding in the skin. This phenomenon was not noticed in other diseases" [10, p. 294]. Furthermore, Leede acknowledged that initially they were unaware of a prior report by Hecht in 1907 of skin bleeding in children with scarlet fever [10]. Hecht's method involved pinching "a skin fold on the back or chest between the forefinger and thumb and holding it in this position under slight pressure for about 5–10 seconds until petechial hemorrhage occurs. Scarlet fever is excluded if bleeding does not occur" [10, p. 294]. The congestion test, described by Leede, is elicited as follows (Fig. 18.1):

> In each case, I determined the systolic and diastolic blood pressure and then filled the cuff to a pressure considerably below the diastolic pressure (usually 45–60 mm of mercury), leave the cuff with the tube disconnected, and examined the area within 5 minutes for bleeding (typically occurs in 5–20 minutes). (…) Only exceptionally has similar bleeding been observed by this method in other diseases which I have examined. Only in the case of measles did I obtain values which approached that of scarlet fever [10, p. 294].

Thus, the finding of petechiae and purpura distal to the sight where the arms are occluded by a tourniquet is a positive test. Leede accounted for the pathogenesis of his finding:

> I had the impression that the capillaries in measles are less altered than in scarlet fever. I believe I have demonstrated that in scarlet fever, almost without exception, there is a pathologically increased vulnerability of the capillaries and that this symptom can be used diag-

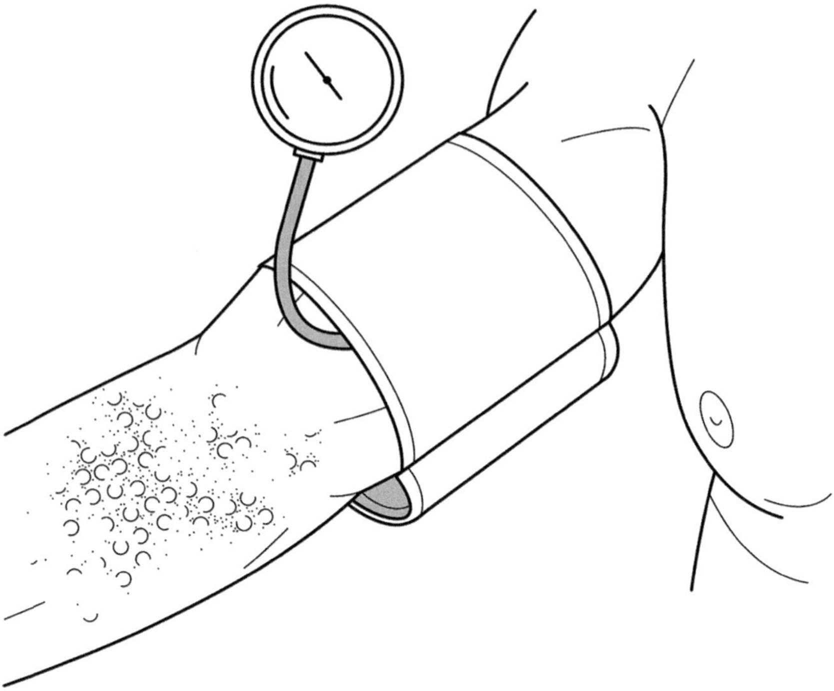

Fig. 18.1 Rumpel – Leede sign (by Ryan Yale)

> nostically. In my experience, a negative stasis test can be used as criteria against scarlet fever, while a positive test should be used jointly with the other symptoms [10, p. 295].

A test for capillary fragility has also been described by Alfred Fabian Hess (1875–1933) and Mildred Fish in 1914 and is referred to as the "Hess Test" or capillary resistance test. It is performed by:

> [s]ubjecting the capillaries and vessels of the arm to increased intravascular pressure, by means of an ordinary blood-pressure band, and observing whether this strain results in the escape of blood through the vessels—the appearance of petechial hemorrhages on the skin. The vessels of normal infants were found to withstand, without apparent disturbance, 90 degrees of pressure for three minutes, whereas the vessels of infants suffering from scurvy gave way under this pressure. The test is not specific for scurvy, but is a method of demonstrating a weakness of the vessel walls, whatsoever may be its cause [11, p. 346].

A positive test may occur in patients with a bleeding diathesis. A false-positive test has been reported in patients undergoing continuous blood pressure monitoring using a small sphygmomanometer cuff [12, 13]. It has also been described in patients with diabetes and hypertensive urgency, diabetic microangiopathy, and a host of infectious diseases such as dengue, rocky mountain spotted fever, meningococcemia, Ebola, and other hemorrhagic viral diseases [13, 14]. In a systematic review and meta-analysis of 9836 patients with suspected dengue, 4043 of which

Table 18.1 Vital sign eponyms

Name	Year	Description of sign
Rumpel-Leede [10]	1909	Using a sphygmomanometer, determine the systolic and diastolic blood pressure in the arm. Inflate the sphygmomanometer to a level below the diastolic blood pressure and leave the cuff in place for 5–20 minutes while examining the forearm for petechiae and purpura.
Grocco-Frugoni [21]	1911	An elastic ligature is placed firmly around the arm. Observe for purpura at flexor surface and limbs folds (popliteal fossa, inguinal canal, and cubital fossa). A characteristic ecchymotic band also forms at the site where the elastic ligature is applied.
Weil-Chalier [32]	1911	Place a band around the arm or thigh and observe for the presence of petechia and purpura.
Lucatello [35]	1913	External (axillary) temperature is 0.2 or 0.3 higher than the internal (oral) temperature in hyperthyroidism.
Brockenbrough [61]	1961	Weak pulse following a premature ventricular contraction in patients with HOCM.
Braunwald [61]	1964	Weak pulse following a premature ventricular contraction in patients with HOCM.

were confirmed by IgM-antigen ELISA laboratory test, the tourniquet test was found to have a sensitivity and specificity of 19.1% and 86.4%, respectively [15]. Based on disease severity, the tourniquet test was found to be positive in 61.7% of patients with classic dengue, 82.9% in complicated, and 82.9% in hemorrhagic dengue. Thus, the tourniquet test in the appropriate clinical setting is useful to support a diagnosis of dengue. However, a negative test does not exclude the diagnosis. Furthermore, the likelihood of a positive study increases with disease severity [15].

Thus, the Rumpel-Leede sign, as well as other signs described in this review including Grocco-Frugoni, and Weill-Chalier, are found in a wide variety of conditions such as scarlet fever, scurvy, or thrombocytopenic disorders causing bleeding diathesis due to impaired function or reduced platelet numbers, or conditions causing damage to the vascular capillary wall (vasculopathies) and increased capillary fragility [16, 17]. Alone, these signs lack sufficient sensitivity and specificity in diagnosis. However, in the appropriate clinical settings, their presence may be useful in supporting a diagnosis (Table 18.1) (See Grocco-Frugoni and Weill-Chalier).

Grocco-Frugoni Sign

Pietro Grocco (1856–1916) was born in Albonese (Lomellina), Italy, and received his medical degree from the University of Pavia in 1879. He continued his studies in Paris serving in Jean-Martin Charcot (1825–1893) Clinic and Vienna, Austria [18]. He was appointed chair of the practice of medicine at the University of Perugia, Italy, from 1884 to 1887 followed by the same position in Pisa and at the Istituto di Studi Superiori (Institute of Higher Studies) in Florence, Italy, in 1892 [19]. In

Florence, he was appointed government inspector and medical director of the balneary center in Montecatini, Italy, in 1892 [19]. His name is perhaps best recognized for the eponymous paravertebral triangle, a dull obtuse region in the form of a right triangle found in the lung base in the side opposite to a pleural effusion described in 1902. As a description of his character:

> The Florentine school enjoyed his special care and generosity, founding as he did, mainly from his own resources, the Istituto Antirabico on the lines of Pasteur. In 1905 he was made a senator of the kingdom, in accordance with Italy's custom to promote men of scientific distinction to the Upper Chamber, and here again his advice on intervention was of public benefit in more than one hygienic departure [19, p. 43].

Cesare Frugoni (1881–1978) was born in Brescia, Italy, initiated his medical studies at the University of Parma, and received his medical degree from the Institute of Practical and Advanced Studies in Florence, Italy, in 1904 [20]. He served at the General Pathology Institute at the University of Pavia, directed by Camillo Golgi (1843–1926), and returned to Florence where he held the title assistant of the medical clinic directed by his prior mentor Pietro Grocco in 1909 [20]. He was an adjunct professor of medical pathology and head of the medical clinic at the School of Medicine at Florence, Italy, in 1911 and served at the Arcispedale of Santa Maria Nuova Hospital in Florence in 1914 [20, 21]. From 1915 to 1919, during World War I, he received the war cross and silver medal for military valor [22]. At the end of the war, he returned to Florence where he taught special medical pathology from 1921 to 1923 [20]. From 1923 to 1926 he was appointed chair of the Institute of Medical Pathology and ordinary professor in Florence, succeeding Luigi Lucatello (1863–1926) for the chair at the Institute of General Medical Clinic, and from 1926 to 1931 as professor at the University of Padova, Italy [20–23]. Here he was instrumental in improving and transforming the postgraduate school of pulmonary medicine and established clinics in the fields of ophthalmology, urology, and pediatrics [20].

He succeeded V. Ascoli, assuming the chair as professor of the General Medicine Clinic at the University of Rome from 1931 to 1951 [23]. In the academic years 1944–1945 he opened the Institute of Medical Semeiotics led by Luigi Gedda (1902–2000) [20]. This program represented the first institute of genetics inaugurated in 1953. In 1952, he chaired the National Health Council to assess the link between vaccination and polio [20]. Among his other accomplishments, he served as the president of the following three societies: Italian Society of Internal Medicine (1942–1958), Superior Council of Health (1950–1966), and Medical Academy of Rome [22]. He was the recipient of the gold medal for Merit of Education and in 1951 was awarded an honorary fellowship in the American Academy of Allergy [20, 24]. Frugoni was the editor of *Minerva medica, La Riforma medica, Il Policlinico, Archivio italiana delle malattie dell'apparato digerente, Cuore e circolazione, Giornale medico del'Alto Adige, Acta medica italica* [20]. In 1953, he chaired the Federazione Nazionale degli Ordini dei Medici Chirurghi e degli Odontoiatri

(FNOMCeO) which was responsible for drafting the code of medical ethics also known as the Code of Medical Deontology. He shared the other obsolete and banished eponym with André Cauchois (1880–1953) and Hans Eppinger Jr. (1879–1946), the later physician who committed crimes against humanity in Dachau concentration camp. The eponym formerly known as Cauchois-Eppinger-Frugoni Syndrome consists of thrombosis, anemia, and thrombosis of the splenic veins or portal vein. He was the coauthor of the *Manuale di pathologia e terapia medica* (Manual of Pathology and Medical Therapy) in 1931 and *e Medicina interna* (Internal Medicine) in 1940 and published three books on clinical lessons (*Lezioni di clinica medica*, 1934; *Attualitá terapeutiche*, 1939) including a two-volume treatise on functional diagnostics (*Diagnostica funzionale*, 1941) [20].

Frugoni and Guigni described in their paper titled "Le signe du lacet dans les maladies à manifestations hémorragiques" (The sign of lace in diseases with hemorrhagic manifestations) a method for detecting diseases with hemorrhagic diathesis (Table 18.1):

> The sign which attracted our attention and which is of interest to us is performed as follows: an elastic ligature placed firmly around the arm causes hemorrhagic manifestations analogous to that occurring spontaneously elsewhere in a patient who presents with the cutaneous phenomenon of hemorrhagic diathesis. This phenomenon occurs during the period of maximum disease activity, decreases and disappears after the cause of the spontaneous hemorrhagic diathesis has resolved. This phenomenon, to which we have given the name the sign of the lace, is not only an excellent prognostic index but also an extremely valuable practical criteria [21, p. 25].

Frugoni and Guigni described the location and predilection for where punctate hemorrhages occur:

> It has been observed that the hemorrhagic findings are more intense and show a greater tendency to occur at sites where friction acts as a mechanical factor. Thus, the flexor surface and limbs folds (popliteal fossa, inguinal canal, and cubital fossa) are particularly prone to these streaks, and a characteristic ecchymotic band forms at the site where a firm elastic ligature is applied [21, p. 25].

They acknowledge the previously reported descriptions of the findings by August Bier (1861–1949) in his book entitled *Hyperämie als Heilmittel* (Hyperemia as a Cure) in 1907:

> It is obvious that the phenomenon described by M. Bier and the sign on which we draw attention differs significantly from the other. First, by the different intensity of the stasis obtained. Our cases were less severe since the lesions appeared when a ligature was applied using moderate pressure. Second, the hemorrhagic manifestations occurred in both otherwise healthy persons and those suffering from an aforementioned or an unknown condition that causes spontaneous cutaneous hemorrhages and comprises the hemorrhagic diathesis [21, p. 25].

They recognized their teacher Professor Grocco, who four year prior drew "attention to the possibility of highlighting this symptom and (…) who instructed us to study it systematically from a clinical and pathological point of view" [21, p. 26].

Weill-Chalier Sign

Edmond Weill (1858–1924) was born in Haguenau, France, and received his medical degree from the University of Lyon, France, in 1882 [25, 26]. He was agrégé to the Faculty of Lyon in 1886 and chief of the Pediatric Clinic at the University of Lyon in 1901 [25, 27]. Weill was a member of the French National Academy of Medicine where he served as a national correspondent to the Division of Anatomy and Physiology from 1920 to 1924 [28]. He was the recipient of the Knight and Officer of the Légion d'honneur (Legion of Honor), France, in 1908 and 1923, respectively [28, 29]. His name should not be confused with a similar sounding one, Edmund Weil (1879–1922) who along with Arthur Felix (1887–1956) described the Weil-Felix reaction as an agglutination test for rickettsia infections [25].

Joseph-Fortuné Chalier (1884–1942) was born in Mende, France, and received his medical degree with his thesis titled *Les ictères hémolytiques* from the Faculty of Medicine and Pharmacy at the University of Lyon, France, in 1909 [30, 31]. That same year he was head of the adjoint laboratory medical clinic and doctor within the Lyon Hospital [31]. During World War I, he served as the divisional ambulance physician (1914–1918) followed by chief medical officer of the army staff [31]. In 1920, he served in the infectious disease service at Croix-Rousse. He was appointed professor of medical pathology from 1937 to 1938 and was named honorary doctor of the hospital and awarded the Silver Medal for Administration in 1937 [31]. From 1938 to 1942, he returned to his work in the Infectious Diseases Clinic [31].

Weill and Chalier in their 1911 publication "Le purpura provoqué par hypertension veineuse" (Purpura caused by venous hypertension) acknowledged the prior publication by Frugoni and Guigni in 1911 of the "lace sign" first identified by Grocco and its prognostic value. The sign is evoked by placing a "lace" or band around the arm or thigh without compressing the artery and observing for the presence of petechiae and purpura. Where both authors differed was the timing and setting where their sign was diagnostic:

> The diagnostic value of this sign appears in cases in which the purpura is preceded by joint manifestations, before any purpuric lesion appears on the integument or hemorrhage of the mucous membranes [32, p. 170]. (…) This sign has particular diagnostic value in the chronic purpura that we have had occasion to observe several times in a very latent form. (…) One of us had the opportunity to observe two cases of scurvy in infants whose only symptom was a painful swelling of one knee. (…) We draw attention to these forms of chronic purpura and articular-type scurvy, the diagnosis of which may perhaps benefit from the search for purpura [32, p. 171].

Thus, Weill and Chalier sign refers to the presence of purpura elicited by the placement of a constricting band around the arm or thigh in patients with joint symptoms in scurvy (Table 18.1).

Lucatello Sign

Luigi Lucatello (1863–1926) was born in Treviso, Italy, and graduated with honors with gold medal distinction from the Faculty of Medicine and Surgery at the University of Genoa, Italy, in 1887 [33]. While a student, he served as a research assistant at the Institute of Pathological Anatomy publishing his work titled "Sulla presenza del bacillo tifoso nel sangue splenico e suo possibile valore diagnostico" (On the presence of the bacillus in the splenic blood and its possible diagnostic value) [33]. He served as a lecturer in microscopy and bacteriology in 1890 and in pathological anatomy from 1890 to 1892 [33]. His primary areas of research interest spanned multiple fields including pathology, infectious diseases, and endocrinology [33]. His other areas of research included studies on pellagra, Banti disease (congestive splenomegaly), and abdominal and pulmonary tuberculosis. In his paper entitled "La puntura del fegato a scopo diagnostico" (The puncture of the liver for purpose of diagnosis) published in 1895, he reported on the design of a needle used for the histological examination of the liver [33]. He was appointed chair of special medical pathology at the University of Naples, Italy, as well as extraordinary professor at the University of Padua, Italy, in 1899, where he also served as the director of the care unit in the pediatric clinic [33]. He was appointed ordinary professor in 1902, selected as chair of the Institute of Medical Clinic in 1916, and served as dean of the Medical Faculty at Padua from 1916 to 1919 [33, 34]. Lucatello described in his paper entitled "Per la sintomatologia endocrina" (The symptoms in endocrinology) the finding of the discrepancy between oral and axillary temperature as a method of diagnosing hyperthyroidism and as a way to distinguish Basedow syndrome (iodine induced hyperthyroidism) from infections:

> In some clinical cases of hyperthyroidism characterized by disturbances in various internal secretions, I observed a discrepancy of the internal compared to the external temperatures, namely a relative or absolute thermal lowering of the oral compared to axillary temperature. (…) The aforementioned thermal phenomenon has helped me in one case to exclude a cryptogenic infection later diagnosed as Basedow syndrome. Therefore, this clinical finding may also assume diagnostic importance. However, from the series of case studies, I can say that this symptom is more easily confirmed when the endocrine imbalance reaches a particular intensity and severity. With regard to pathogenesis, it is probable that this alteration of the relationship between the temperature of the external and internal body locations is linked to vascular mechanisms variously influenced by endocrine secretions [35].

In patients with hyperthyroidism the external (axillary) temperature is 0.2 or 0.3 higher than the internal (oral) temperature (Table 18.1). The difference in temperature is, as postulated by Lucatello, caused by peripheral vasodilation in patients with hyperthyroidism. Marañón and Bonilla studied this phenomenon in 17 patients with hyperthyroidism and found Lucatello sign to be present in two patients [36]. This small study suggests that the sign lacks sufficient sensitivity or specificity to be clinically useful in diagnosing hyperthyroidism.

Pende Sign

Nicola Pende (1880–1970) was born in Noicattaro (Bari), Italy, and received his medical degree from the faculty of medicine at the University of Rome in 1903 with the thesis titled *Alterazione della ghiandola surrenale dopo la resezione del nervo splancnico* (Alteration of the adrenal gland after resection of the splanchnic nerve) [37, 38]. In the 1902–1903 academic year, he received one of two awards from the Girolami Foundation for the best degree dissertation [39]. After graduation, he worked as a physician assistant at the hospital of Rome followed by an internship at Institute of General Pathology where he conducted research in endocrinology from 1903 to 1909. In 1907 he taught special medical pathology and was recognized as adjunct professor of internal pathology in 1908 [38, 40].

In 1909, he coined the term "endocrinology" and served as assistant to Giacinto Viola (1870–1943) at the Institute of Special Medical Pathology at the University of Palmero until 1912. In 1914, he served at medical clinics in Berlin, Germany, and Naples, Italy, under the aegis of Friedrich Kraus (1858–1936) and Pietro Castellino (1864–1933) [38].

During World War I in 1915, he was a medical captain at the military hospitals in Bari, Italy. The following year he was major and director of the military hospital for disabled men in Rome and led the Vittorio Emanuele Hospital in Padua [38]. He published the first edition of his treatise on *Endocrinologia: Patologia e Clinica degli Organi a Secrezione Interna* (Endocrinology: Pathology and Clinics of the Glands with Internal Secretion) in 1916 [41]. Pende was assistant in medical pathology in 1919 and from 1921 to 1923 led the General Medical and Semiotic Medicine Clinic at the University of Messina [38]. He was awarded the title of extraordinary professor followed by ordinary professor of the clinic and specialist in clinical and special medical pathology in 1923 [38]. In 1924, he was founder and first rector of the Faculty of Medicine and Surgery at the University of Bari, renamed after Benito Mussolini in 1925 [38].

In 1924, he joined the National Fascist Party and founded the first institute of biotypology and human orthogenesis in Genoa [38]. This concept was based on the conceptualization and study of the relationship between endocrine-vegetative system and biotypical aspects in which hormone secretion is the determinant link between morphology, psychology, and characters of the individual. Hence, through endocrinology he believed that he was able to identify a biotypological profile or psycho-physical personality of an individuals, family, and racial inheritances, as well as the phenomenal aspects of individuality (morphological, physiological, ethical and affective, and intellective) [38]. Based on these concepts, Pende conceived of a political and social biology theory in which social class were the result of a biotypological characteristic that determined social role. Thus, Pende's endocrinology "became the fundamental instrument of the eugenic and demographic policies of the fascist regime" [42]. The orthogenic clinics were designed on the basis of improving the biological and psychological aspects of individuals and to develop an individual "orthogenetic biotypical profile" aligned with the principles set forth by the fascist state [38]. Thus, the goals were the improvement of the physical, moral, and intellectual aspect of Italians [43].

He was appointed Senator of the Kingdom for scientific merit of Italy in 1933 and was appointed by Benito Mussolini as chair of medical pathology and clinical methodology at the University of Rome in 1935 [38]. There he directed the Institute of Medical Pathology and established another biotypological-orthogenetic institute [38]. He directed the medical sciences section of the Italian encyclopedia and was appointed head of the eugenic section of the National Research Center in 1937 [38].

Pende was appointed rector of the Italian Academy of Littorio in 1941 and received the first-class gold medal awarded of merit by the President of the Republic, Giovanni Gronch, in 1956 [38, 44]. He was also the recipient of the Balbi-Valier Prize for his work on the organs of internal secretion and for the best medical work published in the preceding year by the Venice Reale Istituto [45, 46]. His last position was as professor of pathology at the University of Palermo, Italy.

Pende was believed to be among 42 other signers of the "Manifesto of Race" also referred to as the Charter of Race in 1938, a document on racial laws in fascist Italy. The anti-Semitic laws stripped the Jews of Italian citizenship, governmental, and professional positions. Pende in his defense claimed that his signature had been affixed without his approval to the document [47, 48]. The commission overseeing this matter exonerated the claim and reinstated Pende to the faculty of medicine and surgery. Despite this, Rome still planned to remove the names of Pende as well as other scientists who signed the manifesto from its street [49].

Pende has two eponymic signs ascribed to his namesake: one related to disease of the cerebellum; the other sign refers to the large pulse pressure observed in patients with hyperthyroidism. Pende described in his article entitled "Sopra una triade sintomatica dell'ipertiroidismo costituzionale: sua importanza diagnostica nelle forme larvate di tireotoxicosi" (On a symptomatic triad of constitutional hyperthyroidism: its diagnostic importance in the larval forms of thyrotoxicosis) a triad of symptoms which he believed to be useful in cases of Basedow disease (hereditary or endogenous hyperthyroidism) which are not clearly defined, or in cases in which there is an early presentations with single symptoms or with mild disease [50]. He believed that this sign was also useful in determining the severity of the clinical syndrome and response to treatment. Pende described this sign as:

> Very high variable pressure, i.e., large distance between the systolic blood pressure and the diastolic. I consider this phenomenon besides aortic insufficiency, characteristic of hyperthyroidism. (…) For the most part, when this exists, we find a high systolic pressure of up to 160–190 mmHg, (Riva Rocci palpatory method) and the diastolic pressure of 50–70 mmHg (Korotkow's listening method) [50, p. 311].

He acknowledged that the finding of an elevated pulse pressure had been previously identified by other authors but not believed to be of diagnostic importance. He reported that this finding was:

> [f]or me one of the cardinal signs of the disease is the characteristic and permissive action of thyroid hormone on the heart and on the arterioles. It is pathognomonic of constitutional hyperthyroidism and in cases where it is absent I doubt that the patient has hyperthyroid and

> suspected the presence of other endocrine abnormalities. From research done in my clinic on this sign in Basedow patients subjected with good results to iodine radiotherapy, there is no relationship between the intensity of the symptom and the seriousness of the morbid picture. However, treatment of this syndrome with x-rays or other therapies, causes the systolic and diastolic pressure pressures to approach those found in normal subjects. This confirms that it is a true thyrogenic effect on the arterial pressure [50, p. 312].

Pende found this sign to be "present in at least 95% of cases of Basedow disease and absent only when this syndrome is complicated by atherosclerosis, nephrosclerosis, or heart failure, in which case the elevation of the diastolic pressure can mask the symptom" [50, p. 312]. We are unaware of any study which confirmed this finding.

Eponyms are honorific terms applied to an individual for scientific accomplishments. These terms should not be used for individuals who committed crimes or atrocities against humanity or were anti-Semitic or racists in their rhetoric [51, 52]. Therefore, the name Pende should be removed from medical discourse and was not included in Table 18.1.

Brockenbrough Sign

This sign is referred to in the literature by the singular name Brockenbrough or Braunwald, the dual names Brockenbrough-Braunwald, or the trio Brockenbrough-Braunwald-Morrow [53–59].

Edwin Chamberlayne Jr. Brockenbrough (1930–) graduated from Johns Hopkins University School of Medicine in 1956 [60]. He described the sign which bears his name along with Braunwald (1929–) and Andrew G. Morrow (1922–1982) in 1961 while at the National Heart Institute, Clinic of Surgery, Bethesda, Maryland [61]. He received further training in thoracic surgery at the University of Washington and was the founding director of the Vascular Laboratory at Harborview Medical Center, Seattle, where he also served as an associate surgeon in chief [62]. He is a clinical professor of surgery at the University of Washington and a member of the Pacific Surgical Association. He served as secretary for the Seattle Surgical Society in 1972, chief of staff at Northwest Hospital, Seattle, and as a member of the Board of Trustees, president of the King County Medical Society, the Washington State Chapter of the American College of Surgeons in 1985, North Pacific Surgical Association, and The American Rhododendron Society (1977–1979) [62–64]. Among his other accolades, he is the recipient of the Honorée Distinguished Worldwide Humanitarian Award, The American Rhododendron Society in 1985, inducted in the Worldwide Lifetime Achievement in 2016, and Fellow of the American College of Surgeons (FACS) [64].

Brockenbrough, Braunwald, and Morrow in 1961 reported their findings of the appearance of the pulse pressure occurring after a premature ventricular contraction in 11 patients with idiopathic hypertrophic subaortic stenosis (currently referred to as hypertrophic obstructive cardiomyopathy or HOCM) on angiography: "[t]he longer filling period following a premature ventricular contraction is followed by a smaller pulse pressure. This paradoxical decrease in pulse pressure is probably an expression of the reduction in orifice size [61, p. 192]."

They found that compared to patients with fixed obstruction caused by aortic stenosis, those with hypertrophic subaortic stenosis were often found to have a lower arterial pressure after a premature ventricular contraction compared to a normal heart beat. That is, "arterial pulse pressure varied inversely with left ventricular systolic pressure and with the duration of diastole" [61, p. 193]. Based on their findings, they concluded:

> In the presence of spontaneously occurring premature contractions, it would be possible to distinguish two forms of obstruction by inspection of direct or indirect arterial pressure tracings obtained without simultaneous intracardiac pressure and perhaps by careful palpation of the peripheral pulse [61, p. 193].

Thus, Brockenbrough, Braunwald, and Morrow sign refers to decreased pulse pressure or palpable pulse occurring after a premature ventricular contraction in patients with HOCM (Table 18.1).

Braunwald Sign

Eugene Braunwald (1929–) was born in Vienna, Austria, and received his medical degree from New York University Medical School in 1952 [65, 66]. He completed his internship at Mount Sinai Hospital, New York, residency training for one year at Johns Hopkins Hospital, Maryland, and postdoctoral cardiology fellowship training at Mount Sinai Hospital, Columbia University, and the intramural training program at the National Heart Institute (renamed the National Heart, Lung and Blood Institute or NHLBI in 1972) [65, 66]. He served as the first chief of the Cardiology Branch in 1961 and subsequently clinical director of National Heart Institute in 1966 [67].

Braunwald was the founding chair in the Department of Medicine at the University of California San Diego School of Medicine from 1968 to 1972 [65, 67]. From 1972 to 1996, he was appointed chairman of the Department of Medicine, physician-in-chief of the Peter Bent Brigham Hospital (Currently the Brigham and Women's Hospital), and Distinguished Hersey Professor of the Theory and Practice of Medicine at Harvard Medical School [65, 68, 69]. He was appointed chairman of the Department of Medicine at Beth Israel Hospital and Blumgart Professor of Medicine at Harvard Medical School from 1980 to 1989 [68]. He founded the TIMI (Thrombolysis in Myocardial Infarction) study group in 1984, serving as its chair until 2011 [65]. This national and international group of researchers has been instrumental in studying interventions and treatments for a variety of cardiovascular conditions. He also chaired the Heart Failure Clinical Trial Network at NHLBI [66, 69]. Braunwald was chief academic officer and founding trustee of Partners HealthCare System, a non-profit hospital and physician network affiliated with Brigham and Women's Hospital and Massachusetts General Hospital in 1996 [67, 68].

He was the editor or editor-in-chief for 12 editions of *Harrison's Principles of Internal Medicine* and the textbook *Braunwald's Heart Disease,* currently in its 11th edition, and is the recipient of numerous accolades including an Honorary Medical Doctorate from the University of Vienna as well as twenty-one other universities worldwide, American College of Cardiology Distinguished Scientist and Lifetime Achievement Award, and member of the National Academy of Sciences [65, 67–69]. The Braunwald Endowed Chair of Medicine was named in his honor at Harvard University in 1996 [65, 67–69].

As a description of Braunwald's character and vision he stated during an interview summarizing his brilliant career:

> It has been my good fortune to have been in the right place, at the right time, and most importantly, with the right people" [66, p. 1351]. (…) It will take intensive training and a powerful commitment to develop the skills required to move the field forward. However, the personal gratification that can come from making an impact on or contributing to preventing and/or treating cardiovascular disease—still the most common cause of death or disability in the world—will be enormous [66, p. 1353].

A subsequent study published by Braunwald, Lambrew, Rockoff, Ross, and Morrow on the pulse pressure in 64 patients with idiopathic hypertrophic subaortic stenosis (IHSS) confirmed findings from their prior study and reported (Table 18.1):

> [i]n 45 of the 57 patients with IHSS the arterial pulse pressure of the postpremature beat was abnormal, i.e. it did not exceed the pulse pressure of a control beat. Ten of the 12 patients with normal post-premature contraction arterial pressure response had no obstruction or only trivial systolic pressure gradients [70].

Gault et al. identified this abnormal response in 18 of 19 patients with hypertrophic subaortic stenosis [71]. Interestingly they found no drop in pulse pressure in eight patients with nonobstructive intraventricular pressure difference caused by catheter entrapment [71]. Other studies found the fall in pulse pressure in patients with IHSS to be present in 33% (4 of 12 patients) and 36% (5 of 14 patients) with IHSS [72, 73]. The sign, despite the findings in some studies which showed it to lack sufficient sensitivity and specificity, is believed to be an important modality in the assessment of patients with hypertrophic cardiomyopathy with dynamic left ventricular outlet obstruction [73].

Thus, Brockenbrough sign, Braunwald sign, or Brockenbrough-Braunwald-Marrow Sign refer to the presence of a palpable weak pulse following a premature ventricular contraction in HOCM. Braunwald and colleagues confirmed prior findings first described by Brockenbrough, himself and Marrow.

Conclusion

The method of naming medical eponyms with more than one name lacks sufficient structure and has a variable convention in the literature. In some instances only the name of the primary author is used while others argue that all names of the persons who contributed to the manuscript should be included. In other instances the author of another manuscript who more thoroughly studied the sign is recognized and given primary attribution. In the case of Grocco-Frugoni sign the name Giugni was dropped and Grocco included as the authors acknowledged his previous recognition of this symptom. It is this confusion of medical terminology which supports the critic's view of the frequent misattribution of credit for the work. Despite these shortcomings, we believe that medical eponymic signs are important to learn and recognize as reading of the original work provides important insights into understanding physiological principles as well as reemphasizes the importance of clinical observation in diagnosing disease. Since eponyms are honorific terms, any name associated with war crimes, anti-Semitic, or racist connotations should be stricken from the literature and discourse. Many of the signs discussed lack sufficient sensitivity or specificity to be clinically useful.

References

1. Seguin E. The use of the thermometer in clinical medicine. Chicago Med J. 1866;23:193–201.
2. Cushing H. On routine determinations of arterial tension in operating room and clinic. Boston Med Surg J. 1903;148(10):250–6.
3. Skinner HA. The Origin of Medical Terms. Baltimore: Williams & Wilkins; 1949.
4. Neff T. Routine oximetry: a fifth vital sign? Chest. 1988;94(2):227.
5. Bruwer AJ. Classic Descriptions in Diagnostic Roentgenology, vol. 2. Springfield: Charles C. Thomas; 1964.
6. B. RW. Medical eponym: Rumpel-Leede sign. N Engl J Med. 1944;230(4):122–3.
7. Kast A, Rumpel T, Fraenkel E. Pathologisch-anatomische Tafeln nach frischen Präparaten mit erläuterndem anatomisch-klinischem Text. Hamburg: Staatskrankenhäusern-Wandsbeck-Hamburg; 1909.
8. Rumpel T. Photographien von Scharlachkranken mit multiplen Hautblutungen. Deutsche med Wchenschr. 1909;35:2297.
9. [No author]. Directory of Medical Specialists Certified by American Boards, vol. 8. Chicago: Advisory Board for Medical Specialties; 1957.
10. Leede C. Hautblutungen, durch Stauung hervorgerufen als diagnostisches Hilfsmittel. München med Wochenshr. 1911;58:293–5.
11. Hess AF, Fish M. Infantile scurvy: the blood, the blood–vessels and the diet. Am J Dis Child. 1914;8(6):385-405.
12. Wang K, Lee J. Rumpel-Leede sign. N Engl J Med. 2014;370(1):e1.
13. Saraf S. Tourniquet induced purpura during hand surgery: a case report. Internet J Hand Surg. 2016;7(1):1–4.
14. Varela D, Tran D, Ngamdu KS, Trullender B, Mukherjee D, Abbas A. Rumple-Leede phenomenon presenting as a hypertensive urgeny. Proc Bayl Univ Med Cent. 2016;29(2):200–1.
15. Antunes AC, Oliveira GL, Nunes LI, Guedes Filho LA, Prado RS, Henriques HR, Vieira AJC. Evaluation of the diagnostic value of the tourniquet test in predicting severe dengue cases in a population from Belo Horizonte, State of Minas Gerais, Brazil. Rev Soc Bras Med Trop. 2013;46(5):542–6.
16. Dubach PI, Mantokoudis G, Lammie B. Rumpel-Leede sign in thrombocytopenia due to Epstein-Barr virus-induced mononucleosis. Br J Haematol. 2010;148(1):2.
17. Duncan SC, Winkelmann RK. Early histopathology of the cutaneous capillary fragility test (Rumple-Leede). J Cutan Pathol. 1979;6(1):1–4.

18. Castiglioni diArture. Grocco, Pietro. Cesare Patrizi. Enciclopedia italiana. 1933. Treccani. http://www.treccani.it/enciclopedia/pietro-grocco_%28Enciclopedia-Italiana%29/. Accessed 2 Oct 2020.
19. [No author]. Notes. Nature. 1916;97:42–3.
20. Fantini B. Polio in Italy. Dynamis. 2012;32(2):329–59.
21. Frugoni C, Giugni E. Le signe du lacet dans les maladies à manifestations hemorragiques. Semaine méd. 1911;31(3):25–8.
22. Italo Vittorio Tondi. Cesare Frugoni Un Principe Della Medicina Clinica. 2000. http://www.bpp.it/Apulia/html/archivio/1995/I/art/R95I028.html. Accessed 2 Oct 2020.
23. Frugoni C. Di Giuseppina Bock Berti. Dizionario Biografico degli italiana, vol. 56. 1998. http://www.treccani.it/enciclopedia/cesare-frugoni_(Dizionario-Biografico)/. Accessed 2 Oct 2020.
24. [No author]. Presentation of honorary fellowship in the American Academy of Allergy to Professor Cesare Frugoni in Rome, Italy. J Allergy. 1951;22(4):381–2.
25. Koren N. Jewish Physicians: A Biographical Index. Jerusalem: Israel Universities Press; 1973.
26. Edmond Weill Geni @ 2019 Geni.com. https://www.geni.com/people/Edmond-Weill/375474846080003021. Accessed 12 Sep 2019.
27. [No author]. Death of Prof. E. Weill. Am J Dis Child. 1924;29(4):523.
28. Barrier G, Weill E. Committee on Historical and Scientific Works. Institute attached to the National School of Charters. Last updated on 20/08/2019. https://cths.fr/an/savant.php?id=4988. Accessed 10 Aug 2019.
29. Weill E. Wikipédia. https://fr.wikipedia.org/wiki/Edmond_Weill. Accessed 10 Jul 2019.
30. Chalier JF. Les ictères hémolytiques. Lyon: Imprimeries Réunies; 1909.
31. [No author]. Joseph Chalier (1884–1942). Presse Méd. 1942;51:573.
32. Weill E, Chalier J. Purpura provoqué par hypertension veineuse. Bull Soc Med d Hosp de Lyons. 1911;10:167–72.
33. Lucatello L. Stefano Arieti Dizionario Biografico degli Italiani. Treccani. 2006. http://www.treccani.it/enciclopedia/luigi-lucatello_(Dizionario-Biografico)/. Accessed 10 Aug 2019.
34. Bonati MR, Zampieri F, Zanatta A. Per una storia della medicina. In: Selezione di Lavori del Gruppo di Medicina Umanistica, Universitá degli studi di Padova, 2010–2011. Padova: Libraria Padovana Editrice; 2012.
35. Lucatello L. Per la sintomatologia endocrina. In: Lavori dei Congressi di medicina interna, XXIII Congresso (1913, Roma). Roma; 1914. p. 328.
36. Gregorio M. The sign of Lucatello. Endocr Surv. 1928;5:399–401.
37. Nicola Pende's birthplace. Himetop: the history of medicine topographical database. http://himetop.wikidot.com/nicola-pende-s-birthplace. Accessed 10 May 2020.
38. Pende, Nicola di Emmanuel Betta-Dizionario Biografico degli Italiani. 2015;82. Treccani. http://www.treccani.it/enciclopedia/nicola-pende_%28Dizionario-Biografico%29/. Accessed 15 May 2020.
39. Assegnazione di premi. Gazzetta degli ospendall e delle cliniche. 1904;25. https://play.google.com/books/reader?id=76rwjXM4ELwC&printsec=frontcover&output=reader&hl=en&pg=GBS.PP855. Accessed 15 May 2020.
40. [No author]. Medical news: foreign university intelligence. Lancet. 1908;1:824.
41. Pende N. Endocrinologia: Patologia e Clinica degli Organi a Secrezione Interna. Milan: Vallardi Endocrinology; 1916.
42. Strategie politiche ed esignenze scientificheL il ruolo di Nicola Pende nel'instituzione e nell'organizzazione dell'Universita di Bari Annali di Storia delle Universita Italiane. 2013;17. http://www.cisui.unibo.it/annali/17/testi/03_Dell_Era_frameset.htm. Accessed 15 May 2020.
43. Nicola Pende, la via italiana al razzismo. Quotidiano di Bari. 2018. https://quotidianodibari.it/nicola-pende-la-via-italiana-al-razzismo/. Accessed 15 May 2020.
44. Gronch G. Bari cancella via Nicola Pende. 2006. http://www.lagazzettadelmezzogiorno.it/news/home/44099/bari-cancella-via-nicola-pende.html?refresh_ce. Accessed 15 May 2020.

45. [No author]. New items: award to Pende. N York M J. 1929,112:197.
46. [No author]. Prize to Pende. JAMA. 1920;75:115.
47. Levi-Montalcini R. Elogio dell'imperfezione. Milano: Garzanti; 1987.
48. Bari cancella via Nicola Pende la Gazzetta del Mezzogiorno.it. Sabato 07 Luglio 2018. http://www.lagazzettadelmezzogiorno.it/news/home/44099/bari-cancella-via-nicola-pende.html. Accessed 15 May 2020.
49. Rome to remove race law signatories. ANSA en Politics. 2018. http://www.ansa.it/english/news/politics/2018/01/22/rome-to-remove-race-law-signatories_da4c7f1b-1743-47d9-8434-52aac7230c0c.html. Accessed 15 May 2020.
50. Pende N. Sopra una triade sintomatica dell'ipertiroidismo costituzionale: sua importanza diagnostica nelle forme larvate di tireotoxicosi. Endocrinol Patol Costit. 1926;1:311–2.
51. Nicola pen scienziato razzista. La Repubblica Archivivio. 2006. http://ricerca.repubblica.it/repubblica/archivivio/repubblica/2006/09/14/nicola-pend-scienziato-razzista.html. Accessed 15 May 2020.
52. ARCA centro di iniziativa democratica. Elimare dalla toponomastica barese via Nicole Pende. 2018. http://wwwarcabari.it/2013/02/eliminare-dalla-toponomastica-barese-via-nicola-pende/. Accessed 15 May 2020.
53. Birrer RB, Birrer CD. Medical Diagnostic Signs: A Reference Collection of Eponymic Bedside Signs. Illinois: Charles C. Thomas Publishers; 1982.
54. Marcucci L. Handbook of Medical Eponyms. Baltimore: Lippincott Williams & Wilkins; 2002.
55. White FA. Physical Signs in Medicine and Surgery: An Atlas of Rare, Lost and Forgotten Physical Signs. Ocala: Museum Press Books; 2009.
56. Pollock SG. Pressure tracings in obstructive cardiomyopathy. N Engl J Med. 1994;331:238.
57. Grossman W. Profiles in dilated (congestive) and hypertrophic cardiomyopathies. In: Grossman W, editor. Cardiac Catheterization and Angiography. Philadelphia: Lea & Febiger; 1986. p. 420–1.
58. Cui H, Nguyen A, Schaff HV. The Brockenbrough-Braunwald-Morrow sign. J Thorac Cardiovasc Surg. 2018;156(4):1614–5.
59. Criley JM, Goldberg SL, French WJ. The Brockenbrough-Braunwald-Morrow sign. N Engl J Med. 1994;331:1589–90.
60. Dorland WAN. Dorland's Illustrated Medical Dictionary. 32nd ed. Philadelphia: Elsevier Saunders; 2012. p. 251.
61. Brockenbrough EC, Braunwald E, Morrow AG. A hemodynamic technic for the detection of hypertrophic subaortic stenosis. Circulation. 1961;23(2):189–94.
62. Edwin C. Brockenbrough, MD, Medical Director, Pacific Vascular/PVICME. Pacific Vascular Incorporated. 2016. http://www.pvicme.com/faculty.htm. Accessed 3 Mar 2020.
63. [No author]. Seattle Surgical Society. Northwest Med. 1972;71:333.
64. Edwin C. Brockenbrough, MD, FACS. Marquis who's who. Humanitarian award. https://worldwidehumanitarian.com/2017/02/20/edwin-brockenbrough/. Accessed 3 Mar 2020.
65. Eugene Braunwald, MD, MACC, A lifetime of achievements and a legend of cardiology. American College of Cardiology Dec 27, 2014. Cardiology magazine. https://www.acc.org/latest-in-cardiology/articles/2014/02/27/13/20/eugene-braunwald-md-macc-a-lifetime-of-achievements-and-a-legend-of-cardiology. Accessed 8 Aug 2019.
66. Nicholls M. Eugene Braunwald MD: an icon of the 20th century still going strong. Eur Heart J. 2015;36(22):1350–1.
67. Cohn LH. Eugene Braunwald, MD. J Thorac Cardiovasc Surg. 2013;146(4):743–4.
68. Dr. Eugene Braunwald, World-renowned cardiologist, to Speak at Miller School on April 18. University of Miami Miller School of Medicine. http://med.miami.edu/news/dr.-eugene-braunwald-world-renowned-cardiologist-to-speak-at-miller-school-. Accessed 30 Aug 2019.
69. Eugene Braunwauld, MD. Executive committee chair, Heart failure network. Heart failure network. https://hfnetwork.org/about-us/our-leadership/eugene-braunwald-md. Accessed 28 Aug 2019.

70. Braunwald E, Lambrew CT, Rockoff SD, Ross J Jr, Morrow AG. Idiopathic subaortic stenosis: a description of the disease based upon an analysis of 64 patients. Circulation. 1964;suppl IV:3–119.
71. Gault JH, Simon AL. Clinical and laboratory findings in patients with nonobstructive intraventricular pressure differences. Circulation. 1970;42(2):235–44.
72. Hancock EW. Arterial pulse contour in mild muscular subaortic stenosis. Clin Res. 1965;13:91.
73. White CW, Zimmerman TJ. Prolonged left ventricular ejection time in the post-premature beat: a sensitive sign of idiopathic hypertrophic subaortic stenosis. Circulation. 1975;52(2):306–12.

Chapter 19
Miscellaneous Physical Signs and Medical Eponyms

Introduction

Described in this section are three signs that may be found on the cardiovascular examination in patients with tuberculosis, malignancy, and in relation to anatomical changes in the right atrium. Of these signs, only the Chiari network has been the most thoroughly studied. In fact, we are unaware of any studies which evaluated the utility of Grossman or Gordon signs, which used percussion of the chest wall to detect heart size in the assessment of patients with tuberculosis or malignancy. We believe that these signs are useful to learn as they provide keen insights into how physicians identified and proposed disease pathogenesis based on key clinical findings.

Signs

Chiari Network Sign

Hans Chiari (1851–1916) was born in Vienna, Austria, and received the Doctor Medicinae Universalis (Dr. Med. Univ.) in 1875 at the University of Vienna [1]. Prior to graduation in 1874, he worked as an assistant to Carl von Rokitansky (1804–1878) and his successor Richard Ladislaus Heschl (1824–1881), Viennese Chair at the Vienna Institute of Pathology [1–3]. In 1876, he habilitated and was awarded venia legendi at the University of Vienna [1–4]. He was promoted as Deputy Prosecutor at K.K. Rudolfspital (K.K. Hospital Foundation Rudolfspital), Vienna, beginning in 1877 and Prosecutor at St. Anna Children's Hospital in Vienna in 1878 [1]. He habilitated in pathological anatomy in Vienna in 1878 and was appointed Associate Professor and Chair of Pathological Anatomy at the German Karl Ferdinand University, Prague, in 1882, the position previously occupied by

S. H. Yale et al., *Cardiovascular Eponymic Signs*,
https://doi.org/10.1007/978-3-030-67596-7_19

Edwin Klebs (1834–1913) [1, 2, 4]. In 1883, he was appointed Ordinarius Professor for Pathological Anatomy and in 1906 accepted the position as Chair of von Recklinghausen at the Kaiser Wilhelm University in Strasburg [1–3]. He was rector magnifico at the University in Prague in 1900 and again in Strasbourg in 1914 [1]. As described by Hermann Dürck (1869–1941) regarding his character:

> All these works from Chiari's first period as a researcher bear those qualities which characterize his later works to such an outstanding degree. Along with extensive knowledge and keen powers of observation he had a very extraordinary thoroughness and extended a sincere effort, even in new cases, to follow up on observations made earlier and to acknowledge wholeheartedly the merit of the past. This characteristic was found in Chiari's works during all periods of his life. He was always immensely sympathetic and evinced by the truth, properly modest and noble in his mode of thinking, a fundamental feature of his nature [1, p. 1080].

His name is perhaps best recognized in the description of the different malformation of the cerebellum (hindbrain herniation) caused by hydrocephalus of the cerebrum published in *Deutsche medizinische Wochenschrift* in 1891 [5]. Chiari identified a network formation in the right atrium that:

> In spite of the very numerous studies on malformation of the heart, the network formation to be discussed in the right atrium of the heart has hitherto received no particular attention, although it is very interesting in morphological and developmental history and may assume pathological significance under certain circumstances. These network formations are not uncommon, so once I became aware of it, I was able to collect a large number of relevant cases and put them in the museum [6, p. 1].

He found 11 patients with a reticulated network in the right atrium and believed that, "All cases of reticulum formation in the right atrium could be reconciled, according to their morphological behavior, based on the assumption that they contain remnants of the septum spurium and right valvular venosa" [6, p. 9]. In a 36-year-old man who died of pleurisy, microscopic examination of the reticulum showed that:

> Most of the fibers of the reticulum which had been cut out immediately at the time of the section consisted only of fibrous connective tissue. Some of them also contained tracts of branched muscle fibers. On the outer surface all threads were covered with endothelium [6, p. 5].

Thus, the Chiari network refers to the embryological remnants of tissue from the valves of the sinus venosus appearing as a mobile fenestrated reticular network-like pattern most commonly occurring in the right atrium (Table 19.1). This network may connect the crista terminalis with margins of the valves of the coronary sinus (Thebesian) and inferior vena cava (Eustachian); part of the lattice network along with other atrial structures [7]. The network is caused by the failure of resorption of the right valvular venosa (sinus venosus valve). It is this embryological structure which develops into the Eustachian and Thesbian valves.

The Chiari network was identified in 3.75% of 80 cadaveric hearts [8]. Although typically a benign incidental finding, it may have pathological significance as reported by Chiari as serving as a nidus for thromboembolism and endocarditis [8–11]. It has also been reported to lead to catheter and guidewire entrapment

Table 19.1 Miscellaneous medical eponymous signs

Name	Year	Description of sign	Method
Chiari [5]	1891	Mobile, fenestrated reticular network-like pattern most commonly occurring in the right atrium.	Observation
Gordon [21]	1904	Patient recumbent: Percussion of the chest normally shows cardiac dullness above at the third costal cartilage with a rightward limit about the mid-sternum, measuring about 3 in. across at the level of the fifth costal cartilage. In patients with malignancy, cardiac dullness begins above about the fourth costal cartilage, has its rightward limit slightly to the left of the left sternal border, and measures across at the level of the fifth costal cartilage less than 2 in., or in many cases, less than 1 in. In some cases, cardiac dullness is absent.	Percussion
Grossman [25]	1916	Slight dilation of the heart and diffuseness of the apex beat seen or felt at the fifth left intercostal interspace.	Observation and palpation

[12–16]. Conversely, its presence has been attributed as having a beneficial effect by acting as a sieve or filter and thereby hindering the propagation of thrombus leading to pulmonary emboli [7, 8, 17, 18].

Gordon Sign

William Gordon (1863–1929) was born in Tyrone County, Ireland and received his medical training in Heidelberg, Germany and the University College Hospital, London, qualifying (MB, BBCh Camb) in 1890 [19, 20]. This was followed by a house appointment at the University College Hospital [20]. He received his medical degree (MD) in 1894 and began practice in Exeter, England, where he served as a physician at Royal Devon and Exeter Hospitals, West of England Eye Infirmary, and Exeter Dispensary in Queen Street [19].

He was elected fellow to the Royal College of Physicians in 1903. During World War I, he served from 1914 to 1918 as medical officer of No. 1 Temporary Hospital, Exeter [19]. He was an active member of the British Medical Association serving as a member from 1893 to 1897 and chairman of the Parliamentary Bills Subcommittee on Army Medical Reform from 1896 to 1898 [19]. In this latter position, he was instrumental in founding the Royal Army Medical Corps. Among his many accolades, he served within the British Medical Association including as honorary secretary of its South-Western Branch (1895–1897), member of Branch Council (1898–1923 and 1927–1929), vice president and president from 1924 to 1925 and 1928 to 1929, respectively [19]. He was active in the Exeter division (member of executive and ethical committees [1915–1921], vice chairman [1920–1922], and chairman [1922–1923]) [19]. Gordon was president of Balneological and Climatological Section of the Royal Society of Medicine from 1915 to 1917 and vice president of the Section of Medicine from 1923 to 1925 [19].

In a description of his character, Mr. Russell Coombe, FRCS said:

> He was the most, loyal of friends, an- upright, courageous, conscientious man; one to be trusted to the uttermost. It is as a great scientific physician that we must think of William Gordon [19, p. 698]. (…) As a surgeon I am unfit to assess his medical achievements, but we frequently met in doubtful and anxious cases, and I never failed to be impressed by the scrupulous care of his methods and by the accuracy of his conclusions. He was invaluable to me as a medical consultant. His scientific methods led to diagnosis by exclusion that were almost uncanny. (…) I wondered at first at his coming to Exeter; it hardly seemed a big enough sphere for his scholarly attainments, and sometime after his arrival I inquired his reasons. He told me of his extremely keen interest in medicine; that the opportunity of getting immediate clinical work attracted him and was not one, to be lost; and that if he only succeeded in laying firmly one brick in the edifice of medical knowledge life would have his reward. Who shall say that he has not so laid-well and truly-and that his life's purpose has not been fully realized? There was no guessing about his methods; his conclusions were all the result of most careful observations. For myself, I have lost the last intimate of my own standing, and it is with a sad heart that I write the word Vale [19, p. 699].

Gordon initially described in 1904 a finding identified during percussion of the heart in several patients with gastric cancer:

> [I] observed that, although no evidence existed of ordinary emphysema, the area of cardiac dullness, mapped out in the recumbent position, was either much reduced or actually obliterated. In some of them, where the dullness was obliterated, the resonant note over the heart was, it is true, slightly higher pitched than over the lung, but it was definitely resonant, not dull. The reduction or obliteration of the cardiac dullness was sometimes associated with a rather surprisingly small and soft pulse [21, p. 327].

He defined diminished cardiac dullness as follows:

> With a patient completely recumbent that is essential a normal cardiac dullness generally begins above at the third costal cartilage, has its rightward limit about the mid-sternum, and measures about 3 in. across at the level of the fifth costal cartilage; but in the condition discussed here the dullness begins above about the fourth costal cartilage, has its rightward limit a little to the left of the left sternal border, and measures across at the level of the fifth costal cartilage, less than 2 in; or in many cases less than 1 in; sometimes there is no cardiac dullness at all [22, p. 299].

Based on his experience and description of findings in 11 patients, Gordon concluded: Putting aside cases where special cause exist, either for the obliteration of the heart dullness or for prevention of such obliteration, the following seem to be true:

1. Great reduction or obliteration of the normal cardiac dullness is common in cases of cancer, particularly in cancers of the alimentary canal and in their late stages.
2. This loss of cardiac dullness does not seem to be found in the earliest stages of a cancerous case, but may precede cachexia, marked wasting, and loss of skin elasticity.
3. It is rarely observed in noncancerous cases.
4. It is rarely absent in the later stages of cases of cancer of the alimentary canal.
5. It does not seem to occur in cases of sarcoma.
6. In doubtful cases, its presence is highly suggestive of cancer; its absence is slightly suggestive of the absence of cancer, if the symptoms under consideration have lasted for several months [21, p. 336].

In a subsequent publication titled "The value of diminished cardiac dullness in the diagnosis of cancer," Gordon reported his experience in 103 patients, 46 without known cancer, of whom only 11 (24%) showed a diminished cardiac dullness [22]. Gordon proposed the following pathogenesis for his findings:

(a) It is possible that the heart, in a case of cancer, may, like other muscles, become more flaccid than normal, and (judging from the anemia and small pulse so often present) may be less well filled than in health. If so, it may perhaps fall away from the front chest wall, on recumbency, more than a normal heart would.
(b) It is possible that the lungs, like the abdominal skin, lose some of their elasticity in cases of cancer, so that a spurious emphysema may perhaps results from ordinary breathing.
(c) Finally, in many cases of cancer, the heart is known to become much reduced in size [22, p. 300].

Gordon described a variety of conditions which may lead to a false-positive or false-negative test result:

> Certain limitations exist to the significance of the sign. Thus when any cause is present, tending, like ordinary emphysema, to reduce the area of cardiac dullness, then a very small dullness naturally conveys no special meaning. On the other hand, when there is any well-known cause of enlargement of heart-dullness, such as albuminuria, valvular heart disease, pericarditis, or retraction of lung from phthisis or past pleurisy, then the absence of the sign is equally without significance. Moreover, where the heart is displaced considerably upwards the absence of the sign is unreliable, since the organ has been moved from a wider into a narrower space, in which it is not so free to fall back from the anterior chest-wall on recumbency. And lastly, where a large oesophageal carcinoma has lain directly behind the heart, I have thought that the absence of the cardiac sign was due to the growth pinning the organ forward against the sternum and rib cartilages [23, p. 21].

Thus, Gordon sign refers to the presence of reduced cardiac dullness on percussion in cases of cancer (Table 19.1). As enumerated by Gordon, this sign is not commonly found in patients with malignancy of the gastrointestinal tract and thus lacks sufficient sensitivity or specificity to be useful in clinical practice.

Grossman Sign

Morris (Max) Grossman (1881–1955) was born in Hungary, graduated from Fordham's Medical School (1905–1921), New York City in 1909, followed by additional postgraduate training in neurology [24]. He was a private practitioner of neurology in New York City and served as a consultant at Monmouth Memorial Hospital, New Jersey. He subsequently continued working as a private practitioner in New Jersey from 1942 to 1955 [24]. Grossman is credited for developing the neurologic clinic at Mt. Sinai Hospital, New York City, and later served as its chief [24]. Grossman described a sign that he observed and palpated in patients with early tuberculosis [25, 26]:

> The writer has noticed, however, that slight dilation of the heart, diffuseness of the apex beat seen or felt at the fifth left intercostal interspace appears very often simultaneously with, or even precedes, the earliest physical signs of incipient pulmonary tuberculosis [25, p. 695].

Thus, Grossman sign refers to the presence of cardiac dilatation and observed and palpable apex beat at the fifth intercostal space in patient with early apical pulmonary tuberculosis (Table 19.1).

Conclusion

Of the miscellaneous sign, Chiari reticulated fibrous network in the right atrium remains an important finding, which when present may have pathological as well as therapeutic benefits. Grossman and Gordon signs remain of interest for historical purposes. They serve as a guide, emphasizing to clinicians about the ability to identify more subtle findings when performing a meticulous, comprehensive, and detailed physical examination.

References

1. Dürck H. Hans Chiari. Münch med Wchnschr. 1916;63:1080–2.
2. Gruber G. Hans Chiari. Zentralbl allg Pathol Anat. 1916;27:289–94.
3. Tubbs RS, Cohen-Gadol AA. Hans Chairi (1851–1916). J Neurol. 2010;257:1218–20.
4. Gruber GB. Hans Chiari. Dtsch med Wchnschr. 1916;42:982–3.
5. Chiari H. Über Veränderungen des Kleinhirns infolge von Hydrocephalie des Grosshirns. Dtsch med Wchnschr. 1891;17:1172–5.
6. Chiari H. Über Netzbildungen im rechten Vorhof des Herzens. Beitr pathol Anat. 1897;22:1–10.
7. Islam AKMM, Sayami LA, Zaman S. Chiari network: a case report and brief overview. JSHA. 2013;25(3):225–9.
8. Jansirani DD, Deep SS, Anandarajha A. Anatomical study of Chiari network and the remnant of left venous valve in the interior of right atrium. 2015. https://www.hindawi.com/journals/ari/2015/247680/. Accessed 15 May 2019.
9. Carrena O, Oluoha O, Wahba A, Eshun D, Endsley M, Okafor H. Complicated infective endocarditis limited to a Chiari network. Case Rep Cardiol. 2018:3837825. https://doi.org/10.1155/2018/3837825.
10. Figueras-Coll M, Sabaté-Rotés A, Cañete-Abajo N, Domènech-Ximenos B. The Chiari network-only an embryonic remnant or a confusing finding? World J Pediatr Congenit Heart Surg. 2020;11:NP47–9.
11. Schwimmer-Okike N, Niebuhr J, Schramek GG, Frantz S, Kielstein H. The presence of a large Chiari network in a patient with atrial fibrillation and stroke. Case Rep Cardiol. 2016;4839315. https://doi.org/10.1155/2016/4839315.
12. Goldschlager A, Goldschlager N, Brewster H, Kaplan J. Catheter entrapment in a Chiari network involving an atrial septal defect. Chest. 1972;62:345–6.
13. Zhu W, Jin Z, Li Q. Entrapment of guide wire by Chiari's network during pacemaker implantation. Cardiol J. 2019;26:607.

14. Nagahama MV, Sakai MH, Souto MCX, Frota ESD, Cirenza C, de Paola AAV. Catheter entrapment in Chiari network: extraction with radiofrequency. IPEJ. 2019;19:195–6.
15. Chu S, Solheim E, Chen J, Hoff PI, Schuster P. Entrapment and retrieval of a diagnostic electrophysiological catheter in the Chiari network. J Arrhythm. 2018;34:647–9.
16. Yoshimura M, Toriumi T. Guidewire entrapment in the Chiari network. J Cardiothorac Vasc Anesth. 2016;30:e24–5.
17. Sonaglioni A, Nicolosi GL, Lombardo M, Anza C. A nonfatal massive pulmonary embolism in a very old patient: the protective filter-effect of the Chiari network. J Cardiovasc Echogr. 2019;29:32–4.
18. Honda K, Yuzaki M, Kunimoto H, Nishimura Y. Right atrial thrombus entrapped in a Chiari's network. J Card Surg. 2018;33:444–5.
19. [No author]. William Gordon M.D., F.R.C.P. Br Med J. 1929;2(3588):698–9.
20. Brown GH. William Gordon. Lives of the fellows. Royal College of Physicians. Available from: http://munksroll.rcplondon.ac.uk/Biography/Details/1830. Accessed 20 Jun 2019.
21. Gordon W. The cardiac dullness in cases of cancer. Med-Chir Tr. 1904;87:327–37.
22. Gordon W. The value of diminished cardiac dullness in the diagnosis of cancer. Br Med J. 1908;2(2484):298–302.
23. Gordon W. On digital percussion and cardiac sign in carcinoma. Bristol M-Chir J. 1914;32:19–26.
24. Grossman M. J M S N Jersey. 1956;53:100.
25. Grossman M. Dilated heart as a sign of apical pulmonary tuberculosis. Med Rec. 1916;89:694–5.
26. Grossman M. A study of the newer physical signs in the diagnosis of early pulmonary tuberculosis. Med Rec. 1916;89:855–6.

Index

S. H. Yale et al., *Cardiovascular Eponymic Signs*,
https://doi.org/10.1007/978-3-030-67596-7

Q

R

S

GPSR Compliance

The European Union's (EU) General Product Safety Regulation (GPSR) is a set of rules that requires consumer products to be safe and our obligations to ensure this.

If you have any concerns about our products, you can contact us on ProductSafety@springernature.com

In case Publisher is established outside the EU, the EU authorized representative is:

Springer Nature Customer Service Center GmbH
Europaplatz 3
69115 Heidelberg, Germany

Batch number: 10726532

Printed by Printforce, the Netherlands